# CARDIAC BIOASSIST

The Bakken Research Center Series
Volume 11

*Editors*

**Alain F. Carpentier, MD, PhD**
Professor, Université de Paris VI
Chief, Department of Cardiovascular Surgery and Organ Transplantation
Hôpital Broussais
Paris, France

**Juan Carlos Chachques, MD, PhD**
Associate Professor Director for Clinical Research
Department of Cardiovascular Surgery and Organ Transplantation
Hôpital Broussais
Paris, France

**Pierre A. Grandjean, MS**
Worldwide Research Manager
Cardiac Assist Systems
Bakken Research Center
Maastricht, The Netherlands

*Associate Editor*

**John Y.M. Relland**
Department of Cardiovascular Surgery
Hôpital Broussais
Paris, France

FUTURA

**Futura Publishing Company, Inc.**

**Library of Congress Cataloging-in-Publication Data**

Cardiac bioassist / edited by Alain Carpentier, Juan Carlos Chachques, Pierre A. Grandjean.
p. cm. — (The Bakken Research Center series ; v. 11)
Includes bibliographical references and index.
ISBN 0-87993-647-9
1. Cardiomyoplasty. I. Carpentier, Alain, M.D. II. Chachques, Juan Carlos. III. Grandjean, Pierre A. IV. Series.
[DNLM: 1. Cardiomyoplasty—congresses. W1 BA4794 v.11 1996 / WG 169 C2659 1996]
RD598.35.C37C35 1996
617.4′12—dc20
DNLM/DLC
for Library of Congress 96-41246
CIP


Futura Publishing Company, Inc.
135 Bedford Road
Armonk, New York 10504-0418
LC#: 96-41246
ISBN: 0-87993-647-9

Every effort has been made to ensure that the information in this book is as up to date and as accurate as possible at the time of publication. However, due to the constant developments in medicine, the author, the editor, or the publisher cannot accept any legal or any other responsibility for any errors or omissions that may occur.



Printed in the United States of America.

This book is printed on acid-free paper.

*Other volumes in the Bakken Research Center Series:*

Volume 1, Part I. The Foundation of Cardiac Pacing: An Illustrated Practical Guide to Basic Pacing, by Richard Sutton, DSc Med, FRCP, FACC and Ivan Bourgeois, MSc, MBA

Volume 2. Transformed Muscle for Cardiac Assist and Repair, edited by Ray Chu-Jeng Chiu, MD, PhD, and Ivan Bourgeois, MSc, MBA

Volume 3. Cardiomyoplasty, edited by Alain Carpentier, MD, PhD, Juan-Carlos Chachques, MD, and Pierre A. Grandjean, MS

Volume 4. Challenges in Cardiology I, edited by Charles E. Rackley, MD

Volume 5. Practical Aspects of Staged Therapy Defibrillators, edited by Lukas J. Kappenberger, MD, and Fred W. Lindemans, PhD

Volume 6. Tachycardias: Mechanisms and Management, edited by Mark E. Josephson, MD, and Hein J. J. Wellens, MD

Volume 7. Vagal Control of the Heart: Experimental Basis and Clinical Implications, edited by Matthew N. Levy, MD, and Peter J. Schwartz, MD

Volume 8. Atrial Fibrillation: Facts From Yesterday—Ideas For Tomorrow, edited by Henri E. Kulbertus, MD, Hein J. J. Wellens, MD, Ivan Bourgeois, MSc, MBA, and Richard Sutton, DSc, Med

Volume 9. Atrial and Ventricular Fibrillation: Mechanisms and Device Therapy, edited by Mauritz A. Allessie, MD, PhD, and Martin Fromer, MD

Volume 10. Neurally Mediated Syncope: Pathophysiology, Investigations, and Treatment, edited by Jean-Jacques Blanc, MD, David Benditt, MD, and Richard Sutton, DSc, Med

# Contributors

**Shamil D. Akhmedov, MD**
Siberian Centre of Cardiac Surgery, Tomsk, Russia

**Ottavio Alfieri, MD**
Cardiac Surgery Department, Civile Hospital, Brescia, Italy

**Gary L. Anderson, PhD**
Division of Plastic and Reconstructive Surgery, Department of Physiology, University of Louisville and The Jewish Hospital Heart and Lung Institute, Louisville, Kentucky

**Rafael A. Avila, MD**
Brookdale Hospital Medical Center, Brooklyn, New York

**William F. Bailey, Jr., MD**
Division of Cardiothoracic Surgery, Department of Surgery, Thomas Jefferson University, Philadelphia, Pennsylvania

**Joaquín Barba, MD**
Department of Cardiology and Cardiovascular Surgery, University Clinic of Navarra, Faculty of Medicine, University of Navarra, Pamplona, Spain

**John H. Barker, MD, PhD**
Division of Plastic and Reconstructive Surgery, Department of Surgery, University of Louisville and The Jewish Hospital Heart and Lung Institute, Louisville, Kentucky

**Giovani Bellotti, MD**
Heart Institute of São Paulo University Medical School, São Paulo, Brazil

**A. Bennett, BS**
The Heart Institute, St. Vincent Hospital and Medical Center, Portland, Oregon

**Michael Beyer, MD**
Department of Cardiac Surgery, University of Ulm, Ulm, Germany

**Richard W. Bianco, BA, BSc**
Cardiovascular Surgery Research, Division of Cardiovascular and Thoracic Surgery, University of Minnesota, Minneapolis, Minnesota

**Pascale Blanc, MD**
Louis Pradel Cardiovascular and Pneumologic Hospital, Department of Anesthesiology and Intensive Care, Lyon, France

**Edimar A. Bocchi, MD**
Heart Institute of São Paulo University Medical School, São Paulo, Brazil

**R. Mortin Bolman, III, MD**
Minnesota Heart and Lung Institute, University of Minnesota, Minneapolis, Minnesota

**June Boon, MS**
Department of Clinical Sciences, College of Veterinary Medicine, Colorado State University, Fort Collins, Colorado

**Valentino Borghetti, MD**
Cardiac Surgery Department, Civile Hospital, Brescia, Italy

**Valéria Bors, MD**
Department of Cardiovascular and Thoracic Surgery, Hôpital La Pitie, Paris, France

**Tuan Bui, PhD**
Telectronics Pacing Systems, Inc., Englewood, Colorado

**John H. Burgess, MD**
Department of Cardiology, The Montreal General Hospital, Montreal, Quebec, Canada

**Ciro Campanella, MD**
University of Edinburgh, Department of Cardiothoracic Surgery, Edinburgh, Scotland

**Alain F. Carpentier, MD, PhD**
Department of Cardiovascular Surgery and Organ Transplantation, Hôpital Broussais, Paris, France

**Jean-Pierre Carteaux, MD**
Department of Cardiovascular Surgery and Organ Transplantation, Hôpital Broussais, Paris, France

**Juan Carlos Chachques, MD, PhD**
Department of Cardiovascular Surgery and Organ Transplantation, Hôpital Broussais, Paris, France

**Catherine Chardigny, MD**
Department of Cardiovascular Surgery, Broussais Hospital, Paris, France

**François Chaussende, BS**
Bakken Research Center, Maastricht, The Netherlands

**Valeri S. Chekanov, MD, PhD**
Sinai Samaritan Medical Center, Milwaukee, Wisconsin

**Wang Cheng, MD, PhD**
Division of Thoracic and Cardiovascular Surgery, Department of Surgery, Maimonides Medical Center, Brooklyn, New York

**Ray C.-J. Chiu, MD, PhD**
Divisions of Cardiovascular and Thoracic Surgery, The Montreal General Hospital/McGill University, Montreal, Quebec, Canada

**Alejandra I. Christen, MD**
Research Department, Institute of Cardiology and Cardiovascular Surgery, Favaloro Foundation, Buenos Aires, Argentina

**William J. Corin, MD**
University of Florida Cardiologists at Leesburg, University of Florida, Leesburg, Florida

**Bobby S. David, MD**
Brookdale Hospital Medical Center, Brooklyn, New York

**François Delahaye, MD**
Department of Cardiology, Hôpitaux de Lyon, Lyon, France

**Vince Doerr, MSEE**
Telectronics Pacing Systems, Inc., Englewood, Colorado

**Richard Dorent, MD**
Department of Cardiovascular and Thoracic Surgery, Hôpital La Pitie, Paris, France

**Changping Duan, PhD**
Cardiothoracic Surgical Research, Allegheny-Singer Research Institute, Pittsburgh, Pennsylvania

**Harald C. Eichstaedt, MD**
Thoracic and Cardiovascular Surgery, Free University, Brussels, Belgium

**Suzanne Estanove, MD**
Louis Pradel Cardiovascular and Pneumologic Hospital, Department of Anesthesiology and Intensive Care, Lyon, France

**Jean-Noel Fabiani, MD**
Department of Cardiovascular Surgery, Broussais Hospital, Paris, France

**Gerard Finet, MD**
Louis Pradel Cardiovascular and Pneumologic Hospital, Lyon, France

**E.I. Cabrera Fischer, MD**
Research Department, Institute of Cardiology and Cardiovascular Surgery, Favaloro Foundation, Buenos Aires, Argentina

**W. Fleischmann, MD**
Department of Traumatology, University of Ulm, Ulm, Germany

**Keith A.A. Fox, MD**
University of Edinburgh, Cardiovascular Research Unit, Edinburgh, Scotland

**David Francischelli, MS**
Medtronic, Inc., Minneapolis, Minnesota

**Johannes M. Frank, MD**
Division of Plastic and Reconstructive Surgery, Department of Surgery, University of Louisville and The Jewish Hospital Heart and Lung Institute, Louisville, Kentucky

**D. Fritzsche, MD**
Clinic for Heart Surgery, University of Leipzig, Leipzig, Germany

**Anthony P. Furnary, MD**
The Heart Institute, St. Vincent Hospital and Medical Center, Portland, Oregon

**Iradj Gandjbakhch, MD**
Department of Cardiovascular and Thoracic Surgery, Hôpital La Pitie, Paris, France

**Kendra K. Gealow, PhD**
Division of Cardiovascular and Thoracic Surgery, University of Minnesota, Minneapolis, Minnesota

**David T. George, PhD**
School of Medicine, Case Western Reserve, Cleveland, Ohio

**Claude Girard, MD**
Louis Pradel Cardiovascular and Pneumologic Hospital, Lyon, France

**Donald H. Glaeser, MD**
Department of Surgery and Department of Medicine, Baylor College of Medicine, Houston, Texas

**Pierre A. Grandjean, MS**
Bakken Research Center, Maastricht, The Netherlands

**Neil R. Grubb, MD**
University of Edinburgh, Cardiovascular Research Unit, Edinburgh, Scotland

**Wei Gu, PhD**
Department of Cardiology, The Children's Hospital, Harvard Medical School, Boston, Massachusetts

**Norbert W. Guldner, MD**
Department of Cardiac Surgery, University of Lübeck, Lübeck, Germany

**Siegfried Hagl, MD**
Department of Heart Surgery, University Hospital, Heidelberg, Germany

**Ardeshir Hakami, MD**
Division of Plastic and Reconstructive Surgery, Department of Surgery, University of Louisville, Louisville, Kentucky

**A. Hannekum, MD**
Department of Cardiac Surgery, University of Ulm, Ulm, Germany

**Jesús Herreros, MD**
Department of Cardiology and Cardiovascular Surgery, Faculty of Medicine, University of Navarra, Pamplona, Spain

**Steven J. Hoff, MD**
Department of Cardiac and Thoracic Surgery, Vanderbilt University Medical School, Nashville, Tennessee

**H. Hoffer, MD**
Department of Cardiac Surgery, University of Ulm, Ulm, Germany

**Timothy L. Hooper, MD**
Department of Cardiothoracic Surgery, Wythenshawe Hospital, University of Manchester, Manchester, England

**Ignacio Iglesias, MD**
Department of Cardiology and Cardiovascular Surgery, Faculty of Medicine, University of Navarra, Pamplona, Spain

**F. Iudicello, PhD**
Thermo-Fluids Engineering Research Centre, City University, London, England

**Gordon B. Jacobs, MSEE**
Telectronics Pacing Systems, Inc., Englewood, Colorado

**Jonathan C. Jarvis, PhD**
Department of Human Anatomy and Cell Biology, University of Liverpool, Liverpool, England

**W. Jaszcz, MD, PhD**
Department of Laboratory Medicine and Pathology, University of Minnesota, Minneapolis, Minnesota

**Adib D. Jatene, MD**
Heart Institute of São Paulo University Medical School, São Paulo, Brazil

**Olivier Jegaden, MD**
Department of Cardiac Surgery, Hôpital de Lyon, Lyon, France

**Wendy S. Johnson, MD**
Division of Cardiothoracic Surgery, Department of Surgery, Medical University of South Carolina, Charleston, South Carolina

**Guillaume Jondeau, MD, PhD**
Cardiology Department, Hôpital Ambroise Pare, Boulogne, France

**Race L. Kao, PhD**
East Tennessee State University, Johnson City, Tennessee

**Patricia C. Keelen, MD**
Division of Plastic and Reconstructive Surgery, Department of Surgery, University of Louisville and The Jewish Hospital Heart and Lung Institute, Louisville, Kentucky

**Peter Klapproth, MSC**
Department of Cardiac Surgery, University of Lübeck, Lübeck, Germany

**R. Krakor, MD**
Clinic for Heart Surgery, University of Leipzig, Leipzig, Germany

**Alexander A. Krakovsky, MD**
Bakulev Institute for Cardiovascular Surgery, Moscow, Russia

**John M. Kratz, MD**
Division of Cardiothoracic Surgery, Department of Surgery, Medical University of South Carolina, Charleston, South Carolina

**M.M.N. Kwende, PhD**
Department of Human Anatomy and Cell Biology, University of Liverpool, Liverpool, England

**Rüdiger Lange, MD**
Department of Heart Surgery, University Hospital, Heidelberg, Germany

**S. Lange, MD**
Clinic for Heart Surgery, University of Leipzig, Leipzig, Germany

**M. Lass, MD**
Department of Cardiac Surgery, University of Ulm, Ulm, Germany

**Robert R. Lazzara, MD**
Department of Surgery, Allegheny General Hospital, Pittsburgh, Pennsylvania

**Robert Leinders, BS**
Bakken Research Center, Maastricht, The Netherlands

**Peter I. Lelkes, PhD**
Department of Medicine, Laboratory of Cell Biology, University of Wisconsin, Milwaukee Clinical Campus, Milwaukee, Wisconsin

**Raymond Limet, MD**
Department of Cardiovascular Surgery, University Hospital of Liège, Liège, Belgium

**Vassyl A. Lonchyna, MD**
Department of Thoracic and Cardiovascular Surgery, Loyola University, Chicago, Illinois

**Roberto Lorusso, MD**
Cardiac Surgery Division, Civile Hospital, Brescia, Italy

**Michael G. Magno, MD**
Division of Cardiothoracic Surgery, Department of Surgery, Thomas Jefferson University, Philadelphia, Pennsylvania

**George J. Magovern, MD**
Department of Surgery, Allegheny General Hospital, Pittsburgh, Pennsylvania

**James A. Magovern, MD**
Department of Surgery, Allegheny General Hospital, Pittsburgh, Pennsylvania

**John D. Mannion, MD**
Division of Cardiothoracic Surgery, Department of Surgery, Thomas Jefferson University, Philadelphia, Pennsylvania

**C.N. Mayne, MD**
Department of Human Anatomy and Cell Biology, University of Liverpool, Liverpool, England

**Lloyd H. Michael, MD**
Department of Surgery and Department of Medicine, Baylor College of Medicine, Houston, Texas

**Philippe Mikaeloff, MD**
Department of Cardiac Surgery, Hôpital de Lyon, Lyon, France

**Eric Monnet, DVM**
Department of Clinical Sciences, College of Veterinary Medicine, Colorado State University, Fort Collins, Colorado

**Luiz Felipe P. Moreira, MD**
Heart Institute of São Paulo University Medical School, São Paulo, Brazil

**Rupak Mukherjee, MD**
Division of Cardiothoracic Surgery, Department of Surgery, Medical University of South Carolina, Charleston, South Carolina

**Hiroshi Niinami, MD, PhD**
The Department of Cardiovascular Surgery, The Heart Institute of Japan, Tokyo Women's Medical College, Tokyo, Japan

**Todd Nixon, MD**
Surgery Department, Medical College of Virginia, Richmond, Virginia

**Jonah N.K. Odim, MD**
Divisions of Cardiovascular and Thoracic Surgery, The Montreal General Hospital/McGill University, Montreal, Quebec, Canada

**E. Christopher Orton, DVM, PhD**
Department of Clinical Sciences, College of Veterinary Medicine, Colorado State University, Fort Collins, Colorado

**Andy Peczalski, PhD**
Honeywell Systems and Research Center, Bloomington, Minnesota

**Kazimierz Peczalski, PhD**
Division of Cardiovascular and Thoracic Surgery, University of Minnesota, Minneapolis, Minnesota

**Vikenty V. Pekarsky, MD**
Siberian Centre of Cardiac Surgery, Tomsk, Russia

**Michel Pellerin, MD**
Montreal Heart Institute, Montreal, Quebec, Canada

**David Peterson, PhD**
Medtronic, Inc., Minneapolis, Minnesota

**Donald F. Pierce, Jr., MD**
Department of Cell Biology, Vanderbilt University Medical School, Nashville, Tennessee

**Roque Pifarre, MD**
Department of Thoracic and Cardiovascular Surgery, Loyola University, Chicago, Illinois

**Marc A. Radermecker, MD**
Department of Cardiovascular Surgery, University Hospital of Liège, Liège, Belgium

**Renato Ruggiero, MD**
Division of Cardiothoracic Surgery, Wayne State University, School of Medicine, Detroit, Michigan

**Falk-Udo Sack, MD**
Department of Heart Surgery, University Hospital, Heidelberg, Germany

**Stanley Salmons, PhD**
Department of Human Anatomy and Cell Biology, University of Liverpool, Liverpool, England

**Luca Sandrelli, MD**
Cardiac Surgery Department, Civile Hospital, Brescia, Italy

**William P. Santamore, PhD**
Division of Thoracic and Cardiovascular Surgery, University of Louisville, Louisville, Kentucky

**Jan Schreuder, MD**
Departments of Anesthesiology and Cardiology, Academic Hospital, Maastricht, The Netherlands

**Konstantin V. Shatalov, MD**
Bakulev Institute for Cardiovascular Surgery, Moscow, Russia

**A.P. Shortland, PhD**
Department of Clinical Engineering, University of Liverpool, Liverpool, England

**Sara J. Shumway, MD**
Division of Cardiovascular and Thoracic Surgery, University of Minnesota, Minneapolis, Minnesota

**James D. Sink, MD**
Philadelphia Heart Institute, Presbyterian Medical Center, Philadelphia, Pennsylvania

**Eric E. Solien, BS**
Division of Cardiovascular and Thoracic Surgery, University of Minnesota, Minneapolis, Minnesota

**Ernesto R. Soltero, MD**
Department of Surgery and Department of Medicine, Baylor College of Medicine, Houston, Texas

**Francis G. Spinale, MD**
Division of Cardiothoracic Surgery, Department of Surgery, Medical University of South Carolina, Charleston, South Carolina

**John A. Spratt, MD**
Surgery Department, Medical College of Virginia, Richmond, Virginia

**Albert Starr, MD**
The Heart Institute, St. Vincent Hospital and Medical Center, Portland, Oregon

**Paul M. Stein, PhD**
Medtronic, Inc., Minneapolis, Minnesota

**Larry W. Stephenson, MD**
The Department of Surgery, Division of Cardiothoracic Surgery, Wayne State University School of Medicine, Detroit, Michigan

**James R. Stewart, MD**
Department of Cardiac and Thoracic Surgery, Vanderbilt University Medical School, Nashville, Tennessee

**Noedir A.G. Stolf, MD**
Heart Institute of São Paulo University Medical School, São Paulo, Brazil

**George R. Sutherland, MD**
Department of Cardiology, Western General Hospital, Edinburgh, Scotland

**H. Sutherland, PhD**
Department of Human Anatomy and Cell Biology, University of Liverpool, Liverpool, England

**Jeffrey S. Swanson, MD**
The Heart Institute, St. Vincent Hospital and Medical Center, Portland, Oregon

**Stanley K.C. Tam, MD**
Cardiac Surgical Unit, Massachusetts General Hospital, Harvard Medical School, Boston, Massachusetts

**Michel Tapia, MD**
The Department of Cardiovascular Surgery, Broussais Hospital, Paris, France

**Gregory A. Thomas, MD**
Division of Cardiothoracic Surgery, Wayne State University School of Medicine, Detroit, Michigan

**Anne-Elise Tobin, MD**
Division of Plastic and Reconstructive Surgery, Department of Surgery, University of Louisville, The Heart and Lung Institute of Jewish Hospital, Louisville, Kentucky

**Gordon R. Tobin, MD**
Division of Plastic and Reconstructive Surgery, Department of Surgery, University of Louisville and The Jewish Hospital Heart and Lung Institute, Louisville, Kentucky

**Hemant Trehan, MD**
The Heart Institute, St. Vincent Hospital and Medical Center, Portland, Oregon

**Dennis R. Trumble, MS**
Cardiothoracic Surgical Research, Allegheny-Singer Research Institute, Pittsburgh, Pennsylvania

**J.M. Tuchek, DO**
Department of Thoracic and Cardiovascular Surgery, Loyola University, Chicago, Illinois

**Vladimir Y. Ussov, MD**
Siberian Centre of Cardiac Surgery, Tomsk, Russia

**F.H. van der Veen, MD**
Department of Cardiology, Academic Hospital, Maastricht, The Netherlands

**Tony J. Verbeuren, PhD**
Division of Angiology, Servier Research Institute, Suresnes, France

**André Waleffe, MD**
Department of Cardiology, University Hospital of Liège, Liège, Belgium

**Jianyi Zhang, PhD**
Department of Cardiology, University of Minnesota, Minneapolis, Minnesota

**Audrius Zibaitis, MD**
Montreal General Hospital; Divisions of Cardiovascular and Thoracic Surgery, McGill University, Montreal, Quebec, Canada

# Preface

Since the publication of our first book, *Cardiomyoplasty,* 5 years have passed during which new techniques have emerged and new data have accumulated. This new work provides an updated state of the art in ventricular assistance by biological means, i.e., cardiomyoplasty and aortomyoplasty, muscle-powered artificial ventricles, and the most recent development of cellular and molecular cardiomyoplasty. A large portion of the book discusses cardiomyoplasty and its satellites, aortomyoplasty and atriomyoplasty. Worldwide, the total number of operations exceeds 1,000 cases with follow-up extending beyond 10 years. After many years of questions and doubts on the efficacy of this operation, the general consensus drawn from the experience of the leading groups is that significant functional improvements were observed in most cases. Evaluation by echocardiography, isotopic studies, and ventricular PV loop analysis has provided objective data underlining the mechanism of these functional improvements. Of particular importance in this book are the studies on muscle function assessed by electrophysiological and histochemical blood flow analysis, and the effects of vasopressors, vasodilators, sympathectomy, new methods of stimulation, and anabolic steroids on this function.

In addition to clinical evaluation, much of the book covers research and development. The clinical use of aortomyoplasty is under investigation; muscle-powered artificial ventricle is progressing and a new promising technique, cellular and molecular cardiomyoplasty, is emerging. These contributions show the continuous dynamics and creativity in the field of cardiac bioassist, dynamics largely explained by the fact that surgeons and cardiologists in their daily practice are confronted with an increasing number of patients with end-stage heart failure and a decreasing number of donors for cardiac transplantation.

Alain Carpentier, MD, PhD

# Contents

# Part I

## Dynamic Cardiomyoplasty: Clinical Experience

Chapter 1

# Dynamic Cardiomyoplasty at Eleven Years

Alain Carpentier, Juan Carlos Chachques, Jean-Pierre Carteaux

## Introduction

Eleven years after the first case of dynamic cardiomyoplasty,[1–3] our experience encompasses 84 patients. The aim of this chapter is to report the results of this series with particular attention to the changes in indications and techniques which have been made since our last reports.[4,5]

## Patients

From January 1985 to December 1995, 84 patients suffering from severe heart failure were operated on at Hôpital Broussais in Paris. Ages ranged from 15 years to 72 years (mean 50 years). There were 70 males and 14 females.

### Etiology

The two main causes of heart failure were chronic myocardial ischemia and dilated cardiomyopathy.

#### *Myocardial Ischemia*

The 45 patients with myocardial ischemia had suffered several myocardial infarctions and seven had had previous coronary artery revascularization. All were considered to be beyond the possibility of efficient myocardial revascularization at the time of cardiomyoplasty. However, 17 patients had a visible but obstructed coronary artery suitable for bypass which, in the absence of pain, raised the question of the need for revascularization.

From Carpentier A, Chachques JC, Grandjean P: Cardiac Bioassist. © Futura Publishing Co, Inc, Armonk, NY, 1997.

Eleven patients had an extensive anteroapical left ventricular aneurysm. Six had mitral valve insufficiency and two had mitral and tricuspid valve insufficiency.

### *Dilated Cardiomyopathy*

Thirty-three patients presented with dilated cardiomyopathy that was either idiopathic (n=30) or from a valvular origin (n=3). The dilated cardiomyopathy involved predominantly the left ventricle in 14, the right ventricle in six, or both ventricles in 13. Associated mitral valve regurgitation was present in three patients.

### *Cardiac Tumor*

Five patients suffered from a cardiac tumor: fibroma 2, lymphoma 1, hemangioma 1, and metastatic sarcoma 1. These tumors involved the right ventricle and extended to the septum 2, the tricuspid valve 2, and the pulmonary valve 1.

### *Congenital Malformation*

One patient aged 27 had elevated pulmonary resistances and severe venous and liver congestion developed 6 years after a Fontan operation done to correct a single ventricle with pulmonary artery stenosis.

## Clinical Status

All patients but one were in New York Heart Association functional Class III or IV before operation (mean 3.3) (Table 1). Most of the patients had been hospitalized several times for congestive heart failure with an average of 2.3 episodes/patient/year. Sinus rhythm was present in 76 patients. Six were in atrial fibrillation, one had a pacemaker, and one an implanted defibrillator. Ventricular extrasystoles were present in 24 patients among whom five had several episodes of ventricular tachycardia. Other clinical or functional data are listed in Table 1.

Mitral valve incompetence (MVI) was present in nine patients, severe in two, and mild to moderate in seven. Assessed by echocardiography, the functional classification of these MVI cases showed normal leaflet motion (type I) in four patients, leaflet prolapse (type II) in two, and restricted leaflet motion during systole (type IIIb) in three. Tricuspid valve insufficiency was present in seven patients. Functional classification showed restricted leaflet motion during systole (type IIIb) in five patients. In the remaining two patients, tricuspid insufficiency resulted from the involvement of the leaflet tissue by a cardiac tumor.

Associated noncardiac diseases precluding heart transplantation were present in the majority of the patients (Table 2).

**Table 1**
Clinical Status of Patients Prior to Cardiomyoplasty

| | |
|---|---|
| Functional Class IV | 25 |
| III | 59 |
| Left heart failure | 45 |
| Right heart failure | 13 |
| Biventricular failure | 26 |
| Cardiothoracic ratio | 57±5% |
| Indexed LV end-diastolic volume | 178±31 mL/m$^2$ |
| Left ventricular ejection fraction (at rest) | 17±3% |

**Table 2**
Associated Pathology

| | |
|---|---|
| Insulin-dependent diabetes | 13 |
| Pulmonary artery hypertension | 16 |
| Respiratory insufficiency | 15 |
| Gastric ulcer | 11 |
| Renal insufficiency | 6 |
| Cancer | 6 |
| Lupus erythematosus | 1 |
| Colonic diverticulitis | 1 |

# Surgical Technique

## Cardiomyoplasty Procedure

The surgical modalities are summarized in Table 3. In order to reduce the operative complications and to increase the efficiency of the operation, the technical procedure described earlier[2,3] has benefited from the following modifications.

*Latissimus dorsi mobilization* is a key factor for the success of the operation. Any injury, distortion, or traction on the vascular and nervous pedicle may lead to some degree of ischemia of the muscle and subsequent fibrosis or fat degeneration of the muscular fibers. On the other hand, a too limited dissection of the pedicle is associated with a reduced amount of muscular flap to wrap the dilated ventricle. With experience, we have the tendency today to dissect more widely the vascular pedicle by ligating all of the posterior collateral branches. The tendon of the muscle is secured to the third rib inside the thorax. Whenever the heart is particularly large, suggesting that the wrapping will be unsatisfactory, the muscular surface is extended by the placement of an implantable balloon (JC Chachques) between the muscle and the ribs. Progressive distention of the balloon over a period of 2 months provided a 30% augmentation of the surface area of the muscle in two patients. Extreme care is mandatory during the introduction of the muscle through the thorax window created by removing a segment of the second rib. The resec-

**Table 3**
Surgical Modalities

| | | |
|---|---|---|
| Reinforcement technique | 69 | (82%) |
| Substitution technique | 15 | (18%) |
| Anterior wrap | 13 | (15.5%) |
| Posterior wrap | 70 | (83.3%) |
| Atrial wrap | 1 | (1.2%) |
| Extracorporeal circulation | 29 | (34.5%) |
| Intra-aortic balloon counterpulsation | 38 | (45.2%) |

tion should be extended anteriorly and the window should be enlarged to four fingerbreadths to avoid compression injury. In order to decrease the amount of fluid in the dead space left by the transferred latissimus dorsi muscle, the subcutaneous tissue is applied to the chest wall with multiple tacking sutures. In addition, a compressive dressing is left in place for 10 days after the operation.

*Extracorporeal circulation* was avoided as often as possible since it proved to be a risk factor associated with a higher incidence of bleeding, infection, difficulty of weaning off bypass, and death. Of 84 patients, only 29 were operated under extracorporeal circulation, most of them in the beginning of our experience or whenever extracorporeal circulation was necessary to perform associated procedures.

*The technique of wrapping* of the heart was guided by the ventricle involved and the shape of the flap, selecting the position that provided the largest covering without distortion of the neurovascular pedicle. The superficial surface of the muscle was placed in contact with the epicardium in 48 patients and the deep fascia in contact with epicardium in 36 patients.

*A posterior wrap* or clockwise rotation (i.e., the muscle flap placed posteriorly in contact with the left ventricle) was used in 70 cases with predominant left ventricular failure. The positioning of the flap was carried out using the "flap sliding technique" which makes it possible to avoid heart mobilization.[2] Two stay sutures, placed on the leading edge of the muscle flap, are used to slide the flap behind the heart. The sliding is facilitated by holding the two sutures at their origin of the muscle with two long clamps (Fig. 1). Posterior and medial displacement of these clamps allows positioning of the free edge of the muscle, first below the apex and then behind the left ventricle. The distal stay suture is secured to the pericardium in front of the inferior vena cava and the proximal suture is secured to the remnant of the pericardium at the level of the left atrial appendage.

*An anterior wrap* was preferred whenever predominant right ventricular insufficiency was present (nine cases) or in right heart reconstruction after tumor resection (four cases). In cases with large LDM surface, the muscle is folded longitudinally so that two layers of muscle are applied to the right ventricle. The extremity of the muscle is sutured to the pericardial sac posteriorly at the junction between the diaphragmatic and the posterior parts of the pericardium (Fig. 2).

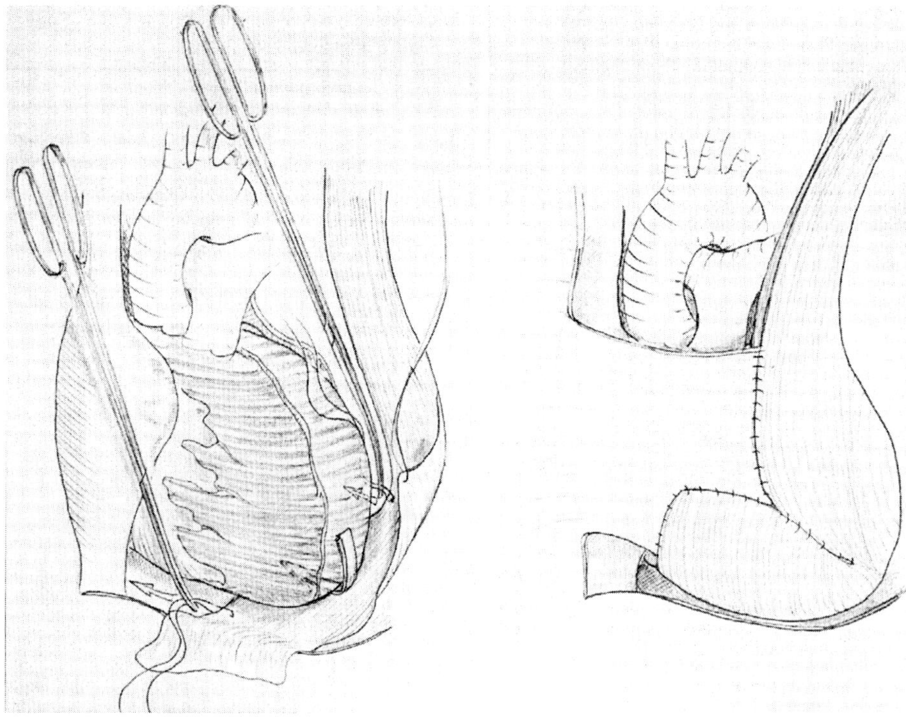

**Figure 1:** *Posterior wrap. The "flap-sliding technique."* Left*: two long clamps hold two stay sutures placed on the leading edge of the flap. Posterior and medial displacement of these clamps allows the free edge of the muscle to slide below the apex and then behind the left ventricle without the heart being mobilized.* Right*: the two stay sutures are secured to the pericardial sac, the wrap is completed, and the pericardial flap (tailored at the beginning of the operation) is sutured to the free edge of the muscle flap so as to maintain its proper position. Reproduced from A. Carpentier et al: Dynamic cardiomyoplasty at seven years.* J Thorac Cardiovasc Surg *106:42–54, 1993.*

This orientation allows coverage of the entire right ventricle and the diaphragmatic wall of the left ventricle.

*An atrial wrap* was used in a patient who developed elevated pulmonary resistance following a Fontan operation. The two atria were dissected and separated, a homograft valve was implanted in the inferior vena cava, and the left latissimus dorsi was used to wrap the right atrium according to a technique previously described.[4,5]

*A two-stage procedure* was used in four patients who developed a significant hypotension, tachycardia or arrhythmia during latissimus dorsi mobilization or ventricular wrapping. The muscular flap was left in place in the left pleural cavity and the wrapping was delayed until the following day. The patients were given small doses of continuous intravenous xylocaine and an intra-aortic balloon counterpulsation was placed. The wrapping of the heart could take place the following day without difficulty. In general, a large use of balloon counterpulsation is recommended whenever one or several risk factors are present or cardiotonic drugs are needed.

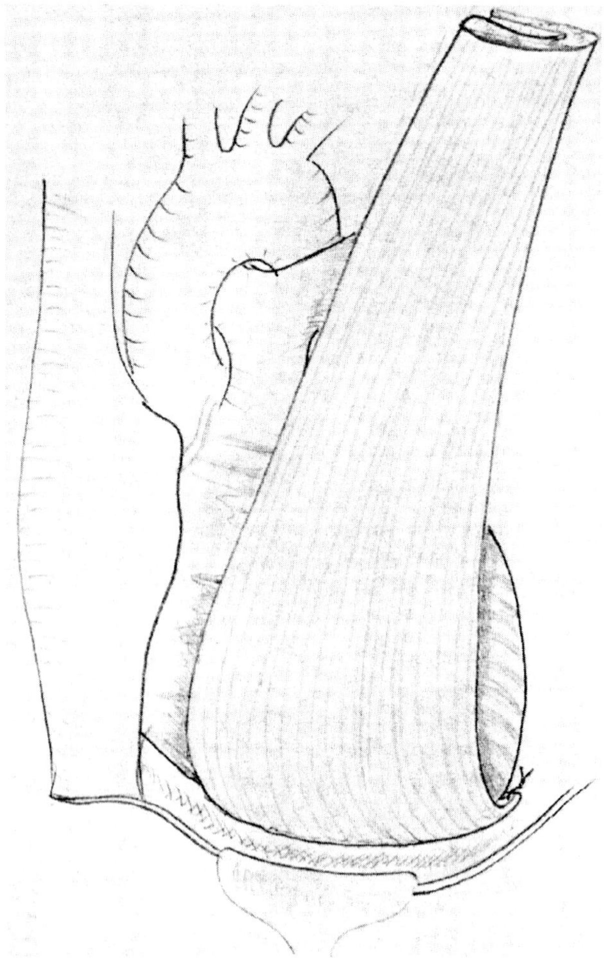

**Figure 2:** *Anterior wrap. The "two-layer technique." The muscle flap is folded longitudinally and its distal end is secured to the pericardial sac as far posterior as possible at the junction between the diaphragmatic and the posterior parts of the pericardium. Reproduced from A. Carpentier et al: Dynamic cardiomyoplasty at seven years.* J Thorac Cardiovasc Surg *106:42–54, 1993.*

## Associated Surgical Procedures and Coronary Artery Revascularization

Mitral valve repair or tricuspid valve repair performed under extracorporeal circulation in a one-stage operation immediately prior to the wrapping have been associated with a high mortality rate and are seen today as a contraindication unless they are carried out in a two-stage operation 1 or 2 weeks before the cardiomyoplasty procedure.

Coronary artery revascularization was carried out in 11 patients; in two patients suffering from a tumor of the right ventricle, the posterior descending artery was revascularized after the right coronary artery had been resected together with the right ventricular wall affected by the tumor. In patients with ischemic heart disease, at the beginning of our experience, revascularization was thought to be unnecessary because these patients had no residual angina and because the visible stenotic coronary arteries were located in infarcted areas. This proved to be an inappropriate policy since two patients died from recurrent myocardial infarction 6 months and 2 years following operation. Revascularization was therefore undertaken thereafter in nine patients with accessible obstructed coronary arteries. Revascularization was performed either prior to the cardiomyoplasty procedure in three cases or during this procedure in six cases. The techniques used were transcutaneous balloon dilatation (three procedures in two patients) and/or coronary artery bypass grafting (eight procedures in eight patients). Coronary artery bypass grafting without extracorporeal circulation was preferred whenever possible because of the frequent difficulty of weaning these very sick patients from bypass. This was possible in one patient on the right coronary artery and in another patient on the anterior descending artery because of the decreased anterior wall motion. In this case, the coronary artery was widely dissected and surrounded by two tapes. After heparin was given, a U-shaped arterial clamp* was applied that occluded the artery and stabilized the anastomotic site. Under these conditions, a bypass graft could be constructed easily.

## Muscle Stimulation

The second sensing electrode is no longer used whenever the first electrode provides adequate signal collection, i.e., at least 5 mV amplitude and 0.5 V/sec slew rate.

The protocol of progressive sequential stimulation, as described in previous papers,[6,7] was used in all patients. The stimulator used was initially the Medtronic® SP 1005 and since December 1993, the Medtronic "Transform" System (16 implants). After a 2-week period of no stimulation (the time necessary for the muscle to adhere to the heart), progressive sequential stimulation was undertaken which after 6 weeks culminated to full stimulation with trains of impulses and maximum pulses amplitude (4 volts ± 0.6). The 1:2 mode was used in most patients since it was associated with better patient comfort and ventricular performances. Echo-Doppler served to assess the proper timing of stimulation since the muscle should contract only after mitral valve closure.

## Results

Results were divided into two periods: (1) the preassist period (first 2 months), which was strongly influenced by the patient's preoperative condition and his capacity to recover from the operation without muscle assistance; and (2) the assist period, which reflected the efficiency of the procedure and the evolution of the underlying heart disease.

*CardioThoracic Systems, 3280 Alpine Road, Portola Valley CA 94028 (USA).

## Preassist Period

### *Mortality*

Sixteen patients (19%) died during the preassist period in spite of pharmacological support in all and intra-aortic balloon counterpulsation in nine. The causes of death were cardiac failure in 6, myocardial infarction in 1, multiorgan failure in 5, sepsis in 2, sudden death in 2.

Multivariate analysis of preoperative risk factors for hospital mortality showed that New York Heart Association (NYHA) functional Class IV, extracorporeal circulation, associated mitral valve procedures, pulmonary artery hypertension, biventricular failure, and respiratory insufficiency were predictors of unfavorable outcome (Table 4). All of the patients with a cardiac index of less than 1.3 L/min/m$^2$ and/or a capillary wedge pressure over 40 mm Hg, and/or a left ventricular end diastolic pressure over 50 mm Hg died during the preassist period. Taking into consideration these risk factors led to an improved selection of the patients and a reduced preassist mortality in the past 8 years: 13% (9/71) in the 1988–1996 period versus 54% (7/13) in the 1985–1987 period.

### *Complications*

Most of the patients experienced a difficult postoperative course due to their severe preoperative condition. Only 23% of the patients remained in the intensive care unit (ICU) for less than 3 days and 42% for less than 6 days.

Low cardiac output, present in 26 patients (31%), was by far the most frequent complication. Eleven patients died of either cardiac failure (six patients) or multiorgan failure (five patients). One patient who died from cardiac failure had necrosis of the latissimus dorsi at autopsy.

**Table 4**
Preoperative Risk Factors Influencing Hospital and Late Mortality (Multivariate Analysis)

| Risk Factors |
|---|
| **Risk Factors Influencing Hospital Mortality** |
| NYHA functional Class IV |
| Biventricular heart failure |
| Pulmonary artery hypertension |
| Respiratory insufficiency |
| Associated surgical procedures |
| **Risk Factors Influencing Long-Term Mortality** |
| LV ejection fraction <15% or filling pressures >45mm Hg |
| Biventricular heart failure |
| Age >65 years |
| Severe ventricular arrhythmias |
| Atrial fibrillation |
| Cardiothoracic ratio >0.60 or LVDD >75mm |

All patients displayed some episodes of arrhythmia during the operation. Ventricular ectopic beats were the most commonly encountered arrhythmia. Severe ventricular arrhythmias were usually associated with hypoxemia and hypotension. In four cases, severe arrhythmia and hypotension produced by the wrapping led to a two-stage operation. The flap was repositioned in the left pleural cavity and the wrapping was carried out the following day without complications. The development of the "noncardiac suture" technique[3] and the "flap sliding maneuver"[2] have been associated with a reduced risk of arrhythmia.

Renal failure, encountered in 10 patients, was caused by poor preoperative clinical condition, low cardiac output, and/or infection. Four patients required renal dialysis and three others died. Six other patients had creatinine elevations and were given dopamine 3 mg/kg/min.

Infection was present in six of 84 cases (7%): septicemia leading to death in two functional Class IV patients and local infection in four patients. The infection was localized to the area of dissection of the latissimus dorsi in two patients and to the pocket of the stimulator in two other patients. All were successfully treated by debridement and long-term antibiotics. One patient with infection of the pocket of the stimulator had the stimulator removed and was subsequently transplanted. In another patient, the stimulator was removed and subsequently replaced.

Five patients had partial necrosis of the skin in the area of dissection of the latissimus dorsi muscle, for which they were successfully treated by skin resection and suture. Three patients with intra-aortic balloon counterpulsation had an ischemia of one leg. One of these patients eventually died.

## Postassist Period

Sixty-eight patients were followed up for from 6 months up to 11 years (mean 4 years, 2 months).

### *Late Mortality*

During this period of follow-up, 19 of 68 patients (28%) died. The causes of death were cardiac failure in nine, gastric bleeding in one, myocardial infarction in two, stroke in one, and sudden death in six. In one patient who died from ischemic heart failure 8 years and 6 months after cardiomyoplasty, histology of the heart showed an extensive fibrosis in contrast with the well-preserved structure of the latissimus dorsi muscle (Fig. 3).

Including hospital mortality, the actuarial survival at 7 years was 52%. Actuarial survival at 7 years was 82% in the group of predominant right ventricular failure, 57% in the group of left ventricular failure, and 48% in the group of biventricular failure. Breaking down the series according to preoperative functional class, the actuarial survival at 7 years including hospital mortality was 28% for the functional Class IV group and 70% for the functional Class III group (Fig. 4). No significant difference was found in the survival rates of patients with ischemic cardiomyopathy versus idiopathic cardiomyopathy.

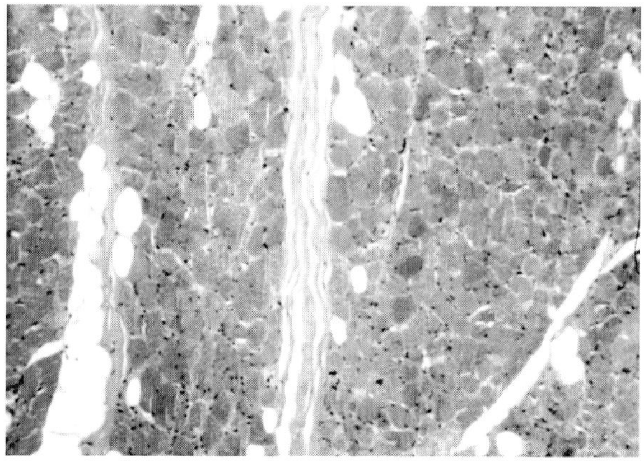

**Figure 3:** *Well-preserved histological structures of the latissimus dorsi 8 years and 6 months following cardiomyoplasty.*

Multivariate analysis of preoperative risk factors showed that left ventricular ejection fraction less than 15%, biventricular failure, severe arrhythmias, atrial fibrillation, cardiothoracic ratio greater than 0.60, and left ventricular diastolic dimension >75mm were predictors of unfavorable outcome (Table 4). The greater the number of risk factors in a given patient, the higher the mortality (Table 5).

*Complications*

Within the 11-year period of follow-up, cardiac failure was encountered in 16 patients (19%). The first cause to evoke whenever a cardiac failure appears rather suddenly is a premature depletion of the battery. This was seen in two patients who were rehospitalized for severe cardiac failure and pulmonary edema 2 and 3 years after the operation. Both improved dramatically after the stimulator had been changed. Except for these two patients, battery depletion was usually progressive and marked by shortness of breath, fatigue, and peripheral edema. The other causes of cardiac failure were: onset of atrial fibrillation in two, battery removal for infection in one, muscular wasting following hepatitis in one, pulmonary insufficiency and infection in one. In the remaining nine cases, cardiac failure was linked to the continuous evolution of the underlying disease. Two of these patients were in functional Class IV at the time of operation with an EF below 14% and one patient developed a recurrent myocardial infarction.

Among the 16 patients with cardiac failure, five underwent successful transplantation at average 29±21 months after cardiomyoplasty and nine died in whom transplantation was contraindicated.

Finally, four patients developed cholecystitis and underwent successful cholecystectomy.

*Functional Improvement*

Among the 68 survivors, the 63 who had not been transplanted displayed a significant functional improvement. The mean NYHA class went from 3.3

**Table 5**
Mortality in Relation to the Number of Risk Factors in a Given Patient

| *Risk Factors* | *Mortality* |
|---|---|
| 0 | 3.5% |
| 1 | 6% |
| 2 | 17% |
| 3 | 32% |
| 4 | 38% |

**Table 6**
Functional Improvement in 63 Patients Surviving Cardiomyoplasty and Not Transplanted

| | *Preoperative* | | *Postoperative* |
|---|---|---|---|
| Functional class (mean) | 3.3 | *p*<0.05 | 1.7 |
| Exercise capacity (Watts) | 60±24 | *p*<0.1 | 96±18 |
| Hospitalizations (nb/pt/year) | 2.3 | *p*<0.05 | 0.4 |

preoperatively down to 1.7 postoperatively ($p<0.05$). In most patients, improvement continued over a period of 8 months after the operation and up to 1 year in nine patients. Functional improvement was associated with increased exercise capacity, significant reduction in the need for drugs in 63% of the patients, and reduction of the number of episodes of hospitalizations for congestive heart failure (Table 6). Daily activities, mental health and quality of interactions scores showed a 80% average 1 year after the operation. The functional improvement persisted throughout the years in 80% of the 63 survivors within the time frame of this study.

*Noninvasive Investigations*

Cardiothoracic ratio in the survivors showed stabilization of heart size (Fig. 4). The mean postoperative LV ejection fraction (Muga) showed an improvement over the preoperative ejection fraction (25% versus 17%) and was stable over years (Fig. 5). Hemodynamic evaluation by aortic flow Doppler study with the cardiomyostimulator turned off and on was performed in the 51 patients surviving more than 2 years after the operation and showed significant improvement in 65% of them.

*Catheterization*

Catheterization obtained in 60 patients followed up for more than 2 years showed no significant changes in capillary wedge pressure, pulmonary artery

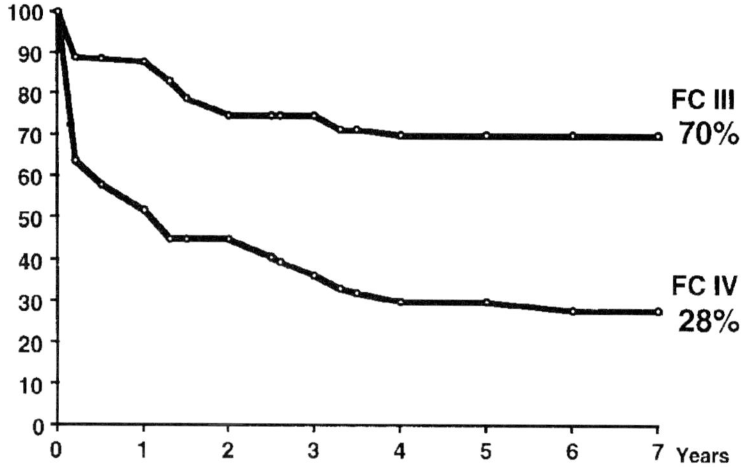


**Figure 4:** *Survival curve in relation to functional class.*

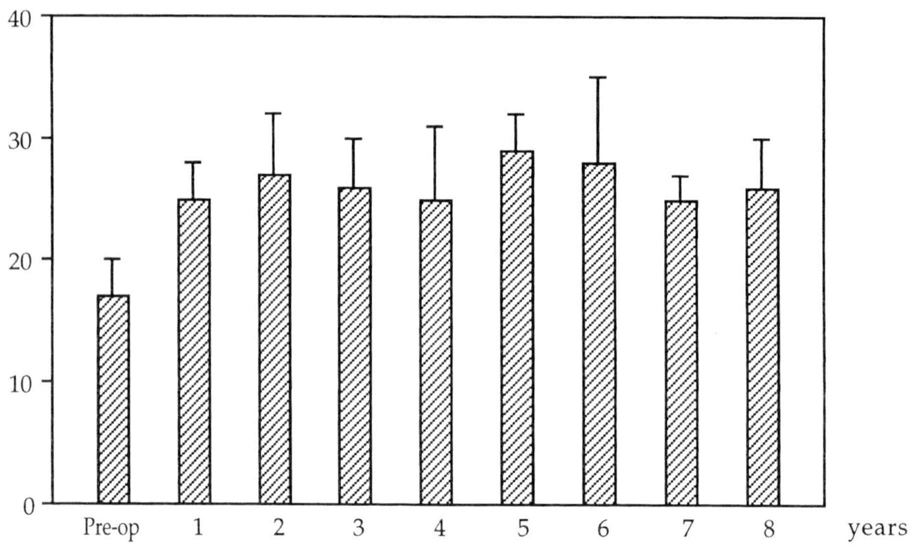


**Figure 5:** *Ejection fraction 1 to 8 years after cardiomyoplasty in 63 survivors.*

pressure, and left ventricular end-diastolic pressure when compared with preoperative values. With the exception of the patients who had a resection of a ventricular aneurysm, postoperative left ventricular end-diastolic volume showed no significant change. However the cardiac index and ejection fraction increased significantly (Table 7).

## Discussion

Despite improved medical management, end-stage heart failure remains a major concern in cardiology because of its prevalence in Western countries

**Table 7**
Hemodynamic Data in 60 Patients at 2 Years

| | *Preoperative* | *Postoperative (2 years)* | |
|---|---|---|---|
| MPAP (mm Hg) | 24.4±6.2 | 26.2±4 | NS |
| MPWP (mm Hg) | 15.8±2.8 | 17.6±3.1 | NS |
| LVEDP (mm Hg) | 20.3±4.2 | 18.7±2.6 | NS |
| CI (L/min/m$^2$) | 2.38±.41 | 2.87±.63 | p=0.049 |
| LVEF (%) | 24±6.2 | 30.6±5 | p=0.043 |
| LVED Vol (mL/m$^2$) indexed | 178±31 | 186±36 | NS |

MPAP = artery pressure; MPWP = wedge pressure; LVEDP = left ventricular end-diastolic pressure; CI = cardiac index; LVEF = left ventricular ejection fraction; LVED = left ventricular end-diastolic.

and the severity of its prognosis. Actuarial survival at 3 years has long been said to be only 20%.[8] Recent medical progress and particularly the use of vasodilators have improved the tolerance to this condition but only slightly modified the survival itself.[9] Heart transplantation is efficient in patients with end-stage heart failure but this technique is limited by shortage of donors, contraindications, and the need for immunosuppressive therapy. Cardiomyoplasty has the advantage of using the patient's own living tissues, thus avoiding rejection and related problems. The hemodynamic effect of this technique had been demonstrated in numerous short-term experiments using skeletal muscle wrapped around the heart.[10–12] Cardiac output was restored when the right or left ventricular walls were partially replaced by the latissimus dorsi muscle.[13] Hemodynamic improvement had also been documented in the presence of acutely induced myocardial dysfunction.[14] However, muscle fatigue was thought to be an insurmountable barrier whenever long-term stimulation was used. The introduction by our group of the concept of progressive sequential stimulation[1] was able to overcome this difficulty as shown by long-term experiments.[15] The first clinical application took place in 1985.[1] Since then, cardiomyoplasty has been used clinically in the treatment of various cardiac diseases: tumor, aneurysm, ischemic cardiomyopathy, dilated cardiomyopathy, and Chagas' disease.[2,16–20] Results have been encouraging so far although variations were found due to the heterogenicity of the patient population and to the techniques used. Therefore, numerous questions remain to be addressed concerning surgical technique, survival, functional benefit, hemodynamic results, and the mechanism of action.

## Surgical Technique

The surgical technique has evolved throughout the years with the aim of reducing preassist mortality and increasing the efficiency of the procedure. In the past 6 years, the use of the "noncardiac suture" technique[3] and the "flap-sliding maneuver"[2] reduced the preoperative mortality to 12%. There are, however, still controversial technical points that must be discussed.

### *Muscle Orientation*

Experimental studies have shown that an anterior positioning of the flap with a counterclockwise wrapping of the heart could be more efficient than the posterior wrapping.[23] However, in patients with enlarged hearts, the anterior positioning of the muscle flap does not allow the left ventricle to be completely covered. A pragmatic approach must take into consideration: the type of ventricular failure, the size of the heart, the size of the flap, and the patient's condition.

In predominant left heart failure, the flap must be positioned posteriorly in contact with the left ventricle. In predominant right heart failure, the flap is positioned anteriorly. Enlarged heart size is a serious limitation to muscle wrapping, particularly when the size of the muscle flap is small. There are three ways to minimize this problem: (1) extensive dissection of the pedicle with ligature of the posterior branches. This technique allows a better mobilization of the muscle and the positioning of the muscle tendon 5 cm below the current level; (2) muscle expansion using the Chachques implantable balloon; and (3) partial excision of the ventricle in order to reduce its size. The latter technique has not been associated with good results in our hands. Poor results were also observed whenever trying to reduce the size of the heart by excess tension on the muscle flap. It seems that severely dilated ventricles have adapted themselves to a given wall tension which cannot be reduced without impairing the residual contractility.

### *Muscle Stimulation and Ventricular Compliance*

Although some hemodynamic benefits have been obtained with single pulse muscle stimulation,[17] it is now widely accepted that the protocol of progressive sequential stimulation and pulse trains are preferable for muscle transformation and cardiac assistance.[12,13,25] The interval between the sensed QRS complex and each pulse train is of paramount importance. Both experimental and clinical data have shown that muscle contraction may affect ventricular filling when no delay was present between the QRS complex and the pulse train.[24] Echocardiography must be used to adjust this delay in order to provide optimal synchronization among muscle contraction, ventricular systole, and mitral valve closure. Tachycardia is another factor that may impair ventricular filling since in the current model of cardiomyostimulator (SP 1005), the pulse train has a fixed duration (185 msec). For this reason, the stimulator automatically increases the heart muscle contraction ratio (2:1, 3:1) with increasing heart rates which results in assisting only 1 systole over 2 or 3 during exercise. In the new stimulator developed by Medtronic (TRANSFORM® system) the pulse train duration depends upon heart rate. The heart muscle contraction ratio must be adapted to each individual patient according to functional improvement. Most of the time the optimal ratio is 2:1. Whenever synchronization between heart and muscle contraction is adequate, the muscle does not impair the ventricular compliance because of the greater wall tension of the dilated ventricles.

## Survival

This study demonstrates that cardiomyoplasty improves long-term survival. The 52% actuarial survival at 7 years contrasts with the 20% survival at 3 years in medically treated patients.[8,9] Improved survival in patients with cardiomyoplasty was also demonstrated by Jatene and Moreira comparing medically treated patients with cardiomyoplasty patients.[21] Survival can further be improved by taking into consideration the risk factors of the preassist and the postassist periods. Indeed, the greater the number of risk factors, the higher the mortality (Table 5). Contrary to the type of ventricular failure and the functional class, the etiology of cardiac disease had little influence on the overall mortality (Table 8).

## Functional Benefit

In addition to improved survival, a significant functional improvement was found in the great majority of the patients. Functional class decreased from an average 3.3 preoperatively to 1.8 postoperatively. Exercise capacity was generally improved, the number of episodes of hospitalizations per patient/year was reduced from 2.4 to 0.4, and in 62% of the patients the need for drugs was significantly reduced. Similar improvements have been described by others.[17–22] Also of interest is the fact that functional improvement was progressive over a period of up to 1 year, which shows the capacity of the muscle to adapt to its new function. Functional improvement varied, however, from patient to patient, the least improvement being seen in patients with preoperative biventricular failure, excessive cardiac enlargement, and ejection fraction below 15%.

**Table 8**

Influence of Pathology and Type of Cardiac Failure on the Overall Mortality (Follow-up 6 Months to 11 Years, Mean 4 Years–2 Months)

| | *Mortality* | |
|---|---|---|
| Ischemic cardiomyopathy | 42% | |
| LV aneurysm | 36% | |
| Idiopathic | 32% | |
| Tumor | 20% | * |
| LV failure | 43% | |
| RV failure | 18% | * |
| Biventricular | 52% | * |
| | | |
| NYHA FC IV | 72% | |
| NYHA FC III | 30% | * |

*$p<0.05$

FC = functional class.

## Hemodynamics

Most disappointing was the fact that functional improvement did not always imply documented hemodynamic improvement. Ejection fraction did increase in the majority of the patients, but no significant changes in filling pressures could be documented in the majority of the patients in this series. Jatene and Moreira, however, reported a significant reduction of the mean pulmonary artery pressure (from 37.4 mm Hg to 26.6 mm Hg) and of the mean pulmonary wedge pressure (from 24.8 mm Hg to 16.6 mm Hg) 12 months after the operation.[20] Patients with greater LV dimensions presented lesser LV ejection fraction improvements. More precisely, significant improvement in left ventricular function was found in patients whose left ventricular diastolic diameter was below 70 mm, whereas no change was found in patients with a ventricular diastolic diameter greater than 75 mm. Both in Jatene's experience and in our experience, LV dimensions throughout the years showed a stabilization in the process of ventricular dilatation in the majority of the patients.

Recent studies analyzing left ventricular pressure-volume relation have shown significant improvements in pressure volume loops after cardiomyoplasty with the stimulator on and off.[26,27]

## Mechanism of Enhanced Heart Function

The improved ejection fraction observed in most cases, although limited, demonstrates that the functional improvement results from enhanced heart function. A placebo effect can therefore be ruled out. This is confirmed by the functional impairment following battery depletion observed in two patients and its complete reversibility after a new battery was implanted. Enhanced heart function involves several mechanisms.

### *Active Reinforcement*

The heart and the wrapped skeletal muscle behave like a cybernetic system with two interactive components: the heart governing the muscle and the muscle reinforcing heart contraction. The efficiency of the system depends on the mechanical characteristics of these two components and the synchronization of their action. According to Laplace's law, the larger the ventricle the greater the tension that must be generated to produce a given pressure. Indeed, greater left ventricular dimension presented lesser left ventricular ejection fraction improvements after cardiomyoplasty. Active reinforcement depends also on the size of the muscle and the amount of wrapping. The power of a transformed muscle has been calculated to be 40 W/kg, identical to the power developed by cardiac muscle during systolic contraction.[25] It is unfortunate that only a portion of this force is used since only a part of the muscle can be wrapped around the heart in order to prevent excessive tension on the neurovascular pedicle. Even though the free portion of the graft may also participate to some extent in cardiac assistance by traction and elevation of the heart during contraction, more than 50% of the force of the muscle is lost. The technique of extensive dissection of the pedicle by ligating the posterior branches underlined in this article has been effective in increasing the mobilization of the muscle flap and the covering of the heart.

### *Passive Reinforcement*

By its intrinsic tension, the muscle reduces the ventricular wall stress, prevents further dilatation of the ventricles, and can restore more orderly cardiac contraction. In our experience, a stabilization of the process of ventricular dilatation was documented as well as reduction in the paradoxical motion of the ventricular septum. Even in the case of passive reinforcement, the stimulation of the muscle is important since it increases the tension of the muscle at an appropriate time and then developed severe heart failure.

### *Biological Effect*

By taking part of the workload of the heart without increasing the myocardial oxygen requirement, the muscle actually increases the oxygen supply to the heart so that some recovery of the cardiac function may result from this mechanism. This "biological effect" is suggested by two patients in our series who kept the full functional benefit of the operation for several days after the battery had been removed for infection and then developed a severe heart failure.

### *Enhanced Coronary Revascularization*

Coronary capillaries have been filled by microspheres, previously injected into the latissimus dorsi artery in experimental animals after cardiomyoplasty. However, this has not been documented in the human thus far.

## Mechanisms of Failure of Cardiomyoplasty

Deterioration of an initially good functional result can be due to several causes that should be identified because some of them can be corrected or prevented.

### *Electrical Stimulation*

The first cause to evoke is the depletion of the battery, which can be easily recognized by electronic testing. The second cause is an improper synchronization between muscle contraction and mitral valve closure.[24] It is easily recognized by echocardiography and corrected.

*Muscular Causes*

Progressive degeneration of the muscle by fibrosis or fat transformation has been described following cardiomyoplasty.[28] One factor that has been identified as a possible cause of muscle damage is muscle ischemia.[29] This may be due to several causes: division of collateral vessels at the time of muscle mobilization, tissue edema following muscle transfer, compression or torsion of the vascular and nerve pedicles, use of vasopressors during the postoperative period, and a 1:1 stimulation mode leading to excess blood flow demand.[30] In our experience, a significant degeneration of the muscle has been documented by electron beam computed tomography in five of the 42 patients studied (12%) with a mean follow-up of 4.3 years. Careful prevention of the causes of ischemia underlined above should further reduce this complication, in particular, careful mobilization and transfer of the muscle, avoidance of vasopressors with generous use of intra-aortic balloon counterpulsation, and a 1:2 mode of stimulation.

*Cardiac Causes*

Progression of the underlying cardiac disease is a major cause of progressive deterioration of an initially good functional result. In ischemic cardiomy-

**Table 9**

Indications and Contraindications for Cardiomyoplasty

**Optimal Indications**

- Patients below 70 years of age
- Dilated cardiomyopathy (idiopathic or ischemic)
- Functional Class III or intermittent Class IV
- Sinus rhythm
- Coronary arteries: good collateral circulation, no pain, no critical stenosis
- Mitral valve regurgitation <++
- LV ejection fraction > 15%
- LV end-diastolic volume <250 ml
- Peak $VO_2$>10 mL/kg/min

**Suboptimal Indications**

- Patients with more than one risk factor listed in Table 4

**Contraindications**

- Hypertrophied and restrictive cardiomyopathies
- Permanent functional Class IV
- Severe, intractable ventricular arrhythmia
- Pulmonary artery hypertension
- Severe biventricular failure
- Mitral valve incompetence >++

- Neurovascular disease, or cachexia
- Left pleura calcifications
- Severe respiratory insufficiency (functional vital capacity <55% predicted)

- Ejection fraction <10%
- Cardiac index <1.5 L/min/$m^2$
- LV end-diastolic volume >300mL. . . diameter >75 mm
- LV end-diastolic pressure >45 mm Hg

opathy, the progression can be delayed by coronary artery revascularization prior to, during, or after cardiomyoplasty. In both ischemic and dilated cardiomyopathy, the onset of atrial fibrillation is the most common cause of functional deterioration. Another cause is the excess weight experienced by some patients after cardiomyoplasty. The patients should be advised to remain in the lower range of the estimated normal weight.

## Indications and Conclusion

Although significant improvements have been achieved in the past few years, numerous points remain obscure and some drawbacks persist. The two most important are the variability of the results and the contrast between functional improvement and the hemodynamics parameters observed after this operation. Numerous factors may explain these drawbacks: heterogeneous patient population, heart size, underlying diseases, suboptimal indications, variable muscle anatomy, and vascularization. Some of these factors have been improved. They may be further improved in the future, especially the selection of the patients (Table 9).

In contrast, some positive points must be recognized that justify and stimulate our continuous effort to develop this operation. The fact that continuous fatigueless contraction of a skeletal muscle at the frequency of the heart has been obtained for periods of more than 8 years in humans is in itself remarkable. The fact that patient survival was increased and that most patients were functionally improved with a significant increase in cardiac output and ejection fraction in many of them is most encouraging. Finally, the fact that similar results have been obtained by various groups throughout the world, provided that they had access to burst train generators, demonstrates that the operation is reproducible. All new operations face uncertainties and shortcomings in their developmental phases. As experience has accumulated, some of them have already been solved. Further progress is necessary, however, in order for this operation to face the challenge of the growing lack of donors for cardiac transplantation.

## References

1. Carpentier A, Chachques JC: Myocardial substitution with a stimulated skeletal muscle: First successful clinical case. *Lancet* 1:1267, 1985.
2. Carpentier A, Chachques JC, Acar C, Relland J, et al: Dynamic cardiomyoplasty at seven years. *J Thorac Cardiovasc Surg* 106:42–54, 1993.
3. Carpentier A, Chachques JC: Surgical technique. In Carpentier A, Chachques JC, Grandjean PA (eds): *Cardiomyoplasty*. Mount Kisco, NY, Futura Publishing Company Inc, 1991, pp 105–122.
4. Chachques JC, Carpentier A, Grandjean PA: Atrial or ventricular assistance using the cardiomyoplasty procedure. In Chiu RC-J, Bourgeois I (eds): *Transformed Muscle for Cardiac Assist and Repair*. Mount Kisco, NY, Futura Publishing Company Inc, 1990, pp 161–178.
5. Loulmet D, Carpentier A, Beaudet RL: Atriomyoplasty. In Carpentier A, Chachques JC, Grandjean PA (eds): *Cardiomyoplasty*. Mount Kisco, NY, Futura Publishing Company Inc, 1991, pp 195–198.

6. Carpentier A, Chachques JC, Grandjean PA, Perier P, et al: Transformation d'un muscle squelettique par stimulation séquentielle progressive en vue de son utilisation comme substitut myocardique. *CR Acad Sciences Paris* 301:581–586, 1985.
7. Chachques JC, Carpentier A: Postoperative management. In Carpentier A, Chachques JC, Grandjean PA (eds): *Cardiomyoplasty*. Mount Kisco, NY, Futura Publishing Company Inc, 1991, pp 131–138.
8. Franciosa JA, Wilen M, Ziesche S, Cohn JN: Survival in men with severe chronic left ventricular failure due to either coronary heart disease or idiopathic dilated cardiomyopathy. *Am J Cardiol* 51:831–836, 1983.
9. Rihal CS, Nishimura RA, Hatle LK, Bailey KR, et al: Systolic and diastolic dysfunction in patients with clinical diagnosis of dilated cardiomyopathy. *Circulation* 90:2772–2779, 1994.
10. Termet H, Chalencon JL, Estour E, et al: Transplantation sur le myocarde d'un muscle strié excité par pace-maker. *Ann Chir Thorac Cardiovasc* 5:270, 1966.
11. Nakamura K, Glenn WL: Graft of diaphragm as a functioning substitute for myocardium. *J Surg Res* 4:435, 1964.
12. Macoviak J, Stephenson LW, Spielman S, et al: Replacement of ventricular myocardium with diaphragmatic skeletal muscle: Short-term studies. *J Thorac Cardiovasc Surg* 81:519, 1981.
13. Dewar ML, Drinkwater DC, Chiu RC-J: Synchronously stimulated skeletal muscle graft for myocardial repair. *J Thorac Cardiovasc Surg* 87:325, 1984.
14. Moreira LFP, Chagas ACP, Camarano GP: Cardiomyoplasty benefits in experimental myocardial dysfunction. *J Cardiac Surg* 4:164–170, 1989.
15. Chachques JC, Grandjean PA, Schwartz K, Mihaileanu S, et al: Effect of latissimus dorsi dynamic cardiomyoplasty on ventricular function. *Circulation* 78(Suppl III): III-203–III-216, 1988.
16. Carpentier A, Chachques JC: The use of stimulated skeletal muscle to replace diseased human heart muscle. In Chiu RC-J (ed): *Biomechanical Cardiac Assist*. Mount Kisco, NY, Futura Publishing Company Inc, 1986, pp 185–192.
17. Magovern GJ, Heckler FR, Park SB, Christlieb IY, et al: Paced skeletal muscle for dynamic cardiomyoplasty. *Ann Thorac Surg* 45:614–619, 1988.
18. Magovern GJ, Park SB, Kao RL, Christlieb IY, et al: Dynamic cardiomyoplasty in patients. *J Heart Transplant* 9:258–263, 1990.
19. Moreira LF, Stolf NA, Bocchi EA, Barretto AP, et al: Latissimus dorsi cardiomyoplasty in the treatment of patients with dilated cardiomyopathy. *Circulation* 82(Suppl IV):IV-257-IV-263, 1990.
20. Jatene AD, Moreira LFP, Stolf NAG, Bocchi EA, et al: Left ventricular function changes after cardiomyoplasty in patients with dilated cardiomyopathy. *J Thorac Cardiovasc Surg* 102:132–139, 1991.
21. Moreira LF, Seferian P, Bocchi EA, Pego-Fernandez PM, et al: Survival improvement with dynamic cardiomyoplasty in patients with dilated cardiomyopathy. *Circulation* 84(Suppl III):III-296-III-302, 1991.
22. Almada H, Molteni L, Ferreira R, Ortega D: Clinical experience with dynamic cardiomyoplasty. *J Cardiac Surg* 5:193–198, 1990.
23. Kao RL, Christlieb IY, Magovern GJ, Park SB, et al: The importance of skeletal muscle fiber orientation for dynamic cardiomyoplasty. *J Thorac Cardiovasc Surg* 99:134–140, 1990.
24. Molteni L, Almada HE, Ferreira RP, Ortega D: Assessment of the optimal time interval between QRS and simple pulse stimulation in dynamic cardiomyoplasty. In Chiu RC-J, Bourgeois I (eds): *Transformed Muscle for Cardiac Assist and Repair*. Mount Kisco, NY, Futura Publishing Company Inc, 1990, pp 189–196.
25. Salmons S, Jarvis JC: Cardiomyoplasty: A look at the fundamentals. In: Carpentier A, Chachques JC, Grandjean PA (eds:) *Cardiomyoplasty*. Mount Kisco, NY, Futura Publishing Company Inc, 1991, pp 3–17.
26. Schreuder JJ, Van der Veen FH, Van der Velde ET, Delahaye F, et al: Beat-to-beat analysis of left ventricular pressure-volume relation and stroke volume by conductance catheter and aortic modelflow in cardiomyoplasty patients. *Circulation* 91:2010–2017, 1995.

27. Kass DA, Baughman KL, Pak PH, Cho PW, et al: Reverse remodelling from cardiomyoplasty in human heart failure. *Circulation* 91:2314–2318, 1995.
28. Moreira LP, Bocchi EA, Stolf NA, Pileggi F, et al: Current expectations in dynamic cardiomyoplasty. *Ann Thorac Surg* 55:299–303, 1993.
29. El Oakley RM, Jarvis JC, Barman D, et al: Factors affecting the integrity of latissimus dorsi muscle grafts: Implications for cardiac assistance from skeletal muscle. *J Heart Lung Transplant* 14:359–365, 1995.
30. Van Doorn CAM, Bhabra MS, Hopkinson DN, Barman D, et al: Latissimus dorsi muscle blood flow during synchronized contraction: implications for cardiomyoplasty. *Ann Thorac Surg* 61:603–609, 1996.

Chapter 2

# Long-Term Results of Cardiomyoplasty in Dilated Cardiomyopathy

Luiz Felipe P. Moreira, Edimar A. Bocchi, Noedir A. G. Stolf, Giovani Bellotti, Adib D. Jatene

## Introduction

Dynamic cardiomyoplasty has been proposed by several authors as an alternative surgical treatment for patients with severe cardiomyopathies. Its primary objectives are to reverse congestive heart failure and to halt the progression of the underlying disease by the increase of ventricular pumping performance and by the reinforcement of ventricular walls.

Initial outcomes demonstrated the improvement of left ventricular function and the reversion of congestive heart failure after cardiomyoplasty in patients with dilated or ischemic cardiomyopathies.[1–6] Nevertheless, mortality varied in these series and the objective documentation of ventricular function changes after this surgical procedure was controversial.[1–6] Furthermore, the accumulated worldwide experience seems to identify potential limitations or risk factors of poor cardiomyoplasty outcome,[1,2,4,6] which may be affected by different heart failure etiologies.

Accordingly, the purpose of this chapter is to outline the long-term results of dynamic cardiomyoplasty in the treatment of patients with advanced heart failure due to idiopathic dilated cardiomyopathy at the Heart Institute of São Paulo University Medical School.

## Patient Selection Criteria

The current indications for dynamic cardiomyoplasty include mainly patients at high risk of dying due to severe cardiomyopathies, which do not essentially differ from heart transplantation criteria.[7] Therefore, candidates for

From Carpentier A, Chachques JC, Grandjean P: Cardiac Bioassist. © Futura Publishing Co, Inc, Armonk, NY, 1997.

this procedure are normally screened based on factors that have been related to mortality in patients with congestive heart failure. These include indexes relating to cardiac pump dysfunction, such as left ventricular (LV) ejection fraction less than 25% and high LV filling pressures,[8,9] as well as the degree of functional impairment assessed by the New York Heart Association (NYHA) as functional Class III or IV, or by the peak oxygen consumption during exercise testing below 16 mL/min/kg.[8,10]

On the other hand, patients submitted to cardiomyoplasty need to be stable enough on medical therapy to withstand a waiting period of 2 to 3 months before effective skeletal muscle flap adaptation. Hence, patients on intravenous inotropic drugs are not candidates for cardiomyoplasty, and persistent functional Class IV has also been recently defined as a contraindication to this procedure.[1,4,6] In addition, patients with important or severe valvular dysfunction, with arrhythmias not controlled by medical therapy, or with pulmonary or multiple organ diseases, are also currently contraindicated for cardiomyoplasty.

Among 32 patients who underwent dynamic cardiomyoplasty at the Heart Institute between May 1988 and March 1993, the indication for this procedure was the idiopathic dilated cardiomyopathy in 27 patients. Twenty of these patients were in NYHA Class III and seven in Class IV despite the use of maximal medical therapy with diuretics, digitalis, and angiotensin-converting enzyme inhibitors.

Patients' ages ranged from 28 to 57 years (mean, 47.8 years) and 21 patients were male. Preoperative laboratory data are summarized in Table 1. In addition, four patients presented with chronic atrial fibrillation and 12 had nonsustained ventricular tachycardia episodes documented by Holter recordings. Cardiac catheterization showed normal coronary arteries in all patients, mild mitral insufficiency in 19, and moderate mitral insufficiency in four. Standard spirometric study documented mild restrictive compromise of ventilatory function in 20 patients.

**Table 1**
Preoperative Laboratory Data

| | |
|---|---|
| *Thorax x-ray:* | |
| Cardiothoracic ratio | 0.58 ± 0.04 |
| *Echocardiography:* | |
| LV diastolic diameter (mm Hg) | 73.3 ± 5.9 |
| LV segmental wall shortening (%) | 11.9 ± 2.1 |
| *Radioisotopic angiography:* | |
| LV ejection fraction (%) | 19.8 ± 2.7 |
| RV ejection fraction (%) | 23.2 ± 5.5 |
| *Right heart catheterization:* | |
| Cardiac index (L/min m$^2$) | 1.8 ± 0.3 |
| Pulmonary wedge pressure (mm Hg) | 25.6 ± 5.7 |
| *Cardiopulmonary exercise test:* | |
| Maximal oxygen consumption (mL/kg/min) | 15.1 ± 4.4 |

LV=left ventricular; RV=right ventricular.
Values are mean ±SD.

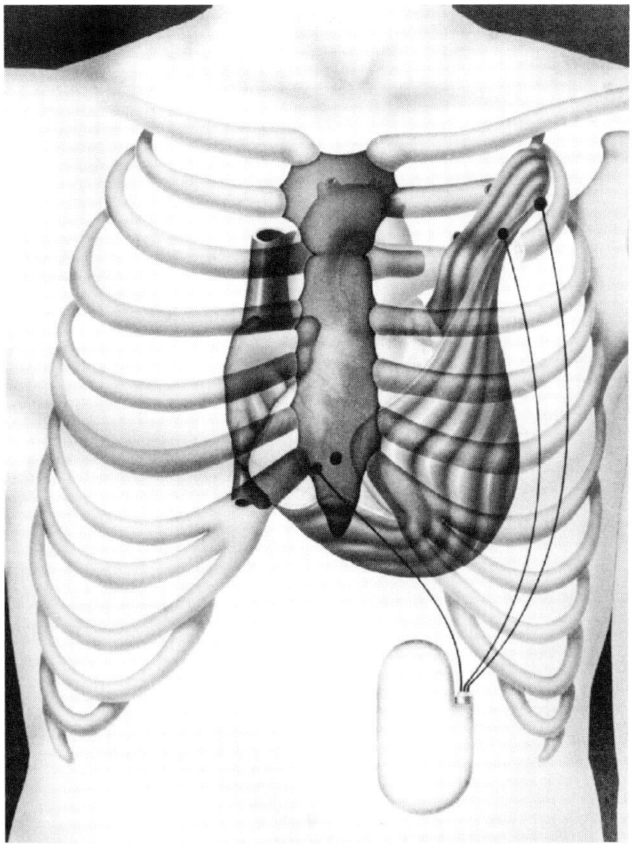

**Figure 1:** *Schematic representation of dynamic cardiomyoplasty providing a left posterior cardiocostal wrapping.*

## Technical Considerations

### Surgical Procedure

Dynamic cardiomyoplasty is normally performed without cardiopulmonary bypass in patients with dilated cardiomyopathies.

At our institution, the left latissimus dorsi (LD) muscle is used and the operation is done by means of two separate incisions: a lateral approach for muscle flap dissection and a subsequent medium sternotomy for cardiac access. Dissection and transposition of skeletal muscle flap follow the technique described by Carpentier and Chachques.[11] Two intramuscular pacing electrodes (Medtronic® SP 5528) are implanted in the proximal portion of LD muscle and an intramyocardial sensing lead (Medtronic® SP 5548) is placed in either the right or left ventricle. The cardiomyostimulator Medtronic® SP 1005 is used for muscle flap stimulation.

The left LD muscle is wrapped around the ventricular surfaces with its scapular and paravertebral edges fixed directly to the myocardium along the posterior atrioventricular line by separated sutures, providing a left posterior cardiocostal wrapping. After its fixation behind the heart, the muscle flap is fixed by additional sutures on the anterior wall of the right ventricle. This approach normally allows left LD muscle to cover up to 90% of the LV free wall and up to 50% of the right ventricular wall, as depicted in Figure 1.

The anesthetic management of cardiomyoplasty includes the systematic use of dopamine, dobutamine, and sodium nitroprusside, associated with maintenance of adequate volume loading, in order to improve the hemodynamic profile and to allow the stability of arterial blood pressure even during the muscle heart wrapping procedure.[12] The prophylactic use of intravenous inotropic support, which is associated with the use of the intra-aortic balloon pump in some cases, is maintained for at least 1 week after the operation.

### Muscle Stimulation Protocol

Skeletal muscle flap stimulation starts 2 weeks after the operation, and a progressive muscle-conditioning protocol is followed.[13] During the late postoperative period, muscle flap is normally paced in 1:1 mode with the heart rate. Pulse train stimulation is used with a burst frequency of 30 Hz and associated with supramaximal pulse amplitude values to avoid ineffective muscle flap contraction. The delay between the ventricular sensed event and the muscle burst is adjusted to provide an exact synchronization between muscle flap contraction and ventricular systole.[5]

## Results

### Immediate Surgical Results

There were no intraoperative or early postoperative deaths in this series. Three patients developed ventricular fibrillation during muscle heart wrapping that required countershock.

The immediate postoperative course was uneventful in general. A transient period of renal failure and mesenteric ischemia developed in one patient, three patients experienced transitory atrial fibrillation or flutter, one patient had pulmonary edema, and one patient had pulmonary infection.

Muscle flap ischemic compromise was monitored by variations in the serum level of creatine kinase enzyme, which showed a mean peak value of 946 $\pm$ 582 IU at 39 $\pm$ 18 hours of follow-up. Four patients had peak values of creatine kinase greater than 1500 IU and these patients presented poor muscle flap contraction at the beginning of the muscle stimulation protocol.

### Late Clinical Results

Twenty-five patients completed the muscle-conditioning period and were followed up from 3 to 60 months (mean, 22.8 months). One patient died at 2 months of follow-up due to severe pulmonary thromboembolism and infection and one patient presented heart failure progression and underwent successful heart transplantation 42 days after the cardiomyoplasty.

Eight patients died during long-term follow-up and the actuarial survival rates are depicted in Figure 2. The causes of death were: progression of heart failure associated with pulmonary infection, cerebral vascular accident, atrial fibrillation, or renal failure in four patients, pulmonary thromboembolism in two patients, and sudden death in two patients. Progression of heart failure occurred in patients without postoperative improvement of LV function, whereas patients who died suddenly were receiving medical therapy for severe ventricular arrhythmias and atrial fibrillation.

Among the 17 surviving patients in long-term follow-up, eight returned to NYHA Class I, and nine are in Class II, some of them using fewer drugs or lower doses than they did in the preoperative period. Ten of these patients resumed their professional activities.

## Left Ventricular Function Changes

At 6 months of follow-up, radioisotopic angiography demonstrated that LV ejection fraction improved from 19.8 ± 2.8 to 24.4 ± 6.3% ($p$<0.01). There was no variation in right ventricular ejection fraction after cardiomyoplasty (22.7 ± 5.5 versus 24.1 ± 7.6%).

Otherwise, LV cineangiographic study, performed on 10 patients at 16 ± 4 months of follow-up,[14] documented that LV ejection fraction increased in patients who survived long term after cardiomyoplasty from 15.1 ± 7.9 to 30.9 ±

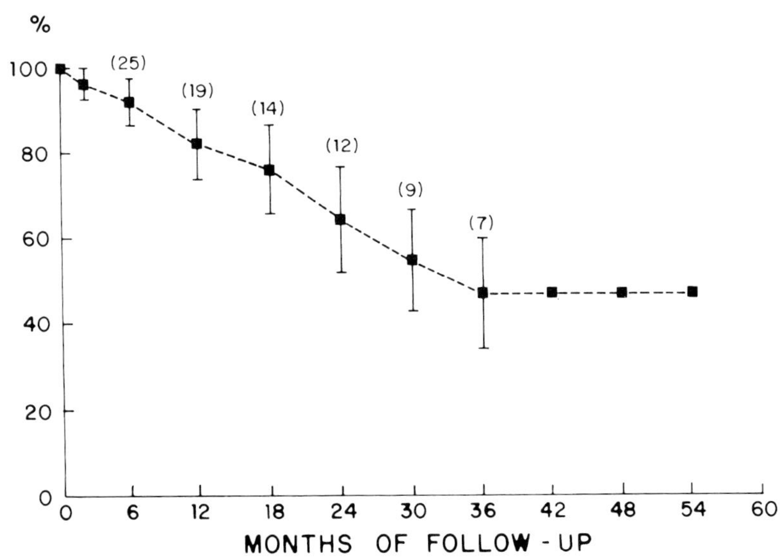


**Figure 2:** *Plots of actuarial survival rates after cardiomyoplasty. Numbers in parentheses indicate patients at risk in the period. Values are mean ±SEM.*

8.3% ($p<0.01$). This improvement resulted from similar modifications of anterobasal, anterolateral, apical, diaphragmatic, and posterobasal LV regional wall motions. This study also showed a decrease in LV ejection fraction to 23.1 ± 13.4% when the myostimulator was turned off for 24 hours ($p=0.06$).

Right heart catheterization demonstrated that stroke index increased from 20.2 ± 3 to 24.9 ± 7.2 mL/m$^2$ at 6 months of follow-up ($p<0.01$) and showed significant improvement of LV stroke work and significant decrease of pulmonary pressures after cardiomyoplasty.[5,6] In addition, more evident changes in cardiac output and global circulatory function after this procedure were documented during a treadmill exercise test in three patients.[15]

Besides these hemodynamic benefits, cardiomyoplasty may also influence LV mechanical properties. That was documented by pressure-volume loops obtained on simultaneous echocardiographic-hemodynamic studies performed on eight patients at 16 ± 4 months of follow-up, with the myostimulator on and turned off for 24 hours.[16] Significant reduction of LV end-systolic stress from 175 ± 12 to 149 ± 10 g/cm$^2$ ($p<0.05$) and of LV end-diastolic stress from 69 ± 8 to 37 ± 5 g/cm$^2$ ($p<0.01$) were demonstrated with myostimulator on compared with myostimulator turned-off data. Significant decrease of LV chamber stiffness from 120 ± 31 to 52 ± 11 mm Hg/cm ($p<0.01$) and significant improvement of LV maximal elastance from 17 ± 1 to 21 ± 1 mm Hg/cm ($p<0.01$) were also observed during skeletal muscle flap stimulation.

The long-term influence of cardiomyoplasty on LV dimension and LV ejection fraction was studied by sequential echocardiographic and radioisotopic evaluations (Table 2). These studies demonstrated the absence of later LV dilatation, despite the tendency of LV ejection fraction to decrease after 2 years of follow-up. On the other hand, sequential right heart catheterization documented the maintenance of cardiomyoplasty hemodynamic benefits for up to 4 years of follow-up, as depicted in Figures 3 and 4.

**Table 2**
Noninvasive Evaluation of Left Ventricular Function

| | | Follow-up | | | | |
|---|---|---|---|---|---|---|
| | *Preop* | *6 mo* | *1 yr* | *2 yr* | *3 yr* | *4 yr* |
| *Doppler echocardiographic data:* | | | | | | |
| LVDD (mm) | 73.3 ± 6.1 | 73.5 ± 7.8 | 73.2 ± 7.4 | 74.1 ± 3.1 | 75.6 ± 5.1 | 76.2 ± 4.7 |
| LVSD (mm) | 64.7 ± 6.6 | 61.9 ± 6.2* | 61.9 ± 6.2* | 63.4 ± 3.5 | 65.6 ± 4.8 | 66.4 ± 3.6 |
| LVSWS (%) | 11.8 ± 2 | 15.7 ± 2.8* | 15.3 ± 3* | 14.3 ± 3.3 | 3.2 ± 1.8 | 12.8 ± 1.6 |
| CO (L/min) | 2.3 ± 0.7 | 2.6 ± 0.4 | 3.1 ± 0.6* | 2.7 ± 0.9 | 3.4 ± 0.9 | 3.5 ± 0.8 |
| *Radioisotopic angiography:* | | | | | | |
| LVEF (%) | 19.8 ± 2.8 | 24.4 ± 6.3* | 24.3 ± 5.9* | 24.9 ± 5.6* | 22.1 ± 3.8 | 22.8 ± 2.2 |
| RVEF (%) | 22.7 ± 5.5 | 24.1 ± 7.6 | 26.4 ± 9.1 | 27.6 ± 8 | 24.6 ± 4.3 | 25.3 ± 5.8 |

LVDD = left ventricular end-diastolic diameter; LVSD = left ventricular end-systolic diameter; LVSWS = left ventricular segmental wall shortening; CO = cardiac output; LVEF = left ventricular ejection fraction; RVEF = right ventricular ejection fraction.

Values are mean ±SD; *$p<0.05$ (in relation to preoperative data).

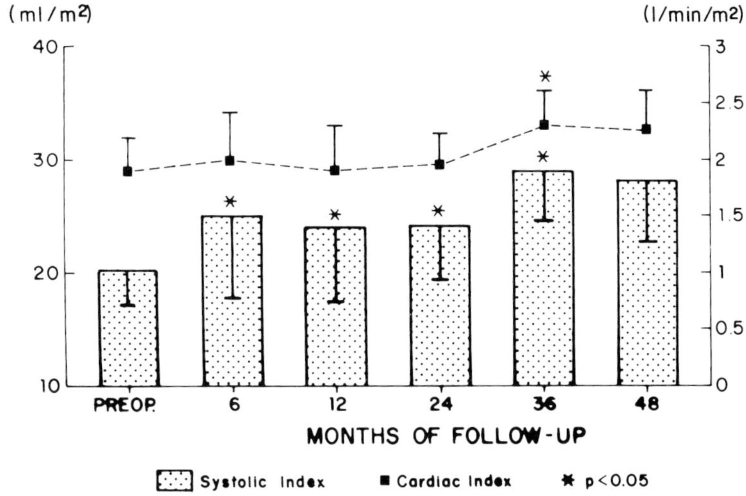


**Figure 3:** *Plots of long-term variations of systolic index and cardiac index documented by right heart catheterization. Values are mean ±SD.*

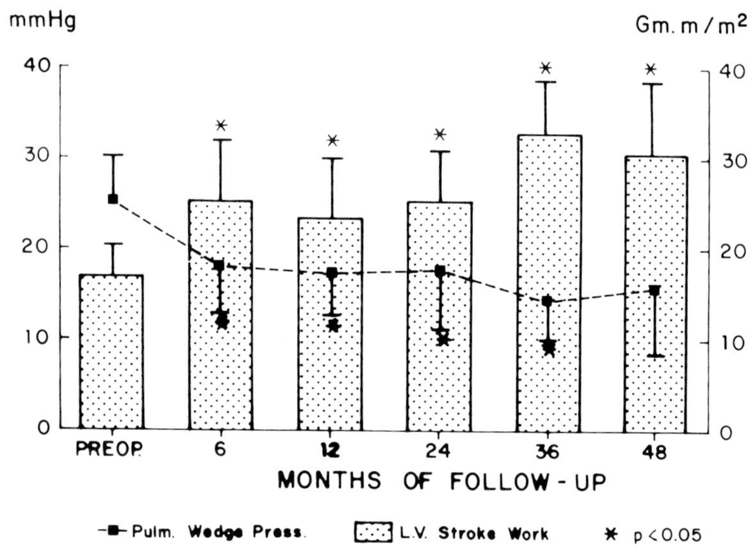


**Figure 4:** *Plots of long-term variations of pulmonary wedge pressure and left ventricular (LV) stroke work documented by right heart catheterization. Values are mean ±SD.*

## Exercise Capacity and Arrhythmias Incidence

Cardiopulmonary exercise test, performed using a Naughton modified protocol, showed significant improvement of maximal oxygen consumption from 14.8 ± 3.6 to 18.2 ± 4.3 mL/min/kg at 6 months of follow-up ($p<0.05$). Significant increment of maximal workload from 77 ± 27 to 113 ± 26 watts ($p<0.05$) was also documented in this study.

Finally, it was observed on sequential Holter recordings that nonsustained ventricular tachycardia episodes and the number of premature ventricular contractions tended to decrease after cardiomyoplasty (Table 3).

## Factors Influencing Prognosis

This experience, as well as others, seems to identify factors influencing the long-term results of cardiomyoplasty.

One-year outcome in this series was influenced by creatine kinase enzyme peak level at the immediate postoperative period, demonstrating the importance of muscle flap ischemic compromise for cardiomyoplasty results.[6,17]

Furthermore, patients who had surgery in NYHA Class IV had lower survival rates than Class III patients until 48 months of follow-up (Fig. 5). Pulmonary vascular resistance values above 5 Wood units were also a significant prognostic factor of poor long-term survival, as shown in Figure 6.

Otherwise, this study did not identify any significant influence of preoperative arrhythmias or of the level of right or left ventricular ejection fraction on cardiomyoplasty long-term outcome.

## Comment

The present experience with dynamic cardiomyoplasty shows that this procedure improves LV function, reverses congestive heart failure, and seems to improve long-term survival of patients with idiopathic dilated cardiomyopathy.

In spite of controversial results regarding cardiomyoplasty influence on LV function and hemodynamic profile,[1–6] selection of patients including only those with dilated cardiomyopathy and severe LV function impairment in this study was advantageous for documenting the beneficial effects of this procedure.

Modest improvement of LV ejection fraction and stroke volume were demonstrated after cardiomyoplasty. Otherwise, this procedure's impact on circulatory function could be better evaluated by its significant influence on LV stroke work and pulmonary pressures.[5,6] In addition, cardiomyoplasty also influenced the mechanical properties of the failing heart itself. Reduction of LV wall stress and LV chamber stiffness were documented under skeletal muscle flap stimulation,[16] indicating that cardiomyoplasty may also decrease myocar-

**Table 3**
Holter Recordings

| | *Follow-up* | | | | | |
|---|---|---|---|---|---|---|
| | *Preop* | *6 mo* | *1 yr* | *2 yr* | *3 yr* | *4 yr* |
| PVC (no/hr) | 131 ± 60 | 91 ± 45 | 53 ± 22 | 57 ± 37 | 71 ± 35 | 59 ± 33 |
| VT (epis/24 hrs) | 3.7 ± 1.7 | 2 ± 0.7 | 0.7 ± 0.5 | 0.6 ± 0.4 | 1.5 ± 1.1 | 0.8 ± 0.6 |

PVC = premature ventricular contractions; VT = ventricular tachycardia; epis = episodes.
Values are mean ±SEM.

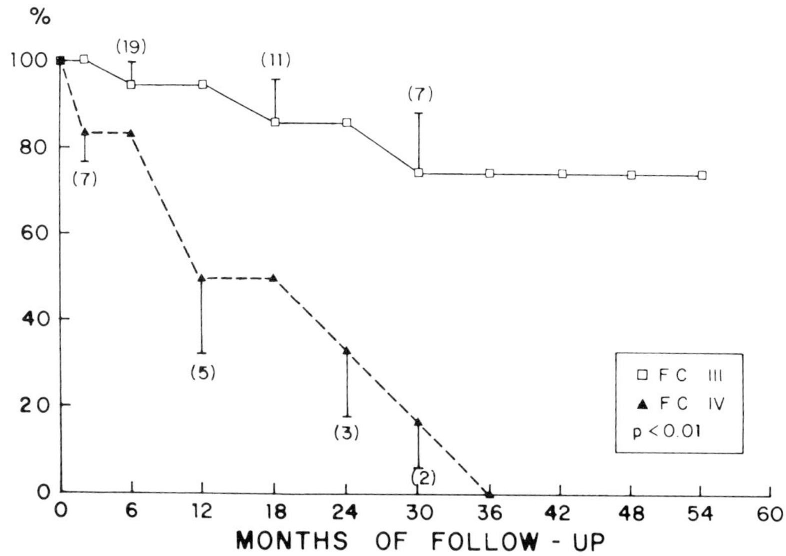


**Figure 5:** *Plots of actuarial survival rates after cardiomyoplasty for patients operated in functional Class (FC) III or IV. Numbers in parentheses indicate patients at risk in the period. Values are mean ±SEM.*

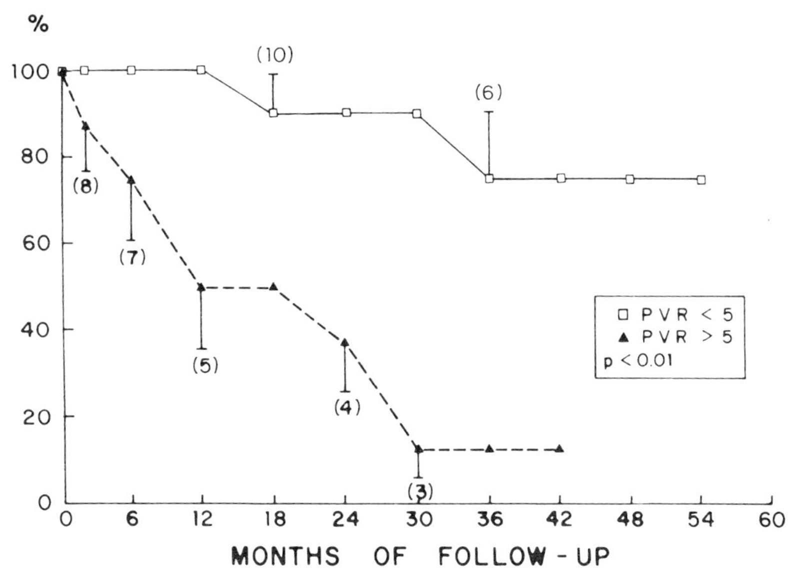


**Figure 6:** *Plots of actuarial survival rates after cardiomyoplasty for patients operated with pulmonary vascular resistance (PVR) below or above 5 Wood units. Numbers in parentheses indicate patients at risk in the period. Values are mean ±SEM.*

dial oxygen consumption.[18] Therefore, in a dilated, failing left ventricle, the primary pathophysiological abnormalities[19] were partially corrected and slow progression of the underlying cardiomyopathy could result from this mechanism. That this may have occurred is indicated by the absence of later LV dilatation and the maintenance of hemodynamic improvement for up to 4 years after cardiomyoplasty.

Improvement in functional class and exercise capacity were also demonstrated after cardiomyoplasty in this series, which is in agreement with the overall clinical experience with this procedure.[1–4]

Furthermore, cardiomyoplasty could be performed in these patients without surgical mortality and the long-term survival after this operation was much more favorable than the survival of a comparable, but not randomized, group of patients maintained on medical therapy.[20] Also, patients operated on in functional Class III presented late survival rates similar to those reported after cardiac transplantation.[21]

Otherwise, patients submitted to cardiomyoplasty in functional Class IV or with elevated pulmonary vascular resistance exhibited a significantly high mortality, suggesting that the degree of cardiac function impairment before the operation plays an important role in the long-term outcome. Other studies also documented the impact of these factors on cardiomyoplasty results,[1,2,4] and other risk factors influencing perioperative and late mortality after this procedure have also been reported.[1,2] The absence of significant influence of preoperative right or left ventricular ejection fractions and atrial fibrillation on cardiomyoplasty results in this study suggests, however, that these factors may not be very important in patients with idiopathic cardiomyopathy. In addition, the analysis of preoperative factors associated with outcome requires further validation with data from a larger and multicenter clinical trial.

Besides these findings, cardiomyoplasty results may also be influenced by technical aspects and by the possibility of skeletal muscle flap damage at the perioperative period. The use of right[22] or left LD muscle, as well as the optimal stimulation protocol for transformation and assist remain controversial. Likewise, specific studies are needed to investigate methods to decrease skeletal muscle flap ischemic compromise.

From these findings, we tend to conclude that dynamic cardiomyoplasty is a promising surgical alternative to the treatment of advanced heart failure due to idiopathic dilated cardiomyopathy, in the presence of some preservation of myocardial function and mild or moderate pulmonary hypertension. In this regard, the absence of surgical mortality in this series ensures a low-risk procedure, and cardiomyoplasty does not preclude future heart transplantation. Further studies are needed, however, to improve technical aspects, as well as to confirm these observations and to establish the efficacy of this procedure in the treatment of patients with other cardiomyopathies.

## References

1. Carpentier A, Chachques JC, Acar C, et al: Dynamic cardiomyoplasty at seven years. *J Thorac Cardiovasc Surg* 106:42–54, 1993.

2. Furnary AP, Magovern JA, Christlieb IY, et al: Clinical cardiomyoplasty: preoperative factors associated with outcome. *Ann Thorac Surg* 54:1139, 1992.
3. Delahaye F, Jegaden O, Montagna P, et al: Latissimus dorsi cardiomyoplasty in severe congestive heart failure: The Lyon experience. *J Cardiac Surg* 6(Suppl):106, 1991.
4. Grandjean PA, Austin L, Chan S, et al: Dynamic cardiomyoplasty: Clinical follow-up results. *J Cardiac Surg* 6(Suppl):80, 1991.
5. Jatene AD, Moreira LFP, Stolf NAG, et al: Left ventricular function changes after cardiomyoplasty in patients with dilated cardiomyopathy. *J Thorac Cardiovasc Surg* 102:132, 1991.
6. Moreira LFP, Bocchi EA, Stolf NAG, et al: Current expectations in dynamic cardiomyoplasty. *Ann Thorac Surg* 55:299, 1993.
7. Vagelos R, Fowler MB: Selection of patients for cardiac transplantation. *Cardiol Clin* 8:23, 1990.
8. Pitt B, Cohn JN, Francis GS, et al: The effect of treatment on survival in congestive heart failure. *Clin Cardiol* 15;323, 1992.
9. Stevenson LW, Tillisch JH, Hamilton M, et al: Importance of hemodynamic response to therapy in predicting survival with ejection fraction <20% secondary to ischemic or nonischemic dilated cardiomyopathy. *Am J Cardiol* 66:1348, 1990.
10. Likoff MJ, Chandler SL, Kay HR: Clinical determinants of mortality in chronic congestive heart failure secondary to idiopathic dilated or to ischemic cardiomyopathy. *Am J Cardiol* 59:634, 1987.
11. Chachques JC, Grandjean PA, Carpentier A: Latissimus dorsi dynamic cardiomyoplasty. *Ann Thorac Surg* 47:600, 1989.
12. Auler JOC Jr, Moreira LFP, Carvalho MJ, et al: Anesthetic management of patients undergoing cardiomyoplasty. *Anesthesiology* 77:379, 1992.
13. Chachques JC, Grandjean PA, Schwartz K, et al: Effect of latissimus dorsi dynamic cardiomyoplasty on ventricular function. *Circulation* 78(Suppl III):III-203, 1988.
14. Bocchi EA, Moreira LFP, Moraes AV, et al: Effects of dynamic cardiomyoplasty on regional wall motion, ejection fraction and geometry of left ventricle. *Circulation* 86(Suppl II):II-231, 1992.
15. Bocchi EA, Moreira LFP, Bellotti G, et al: Hemodynamic study during upright isotonic exercise before and six months after dynamic cardiomyoplasty for idiopathic dilated cardiomyopathy or Chagas' disease. *Am J Cardiol* 67:213, 1991.
16. Bellotti G, Moraes AV, Bocchi EA, et al: Late effects of cardiomyoplasty on left ventricular mechanics and diastolic filling. *Circulation* 88(Suppl):II304-II308, 1993.
17. Bocchi EA, Moreira LFP, Barreto ACP, et al: Creatinokinase levels may be a determinant of prognosis after cardiomyoplasty: Preliminary results. *JAAC* 19(Suppl): 98A, 1992.
18. Kawaguchi O, Goto Y, Futaki S, et al: Mechanical enhancement and myocardial oxygen saving by synchronized dynamic left ventricular compression. *J Thorac Cardiovasc Surg* 103:573, 1992.
19. Packer M: Pathophysiology of chronic heart failure. *Lancet* 340:88, 1992.
20. Moreira LFP, Seferian P Jr, Bocchi EA, et al: Survival improvement with dynamic cardiomyoplasty in patients with dilated cardiomyopathy. *Circulation* 84(Suppl III):III-296, 1991.
21. The registry of the International Society of Heart and Lung Transplantation: Ninth official report, 1992. *J Heart Lung Transpl* 11:599, 1992.
22. Magovern JA, Furnary AP, Christlieb IY, et al: Right latissimus dorsi cardiomyoplasty for left ventricular failure. *Ann Thorac Surg* 53:1120, 1992.

Chapter 2

# Discussion

**Dr. Carpentier:** Did you anticoagulate your patients?

**Dr. Moreira:** We only anticoagulated patients in atrial fibrillation and patients who had previous pulmonary thromboembolic episodes.

**Dr. Lazarra (Pittsburgh):** Your improvement in end-systolic pressure is very impressive. I have a question with regard to your cardiomyostimulator parameters. In particular, what was your burst duration and frequency and what was your pulse amplitude at the time you were stimulating?

**Dr. Moreira:** We are using the Medtronic® stimulator and the burst ratio is around 180 msec. Therefore, I think that we are using bursts of 30 Hz and we try using supramaximal voltage, in order to obtain a full recruitment of the muscle.

**Dr. Lazarra:** What would that number be? Supravoltage?

**Dr. Moreira:** You have the full recruitment with 2 to 2.5 times more voltage than the threshold.

**Dr. Brady (Sydney):** Could you please elaborate on the patients who had a high CPK rise. You said that they didn't do so well postoperatively at 12 months. Did you notice in the initial postoperative period that hemodynamically they hadn't improved?

**Dr. Moreira:** Well, the problem with CPK enzymes was that it took one year of follow-up. Almost all patients who had a greater increase of CPK levels in the immediate postoperative period either died or were in Class III or IV. Only patients who had no increase in CPK levels were alive and in Class I or II. This was what we observed and therefore I think that it is a very important parameter because if we have problems with the muscle in the immediate postoperative period, if we have muscle damage, it is obvious that cardiomyoplasty will not work.

**Dr. Carpentier:** I would like to make a comment before closing. It seems to me a little bit hazardous to use the so-called supramaximal voltage and the 1:1 mode. I wonder whether this could lead to an increased risk of muscle damage?

Chapter 3

# Clinical Cardiomyoplasty: Analysis of Results

Hemant Trehan, Jeffrey S. Swanson, Anthony P. Furnary, Andy Bennett, Albert Starr

## Introduction

The idea of using skeletal muscle to augment or replace cardiac muscle has evolved from the laboratory to clinical practice.[1] This was made possible by the stimulation protocol proposed by Carpentier and Chachques[2] and successfully carried out in 1985. It has subsequently been used to treat an increasing population of patients with end-stage heart disease in the New York Heart Association (NYHA) Class III and Class IV.

## Material and Methods

Left latissimus dorsi (LD) cardiomyoplasty has been done in 13 patients at our institution between July 1991 and April 1993. All of the patients were in NYHA Class III at the time of surgery. Eleven patients had idiopathic cardiomyopathy and two patients had ischemic cardiomyopathy. The mean age was 66 ± 8.64 years for the nine males and four females in our series.

Preoperatively, all patients had extensive testing including a clinical examination, laboratory tests, ECG, chest x-ray, 24-hour Holter monitoring, right and left heart catheterization, Doppler echocardiography, pulmonary function tests, metabolic exercise tests, and more recently a signal-averaged ECG. If any abnormality was detected in any of the tests, further follow-up tests were done. These tests were repeated at 6-month intervals for all the survivors.

## Anesthetic and Surgical Techniques

Intraoperatively, we put all patients on a small dose of dobutamine and adjusted it as necessary to maintain an adequate cardiac index (>2 L/m$^2$/min). All

From Carpentier A, Chachques JC, Grandjean P: Cardiac Bioassist. © Futura Publishing Co, Inc, Armonk, NY, 1997.

**Table 1**
Summary of Operative Data

| | | |
|---|---|---|
| Posterior Cardiocostal | 4 (31%) | |
| Posterior Cardiosubcutaneous | 9 (69%) | |
| Total flap time | 120 ± 20.9 minutes | |
| Total wrap time | 98.3 ± 20.6 minutes | |
| Number of days in ICU | 5.9 ± 7.7 (all) | 3.5 ± 2.1 (surv) |
| Number of days in hospital | 12.2 ± 6.4 (all) | 11.1 ± 4.0 (surv) |

operations involved left LD muscle takedown and subsequent wrapping of the heart. The muscle was mobilized through a standard incision from the axilla to the middle of the iliac crest. Pacing electrodes (Medtronic® SP 5528) were placed 5 cm apart at the proximal end of the muscle and the contraction was checked. The second rib was resected and the muscle was placed in the left pleural cavity. The muscle was detached from its humeral insertion, which was then tacked to the upper border of the resected rib. The incisions were closed with multiple tacking sutures and two Jackson Pratt drains. The patient was then positioned supine and a standard median sternotomy was done. The pericardium and the left pleura were opened and the muscle was wrapped posterior to the heart, taking care to cover as much as possible of both ventricles. Pericardial augmentation was done routinely to obtain complete coverage of both ventricles. Cardiopulmonary bypass was only used once for concomitant bypass grafts. Two sensing electrodes (Medtronic® SP 5567) were placed on the right ventricle and their thresholds were checked before and after wrapping. The leads were tunneled to the left subcostal generator pocket and connected to a Medtronic® SP 1005 generator. Our operative data are summarized in Table 1.

A standard muscle stimulation protocol was used (Medtronic®) beginning 2 weeks after surgery and achieving maximum stimulation at 10 weeks. At completion, all patients had a frequency of 30 Hz and a pulse duration of 185 msec. The muscle contraction was checked manually and spikes on the ECG were noted. The AV delay was individually programmed echocardiographically to coincide with mitral valve closure.

## Results

### Early Mortality

We had three early deaths. Two of these were due to cardiac failure and one was due to septicemia. One patient required intra-aortic balloon pump support, from which she was successfully weaned. She required antiarrhythmic therapy for malignant ventricular tachyarrhythmias and could not be weaned off the ventilator. She died of cardiac failure on the 29th postoperative day. Our second patient went into progressive cardiac and renal failure and died on the ninth postoperative day of multiorgan failure. Our third patient was successfully discharged and came back 4 days later with generator pocket infection, which was subsequently found to be an empyema. Her pleural cavity was drained. She developed fulminant septicemia and multiorgan failure and died.

## Postoperative Complications

Postoperative complications were observed in four patients. Two patients had postoperative seromas that responded to aspiration. Following a modification in the operative technique, no further seromas were noted. One patient had subcutaneous emphysema. Three patients had superficial necrosis in the middle part of their muscle incision which was allowed to heal by secondary intention. One patient required a new sensing lead placement because the previous lead had been displaced by the muscle wrap. We subsequently place two sensing leads and check their threshold both before and after the muscle wrap is in place.

## Late Mortality

Ten patients who were operative survivors were followed-up for 6-18 months (mean follow-up = 11.59 ± 8.58 mos). During this period there were three late deaths at 3 months, 6 months, and 12 months of follow-up.

The patient who died at 3 months had an episode of ventricular fibrillation (VF) at home. He was successfully resuscitated but continued to be in a semiconscious condition. He was shifted back to his hometown as per his family's wishes and died upon arrival.

WD was a patient who went into atrial fibrillation 3 months after surgery. He successfully completed his 6-month follow-up and died suddenly at home, presumably due to VF. The third death at 12 months was in a patient who had ventricular tachycardia for which she was hospitalized and put on amiodarone. She developed intestinal obstruction and died.

## Device-Related Morbidity

One patient had early generator failure 8 months after surgery and required a generator replacement.

## Patient-Related Morbidity

Four patients had congestive heart failure. Three required an increased dosage of diuretics. In two patients the pulse generator was reprogrammed to deliver a 33-Hz frequency in an attempt to further stimulate the muscle. One patient had VF at home, which was successfully cardioverted. He was started on amiodarone therapy, which had to be discontinued after 6 months because of lung fibrosis. An AICD was implanted successfully. Following the surgery, he developed noncardiogenic pulmonary edema from which he is recovering.

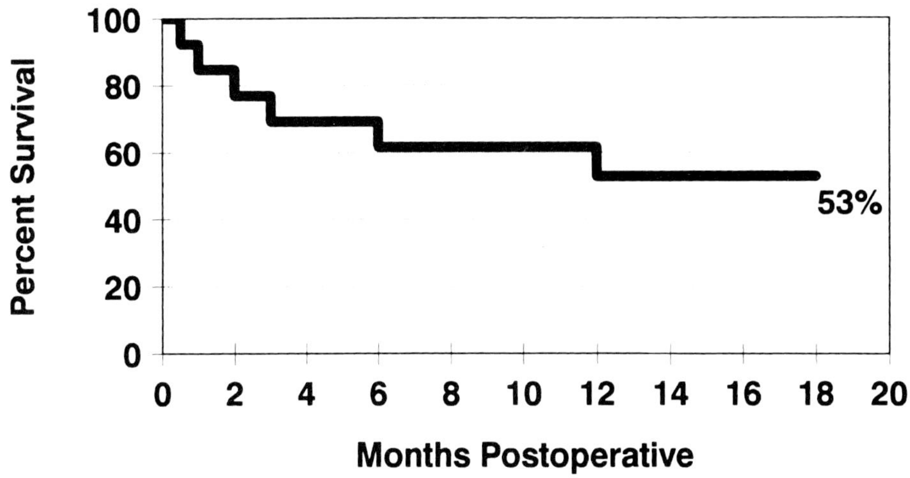


**Figure 1:** Actuarial survival rates after cardiomyoplasty (Kaplan-Meier method).

## Survival

There are seven survivors at 18 months, giving us an actuarial survival rate of 52.75 ± 14.1% (Fig. 1). Five have completed their 18-month follow-up studies and one each have recently completed their 6- and 12-month follow-up study. Eighteen-month data are available for three patients and are summarized in Table 2. We analyzed the results statistically using the Kaplan-Meier method of actuarial survival, Cox univariate regression analysis, and Student's $t$ and paired tests where applicable.

# Discussion

Cardiomyoplasty was initially tried as an alternative to transplantation in Class IV patients. The very high mortality associated with this group restricted its use to Class III patients with end-stage heart disease.[3] The ability to prevent fatigue in skeletal muscle[4] has been a significant impetus to the clinical use of this operation. Subsequent work has focused on refining the technique,[5] the use of right[6] and bilateral muscle flaps,[7] and more recently on a closer look at stimulation protocols to prevent fatigue.

The efficacy of cardiomyoplasty should be judged by its impact on survival, exercise tolerance, and functional class. In addition, its effect on improving quality of life, reducing drug dosage, and reducing the incidence of arrhythmias are factors that need to be considered.

## Analysis of Early Mortality

The mortality in cardiomyoplasty is a direct function of NYHA Class. In the earlier part of the experience with cardiomyoplasty, significantly greater

**Table 2**
Criteria for Selection of Patients

| | |
|---|---|
| RVEF | >30% |
| LVEF | >15% |
| EDVI | <170 mL/$m^2$ |
| ESVI | <140 mL/$m^2$ |
| $O_2$UEI | 4–5 times resting values |

LVEF = left ventricular ejection fraction; RVEF = right ventricular ejection fraction; EDVI = end-diastolic volume index; ESVI = end-systolic volume index; $O_2$UEI = oxygen utilization with exercise index.

early and late mortality was observed in Class IV patients. This has restricted the use of this operation for NYHA Class III patients. We analyzed early mortality in our series. Left and right ventricular ejection fractions, end-systolic and end-diastolic cardiac indices, and oxygen uptake with exercise were significant predictors of operative risk. We currently use the selection criteria in Table 2. Although these numbers are not absolute, deviation from them does tend to enhance mortality. Currently, we believe that the absence of sinus rhythm and specifically the presence of atrial fibrillation are absolute contraindications to surgery as these patients tend to have a much poorer survival rate.

## Late Survival

A high right ventricular ejection fraction (>30%), the absence of atrial fibrillation, and oxygen utilization at exercise ($O_2$UEI) were significant predictors of survival at 18 months. Left ventricular stroke work index, which was significant at 12 months follow-up, was only suggestive at 18 months ($p<0.1$). There is a significant difference between the systolic blood pressure at rest and the diastolic presence with exercise in survivors at 18 months, possibly reflecting a better cardiac output and lowered systemic vascular resistance.

## Functional Class

All patients showed initial improvement in functional class as assessed by NYHA Class (mean improvement 1.3). At 18 months of follow-up, the mean NYHA Class was 2.2 $\pm$ 0.84 ($p=0.028$) (Fig. 2). Two of our patients are in NYHA Class I. Two patients have deteriorated from Class II to Class III due to onset of cardiac failure and lung fibrosis secondary to amiodarone therapy, respectively. One patient remains in Class I.

## Exercise Tolerance and Hemodynamic Parameters

There is no significant change in ejection fractions, cardiac index, systolic and diastolic volumes, or improvement in exercise tolerance (Table 3).

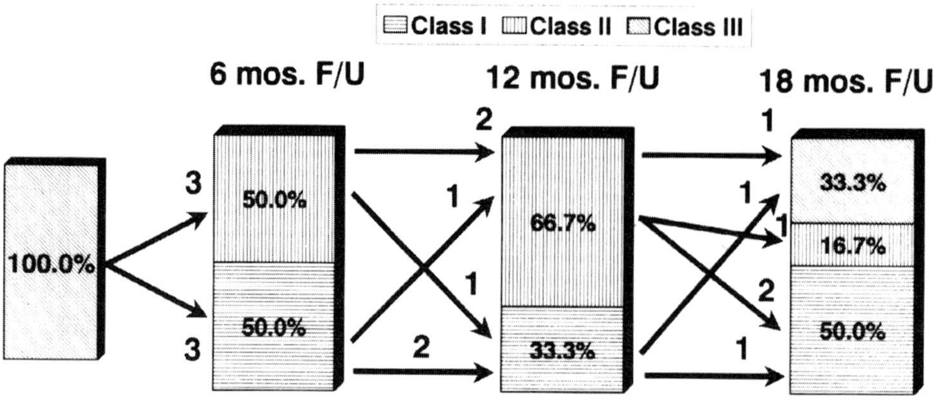


**Figure 2:** NYHA functional class assessment following cardiomyoplasty.

**Table 3**
Hemodynamic Parameters

| | *Preop* | *18 months* | *p* |
|---|---|---|---|
| RVEF | 29.14 ± 9.74 | 23.3 ± 7.64 | 0.39 |
| LVEF | 20.86 ± 6.52 | 23.0 ± 6.98 | 0.65 |
| EDVI | 132.43 ± 71.38 | 191.67 ± 44.16 | 0.23 |
| ESVI | 106.71 ± 60.62 | 152.33 ± 34.93 | 0.27 |
| PCWP | 17.86 ± 8.00 | 19.25 ± 9.20 | 0.81 |
| PA (mean) | 28.30 ± 9.30 | 30.00 ± 11.50 | 0.80 |
| CI (therm) | 2.27 ± 0.70 | 2.45 ± 0.70 | 0.64 |

LVEF = left ventricular ejection fraction; RVEF = right ventricular ejection fraction; EDVI = end-diastolic volume index; ESVI = end-systolic volume index; PCWP = pulmonary capillary wedge pressure; PA (mean) = mean pulmonary artery pressure; CI (therm) = thermodilution cardiac index.

## Effect on Drug Dosages and Arrhythmias

Although some patients have shown a minor decrease in drug requirements and arrhythmias, there has been no significant difference when compared to preoperative values. Keeping in mind our small sample size, further large-scale studies are needed to bring out any differences.

## Quality of Life

In all of our patients there has been a marked improvement in the quality of life as assessed by a standardized questionnaire. After being incapacitated, most patients have returned to their former occupations and are able to be ambulatory. This has resulted in a positive feeling and has minimized dependence on others. Most of our patients are doing productive work in contrast to their condition prior to operation. In some, after initial improvement, their activities have recently been restricted due to the onset of complications.

## Conclusion

We feel that cardiomyoplasty in its current stage of evolution is a valuable palliative procedure to improve functional class and the quality of life in selected NYHA Class III patients with end-stage heart disease. Its impact on survival and improvement of exercise tolerance remains to be elucidated.

## References

1. Bridges CR, Stephenson LW: The mechanics of skeletal-muscle ventricles: a model based on elasticity theory. In Chiu RC-J, Bourgeois IM (eds): *Transformed Muscle for Cardiac Assist and Repair*. Mount Kisco, NY, Futura Publishing Co, 1990, pp 255–265.
2. Carpentier A, Chachques JC: Myocardial substitution with a stimulated skeletal muscle: first successful clinical case. *Lancet* 1:1267, 1985.
3. Grandjean PA, Austin L, Chan S, et al: Dynamic cardiomyoplasty: clinical follow-up results. *J Cardiac Surg* 6:80, 1991.
4. Eisenburg BR, Salmons S: The reorganization of subcellular structure in muscle undergoing fast-to-slow type transformation: a stereological study. *Cell Tissue Res* 220:449, 1981.
5. Carpentier A, Chachques JC: Clinical dynamic cardiomyoplasty: method and outcome. *Semin Thorac Cardiovasc Surg* 3:136, 1991.
6. Furnary AP, Magovern JA, Christlieb IY, Trumble DR: Improved ventricular augmentation with right latissimus cardiomyoplasty. *Surg Forum* 42:307, 1991.
7. Furnary AP, Magovern JA, Christlieb IY, Trumble DR: Component analysis of bilateral cardiomyoplasty. *Ann Thorac Surg* 55:72, 1993.

Chapter 4

# Preoperative Risk Factors Affecting Survival after Cardiomyoplasty

Anthony P. Furnary, James A. Magovern, Jeffrey S. Swanson, Albert Starr, George J. Magovern*

## Introduction

Ventricular assist with autologous skeletal muscle tissue is rapidly gaining popularity as a surgical tool for the treatment of chronic heart failure. The disadvantages of mechanical circulatory assistance, including thromboembolism, infection, and cost, and the shortcomings of cardiac transplantation, such as donor availability and immunosuppression, have led to the search for a more practical surgical treatment for heart failure. Dynamic cardiomyoplasty is at present positioned to fulfill that need. Since its clinical inception by Carpentier and Chachques[1] in 1985, the clinical application of this surgical technique has experienced exponential growth.

The combined world experience with cardiomyoplasty has been divided into two phases. Phase I represents all operations that took place between July 17, 1985, and April 30, 1991.[2] This cohort included 118 patients, 112 of which were left heart failure patients from 14 centers worldwide. Phase II of the cardiomyoplasty project began in May 1991 and is continuing at the time of this writing with over 130 patients enrolled (personal communication: M. Colson, Medtronic®, Inc.). Survival analysis performed on all patients who completed the Phase I study[3] revealed that operative mortality was higher in New York Heart Association (NYHA) Class IV patients as compared to NYHA Class III patients (38.5% vs. 12.3%, $p<0.05$). This operative risk factor continued to show significance in survival following hospital discharge, with a 12-month actuarial survival of 60% for NYHA Class IV patients compared to 93% for NYHA Class III patients.

A univariate analysis of preoperative factors associated with outcome has been published from the Pittsburgh experience.[4] This study attempted

From Carpentier A, Chachques JC, Grandjean P: Cardiac Bioassist. © Futura Publishing Co, Inc, Armonk, NY, 1997.

*With the cooperation of Robert Lazzara, Gary L. Grunkemeier, and Hemant Trehan.

to quantify some of the specific preoperative factors that would cause an NYHA Class IV patient to have a higher risk of death following cardiomyoplasty.The analysis revealed that nonsurvivors had lower right ventricular ejection fraction, higher pulmonary artery mean pressures, higher pulmonary artery diastolic pressures, and higher pulmonary vascular resistance. The shortcoming of this study, however, was the lack of a multivariate analysis of risk due to the small number of patients enrolled. Therefore, the findings were presented with the caveat that further validation was required with analysis of data from a larger clinical trial.

In order to achieve that goal, the perioperative data from all cardiomyoplasty patients at our two centers (Allegheny General Hospital, Pittsburgh, Pennsylvania, and St. Vincent Heart Institute, Portland, Oregon) were combined for analysis. This was facilitated since one of the authors (APF) was involved in the selection, treatment, and care of both groups of patients over the course of the last 4 years. All patient variables were prospectively entered into the database. This included preoperative evaluation variables, intraoperative procedural data, and 6- and 12-month postoperative follow-up data. A univariate as well as a forward stepwise multivariate Cox regression was then performed to determine the relationship of any of these variables to postoperative survival. Statistical analyses were performed with the Statistical Package for the Social Sciences (SPSS) and a statistically significant result was considered to be $p<0.05$. Results are reported as mean ±SEM.

## Demographics

Forty-five patients were entered into the cardiomyoplasty study between September 1985 and January 1993. Patients were selected from the population referred to each hospital for management of congestive heart failure. All patients had progression of heart failure despite maximal medical therapy, including digoxin, diuretics, vasodilators, and angiotensin-converting enzyme inhibitors. None of the patients were suitable transplant candidates because of age, associated medical problems, or patient preference. The standard workup for cardiomyoplasty was done for each patient including right and left heart catheterization, assessment of NYHA class, echocardiography, rest and exercise multigated acquisition scans, and an exercise test with thallium scan. All patients since 1991 underwent metabolic testing as well.

Thirty-two patients were evaluated and treated at Allegheny General Hospital and 13 were evaluated and treated at St. Vincent Hospital and Medical Center. Patients had a mean age of 59 ± 9 years, were predominantly male (67%), and were equally divided between ischemic (49%) and idiopathic (51%) cardiomyopathies. Preoperative mean NYHA class was 3.2 ± 0.1 and mean left ventricular ejection factor (LVEF) was 24 ± 7%.

## Operative Technique

The majority of patients (29) underwent left latissimus cardiomyoplasty. Of the left cardiomyoplasty configurations, 10 were left posterior cardiocostal, 11 were left posterior cardiosubcutaneous, and eight were left anterior cardiocostal.[5] Fifteen patients underwent a right anterior cardiocostal cardiomyoplasty sling at Allegheny General Hospital following compelling experimental evidence that this configuration was superior.[6] Nineteen of the 45 operations were performed using cardiopulmonary bypass. In 18 (95%) of these, cardiopulmonary bypass was used in order to perform a concomitant cardiac procedure such as ventricular aneurysmectomy or coronary artery bypass grafting. In the remaining one patient, cardiopulmonary bypass was used for intraoperative surgical stabilization and decompression of a massive and irritable heart during the wrapping procedure itself.

## Results

There were seven deaths within 30 days of operation for an overall operative mortality of 15.6%. Six (86%) of these early deaths were due to progressive biventricular failure. One (14%) other was due to sudden ventricular arrhythmia. Immediately following the operation, 30/45 (67%) patients required hemodynamic support with inotropes, 13/45 (29%) required an intra-aortic balloon pump, and 2/45 (4%) required the insertion of a left ventricular assist device. The average hospital stay for operative survivors was 12 ± 6 days at St. Vincent and 37 ± 20 days at Allegheny General Hospital.

Actuarial survival at 12, 24, and 36 months was 58 ± 8%, 54 ± 8%, and 23 ± 11%, respectively (Fig. 1). The total follow-up was 648 patient/months with a mean of 14 ± 3 months and a median of 8 months. The etiology of late death was equally divided between progressive heart failure and sudden death.

## Risk Analysis

All preoperative and intraoperative variables were analyzed for their effect on the postoperative risk of death. These variables were analyzed in both a univariate and a multivariate fashion (Tables 1 and 2).

Univariate analysis of the preoperative data (Table 1) revealed that nonsurvivors were more likely to have preoperative atrial fibrillation (6/22 vs. 1/23, $p<0.002$), low right ventricular ejection fractions (39 ± 4% vs. 52 ± 4%, $p<0.004$), and high mean pulmonary artery pressures (31 ± 3 vs. 26 ± 2 mm Hg, $p<0.04$).

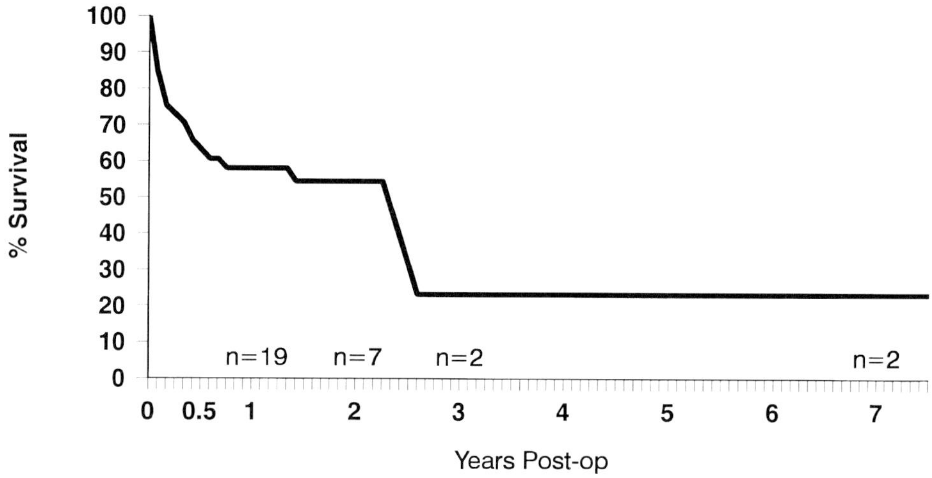


**Figure 1:** *Kaplan-Meier actuarial survival for patients undergoing cardiomyoplasty.*

Using a forward stepwise Cox regression method of survival analysis (Table 2), it was determined that atrial fibrillation ($p$=0.002), low right ventricular ejection fraction (RVEF) ($p$=0.008), and Phase I of the study ($p$=0.029) were significant preoperative predictors of mortality. A Cox model predictive of postoperative death following cardiomyoplasty was developed and is as follows:

$$\text{relative risk} = \exp(1.81 * \text{afib} + 1.2 * \text{Phase I} - 0.038 * \text{RVEF})$$

This allowed the calculation of an overall risk compared to the underlying baseline hazard over time for any individual patient using the variables described above (Fig. 2). When plotted as a scattergram of risk versus survival time according to death status, the risk score is seen to delineate the survival experience fairly well (Fig. 2). This separation is better than that with any single risk factor alone.

For example, a patient with atrial fibrillation would have a risk 6.1 times higher (=exp [1.81]) than a similar patient in normal sinus rhythm at the time of operation. Likewise, each 10% decrease in RVEF would correspond to an increase in relative risk by 1.47 times. This is supported by an examination of median survival in relation to RVEF. For patients with RVEF less than 30% (n=14) median survival was only 3±3 months, for those with RVEF from 30-45% (n=7) median survival was 9±2 months, and for an RVEF greater than 45% (n=24) median survival was 30±1 months ($p$<0.05).

As right ventricular ejection fraction entered the equation, the significance of study phase, which was not predictive ($p$=0.3) on univariate analysis, became important in the multivariate analysis. Specifically, patients who were in Phase I of the study had a higher risk of death than patients entered in Phase II of the study. This risk factor became apparent *only* after adjusting for atrial fibrillation and RVEF.

**Table 1**
Preoperative and Intraoperative Variables: Univariate Analysis

| *Variable* | *Survivors Mean ± SE* | *Nonsurvivors Mean ± SE* | *Univariate p Value* |
|---|---|---|---|
| Age | 62±2 | 56±2 | 0.3 |
| Atrial Fibrillation | 1/22 | 6/23 | 0.01 |
| AGH | 14/22 | 18/23 | 0.8 |
| Right Latissimus CMP | 10/22 | 6/23 | 0.6 |
| Concomitant Surgery | 15/22 | 13/23 | 0.6 |
| CPB | 8/22 | 10/23 | 0.9 |
| Ischemic Etiology | 12/22 | 11/23 | 0.4 |
| NYHA FC | 3±0.1 | 3±0.1 | 0.2 |
| Phase II | 19/22 | 10/23 | 0.3 |
| Male | 15/22 | 15/23 | 0.9 |
| Cardiac Index | 2±0.2 | 3±0.2 | 0.8 |
| LVEF | 25±1 | 23±1 | 0.4 |
| RVEF | 52±4 | 39±4 | 0.01 |
| EDVI | 154±13 | 204±13 | 0.1 |
| ESVI | 114±11 | 165±11 | 0.01 |
| LVSWI | 28±2 | 24±3 | 0.1 |
| RVSWI | 8±0.6 | 8±0 | 0.9 |
| LVEDP | 21±2 | 24±3 | 0.3 |
| PA Diastolic | 20±2 | 23±2 | 0.04 |
| PA Mean | 26±2 | 31±3 | 0.02 |
| PA Systolic | 40±3 | 45±4 | 0.1 |
| PCW | 18±2 | 22±2 | 0.1 |
| SBP at Rest | 137±6 | 108±4 | 0.1 |
| SBP at Exercise | 119±5 | 125±6 | 0.1 |
| DBP at Exercise | 73±2 | 72±3 | 0.4 |
| DBP at Rest | 68±3 | 64±2 | 0.3 |
| HR at Exercise | 140±4 | 151±8 | 0.4 |
| HR at Rest | 96±3 | 104±6 | 0.2 |
| RPP at Exercise | 10634±2281 | 11088±3758 | 1.0 |
| RPP at Rest | 6161±1301 | 5247±1833 | 0.7 |
| METS Exercise | 4±0.4 | 4±0.5 | 0.3 |
| METS Rest | 1±0.1 | 1±0 | 0.3 |

See text for abbreviations.

Among the variables that were not shown to affect outcome by this multivariate analysis were NYHA functional class, hospital, etiology, age, gender, cardiac index, left ventricular ejection fraction, left ventricular stroke work index, systolic or diastolic pulmonary artery pressures, latissimus muscle used, wrap type, cardiopulmonary bypass, and concomitant surgery.

## Discussion

This multivariate analysis of risk following cardiomyoplasty is the first of its kind in this relatively new field. As such, there may be other factors not tracked in our analysis that correlate highly with the variables presented here

**Table 2**
Preoperative and Intraoperative Variables

| *Variable* | *p Value* | *β Coef.* | *Relative Risk (=e^β)* |
|---|---|---|---|
| Age | 0.3 | | |
| Atrial Fibrillation | 0.002 | 1.8 | 6.1 |
| Cardiac Index | 0.7 | | |
| CMP Surgery | 0.4 | | |
| Concomitant Surgery | 0.1 | | |
| CPB | 0.8 | | |
| Etiology | 0.5 | | |
| LVEF | 0.4 | | |
| PA Mean | 0.0 | | |
| Phase 1 | 0.03 | 1.2 | 3.3 |
| RVEF | 0.008 | −0.04 | 0.96 |
| Sex | 1.0 | | |

See text for abbreviations.

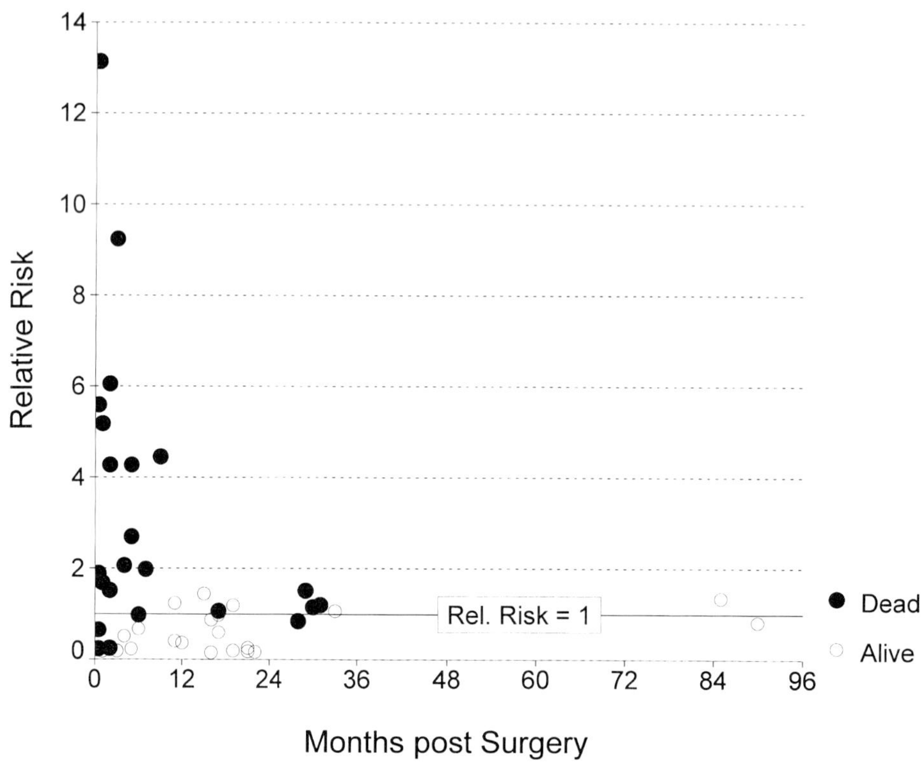


**Figure 2:** *Scattergram of relative risk of death versus length of survival for each individual patient as predicted by the Cox model equation shown. Y axis = predicted risk; x axis = months survival; black dots = nonsurvivors; circles = survivors.*

but may be stronger predictors of risk. This hypothesized situation might eventually allow other covariates of risk into the overall equation. Thus, the risk model described herein cannot be considered absolute dogma. It is only a first-pass model based on the variables considered. In the future we may find other risk factors that outweigh these presented here and make the latter moot.

Our analysis presents an overall relative risk of an individual compared to the baseline hazard function. This risk model is based on the presence of atrial fibrillation, the extent of right ventricular dysfunction, and the cardiomyoplasty study phase under which the operation took place.

Since all future patients will be in Phase II or beyond, this portion of the risk model becomes moot for future calculations. However, it dramatically points out that a significant learning curve exists for patient selection and technical application of this operation (Fig. 3). There were, most definitely, subtle lessons learned during the course of Phase I that were successfully applied in Phase II. This intangible learning curve was independent of the risk factors? atrial fibrillation and poor RVEF. The importance of phase as a risk factor probably reflects the advances in technology in general, the refinements in surgical technique in particular, and subtle selection biases. This would suggest that the field of cardiomyoplasty cannot be entered into half-heartedly by any and all cardiac surgeons. It should continue to be performed under close scrutiny with a constant and cautious learning process.

Poor RVEF most likely represents end-stage biventricular failure unamenable to correction by a muscle wrap designed to assist only the left ventricle. Patients with biventricular failure (low RVEF as well as poor LVEF) are at higher risk of death following cardiomyoplasty (Fig. 4). However, these patients also have a poor prognosis with angiotensin-converting enzyme inhibitor medical therapy.[8]

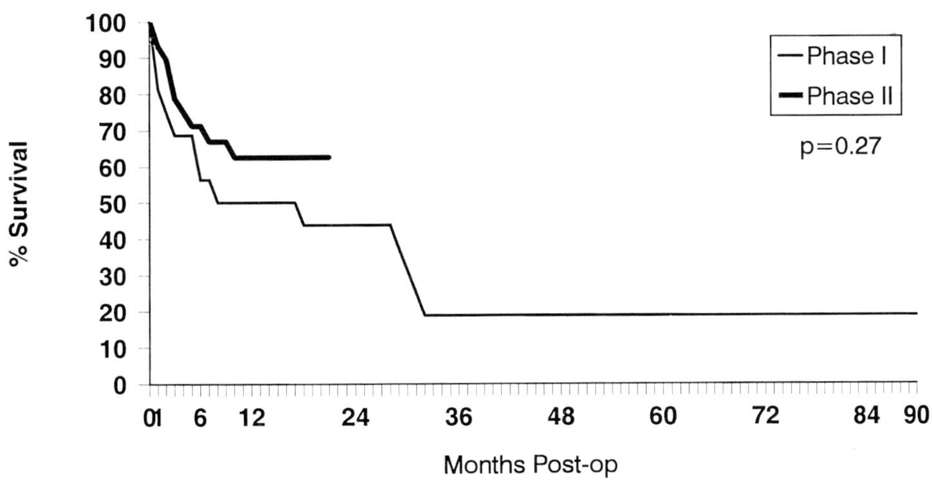


**Figure 3:** *Cumulative hazard of death over time as it relates to phase of the study. Phase I hazard represents a historical comparison only, as all future patients will be in Phase II or beyond (p value shown is for univariate comparison).*

The strong significance of atrial fibrillation and decreasing RVEF on patient survival is compelling evidence for these factors to be considered in the patient selection process. At present, NYHA Class IV is considered the only "hard" exclusion criterion. However, in this analysis NYHA Class as a risk factor was outweighed by RVEF and atrial fibrillation. Perhaps the NYHA Class IV patient in normal sinus rhythm with preserved right ventricular function could safely undergo this procedure.

It is logical that the loss of the "atrial kick" and its associated 15–20% increase in ventricular filling would be a poor prognosticator of long-term survival for any patient in heart failure. This is certainly the case with patients who have had a cardiomyoplasty (Fig. 5). The wrap itself is designed to aug-

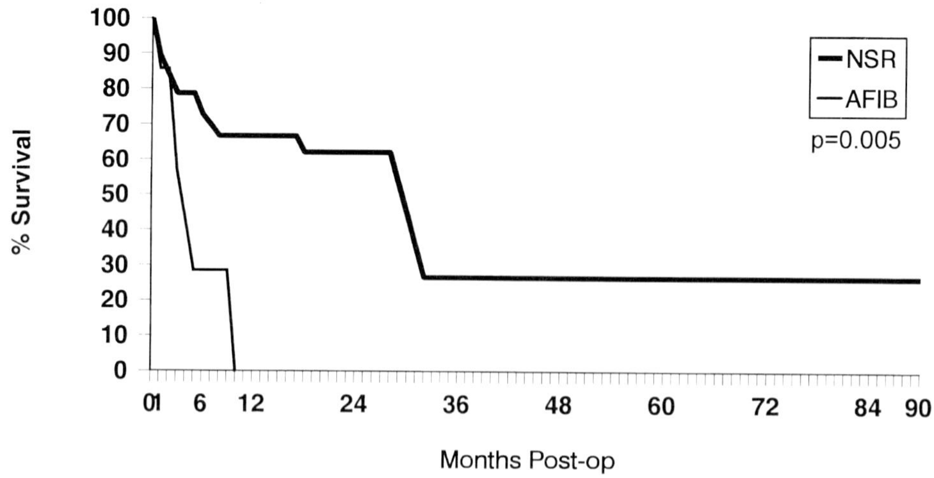


**Figure 4:** *Survival comparison of atrial fibrillation versus normal sinus rhythm.*

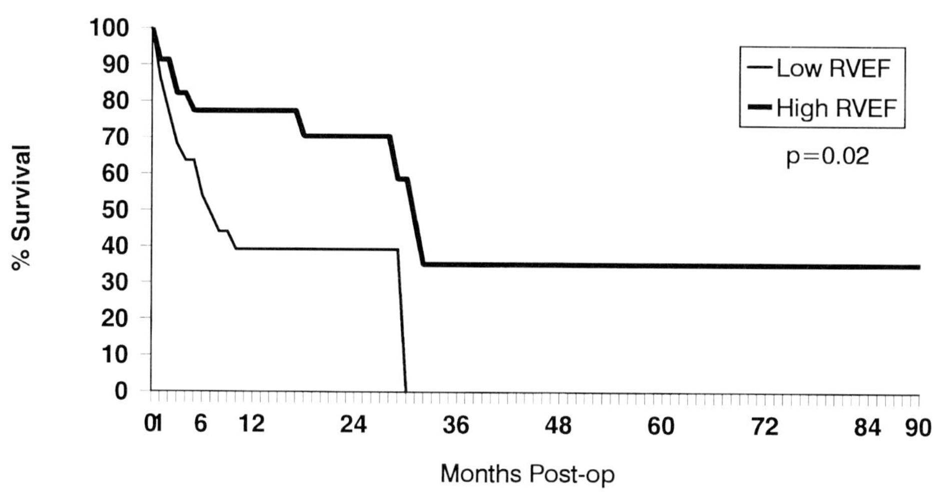


**Figure 5:** *Survival as a function of RVEF.*

ment systolic function and may do so at the expense of impaired diastolic filling.[7] Therefore, both experimental and clinical data suggest that the operation may be contraindicated in the absence of an atrial kick.

## Summary

Cardiomyoplasty remains an evolving option for the treatment of end-stage heart disease. Its high early and late mortality rates in NYHA Class IV patients has previously restricted its use to Class III. Risk of postoperative death following cardiomyoplasty can now be more specifically related to atrial fibrillation and poor RVEF. These specific factors should be considered in the patient selection process for the procedure. In so doing, we may open up a safe surgical option for selected NYHA Class IV patients. As risk factors are honed and applied to the selection process, the risk-benefit ratio for dynamic cardiomyoplasty will improve.

## References

1. Carpentier A, Chachques JC: Myocardial substitution with a stimulated skeletal muscle: first successful clinical case. *Lancet* 1:12–67, 1985.
2. Medtronic Cardiomyoplasty Phase I Study Group: *Phase I Clinical Results through October 1991,* prepared by Medtronic CAS Venture, April 1992.
3. Medtronic dynamic cardiomyoplasty system summary of phase I clinical results, Medtronic, Inc., Minneapolis, Minnesota.
4. Furnary AP, Magovern JA, Christlieb IY, et al: Clinical cardiomyoplasty: preoperative factors associated with outcome. *Ann Thorac Surg* 54:(11)39–43, 1992.
5. Furnary AP, Christlieb IY, Magovern JA, Magovern GJ: A standardized nomenclature for latissimus dorsi cardiomyoplasty. *J Cardiac Surg* 6:74–79, 1991.
6. Furnary AP, Magovern JA, Christlieb IY, et al: Improved ventricular augmentation with right latissimus cardiomyoplasty. *ACS Surg Forum* 42:307–309, 1991.
7. Corin WJ, George DT, Sink JD, et al: Dynamic cardiomyoplasty acutely impairs left ventricular diastolic function. *J Thorac Cardiovasc Surg* 104(6):1662–1671, 1992.
8. The Consensus Trial Study Group: Effects of enalapril on mortality in severe congestive heart failure. *N Engl J Med* 316:1429–1435, 1987.

Chapter 5

# Long-Term Myocardial Assistance by a Wrapped Skeletal Muscle:

## A Clinical Experience

Roberto Lorusso, Luca Sandrelli, Valentino Borghetti, Jan Schreuder, Ottavio Alfieri*

### Introduction

In the past few years, long-term cardiac support has been shown to be feasible by using a transformed and synchronously stimulated skeletal muscle following a ventricular wrapping procedure. We present our preliminary experience consisting of 10 patients affected by progressive heart failure. All patients were male and the mean age was 56.7 years (51–61 years). Preoperative patient data included a mean ejection fraction (EF) of 21% (14%–28%), functional NYHA Class III in seven patients and intermittent Class IV in three patients, and a mean left ventricular end-diastolic diameter of 75 mm (61–86 mm). The etiology of the dilated cardiomyopathy was ischemic in six patients and idiopathic in four patients. No patient was suitable for heart transplantation because of medical or social reasons. All patients underwent dynamic cardiomyoplasty (DC) according to the technique described by Carpentier and Chachques. No additional surgical procedure was performed. There was no intraoperative death. One patient died 2 weeks following DC due to sudden arrythmia. There were two late deaths. Current follow-up ranges from 7 to 22 months. Seven patients underwent postoperative echo-Doppler evaluation at 6 months after surgery which documented beneficial skeletal muscle assistance (EF from 21% to 33%). Four patients were submitted to pressure/volume loop analysis (conductance catheter), which confirmed myocardial improvement during cardiac support (stroke volume increase up to 21%). Three patients underwent right heart catheterization and positive hemodynamic changes were observed (cardiac output from 4.6 ± 0.6 L/min to 5.8 ± 1.1 L/min, and cardiac index went

From Carpentier A, Chachques JC, Grandjean P: Cardiac Bioassist. © Futura Publishing Co, Inc, Armonk, NY, 1997.

*With the cooperation of Edoardo Tulumello, Giovanni La Canna, Marco Metra, Frederick van der Veen.

from 2.5 ± 0.5 L/min/m$^2$ to 3.1 ± 0.7 L/min/m$^2$). Our preliminary data confirm DC as a valuable option in selected patients to treat end-stage heart failure.

Natural history of severe chronic heart failure is characterized by a poor survival rate.[1] Pharmacological treatment achieved outstanding results in recent years[2,3]; nevertheless it does not represent the ultimate solution of progressive ventricular dysfunction and dilatation. Heart transplantation has represented the surgical challenge showing remarkable improved outcome in the past few years, but recently it has been hampered by a marked shortage of donors and a clearer appraisal of immunosuppressive therapy shortcomings and long-term results.[4] Mechanical support and total artificial heart still deserve caution and currently present economical and technical limitations.[5] Following extensive experimental studies, in 1985 Carpentier and Chachques introduced in the clinical practice a new operative approach, dynamic cardiomyoplasty (DC), which consisted of a properly mobilized, transposed, wrapped, and finally synchronously stimulated skeletal muscle to act in a cardiaclike fashion.[6] After further clinical series showing beneficial latissimus dorsi (LD) support, we adopted this technique in selected patients affected by refractory chronic heart failure who were not suitable for heart transplantation. Our preliminary results as well as specific findings are presented here.

## Methods

Ten male patients affected by severe chronic left ventricular dysfunction were referred by our institution. Mean age was 56.7 years (51–61 years). All patients fulfilled the selection criteria for DC, namely a left ventricular end-diastolic diameter (LVEDD) $<$90 mm, a mitral insufficiency $<$grade 2, no major or symptomatic arrhythmia, ventilatory vital capacity $>$60%, a left ejection fraction (EF) $>$10%, and a right EF $>$30%. Preoperative patient data included a mean EF of 21% (14%–28%), NYHA Class III in six patients and intermittent Class IV in four patients, and a mean LVEDD of 75 mm (61–86 mm). Heart transplantation was not indicated in these patients due to insulin-dependent diabetes (three patients), severe peripheral vascular disease (four patients), refusal of heart transplantation waiting list (one patient), and age (two patients). All patients had had several episodes of acute pulmonary edema (from one to six episodes) in the previous year despite maximal medical therapy (digitalis, ACE inhibitors, vasodilators, and diuretics). In some patients serial echo-Doppler studies clearly showed a progressive left ventricular dilatation, predicting an impairment of the Frank-Starling compensatory mechanism. Atrial fibrillation was present in two patients and was not considered a contraindication. One patient had had a pacemaker implantation due to severe second-degree AV block. The etiology of the underlying dilated cardiomyopathy was ischemic in six patients. In these patients conventional coronary bypass grafting was not considered indicated following dobutamine stress-test echocardiography and rest-redistribution myocardial scintigraphy to assess any myocardial viability and its extent.

Dynamic cardiomyoplasty surgery was accomplished according to the technique described by Carpentier and Chachques.[7] The left LD muscle was properly harvested and mobilized from the distal insertions. Two intramuscular electrodes (Medtronic® 5528) were thereafter implanted in the proximal portion of the muscle belly, perpendicularly to the thoracodorsal nerve course and maintaining 4–6 cm in between. Following LD transposition into the left thoracic cavity and careful closure of the muscle mobilization area, the patients were placed in a supine position to enable median sternotomy and the exposure of the cardiac chambers. Since the very first case at our institution, we have been adopting transesophageal echo monitoring during DC in order to optimize wrapped muscle tension as well as AV groove lining of the LD posterior edge. Furthermore, any cardiac geometry distortion or any sign of constriction are looked for during the accomplishment of the surgical technique which consists of a ventricular wrapping by means of the "sutureless technique."[7] Synchronously wrapped LD muscle contraction has been obtained by using an appropriate cardiomyostimulator positioned in the left abdominal wall pocket (Medtronic® SP 1005A) according to the postoperative progressive training protocol proposed by Chachques and Carpentier.

After surgery all patients were submitted to traditional means of hemodynamic assessment. Moreover, an innovative technique was performed on four patients. In these patients a beat-to-beat analysis of the DC effects was recorded by a conductance catheter (Baan's catheter) placed in the left ventricle measuring the volume changes during the cardiac cycle (Fig. 1). The concomitant measurement of pressure (Millar catheter) and volume (P/V) data by

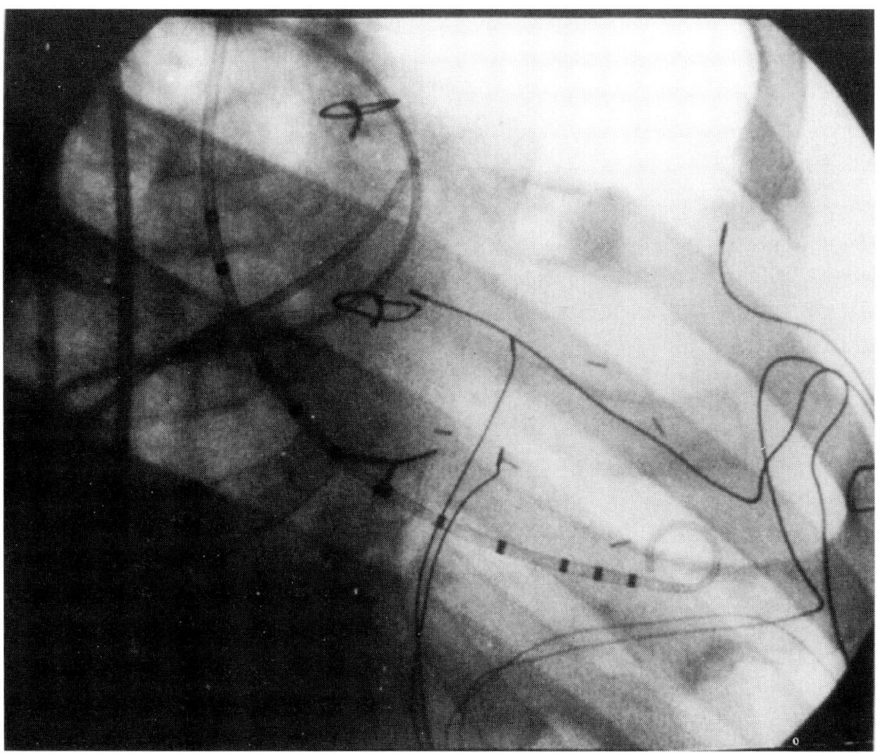

**Figure 1:** *The conductance catheter (Baan's catheter) is located inside the left ventricle up to the apex. The electrodes along the catheter to measure the conductance changes (volume changes) are visible.*

means of computer processing allowed us to have an on-line display of assisted beats, unassisted beats, and basal hemodynamics. Echo-Doppler and P/V loop analyses are performed by varying the stimulation parameters (burst duration, pulse amplitude, and LD activation time) in order to assess the optimal setting for achieving the best hemodynamic improvement. These measurements are accomplished by comparing basal values (cardiomyostimulator off for 1 hour) with unassisted and assisted data since we always adopt a 2:1 LD/heart contraction ratio. During P/V loop recording, a breath-holding maneuver is adopted to avoid any influence of the respiratory cycle on cardiac volumes.

The results are presented as mean values ± standard deviation (SD). Statistical analysis was obtained with the paired Student's *t*-test and a $p$ value $<0.05$ was considered significant.

## Results

No intraoperative deaths occurred. One patient developed low cardiac output syndrome soon after an uneventful surgery. Such a clinical status was successfully controlled by the positioning of an intra-aortic balloon counterpulsation (IABP). At the achievement of stable hemodynamics, IABP was removed and the patient was extubated. Nonetheless, this patient developed a sudden arrhythmia at the 15th postoperative day and was unresponsive to any pharmacological treatment as well as to resuscitation maneuvers. One patient suffered from a sudden deterioration of a previously present arterial vascular disease. This patient developed an acute occlusion of a previously implanted aortic-femoral prosthetic graft requiring three surgical interventions. He subsequently developed an adult respiratory distress syndrome and died 1.5 months from DC surgery. A third patient experienced sudden death 7 months postoperatively despite clear evidence of marked improvement in functional as well as hemodynamic status.

Patient follow-up ranges from 7 to 23 months (mean 18.7). Preliminary postoperative evaluation documented promising results in the majority of treated patients. Right heart catheterization was performed in three patients from 6 to 9 months post DC and showed effective LD support. Cardiac output increased from 4.6 ± 0.6 L/min to 5.8 ± 1.1 L/min-$p$>0.005, stroke volume (SV) from 30.7 ± 8.0 mL to 34.7 ± 10.1 mL-$p$>0.005, and cardiac index from 2.5 ± 0.5 L/min/m$^2$ to 3.1 ± 0.7 L/min/m$^2$-$p$>0.005. Postoperative complications included arrhythmia (atrial fibrillation, supraventricular tachycardia, and frequent premature ventricular beats) and cardiomyostimulator pocket infection (currently under treatment).

The LD contraction was assessed by standard postoperative evaluation tools (echo and MUGA) (Figs 2a,b). Echo-Doppler assessment showed the efficacy of LD contraction in terms of cardiac performance (EF increased from 21% to 33%). Detailed evaluation of heart/LD interaction at different stimulation parameters allowed us to detect a wide range, from suboptimal increase to even unexpected deterioration, of hemodynamic response just varying the LD contraction timing during the systolic phase. Indeed, significant hemodynamic improvements were detected during the assisted circulation in comparison with

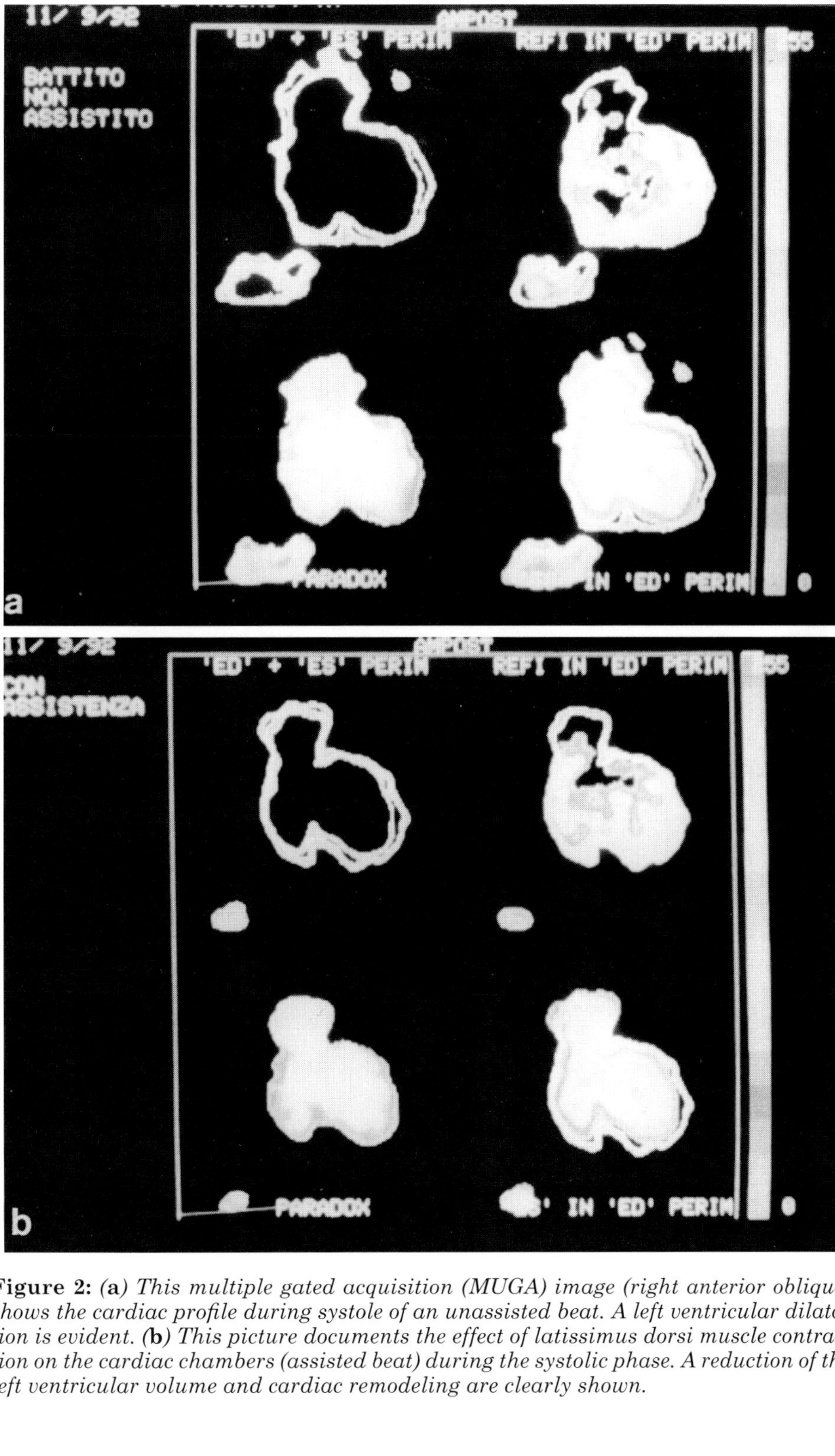


**Figure 2:** *(***a***) This multiple gated acquisition (MUGA) image (right anterior oblique) shows the cardiac profile during systole of an unassisted beat. A left ventricular dilatation is evident. (***b***) This picture documents the effect of latissimus dorsi muscle contraction on the cardiac chambers (assisted beat) during the systolic phase. A reduction of the left ventricular volume and cardiac remodeling are clearly shown.*

the basal data (cardiomyostimulator off), showing an EF increase from 19.4 ± 8.6% to 32.6 ± 13.8%-$p$=0.043, and an SV increase from 51.6 ± 20.6 mL to 63.0 ± 22.0 mL-$p$=0.014.

This finding was totally validated by beat-to-beat analysis by means of P/V loop evaluation. Improved systolic function was strikingly evident (Fig. 3), showing an increase of stroke volume ranging from 9% to 21% during assisted beats. Beat-to-beat analysis furthermore pointed out the importance of LD activation timing in terms of potential hemodynamic deterioration or of suboptimal improvement because of incorrect LD/heart coupling.

## Discussion

The use of an autologous power source to sustainingly assist the chronically impaired heart has been the dream of the majority of researchers and cardiac surgeons since the early decades of this century.

The attractive concept of educating a skeletal muscle to perform a cardiac-like workload was nonetheless always hampered in the first attempts due to naturally occurring muscle fatigue.[8] The outstanding experiments of Buller and Salmons disclosed the unexpected and marvellous world of "muscle plasticity."[9,10] Skeletal muscle eventually assured the new task of potential cardiac assist device capable of chronically supporting the impaired ventricular function.

Another key feature of the development of DC has been represented by the assembly of a pulse generator allowing a train of stimuli, namely a burst, with

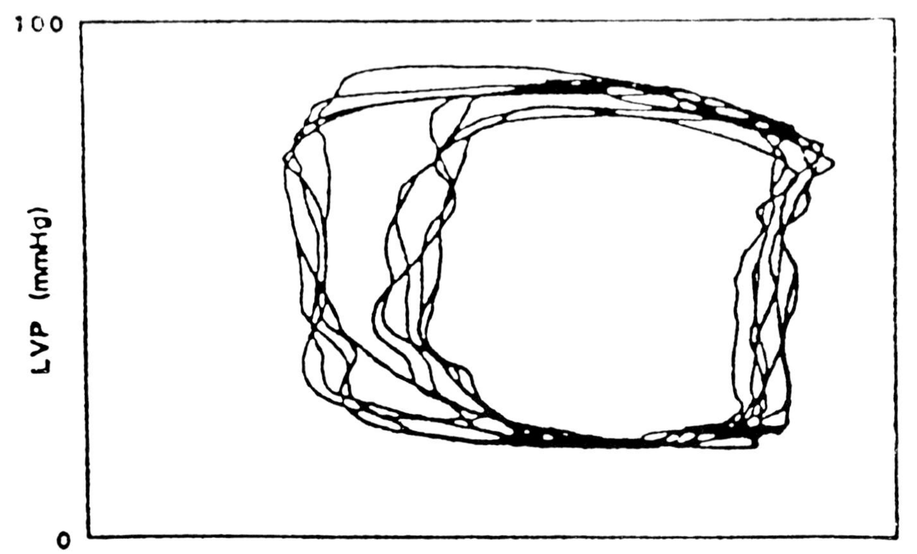


**Figure 3:** *This pressure/volume loop documents the effects of LD contractions. During the assisted beats, a clear increase in stroke volume is observed. A slight increase of the left ventricular pressure (LVP) during systole is shown. LVV = left ventricular volume.*

subsequent achievement of a tetanic contraction, generating more muscle power per contraction and increased hemodynamic assistance.[11]

The use of skeletal muscle to improve the failing heart was first introduced in clinical practice by Carpentier and Chachques in 1985.[6] Since that pioneer experience, we have been witnessing an increasing number of centers involved in the DC program. The dramatic need for alternatives to medical therapy and heart transplantation may be imputed as the rationale for approaching such a new surgical technique.

The first phase of the DC worldwide experience was characterized by controversial results likely related to the heterogenicity of the candidates, to the severely impaired preoperative clinical conditions (NYHA Class IV patients), and to the complexity of postoperative course of associated surgical procedures. Moreira and colleagues clearly documented the improved survival rates of patients submitted to DC because of end-stage heart failure.[12] Other clinical reports have shown improvement in systolic and diastolic functions, quality of life, and functional capacity in patients following DC.[13,14]

These preliminary findings prompted us to consider DC as a potentially useful therapeutic tool in the management of patients affected by medically refractory heart failure who are not candidates for heart transplantation. We do believe that the observations of several episodes of acute pulmonary edema in spite of full medical support and/or the evidence of progressive ventricular dilatation uncontrolled by standard pharmacological treatment are strong predictors of future cardiac decompensation and the impossibility to provide any kind of care.

Taking into consideration the above-mentioned criteria and the worldwide shortcoming represented by the donor shortage in heart transplantation, DC might be considered as a complementary therapy in end-stage heart failure. Our series included patients solely treated by DC procedure, and no extracorporeal circulation or associated surgical procedures were performed. Negligible operative mortality is, adopting such a management, an achievable goal. Perioperative morbidity as well as long-term results can probably benefit from a limited surgical trauma or procedure-related complications and DC might eventually be carried out with a reasonable operative risk.

At our institution, our main goal consists of clearly documenting LD contraction extent postoperatively and the effects of hemodynamics. The wrapped LD muscle contraction appeared to positively remodel the cardiac geometry in some patients. Moreover, marked hemodynamic improvements were observed in some patients while slight improvements were observed in others. Our efforts are therefore being addressed towards a better understanding of the primum movens of such a disparity in postoperative results. It is our opinion that this difference is likely related to the individual skeletal muscle response to training protocol and fiber transformation. Furthermore, the influence of the skeletal muscle derangement in chronic heart failure patients on DC results is still to be elucidated. We have just started preoperative physical training aimed at improving LD conditions, and preliminary results in terms of functional performance and histological changes are promising. Ongoing experimental studies are documenting that a fully transformed type I muscle is not ideal since in order to achieve a complete fatigue resistance, a considerable amount of the original power is lost.

In the clinical setting, the lack of homogeneous results in terms of hemodynamic improvement is still a major source of controversy and debate. This explains the rationale to adopt highly innovative technology in our series to evaluate any change in cardiac geometry or performance following DC. Pressure/volume analysis by means of conductance and micromanometer catheters ensured a beat-to-beat analysis of the cardiac cycle during LD assistance and the appraisal of the efficacy of LD contribution. This study showed the importance of correct heart/LD coupling in terms of proper timing of LD contraction to optimize systolic effects and prevent any potential impairment of the diastolic filling. These findings have already been validated by echo-Doppler assessment by our group as well as by Almada and colleagues.[15,16] Pressure/volume assessment clearly documented the beneficial effects of the LD contribution and allowed the appraisal of the hemodynamic changes, even if subtle. Further studies are required to refine our results (data evaluation and interpreting are under way) and ultimately a pre- and postoperative comparison would be desirable to better analyze the DC results.

In conclusion, we approached the management of refractory heart failure using a biomechanical technique since previous experiences have shown the benefits of such a procedure and the limited options to treat such a clinical syndrome. However, there is increasing evidence that our current knowledge in skeletal muscle assistance is too limited. Many factors can still be varied in the DC management as well as in postoperative evaluation that would lead to a better understanding of the DC mechanisms of action and a more precise appraisal of the actual unknown resources of the skeletal muscles.

## References

1. Kannel WB, Belanger AJ: Epidemiology of heart failure. *Am Heart J* 121:951–957, 1991.
2. The CONSENSUS Trial Study Group: Effects of enalapril on mortality in severe congestive heart failure: results of the Cooperative North Scandinavian Enalapril Survival Study (CONSENSUS). *N Engl J Med* 316:1429–1435, 1987.
3. The SOLVD Investigators: Effects of enalapril on survival in patients with reduced left ventricular ejection fractions and congestive heart failure. *N Engl J Med* 325:293–302, 1991.
4. Stevenson LW, Laks H, Terasaki PI, et al: Cardiac transplantation: selection, immunosuppression, and survival. *Western J Med* 149:572–582, 1988.
5. Davis PK, Rosenberg G, Snyder AJ, Pierce WS: Current status of permanent total artificial heart. *Ann Thorac Surg* 47:172–178, 1989.
6. Carpentier A, Chachques JC: Myocardial substitution with a stimulated skeletal muscle: first successful clinical case. *Lancet* 1:1267, 1985.
7. Carpentier A, JC Chachques: Cardiomyoplasty: surgical technique. In Carpentier A, Chachques JC, Grandjean P (eds): *Cardiomyoplasty.* Bakken Research Center Series, Mount Kisco, NY, Futura Publishing, Inc., 1991, pp 105–122.
8. Kantrowitz A, McKinnon W: The experimental use of the diaphragm as an auxiliary myocardium. *Surg Forum* 9:266–268, 1959.
9. Buller AJ, Eccles JC, Eccles RM: Interaction between motorneurons and muscles in respect of the characteristic speeds of their response. *J Physiol* 150:417–439, 1960.
10. Salmons S, Vroba G: The influence of activity on some contractile characteristics of mammalian fast and slow muscles. *J Physiol Lond* 210:429–439, 1969.
11. Dewar ML, Drinkwater DC, Wittnich C, Chiu RC-J: Synchronously stimulated

skeletal muscle graft for myocardial repair. *J Thorac Cardiovasc Surg* 87:325–331, 1984.
12. Moreira LF, Sefarian P Jr, Bocchi EA, et al: Survival improvement with dynamic cardiomyoplasty in patients with dilated cardiomyopathy. *Circulation* 84(Suppl III):III-296–III-302, 1991.
13. Chachques JC, Acar C, Portoghese M, et al: Dynamic cardiomyoplasty for long-term cardiac assist. *Eur J Cardiothorac Surg* 6:642–648, 1992.
14. Jatene AD, Moreira LFP, Stolf NAG, et al: Left ventricular function changes after cardiomyoplasty in patients with dilated cardiomyopathy. *J Thorac Cardiovasc Surg* 102:132–139, 1991.
15. Almada H, Molteni L, Ferreira R, et al: The value of echo-Doppler in cardiomyoplasty procedures. *J Cardiac Surg* 6(Suppl):113–118, 1991.
16. Lorusso R, Sandrelli L, Maisano F, et al: Echo-Doppler assessment to optimize wrapped skeletal muscle activation time following cardiomyoplasty procedure. *Eur Heart J* 13(Suppl):230, 1992.

# Chapter 5

# *Discussion*

**Unidentified:** Dr. Lorusso, in our experimental work, we found out that delayed time of exercise to transposed muscle around the heart reverses fibers back to type 2 again. What is the time interval between the exercise and the transposition? Also, we have seen angiogenesis following transposition without exercise. I was wondering whether the transposition of LD produces angiogenesis or other factors that may be involved with angiogenesis.

**Dr. Lorusso:** Our three patients were trained for almost 2 months prior to surgery and, unfortunately, we cannot see any results after muscle transposition because we don't do muscle biopsy after surgery unless they die. What we saw, after physical training, was that the muscle improved after physical training. We didn't see any angiogenesis per se, but we saw a marked increase in capillary diameter per fiber ratio. Of course, training improves the vascularization of the skeletal muscles. This could be important to prevent any muscle damage after muscle harvesting because we all know that we have to sever collateral vasculature during muscle dissection, so if you have more blood coming from other capillaries into the muscles, this could of course be of great help to the muscle to be in better shape and be prepared for the stimulation protocol. I cannot give you any answers concerning this kind of muscle structure.

**Unidentified:** I would like to ask Dr. Lorusso this: You showed the effect of a proper or improper synchronization delay. My first question is: how do you determine the proper timing? and the second question is: do you continue the exercise after the cardiomyoplasty is completed to gain the indirect beneficial effects of exercise on cardiac function?

**Dr. Lorusso:** Concerning the first question, we always monitor our patient in the same way and we change the delay between the R-wave and the moment of the LD contraction during systole. And as soon as we have the best hemodynamic value, that is the right setting. But the fact that we observed detrimental effects at some settings means that this can be crucial to patient outcome.

**Unidentified:** Does this change with time?

From Carpentier A, Chachques JC, Grandjean P: Cardiac Bioassist. © Futura Publishing Co, Inc, Armonk, NY, 1997.

**Dr. Lorusso:** No, it has to be tailored to each individual. Of course, we have a range from 25 msec to 100 msec. This was studied and evaluated and documented even by pressure-volume loops at our center and at the centers of Dr. Mikaeloff and Dr. Jegaden. So we have strong evidence that this is a crucial factor.

**Unidentified:** When I say time, I mean 6 months versus 18 months. Is it the same synchronization timing?

**Dr. Lorusso:** No, it changes, of course, because skeletal muscle performs in a different way over time so you can have a longer contraction time, a longer relaxation time and so it means you have to follow your patients and you will see the change in this synchronization delay. But you have to change it, otherwise you would have a tremendous range of hemodynamic changes.

**Unidentified:** The second question is do you continue to exercise them?

**Dr. Lorusso:** You mean after training? Yes, we do.

**Dr. Rebecca** (Medical College of Virginia): I have a question for Dr. Lorusso concerning both your morning and afternoon presentations. From a cardiologist's standpoint, I am very pleased to see some of you are looking at neurohormonal aberrations, especially since norepinephrine levels probably correlate better with prognosis than left ventricular ejection fraction. Your results were somewhat disappointing. I was wondering if you subset those patients, which appears to be about four patients, who were completely withdrawn from angiotensin-converting enzyme inhibitors. Were these the patients who had elevation of vasoconstrictor hormones or was it across the board?

**Dr. Lorusso:** All of the patients are now receiving ACE inhibitors and they are on the same therapy as preoperatively. But it could be decreased. If we look at the response hormone by hormone, norepinephrine increased a lot but the plasma renin activity decreased. If we look at the literature, we can see that the plasma renin activity is considered a strong predictor as well as norepinephrine. Probably none is higher as a predictor of patient survival. The results I presented this morning were the preliminary data and they could suggest new criteria for patient selection. For instance, candidates with unfavorable neurohormonal levels preoperatively could be refused. I don't know yet since we are still collecting data. But I do think that cardiomyoplasty does something. In fact, we had a reduction in plasma renin activity despite the use of diuretics and ACE inhibitors which usually increases the plasma renin activity. So we had controversial results. That is the reason I ask the audience whether there is any willingness among you to cooperate in a multicenter study? Out of 10 patients, we have only seven patients at 2 years follow-up. That's nothing compared with huge medical trials as have been done in the past. Also, we could probably learn a little bit more from the neurohormonal response during chronic cardiac assistance.

**Sir Magdi Yacoub (London):** I have three questions for Dr. Lorusso. One has to do with neuroendocrine changes. Looking at AMP, have you looked at AMP isoenzymes or brain peptides, which could be more predictive? The second is: what is the source of increased NA after cardiomyoplasty? And third: when you looked at the effects of exercising the LD, have you quantified the increased power of the muscle? Did you look at the effect of that program of exercise on the physical capacity and/or the neuroendocrine levels because rehabilitation has shown to improve patients in heart failure?

**Dr. Lorusso:** Regarding the first question, we are studying the brain nutriopeptides. Our research cardiologists are quite skilled in this field. Concerning the source and the cause of these releases, I told you this morning that we are now trying to understand why the plasma renin activity decreases and why the norepinephrine increases. Now I am working with a muscle group in the Netherlands. We are now doing studies in animals concerning the wrapping procedure without stimulation and the wrapping procedure plus stimulation to see whether skeletal muscle usage can induce a release of catecholamines.

**Sir Magdi Yacoub:** But have you looked at different parts of the circulation? Arterial versus coronary sinus. Is it the heart or the skeletal muscle—what is it?

**Dr. Lorusso:** No, unfortunately ours were venous samples, not from the coronary sinus. And as for the last question: our three patients, trained physically, improved dramatically as far as the power force and total work done. I had a patient who increased 190% of power. We trained the LD and the upper thorax muscles. But we have started a program with general physical training looking at the catecholamines. So we're doing quite an extensive study of skeletal muscle performance.

Chapter 6

# Operative and Perioperative Hemodynamic Management

Pascale Blanc, Claude Girard, Olivier Jegaden, Suzanne Estanove*

## Introduction

Dynamic cardiomyoplasty (CMP) is a recent surgical technique that was conceived either to provide a substitute for myocardium[1] or to assist ventricular function in dilated or ischemic cardiomyopathies.[2–5]

The idea of using a skeletal muscle for repair of the heart was reported by Leriche and Fontaine[6] in 1933. However, all initial experimental studies[7,8] of stimulated skeletal muscle flaps for cardiac assistance were limited by the fatigue characteristics of skeletal muscle in contrast with cardiac muscle. Later experiments showed that slow-rate electrical stimulation of skeletal muscle, specifically, induces the transformation of type II or fast-twitch muscle fibers (highly anerobic and fatigable) into type I or slow-twitch muscle fibers (highly aerobic and resistant to fatigue), myocardial fibers.[9–14]

The first clinical experience with dynamic cardiomyoplasty by Carpentier and Chachques in 1985[1] was made possible by the introduction of the progressive sequential stimulation protocol, which solved the problem of muscle fatigue for high-rate electrical stimulation of the muscle. The surgical procedure involves wrapping the left latissimus dorsi (LD) muscle around the failing heart and subsequently providing muscle electrostimulation in synchrony with ventricular systole. The LD muscle is used because of its suitable size and location close to the heart, allowing transfer into the chest with an intact neurovascular bundle without significant functional impairment.

Our team started to use this technique in November 1989. The challenge for us was to decide on the best perioperative management for patients with advanced cardiomyopathy undergoing this complex operation without immediate benefit to cardiac function. Therefore, our aim was to prepare the patient to face every stage of the surgical procedure.

From Carpentier A, Chachques JC, Grandjean P: Cardiac Bioassist. © Futura Publishing Co, Inc, Armonk, NY, 1997.

*With the cooperation of Catherine Vedrinne and Philippe Mikaeloff

## Materials and Methods

### Study Population (Table 1)

After ethical committee approval and informed patient consent, 12 men, aged 45 to 69 years (mean ±SD:59 ± 7) were operated on between November 1989 and September 1990.

Cardiac lesions were ischemic in nine patients, idiopathic in two patients, and mixed cardiomyopathy in one. All patients were New York Heart Association (NYHA) Class III or IV despite maximal therapy with diuretics, digitalis, and vasodilators. The preoperative cardiac index (CI) ranged from 1.36 to 2.82 L/min/$m^2$ (1.96 ± 0.47), the angiographic ejection fraction (EF) from 15% to 47% (25 ± 10) and the isotopic EF from 7% to 32% (18 ± 7). Two patients had chronic obstructive lung disease, four had diabetes mellitus, and creatinine level was over 150 μmol/L in three patients.

### Surgical Procedure

Surgical procedure consisted of two separate stages.

#### *Stage 1: Liberation of Muscle*

With the patient in the right lateral decubitus position, through a wide cutaneous incision between the left axillary region and the posterior iliac crest, the LD muscle was dissected and released from its humeral and thoracolumbar insertions while preserving its neurovascular pedicle.

Two flexible wire electrodes were then attached to the LD flap: a proximal one (negative) nearest to the main nerve branches and a second electrode (positive) 6–8 cm downstream from the cathode.

During this stage of the procedure, muscle relaxants were avoided in order not to disturb electrophysiological testing for threshold and impedance which are necessary to confirm the correct positioning of the electrodes. Next, the LD muscle graft was transferred into the left pleural cavity through a window obtained by partial resection of the second rib. Finally, a chest drain was inserted before suturing the skin.

#### *Stage 2: Insertion of Muscle*

Cardiomyoplasty was performed with the patient in the supine position. The heart was exposed through a median sternotomy and the muscle flap wrapped around the ventricles. Individual myocardial stitches were used for fixation of the muscle flap behind the heart and the procedure was completed, if necessary, by a pericardial patch covering the front side of the right part of the heart up to the aortic root.

A sensing epicardial electrode was implanted into the right ventricle and finally muscle and cardiac electrodes were tunneled through the subcutaneous

**Table 1**
Characteristics of the Patients

| *Patient* | *Age yr* | *Cardiomyopathy* | *Ejection Fraction* | | *Associated Surgical Procedure** |
|---|---|---|---|---|---|
| | | | *Angiographic* | *Isotopic* | |
| 1 | 66 | Ischemic | 24% | 13% | AR |
| 2 | 53 | Idiopathic | 47% | 19% | 0 |
| 3 | 58 | Ischemic | 24% | 14% | 0 |
| 4 | 45 | Ischemic | 23% | 10% | CABG (1) |
| 5 | 64 | Idiopathic + mitral insufficiency | 39% | 32% | CABG (1) + mitral valvuloplasty |
| 6 | 51 | Ischemic | 28% | 17% | AR + CABG (3) |
| 7 | 62 | Ischemic | 17% | 7% | AR |
| 8 | 54 | Ischemic | 16% | 17% | CABG (1) |
| 9 | 64 | Ischemic | 35% | 27% | CABG (1) |
| 10 | 65 | Ischemic | 18% | 17% | AR + CABG (1) |
| 11 | 60 | Ischemic | 15% | 22% | 0 |
| 12 | 69 | Idiopathic | 20% | 26% | 0 |

*Number in parentheses indicates number of coronary artery bypass grafts (CABG).
AR = aneurysm resection.

tissue and respectively connected to the "pacing channel" and the "sensing channel" of the cardiomyostimulator (Medtronic® SP1005 BV, Medtronic Inc., Maastricht, the Netherlands) implanted in the abdominal wall.

Generally, the wrapping procedure does not need extracorporeal circulation (ECC); however, it was always kept on standby in the operating room for potential complications requiring its use.

Eight patients (66%) underwent a mandatory cardiopulmonary bypass (CPB) to treat associated cardiac lesions: aneurysm resection: AR (n=2), coronary artery bypass graft: CABG (n=3), AR + CABG (n=2), mitral valvuloplasty + CABG (n=1).

## Anesthesia and Intraoperative Management

After oral premedication with flunitrazepam and hydroxyzine, general anesthesia was induced by flunitrazepam (0.02 mg/kg) and fentanyl (20 μg/kg). Initially, muscle relaxation was obtained with atracurium (0.6 mg/kg) for intubation with a "high volume-low pressure" endotracheal tube. Then the patient was mechanically ventilated ($V_T$=12 mL/kg) with air/oxygen ($FiO_2$=50%) and an additional positive end-expiratory pressure (PEEP) of 5 cm $H_2O$ was applied at the end of the thoracic stage in patients without obstructive airway disease. Anesthesia was maintained with flunitrazepam (0.01 mg/kg/h) and fentanyl (10–12 μg/kg/h). Only after LD stimulation tests was muscle relaxation reintroduced with pancuronium (0.1 mg/kg).

Besides our usual oxygenated crystalloid cold cardioplegia (FRESENIUS®, Bad Homburg, Deutschland), nondiabetic patients requiring ECC were administered a "glucose-insulin-potassium" (GIK) infusion before aortic cross-clamping (glucose=0.5 g/kg/h, insulin=1 U/kg/h, $K^+$=0.25 mmol/kg/h).

High-dose aprotinin was always used when ECC was required: 3 mg/kg intravenously (IV) before sternotomy, 3 mg/kg in the priming solution of ECC, and 2 mg/kg IV following the injection of protamine sulfate after emergence from ECC.

Hemodynamic assessment included heart rate (HR), mean arterial (MAP), central venous (CVP), pulmonary artery (PAP), and capillary wedge (CWP) pressures, and thermodilution cardiac output through a fiberoptic (7,5F) Swan-Ganz catheter (Opticath®, Abbott, Oximetrix, Mountain View, CA).

Hemodynamic data, arterial/venous blood gases, mean cardiac index (CI), mixed venous oxygen saturation ($SvO_2$), oxygen consumption ($O_2$ CONS) and delivery ($O_2$ DEL) and arteriovenous oxygen difference ($avDO_2$) were recorded while systemic (SVR) and pulmonary (PVR) vascular resistances, left (LVSWI) and right (RVSWI) ventricular stroke work index were calculated at each of the following times:

$T_1$ after induction of anesthesia
$T_2$ at the beginning of the thoracic procedure
$T_3$ after opening the left pleural cavity
$T_4$ just before median sternotomy
$T_5$ after emergence from ECC
$T_6$ at the end of the operation
$T_7$ 60 minutes after arrival in ICU.

Because of their impaired cardiac function, a dobutamine infusion was systematically commenced in all patients after $T_2$, if it had not previously been started.

## Statistics

Results were expressed as the mean (x) and standard deviation (SD). Statistical interpretation was performed with analysis of variance and Newman-Keuls test. Resulting *P* values <0.05 were regarded as significant.

# Results

## Intraoperative Data (Table 2)

At $T_1$, cardiac index was less than 2 L/min/m$^2$ (1.49 ± 0.41) in 11 patients showing a 24% decrease when compared with their preoperative status. Inotropic support was started after $T_1$ in five patients and immediately after $T_2$ in

**Table 2**

Perioperative Hemodynamic and Oxygenation Data in 12 Patients/Mean (SD)

| *Time* | $T_1$ | $T_2$ | $T_3$ | $T_4$ | $T_5$ | $T_6$ | $T_7$ |
|---|---|---|---|---|---|---|---|
| HR | 59 | 63 | 86* | 89* | 105* | 107* | 102* |
| (beats/min) | (12) | (16) | (21) | (22) | (13) | (17) | (16) |
| MAP | 68 | 69 | 73 | 71 | 64 | 73 | 76 |
| (mm Hg) | (10) | (5) | (8) | (7) | (6) | (8) | (8) |
| CVP | 11 | 13 | 16 | 11 | 11 | 12 | 14 |
| (mm Hg) | (5) | (5) | (3) | (5) | (5) | (5) | (4) |
| MPAP | 23 | 28* | 32* | 27 | 23 | 24 | 28* |
| (mm Hg) | (8) | (7) | (8) | (9) | (6) | (7) | (6) |
| PCWP | 15 | 17 | 20* | 16 | 13 | 15 | 16 |
| (mm Hg) | (6) | (6) | (6) | (6) | (5) | (6) | (7) |
| CI | 1.49 | 1.72 | 3.02* | 3.04* | 3.21* | 2.75* | 3.24* |
| (L/min/m$^2$) | (0.41) | (0.48) | (1.24) | (1.03) | (0.67) | (0.78) | (0.51) |
| SVR | 1706 | 1478 | 963* | 905* | 713* | 1026* | 824* |
| (dyn.sec/cm$^5$) | (540) | (419) | (459) | (286) | (137) | (432) | (200) |
| PVR | 255 | 271 | 183* | 169* | 135* | 149* | 157* |
| (dyn.sec/cm$^5$) | (125) | (113) | (58) | (86) | (23) | (61) | (27) |
| LVSWI | 19.6 | 20.0 | 26.4 | 26.1 | 21.6 | 20.8 | 26.2 |
| (g.m/m$^2$) | (8.4) | (6.0) | (11.4) | (10.7) | (7.0) | (8.4) | (6.7) |
| RVSWI | 3.26 | 4.41 | 6.71* | 5.70 | 4.35 | 3.17 | 5.35 |
| (g.m/m$^2$) | (2.55) | (3.95) | (4.24) | (3.11) | (1.81) | (1.20) | (2.32) |
| $SvO_2$ | 67 | 71 | 77* | 79* | 70 | 67 | 68 |
| (%) | (7) | (10) | (6) | (6) | (10) | (9) | (7) |
| $O_2$DEL. | 497 | 567 | 894* | 891* | 803* | 722* | 909* |
| (mL/min) | (115) | (127) | (296) | (255) | (194) | (195) | (160) |
| $O_2$CONS. | 165 | 162 | 183 | 178 | 220* | 242* | 291* |
| (mL/min) | (47) | (45) | (49) | (64) | (44) | (64) | (69) |
| $avDO_2$ | 6.04 | 5.24 | 3.69* | 3.16* | 3.62* | 4.79 | 4.78 |
| (mL/dL) | (1.46) | (1.91) | (1.47) | (0.83) | (1.00) | (1.06) | (0.99) |

*Significantly ($p$<0.05) difference from $T_1$. See text for abbreviations.

the others. After $T_2$, all patients were administered dobutamine (less than 8 μg/kg/min), increasing CI by nearly 100% (3.02 ± 1.24 L/min/m$^2$), mainly by reducing systemic vascular resistances by the same proportion (Fig. 1) with a limited increase in myocardial work (+20%) (Fig. 2). Six patients also received sodium nitroprusside and/or nitroglycerin to decrease SVR or PAP. Mean $SvO_2$ remained over 67% during the whole surgical procedure (Fig. 3).

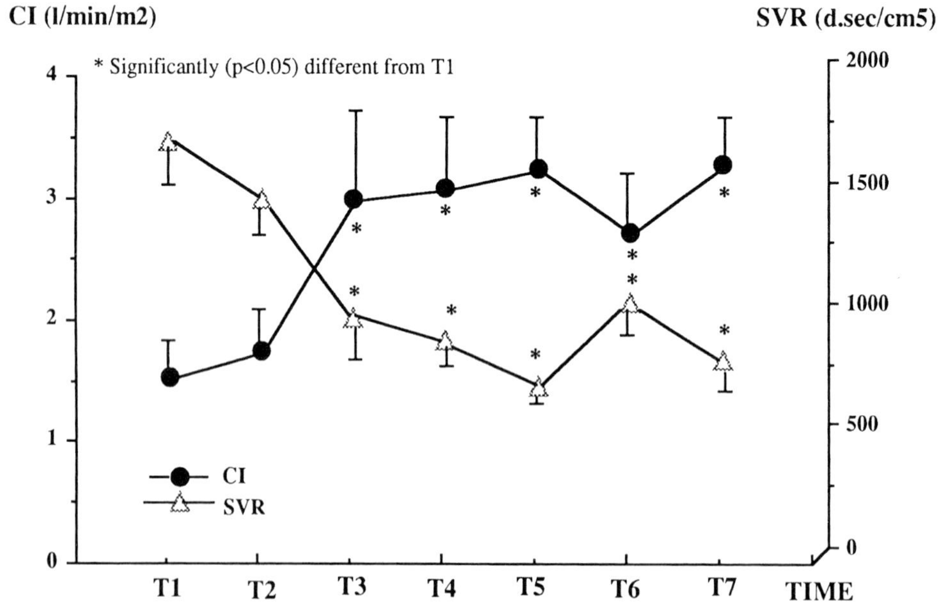


**Figure 1:** *Evolution of cardiac index (CI) and systemic vascular resistances (SVR) throughout surgery. (Used with permission from Chest 103:214–220, 1993.)*

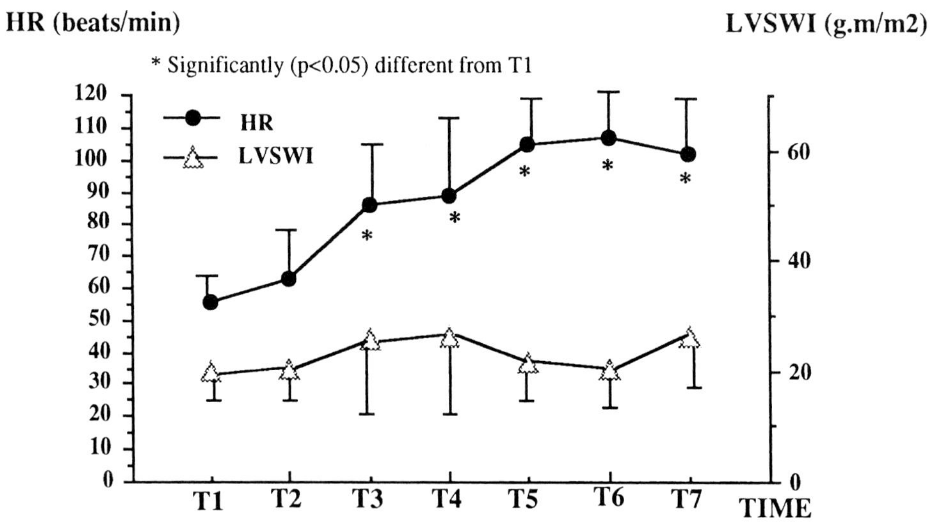


**Figure 2:** *Perioperative relationship between heart rate (HR) and left ventricular stroke work index (LVSWI). (Used with permission from Chest 103:214–220, 1993.)*

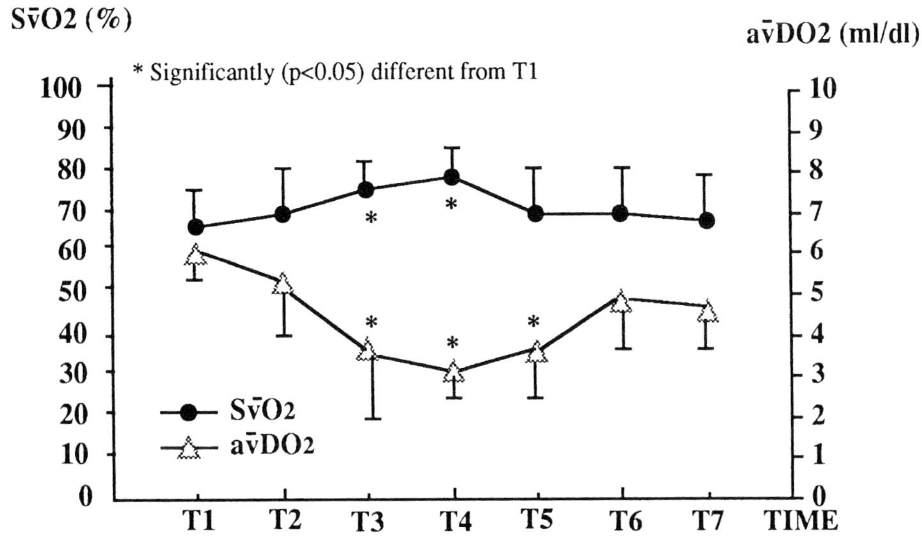


**Figure 3:** *Evolution of mixed venous oxygen saturation ($S\bar{v}O_2$) and arteriovenous oxygen difference ($a\bar{v}DO_2$) throughout surgery. (Used with permission from Chest 103:214–220, 1993.)*

At the end of the thoracic stage (mean duration = 186 ± 32 min), a decrease in $paO_2$ was always noticed, which was lower than 85 mm Hg in four patients.

Arrhythmias occurred on three occasions: atrial fibrillation and nodal tachycardia during venous cannulation before onset of ECC in two patients, and ventricular fibrillation during the wrapping procedure in one patient undergoing CMP without CPB. Spontaneous defibrillation was observed in seven out of eight patients at the end of CPB, and none of the patients required intra-aortic balloon counterpulsation. The mean thoracic time was 186 ± 32 minutes. The average CPB duration was 85 ± 40 minutes. The mean operating time was 438 ± 75 minutes. All patients survived the procedure.

## Early Postoperative Data

The average blood loss during the first 24 hours was 601 ± 210 mL and none of the patients required surgical re-exploration. The average amount of blood transfused was 1.25 ± 1.21 units intraoperatively and 1.09 ± 1.30 units postoperatively. Each patient was administered a ketoprofen infusion (10 mg/kg/day) for analgesia during the first 2 postoperative days, except for one with a history of peptic ulceration. Supraventricular arrhythmia occurred in two cases, and was poorly tolerated in one patient who needed reintubation.

Despite systematic continuation of the inotropic support, most often with dobutamine, low cardiac output syndrome occurred in five cases, mostly during weaning from mechanical ventilation, requiring increasing doses. Two of them also developed right ventricular failure, successfully treated by epinephrine associated with a pulmonary $PGE_1$ infusion.

Apart from two cases of pneumothorax after pleural drain removal and three cases of pneumonia, the pulmonary follow-up of the other patients was uneventful with an average duration of mechanical ventilation of 47 ± 28 hours (range, 15–115).

The average time spent in the intensive care unit (ICU) was 6.8 ± 4.0 days (range, 3–17) for 11 of the patients. The other patient left spent 35 days in the ICU due to a sequence of complications involving pneumothorax, extensive emphysema, pulmonary infection, and renal failure requiring continuous venovenous hemodialysis for 6 days. Six months after the surgical procedure, all patients were alive.

## Discussion

### Intraoperative Management

In this operation, the anesthesiologist had to manage patients with advanced cardiomyopathy, undergoing a long surgical procedure (mean time, 7 to 8 hours, due to the associated surgical procedures) of which the first stage was performed in the right decubitus position. In the closed-chest anesthetized patient, this position is known to be detrimental because the mediastinum rests on the lower lung and impedes its expansion. As gravity causes a vertical gradient in the distribution of pulmonary blood flow, the upper lung is well ventilated but poorly perfused and the lower lung is well perfused but poorly ventilated, creating a marked mismatch of the ventilation-perfusion ratio. Opening the chest wall to introduce the LD muscle in the pleural space may result in a further mismatching of ventilation with perfusion.[15]

In patients without obstructive lung disease, a 5-cm $H_2O$ PEEP was applied in an attempt to restore the ventilation to the dependent (right) lung and was maintained until the end of the surgical procedure to avoid atelectasis. Despite $FiO_2$ of 50% and the application of a PEEP, a decrease in $PaO_2$ was always noticed at the end of the thoracic stage, leading to values less than 85 mm Hg in four patients.

This thoracic time consisted of a large and meticulous dissection with two main consequences: (1) a rather long duration (3 hours) because the surgeon preferred manual hemostasis to electrocoagulation in order to preserve the LD muscle vascular vitality; and (2) a significant risk of bleeding, especially when a CPB was required: hence, to improve the surgical hemostasis, high-dose aprotinin was always used in these cases, with a good result attested by the absence of surgical re-exploration and a low blood transfusion need.[16]

In the absence of CPB, the major problem during the second stage of the procedure, consisting of wrapping the muscle flap around the heart, was a high incidence of arrhythmias which caused hemodynamic instability. All patients were preventively administered 1 to 1.5 mg/kg lidocaine after sternotomy, and in most patients, only isolated drops in $SvO_2$ were noticed, coinciding with a prolonged arrhythmic episode. However, in one patient undergoing simple CMP, ventricular fibrillation occurred during the wrapping procedure, but this was easily reversible with a single shock. Apart from lidocaine and optimal kalemia, the ideal attitude to prevent severe arrhythmias was gentle surgical manipulation, while the anesthesiologist observes the cardiac monitor to inform the surgeon when release of the heart becomes necessary for it to recover.

As most of our patients (66%) required a CPB for treatment of associated cardiac lesions, the major problem was to wean from ECC such patients with prior impaired myocardial function, which could have been still worsened during the aortic cross-clamping. Moreover, as the LD muscle flap was left unstimulated until the third postoperative week in order to allow time for adhesion formation between the muscle and the epicardium, no benefit was expected from the surgical procedure during the initial postoperative course. This is the reason why a rigorous myocardial protection was of the utmost importance. Hence, besides our usual oxygenated crystalloid cardioplegia (FRESENIUS®), nondiabetic patients were administered "glucose-insulin-potassium" (GIK) between sternotomy and aortic cross-clamping. It has been reported that preventive administration of GIK leads to increased myocardial glycogen and adenosine triphosphate and a maintained energy charge during coronary ischemia, thus improving ischemic tolerance and myocardial protection.[17–19] Possibly due to this double myocardial protection, spontaneous defibrillation was observed in seven out of eight patients, despite their prior impairment in myocardial function (mean isotopic LVEF <20%).

With regard to hemodynamic management, our reasoning was based on the fact that because of the myocardial impairment of these patients, confirmed by preoperative low cardiac index at rest, any increase in oxygen consumption could not be obtained by an important increase in myocardial work. Therefore, the rise in cardiac output required by increased oxygen consumption should be absolutely obtained at the expense of a minimal cardiac work. By using an $SvO_2$ Swan-Ganz catheter and the early use of moderate doses of beta inotropic agents, we were able to balance oxygen delivery and consumption, thus avoiding any situation of myocardial and general oxygen deficit during every stage of the surgical procedure. First of all, increased oxygen consumption due to pain and posture was limited by deep anesthesia and analgesia, associated with muscle relaxation as soon as the electrophysiological tests of the LD muscle were performed. This increased oxygen consumption (+35%) was easily covered by a great increase (+70%) in oxygen delivery that allowed the myocardium to become adapted to the metabolic requirements resulting from the different stages of the surgical procedure (Fig. 4). Due to the preferred use of dobutamine, which is known among the inotropic agents to provide the more favorable oxygen supply/demand ratio,[20] the cardiac output allowing this improved oxygen delivery increased by 100% with a limited rise in myocardial work (+20%). The downward trend of the arteriovenous difference and the stability of the mixed venous oxygen saturation over 67% confirmed the absence of tissue deficit in oxygen during the operation (Fig. 3).

This pharmacologically induced improvement in myocardial function remained stable during the whole surgical procedure, being optimal at $T_5$, after emergence from bypass, probably because the well-preserved myocardium was still benefiting from the vasodilating effect of GIK.

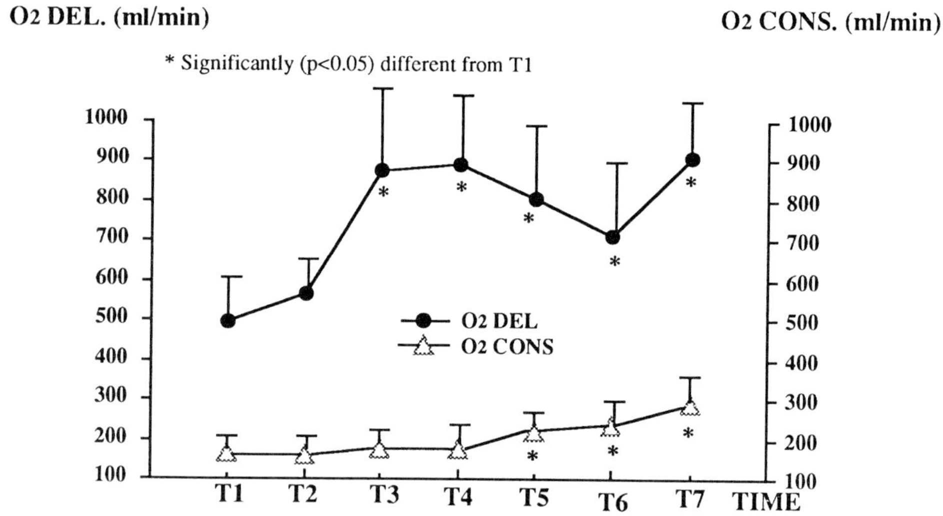


**Figure 4:** *Perioperative relationship between oxygen consumption ($O_2$ CONS) and delivery $O_2$ DEL). (Used with permission from Chest 103:214–220, 1993.)*

## Postoperative Management

Due to the length of the operation, all patients were mechanically ventilated for the first 24 hours. Weaning from assisted ventilation was started with analgesia provided by high-dose ketoprofen, so as not to limit vital capacity because, in addition to the length of the scars, the left lung can be hampered by the LD muscle flap. Most of the patients were extubated within 2 days. The two major problems encountered postoperatively were arrhythmias and low cardiac output syndrome.

After extubation, the third patient of the study presented with prolonged supraventricular tachycardia, poorly tolerated hemodynamically because of the myocardial impairment, needing reintubation. Cardioversion was generally avoided because of the risk of inactivation of the new implanted cardiomyostimulator, except in case of ventricular tachycardia or fibrillation. This was the reason why the next patients planned for CMP were administered amiodarone preoperatively, to reduce the likelihood of arrhythmias postoperatively.

Among the five patients treated for low cardiac output syndrome, mostly revealed at the time of weaning from mechanical ventilation, two of them had right ventricular failure requiring epinephrine to improve the perfusion pressure, associated with a $PGE_1$ infusion into the pulmonary artery to decrease the right ventricular afterload. In one case, this failure was not foreseen (patient no. 7, mean PAP = 25 mm Hg), but in the other case (patient no. 8), this complication could have been expected because of preoperative pulmonary hypertension (mean PAP = 56 mm Hg).

After resolving these acute hemodynamic problems, continued treatment of low cardiac output syndrome consisted of a regimen of a beta-inotropic agent and a vasodilator, associated if necessary with a phosphodiesterase inhibitor (enoximone). This IV treatment was progressively reduced to be replaced by oral captopril and digitalis.

## Conclusion

Cardiomyoplasty is, for selected cases of cardiomyopathy, considered as an alternative treatment providing contractile assistance to the impaired myocardium. However, the surgical conditions induce myocardial stress on a failing heart. The early conditioning of the patients involving on the one hand, a safe anesthesia with deep analgesia, and on the other hand, systematic beta-inotropic support possibly combined with a vasodilator, allows adequate rise in cardiac index to meet metabolic requirements at the expense of a minimal cardiac work. With this protocol, $SvO_2$ remains always over 60%, providing optimum conditions for the patient to overcome this long surgical procedure, despite no immediate improvement in cardiac function.

## References


1. Carpentier A, Chachques JC: Myocardial substitution with a stimulated skeletal muscle: first successful clinical case (letter). *Lancet* 1:1267, 1985.
2. Chachques JC, Grandjean P, Schwartz K, et al: Effect of latissimus dorsi dynamic cardiomyoplasty on ventricular function. *Circulation* 78(Suppl III):III-203-III-216, 1988.
3. Hill AB, Chiu RCJ: Dynamic cardiomyoplasty for treatment of heart failure (review). *Clin Cardiol* 12:681–688, 1989.
4. Magovern GJ, Heckler FR, Park SB, et al: Paced latissimus dorsi used for dynamic cardiomyoplasty or left ventricular aneurysms. *Ann Thorac Surg* 44:379–388, 1987.
5. Macgovern GJ, Park SB, Kao RL, et al: Dynamic cardiomyoplasty in patients. *J Heart Transplant* 9:258–263, 1990.
6. Leriche R, Fontaine R: Essai expérimental de traitement de certains infarctus du myocarde et de l'anévrisme du coeur par une greffe de muscle strié. *Bull Soc Nat Chir* 9:229–232, 1933.
7. Kantrowitz A, McKinnon WHP: The experimental use of the diaphragm as an auxiliary myocardium. *Surg Forum* 9:266–268, 1959.
8. Termet H, Chalencon JL, Estour E, et al: Transplantation sur le myocarde d'un muscle strié excité par pace-maker. *Ann Chir Thorac Cardiovasc* 5:568–571, 1966.
9. Dewar ML, Chiu RCJ: Cardiomyoplasty and the pulse-train stimulator. In Chiu RCJ (ed): *Biomechanical Cardiac Assist.* Mount Kisco, NY, Futura Publishing Company, Inc., 1986, pp 43–58.
10. Salmons S, Sreter FA: Significance of impulse activity in the transformation of skeletal muscle type. *Nature* 263:30–34, 1976.
11. Eisenberg BR, Salmons S: The reorganization of subcellular structure in muscle undergoing fast-to-slow type transformation. *Cell Tissue Res* 220:449, 1981.
12. Chiu RCJ, Kochamba G, Walsh G, et al: Biochemical and functional correlates of myocardium-like transformed skeletal muscle as a power source for cardiac assist devices. *J Cardiac Surg* 4(2):171–179, 1989.
13. Carpentier A, Chachques JC, Grandjean P: Transformation of skeletal muscle by sequential stimulation with a view toward its use as a myocardial substitute. *C R Acad Sci Paris* 301(11):581–586, 1985.
14. Chagas ACP, Moreira LFR, Luz PL, et al: Stimulated preconditioned skeletal muscle cardiomyoplasty: an effective means of cardiac assist. *Circulation* 80(Suppl III):III-202-III-208, 1989.

15. Benumof JL: *Anesthesia for Thoracic Surgery.* Philadelphia, WB Saunders Company, 1987.
16. Bidstrup BP, Royston D, Sapsford RN, et al: Reduction in blood loss and blood use after cardiopulmonary bypass with high dose aprotinin. *J Thorac Cardiovasc Surg* 97:364–372, 1989.
17. Haider W, Eckersberger F, Wolner E: Preventive insulin administration for myocardial protection in cardiac surgery. *Anesthesiology* 60:422–429, 1984.
18. Haider W, Benzer H, Schutz W, et al: Improvement of cardiac preservation by preoperative high insulin supply. *J Thorac Cardiovasc Surg* 88:294–300, 1984.
19. Girard C, Quentin P, Bouvier H, et al: Glucose and insulin supply before cardiopulmonary bypass in cardiac surgery: a double-blind study. *Ann Thorac Surg* 54:259–263, 1992.
20. Goldstein RA: Dobutamine in acute myocardial infarction. In Chatterjee K (ed): *Dobutamine: A Ten-Year Review.* New York, NCM Publishers, Inc., 5:83–95, 1989.

Chapter 7

# Cardiomyoplasty in Congestive Heart Failure

## Late Hemodynamic Results

Olivier Jegaden, François Delahaye, Gerard Finet, Philippe Mikaeloff*

### Introduction

The principle of cardiomyoplasty is to transfer the left latissimus dorsi muscle, wrap it around the heart cavities, and stimulate it in synchronization with the ventricular systole in order to increase the contraction ability of the ventricular cavities. Since the first clinical application by Carpentier and Chachques in 1985,[1] cardiomyoplasty has become a therapeutic possibility in the management of severe congestive heart failure. The results reported by various teams show that cardiomyoplasty may provide effective functional improvement in the patient with severe congestive heart failure, while hemodynamic improvement is inconstant and controversial.[2–5]

Based on a preliminary series of 12 patients who underwent cardiomyoplasty and were followed-up for more than 2 years postoperatively, the purpose of this work is to try to answer two questions: In severe congestive heart failure treated by cardiomyoplasty, what degree of hemodynamic improvement can be expected in the long term postoperatively? What is the ideal profile of the patient amenable to cardiomyoplasty?

### Material and Methods

Between November 1989 and September 1990, 12 patients underwent cardiomyoplasty at our institution. All patients were males, NYHA Class III, of mean age 59 ± 7 years (range, 45–69). Nine patients presented with ischemic

From Carpentier A, Chachques JC, Grandjean P: Cardiac Bioassist. © Futura Publishing Co, Inc, Armonk, NY, 1997.

*With the cooperation of Armand Eker and Pietro Montagna.

myocardiopathy, two patients with primary dilated cardiopathy, and one patient with complex heart pathology associating organic mitral incompetence with primary and ischemic cardiopathy.

The surgical technique used was the one described by Carpentier and Chachques.[6] Four patients had isolated cardiomyoplasty without extracorporeal circulation and eight patients had cardiomyoplasty associated with heart surgery requiring extracorporeal circulation, six patients had coronary bypass, three had resection of a left ventricular akinetic plaque, and one patient had mitral valve repair (Table 1). Medtronic® electrostimulation equipment was used (SP 5528, SP 5548, SP 1005). The protocol of stimulation of the latissimus dorsi[6] began 16 ± 3 days after surgery, i.e., by time suitable adhesions of the latissimus dorsi to the heart had developed. Effective stimulation (burst of six impulses, one heart beat in two) was obtained at 65 ± 18 days postoperatively. The contraction of the proximal portion of the latissimus dorsi was felt manually in the axillary area. The kinetics of the stimulated latissimus dorsi, covered with metal clips during the surgical procedure, was studied by radiocinema. Echocardiography-Doppler was used to set the start of the muscle stimulation in synchronization with the closure of the mitral valve.

Preoperatively, each patient had complete ECG, chest x-ray, echocardiography-Doppler, radionuclide left ventriculography at rest and during exercise (technetium-99m), exercise stress testing (on bicycle, consisting of 2-minute stages, with increments of 20 watts), 24-hour Holter recording, and right and left cardiac catheterization performed by the Seldinger technique in femoral vessels; left ventriculography was done in 30°-right and 60°-left anterior oblique positions. All of these investigations were performed again postoperatively: at 6 months in 11 patients, at 1 year in eight patients and at 2 years in seven patients. In four patients who underwent the 2-year follow-up evaluation, a beat-to-beat analysis of left ventricular volume and stroke volume was performed by conductance catheter and aortic pulse contour.[7,8]

**Table 1**
Surgical Procedures in 12 Patients

| *Patients* | *Surgical Procedure* |
|---|---|
| Pt 1 | LV resection and CMP |
| Pt 2 | CMP |
| Pt 3 | LV resection, CABG, and CMP |
| Pt 4 | LV resection and CMP |
| Pt 5 | LV resection, CABG, and CMP |
| Pt 6 | CABG and CMP |
| Pt 7 | CMP |
| Pt A | CMP |
| Pt B | CABG and CMP |
| Pt C | CABG, MV repair, and CMP |
| Pt D | CABG and CMP |
| Pt E | CMP |

CMP = cardiomyoplasty; CABG = coronary artery bypass grafting; MV = mitral valve; LV = left ventricular; Pt = patient.

Prior to surgery, the cardiothoracic index was 54 ± 7%. Two patients had atrial fibrillation (Pt C, Pt E), another had had episodes of ventricular tachycardia (Pt 5) and eight patients had a left bundle branch block. Pre- and postoperative data were analyzed patient to patient and recorded in Tables 2 and 3.

## Statistical Analysis

Student's paired *t*-test was used for comparison of preoperative and postoperative quantitative data. Results are given as mean ± standard deviation.

## Results

No perioperative deaths were observed. During the early postoperative course, two patients suffered from low cardiac output, one because of bradycardia, and one because of atrial fibrillation (with acute pulmonary edema, necessitating assisted ventilation). One patient suddenly had massive aortic bifurcation embolism, which was successfully removed. One patient had severe pneumonia due to *Legionella,* with acute renal failure necessitating dialysis, and heart failure; despite stimulation, the muscle contraction was not felt,

**Table 2**
Preoperative and 6-Month, 1-Year Postoperative Data in Five Patients with Cardiomyoplasty Failure

| | *Pt $A_i$* | *Pt B* | *Pt C* | *Pt D* | *Pt$E_i$* | *Mean ±SD* |
|---|---|---|---|---|---|---|
| PCWP mm Hg | | | | | | |
| preop | 9 | 18 | 10 | 28 | 25 | 18 ± 8 |
| 6-month/1-year | 29 | 15/30 | 21 | 30 | | 24 ± 7 |
| PAP mm Hg | | | | | | |
| preop | 18 | 28 | 15 | 42 | 32 | 27 ± 11 |
| 6-month/1-year | 35 | 25/44 | 30 | 38 | | 32 ± 6 |
| CI L/mn/m$^2$ | | | | | | |
| preop | 1.9 | 1.8 | 1.6 | 2.1 | 2.0 | 1.9 ± 0.2 |
| 6-month/1-year | 1.8 | 1.9/2.1 | 1.7 | 2.0 | | 1.8 ± 0.1 |
| LVEDP mm Hg | | | | | | |
| preop | 20 | 30 | 3 | 30 | 16 | 20 ± 11 |
| 6-month/1-year | 27 | 15/24 | 12 | 25 | | 20 ± 7 |
| LVEF % preop | 33 | 23 | 35 | 18 | 20 | 27 ± 6 |
| 6-month/1-year | 16 | 27/24 | 33 | 23 | | 25 ± 7 |
| Rd LVEF % | | | | | | |
| preop | 14 | 7 | 32 | 17 | 26 | 19 ± 10 |
| 6-month/1-year | 13 | 13/12 | 13 | 12 | | 13 ± 1 |
| | Transplanted at 8 months alive | Dead at 24 months | Dead at 13 months | Transplanted and Dead at 11 months | Dead at 7 months | |

PT = patient; i = isolated cardiomyoplasty; PCWP = pulmonary capillary wedge pressure; PAP = mean pulmonary artery pressure; CI = cardiac index; LVEDP = left ventricular end-diastolic pressure; LVEF = LV ejection fraction; Rd = radionuclide.

**Table 3**
Preoperative and 6-Month, 1-Year, 2-Year Postoperative Data in Seven Survivors 2 Years after Cardiomyoplasty

| | *Pt 1 (II)* | *Pt 2 (II) i* | *Pt 3 (II)* | *Pt 4 (II)* | *Pt 5 (II)* | *Pt 6 (II)* | *Pt 7 (III)i* | *Mean ±SD* |
|---|---|---|---|---|---|---|---|---|
| PCWP mm Hg | | | | | | | | |
| preop | 8 | 14 | 8 | 18 | 21 | 5 | 10 | 12 ± 6 |
| 6-month | 18 | 16 | 8 | 17 | 8 | 9 | 22 | 14 ± 6 |
| 1-year | 26 | 13 | 7 | 19 | 13 | 15 | 30 | 17 ± 8 |
| 2-year | 16 | 14 | 8 | 12 | 14 | 14 | 24 | 14 ± 5 |
| PAP mm Hg | | | | | | | | |
| preop | 12 | 19 | 14 | 25 | 29 | 9 | 20 | 18 ± 7 |
| 6-month | 27 | 22 | 14 | 20 | 15 | 12 | 40 | 21 ± 10 |
| 1-year | 32 | 20 | 14 | 24 | 20 | 18 | 41 | 24 ± 9 |
| 2-year | 25 | 22 | 12 | 20 | 22 | 20 | 44 | 24 ± 10 |
| CI L/mn/m$^2$ | | | | | | | | |
| preop | 2.4 | 2.8 | 1.4 | 1.8 | 1.7 | 1.6 | 2.6 | 2.0 ± 0.5 |
| 6-month | 2.9 | 2.0 | 1.7 | 1.9 | 1.7 | 1.9 | 1.8 | 2.0 ± 0.4 |
| 1-year | 2.3 | 2.0 | 1.9 | 1.5 | 1.9 | 1.3 | 1.8 | 1.8 ± 0.3 |
| 2-year | 2.6 | 2.3 | 1.9 | 2.1 | 2.3 | 1.6 | 1.8 | 2.1 ± 0.3 |
| LVEDP mm Hg | | | | | | | | |
| preop | 28 | 16 | 18 | 30 | 24 | 14 | 12 | 21 ± 7 |
| 6-month | 28 | 10 | 10 | 23 | 20 | 10 | 16 | 15 ± 6 |
| 1-year | 28 | 13 | 12 | 24 | 20 | 14 | 20 | 18 ± 6 |
| 2-year | 12 | 8 | 7 | 13 | 8 | 9 | 20 | 11 ± 5* |
| LVEF % | | | | | | | | |
| preop | 20 | 40 | 28 | 17 | 18 | 35 | 15 | 24 ± 9 |
| 6-month | 25 | 27 | 43 | 27 | 51 | 55 | 36 | 37 ± 12 |
| 1-year | 29 | 56 | 50 | 32 | 49 | 46 | 24 | 39 ± 13 |
| 2-year | 41 | 54 | 52 | 23 | 47 | 49 | 15 | 40 ± 15* |
| Rd LVEF % | | | | | | | | |
| preop | 13 | 19 | 17 | 7 | 25 | 25 | 22 | 18 ± 7 |
| 6-month | 16 | 11 | 18 | 20 | 17 | 14 | 18 | 16 ± 3 |
| 1-year | 15 | 13 | 20 | 19 | 16 | 22 | 19 | 18 ± 3 |
| 2-year | 10 | 17 | 22 | 25 | 22 | 25 | 19 | 20 ± 5 |
| Peak exercise watts | | | | | | | | |
| preop | 40 | 80 | 80 | 60 | 60 | 60 | 60 | 62 ± 13 |
| 6-month | 60 | 80 | 100 | 80 | 60 | 60 | 80 | 74 ± 15 |
| 1-year | 80 | 80 | 100 | 100 | 100 | 60 | 80 | 86 ± 15* |
| 2-year | 60 | 100 | 100 | 100 | 80 | 60 | 80 | 83 ± 17* |
| Double product | | | | | | | | |
| preop | 15625 | 23360 | 22560 | 17360 | 13000 | 19200 | 32560 | 20523 ± 6447 |
| 6-month | 28050 | 27000 | 32300 | 34560 | 17670 | 19775 | 40560 | 28559 ± 8087* |
| 1-year | 26887 | 24650 | 32400 | 25560 | 22860 | 24990 | 36960 | 27758 ± 5051 |
| 2-year | 22650 | 31000 | 32000 | 25500 | 11310 | 20800 | 29200 | 24632 ± 7217 |

Pt = Patient; () = NYHA class at 2-year; i = isolated cardiomyoplasty, PCWP = pulmonary capillary wedge pressure; PAP = mean pulmonary artery pressure; CI = cardiac index; LVEDP = left ventricular end-diastolic pressure; LVEF = LV ejection fraction; Rd = radionuclide; * = $p<0.05$.

probably because of edema or ischemia. The muscle finally recovered. All patients recovered well.

In time, however, failure of the cardiomyoplasty was observed in five patients: three patients died of terminal congestive heart failure at 7, 13, and 24 postoperative months, respectively; two patients underwent heart transplantation at 8 and 11 postoperative months, respectively, made necessary by the recurrence of disabling congestive heart failure. One of these patients died immediately after transplantation due to primary dysfunction of the graft; the other patient is still alive. The two patients with preoperative atrial fibrillation had cardiomyoplasty failure.

Table 2 summarizes the pre- and postoperative hemodynamic data obtained for these five patients. Patient E, who died earliest, presented preoperatively with signs of right ventricular failure combined with stage II pulmonary arterial hypertension. No postoperative functional improvement was observed in this patient. Retrospectively, we think that the preoperative condition of this patient was too severe to be amenable to cardiomyoplasty. The other four patients showed obvious but transient signs of functional improvement postoperatively. The aggravation of their heart failure, which led either to death or to the indication of heart transplantation, was accountable either to repeated episodes of ventricular rhythm disorders or to the consequences of severe pneumopathy. At 6 months of follow-up, hemodynamic changes in these patients showed aggravation instead of improvement, with elevation of pulmonary arterial and capillary pressures, and no change of LV end-diastolic pressure and ejection fraction. In this series, the survival rate was 82% at 1 year and 73% at 2 years (Fig. 1).

Two years after surgery, seven nontransplanted patients are surviving, with a significant functional improvement (NYHA Class II) and reduced medical treatment in six patients. The first signs of functional improvement appeared during the third postoperative month, progressed steadily during the first year, and stabilized later on. The functional improvement of these patients was combined with an improvement of their exercise ability marked by a significant increase in workload at exercise stress testing at 1 year and at 2 years (Table 3). Repeated postoperative hemodynamic investigations showed no change in the cardiac index, pulmonary arterial pressure, and pulmonary capillary wedge pressure. In contrast, there was a significant improvement of the left ventricular function at 2 years, with decreased LV end-diastolic pressure and increased LV ejection fraction. The analysis of the patient-to-patient results (Table 3) shows that the patient with no clinical improvement (patient 7) was clinically and hemodynamically stable until the 16th postoperative month, then he had two episodes of cardiac decompensation. His functional condition was stabilized by increased medical treatment, but at 2 years there were hemodynamic signs of aggravation, with increased pulmonary pressures, increased LV filling pressures, and diminished LV ejection fraction. The outcome of this patient seems to be compromised.

The results of isotopic investigations did not confirm the changes in hemodynamic data since there was no improvement of the radionuclide LV ejection fraction in all cases (Table 3).

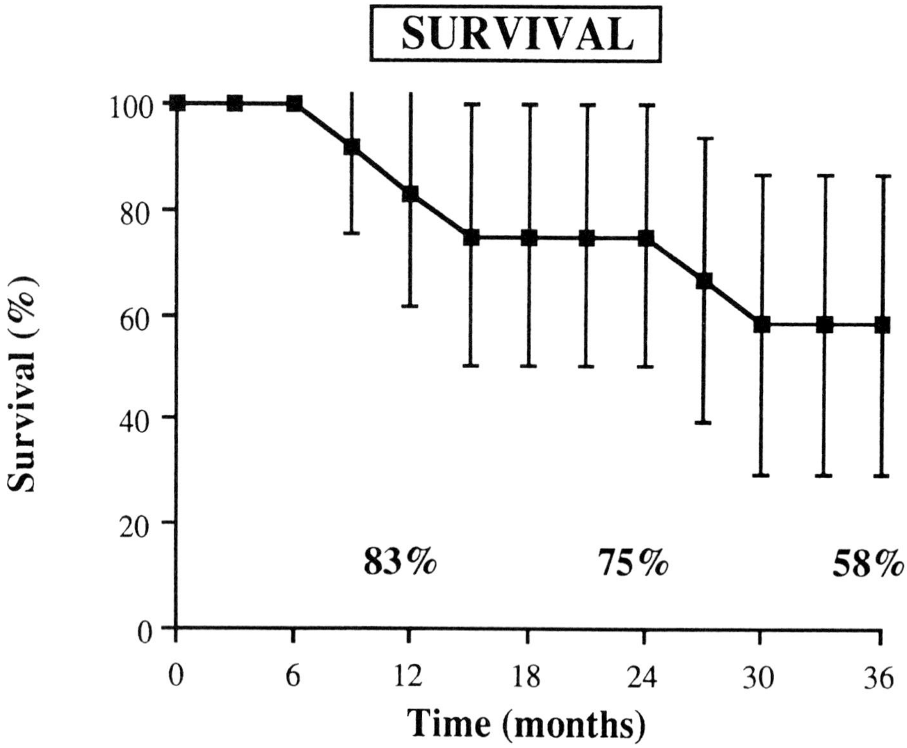


**Figure 1:** *Actuarial survival following cardiomyoplasty. Early mortality is included.*

The analysis of hemodynamic data before surgery and at 6-month follow-up does not show any significant difference between deceased or transplanted patients and nontransplanted survivors at 2 years (Table 4). However, in the cases where cardiomyoplasty failed, the preoperative pulmonary pressures and LV end-diastolic diameter were found to be higher and, at 6 months, there was no hemodynamic change in the left ventricular function, with an increase of pulmonary pressures. Conversely, in the seven nontransplanted survivors at 2 years, preoperative pulmonary pressures were lower and, at 6 months, improvement of the LV function was observed, with no change in pulmonary pressures.

Moreover, the beat-to-beat analysis of LV volume and pressures performed at 2-year follow-up in four patients (Pt 1–Pt 4), showed that during the beats assisted by latissimus dorsi stimulation, LV stroke volume increased while LV end-systolic volume decreased and both LV and aortic pressure increased (Figs. 2, 3). There was no change of LV end-diastolic volume. Figures 2 and 3 illustrate that in the case of cardiomyoplasty with associated procedure (Pt 3), the hemodynamic effect of cardiomyoplasty is real: synchronized with the mitral valve closure, assisted beats (a) improved LV performances; desynchronized, assisted beats (b) decreased LV performances. In the four patients, LV stroke volume increased by 7% to 35% while aortic end-systolic pressure increased by 5% to 9% (Table 5).

**Table 4**
Comparative Analysis of Preoperative and 6-Month Postoperative Data in 12 Patients after Cardiomyoplasty

| | *Patients Dead or Transplanted n=5* | *Patients Alive at 2 Years n=7* |
|---|---|---|
| Age (years) | 58 ± 9 | 60 ± 5 |
| Isolated CMP | 2 | 2 |
| PCWP mm Hg | | |
| preop | 18 ± 8 | 12 ± 6 |
| 6-month | 24 ± 7 | 14 ± 6 |
| PAP mm Hg | | |
| preop | 27 ± 11 | 18 ± 7 |
| 6-month | 32 ± 6 | 21 ± 10 |
| CI L/mn/m$^2$ | | |
| preop | 1.9 ± 0.2 | 2.0 ± 0.5 |
| 6-month | 1.8 ± 0.1 | 2.0 ± 0.4 |
| LVEDP mm Hg | | |
| preop | 20 ± 11 | 21 ± 7 |
| 6-month | 20 ± 7 | 15 ± 6 |
| LVEF % | | |
| preop | 27 ± 6 | 24 ± 9 |
| 6-month | 25 ± 7 | 37 ± 12 |
| LVED Diameter mm | | |
| preop | 75 ± 9 | 70 ± 8 |
| 6-month | 74 ± 7 | 68 ± 8 |

CMP = cardiomyoplasty; PCWP = pulmonary capillary wedge pressure; PAP = mean pulmonary artery pressure; CI = cardiac index; LVEDP = left ventricular end-diastolic pressure, LVEF = left ventricular ejection fraction; LVED diameter = echocardiographic left ventricular end-diastolic diameter.

One of the seven survivors (Pt 4) experienced sudden death at 29 months of follow-up despite functional and hemodynamic improvement.

## Discussion

Since the first clinical application of cardiomyoplasty by Carpentier and Chachques in 1985,[1] several teams have been studying this new technique and the evaluation of its results in the management of severe congestive heart failure.[9–13] The published series consist of small numbers of patients but the results are in mutual agreement: there is postoperative functional and clinical improvement but absence of hemodynamic improvement.[3–5,14] Even when some degree of hemodynamic improvement is observed, such improvement is disputable since it lies within the confidence range of the measurement techniques.[14,15] As a consequence, two questions continue to emerge: Is cardiomyoplasty actually effective in the treatment of severe congestive heart failure? Can this effectiveness be objectively quantified?

Our series consists of 12 patients, operated consecutively, followed-up postoperatively for up to 2 years, with postoperative hemodynamic evaluations at 6 months, 1 year, and 2 years. This series emphasizes two important points:

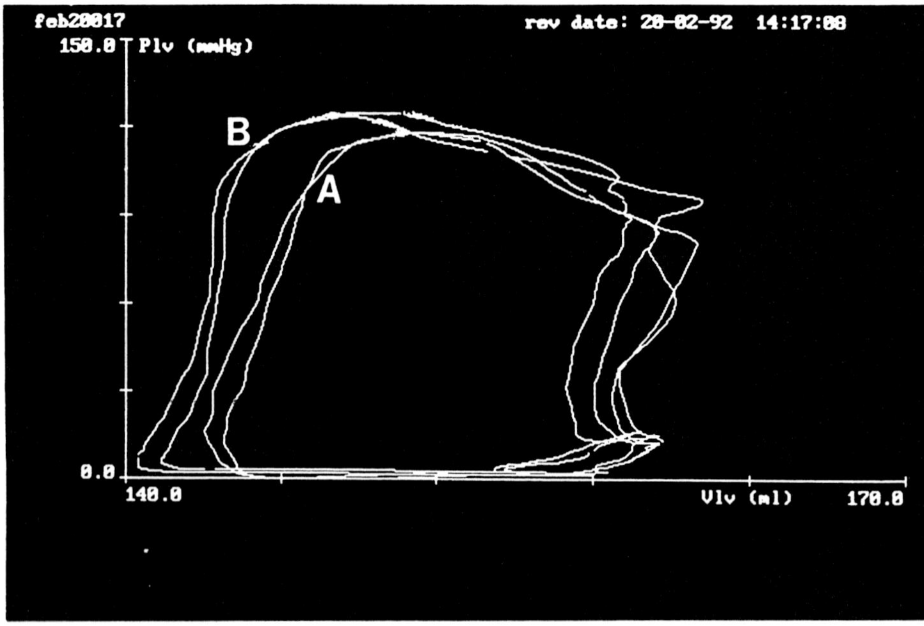


**Figure 2:** *Left ventricular pressure/volume relationship in patient 3, 2 years after cardiomyoplasty. Comparative analysis of two unstimulated (A) and two stimulated (B) loops. Vlv = left ventricular volume; Plv = left ventricular pressure.*

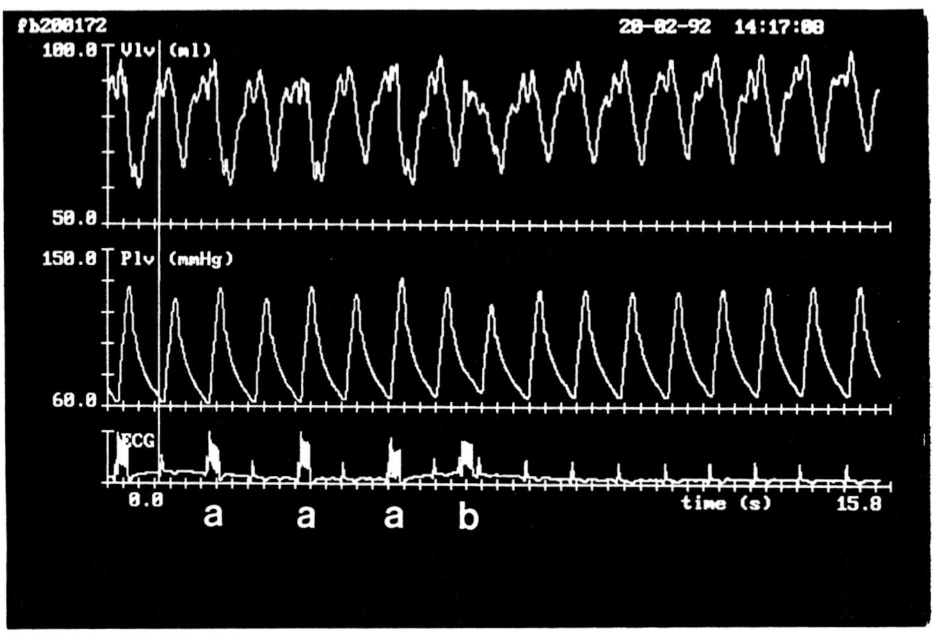


**Figure 3:** *Beat-to-beat analysis of left ventricular pressures and volumes in patient 3, 2 years after cardiomyoplasty. Assisted beats (a) with larger stroke volume and higher end-systolic pressure are present. a = assisted beats synchronized with the mitral valve closure; b = assisted beats desynchronized with the mitral valve closure; ECG = muscle stimulation one heart beat in two; Vlv = left ventricular volume; Plv = left ventricular pressure.*

**Table 5**
Beat-to-Beat Analysis of Left Ventricular Pressures and Volumes in Four Patients 2 Years after Cardiomyoplasty

| | *SVpc* | *SVcond* | *Pao* |
|---|---|---|---|
| Pt 1 | +10% | +10% | +5% |
| Pt 2 | +35% | +32% | +9% |
| Pt 3 | +9% | +14% | +5% |
| Pt 4 | +7% | +9% | +5% |

Improvement in %, between unstimulated beat and stimulated beat, of stroke volume pulse contour (SVpc), stroke volume conductance (SV cond), and aortic end-systolic pressure (Pao).

(1) cardiomyoplasty can be performed without operative mortality despite the severity of the disease observed before surgery; and (2) cardiomyoplasty is not a therapeutic deadlock, as in the case of failure it is possible to resort to heart transplantation.[16]

In this series, our patients presented with ischemic cardiopathy (9 out of 12) and eight patients underwent cardiomyoplasty associated with other cardiac surgery: parietal resection of the left ventricle concerned akinetic plaques and not aneurysms; its purpose was to reduce the volume of the left ventricular cavity rather than to improve left ventricular kinetics. Coronary bypass was preferentially applied to the left anterior descending coronary artery; its purpose was to prevent sudden death at a later date. No patient presented with angor at the time of surgery.

The five observed cardiomyoplasty failures occurred independently of the etiology of the cardiopathy, or of whether or not cardiomyoplasty alone was performed; they involved patients who presented with biventricular heart failure or incipient right ventricular dysfunction or very dilated heart disease. One patient died of terminal heart failure soon after surgery (Pt E): retrospectively, his condition was so severe that he was not amenable to cardiomyoplasty. In contrast, the postoperative evolution of the other four patients occurred in two stages. One period was marked by stability, with functional improvement associated with stabilized hemodynamic LV function, but also with elevation of pulmonary pressures. The second period was marked by functional degradation, caused by rhythm disorders or infection, which prompted the indication of heart transplantation or led to the patient's death. Heart failure in these patients appeared to be stabilized only very transiently by cardiomyoplasty. Above all, cardiomyoplasty proved unable to avoid aggravation of cardiac insufficiency during rhythmic or intercurrent complications and prevent aggravation of the underlying cardiopathy, although the stimulated latissimus dorsi was functional. Cinefilms showed effective stimulation of the muscle, perioperative anatomical findings in the transplanted patients, and postmortem findings in the other patients showed a live latissimus dorsi, without fibrosis or atrophy.[16] Cardiomyoplasty failure occurred in all patients with preoperative atrial fibrillation: it is a sign of advanced cardiomyopathy that is not amenable to cardiomyoplasty.[17]

Two years after surgery, the seven untransplanted surviving patients indisputably showed signs of functional improvement, increased resistance on exertion, and certainly an extended life expectancy, with an 83% survival rate at 1 year and 73% at 2 years, as shown by Moreira's study.[14] This clinical improvement made it possible to reduce medical treatment. Hemodynamic results showed a tendency toward improvement of the left ventricular function together with decreased LV end-diastolic pressure, increased LV ejection fraction, and stabilized pulmonary pressures. However, in this study, the variations affecting hemodynamic data remain within the confidence range of measurement techniques and it is difficult to make a conclusive evaluation of long-term postoperative hemodynamic improvement. However, it should be emphasized that there was a discrepancy between the five patients with failed cardiomyoplasty and the seven untransplanted survivors at 2 years with regard to hemodynamic changes at 6 months: aggravated hemodynamics in the former, improved hemodynamics in the latter. This finding shows that functional condition in this series is consistent with hemodynamic results and suggests that the hemodynamic variations observed should be considered significant.

The study of the LV pressure/volume relationship in these patients enabled us to make a finer hemodynamic study and particularly a study of the LV diastolic function, which is doubtlessly the main target of the mechanism of action of cardiomyoplasty.[17] The results of beat-to-beat analysis confirmed the late hemodynamic efficiency of the latissimus dorsi stimulation with increase of LV stroke volume, decrease of LV end-systolic volume, and increase in both LV and aortic end-systolic pressures, even in cases with an associated procedure. On the other hand, there was no change of LV end-diastolic volume. The hemodynamic effect of cardiomyoplasty is subordinated to the synchronization of the latissimus dorsi stimulation with the mitral valve closure.

However, the improvement of LV function is limited and explains the less than expected improvement of classic hemodynamic data. Despite LV function improvement, cardiomyoplasty does not preclude late sudden death, as in one of our patients.

Analysis of this preliminary series at 2 years postoperatively allows us to define more accurate indications for cardiomyoplasty and reserve this new surgical technique for patients presenting with disabling heart failure and moderately dilated cardiopathy without right ventricular dysfunction or pulmonary arterial hypertension.[17] In such patients, late functional and hemodynamic results are satisfactory.[18]

In disabling congestive heart failure, the indications for cardiomyoplasty lie between medical treatment and heart transplantation.[19] This accounts for the reduced number of indications. At the present time, we perform cardiomyoplasty, without associated procedure if possible, but only in patients with preoperative isolated left ventricular dysfunction. The technical modifications suggested by Magovern,[20] based on the use of the right latissimus dorsi, and even of both left and right latissimus dorsi muscles, could make it possible to extend the indications of cardiomyoplasty to more severely diseased patients.

## References

1. Carpentier A, Chachques JC: Myocardial substitution with a stimulated skeletal muscle: First successful clinical case. *Lancet* 1:1267, 1985.

2. Delahaye F, Jegaden O, Montagna P, et al: Latissimus dorsi cardiomyoplasty in severe congestive heart failure: The Lyon experience. *J Cardiac Surg* 6(Suppl):106–112, 1991.
3. Hagege AA, Desnos M, Chachques JC, et al: Preliminary report: Follow-up after dynamic cardiomyoplasty. *Lancet* 335:1122–1124, 1990.
4. Jatene AD, Moreira LFP, Stolf NAG, et al: Left ventricular function changes after cardiomyoplasty in patients with dilated cardiomyopathy. *J Thorac Cardiovasc Surg* 102:132–139, 1991.
5. Lee KF, Dignan RJ, Parmar JM, et al: Effects of dynamic cardiomyoplasty on left ventricular performance and myocardial mechanics in dilated cardiomyopathy. *J Thorac Cardiovasc Surg* 102:124–131, 1991.
6. Carpentier A, Chachques JC: Cardiomyoplasty: surgical technique. In Carpentier A, Chachques JC, Grandjean P (eds): *Cardiomyoplasty*. Mount Kisco, NY, Futura Publishing Co., 1991, pp 105–122.
7. Baan J, Van Der Velde ET, De Bruin HG, et al: Continuous measurement of left ventricular volume in animals and humans by conductance catheter. *Circulation* 70:812–823, 1984.
8. Schreuder JJ, Biervliet JD, Van Der Velde ET, et al: Systolic and diastolic pressure-volume relationships during cardiac surgery. *J Cardiothorac Vasc Anesthesia* 5:539–545, 1991.
9. Magovern GJ, Heckler FR, Park SB, et al: Paced latissimus dorsi used for dynamic cardiomyoplasty of left ventricular aneurysms. *Ann Thorac Surg* 44:379–388, 1987.
10. Magovern GJ, Heckler FR, Park SB, et al: Paced skeletal muscle for dynamic cardiomyoplasty. *Ann Thorac Surg* 45:614–619, 1988.
11. Molteni L, Almada H, Ferreira R: Synchronously stimulated skeletal muscle graft for left ventricular assistance: case report. *J Thorac Cardiovasc Surg* 97:439–446, 1989.
12. Moreira LP, Stolf NAG, Bocchi EA, et al: Latissimus dorsi cardiomyoplasty in the treatment of patients with dilated cardiomyopathy. *Circulation* 82(Suppl IV): IV-257–263, 1990.
13. Rossi MA, Braile DM, Souza DRS, et al: Dynamic cardiomyoplasty in chronic Chagas' heart disease: clinicopathological data. *Ann Thorac Surg* 51:649–651, 1991.
14. Moreira LF, Seferian P Jr, Bocchi EA, et al: Survival improvement with dynamic cardiomyoplasty in patients with dilated cardiomyopathy. *Circulation* 84(Suppl III):III-296–302, 1991.
15. Silverman NA: Left ventricular function changes after cardiomyoplasty in patients with dilated cardiomyopathy. *J Thorac Cardiovasc Surg* 102:156–157, 1991.
16. Jegaden O, Delahaye F, Montagna P, et al: Cardiomyoplasty does not preclude heart transplantation. *Ann Thorac Surg* 53:875–881, 1992.
17. Chachques JC, Acar C, Portoghese M, et al: Dynamic cardiomyoplasty for long-term cardiac assist. *Eur J Cardiothorac Surg* 6:642–648, 1992.
18. Furnary AP, Magovern JA, Christlieb IY, et al: Clinical cardiomyoplasty: preoperative factors associated with outcome. *Ann Thorac Surg* 54:1139–1143, 1992.
19. Magovern JA, Magovern GJ Jr, Palumbi MA, Orie JE: Surgical therapy for congestive heart failure: indications for transplantation versus cardiomyoplasty. *J Heart Lung Transplant* 11:538–544, 1992.
20. Magovern JA, Furnary AP, Christlieb IY, Kao RL, Magovern GJ: Right latissimus dorsi cardiomyoplasty for left ventricular failure. *Ann Thorac Surg* 53:1120–1122, 1992.

Chapter 7

# *Discussion*

**Dr. Jacobovitz (Brooklyn, New York):** This is to all the panelists. You showed a consistent improvement in ejection fraction, while the cardiac indices, capillary wedge pressure, and left ventricular end-diastolic pressure were unchanged. I wonder whether the ejection fraction is more reflective of changes in end-diastolic volume or restriction rather than of true functional improvement. Is ejection fraction the best way to measure functional improvement?

**Dr. Jegaden (Lyon):** In our experience, we have been studying the level of ejection fraction by angiography and by isotopes. We have shown some improvement in left ventricular ejection fraction by angiography, but there was no correlation with the isotopic measure. Beat-to-beat analysis of cardiac output confirms that left ventricular function improvement is probably a consequence of the end-systolic volume decrease. During the surgical procedure, we used metal clips for hemostasis of the muscle and after cardiomyoplasty it was possible to film muscle contraction. Muscle contraction was greater in the proximal part of the muscle than in the distal part. During angiography, we looked at the effect of the better contraction of the proximal part of the muscle. We saw an upward motion of the heart. Left ventricular improvement is limited after cardiomyoplasty with important loss of the contraction of the muscle.

**Dr. Carpentier:** I would like to mention that the upward motion of the heart during muscle contraction can be minimized by careful suturing of the two layers of the muscle above the upper border of the left ventricle.

Chapter 8

# Range of Responses to Dynamic Cardiomyoplasty in Dilated Cardiomyopathy Patients*

Jonah N.K. Odim, John H. Burgess, Ray C.-J. Chiu, and the McGill Cardiomyoplasty Group**

## Introduction

Dynamic cardiomyoplasty is an experimental surgical procedure whereby a patient's native skeletal muscle is wrapped around the failing ventricles for circulatory support. After transforming this skeletal muscle pedicle flap with low-frequency electrical stimulation, to highly fatigue-resistant, predominantly type I fibers, a synchronized burst stimulator coordinates contraction during systole, thus assisting the enfeebled heart.[1,2] Interest in this new therapeutic approach to managing patients with advanced heart failure is in part related to the increasing waiting period for cardiac transplantation, due to a shortage of donor organs, and the rising prevalence of congestive heart failure.

This procedure is in the developmental stage. Case selection, surgical technique, and follow-up end-points are still evolving. In this report, we review four patients, afflicted with dilated cardiomyopathy, who underwent cardiomyoplasty in a single institution. Although the number is small, these patients are unique since they were all turned down for heart transplantation and received no additional surgical intervention other than dynamic cardiomyoplasty. Our evolving pathophysiological concept underlying this operation is discussed in light of the postoperative findings in our series.

Supported by grants from the Medical Research Council of Canada and the Canadian Heart and Stroke Foundation.

*Data published in part in the *American Journal of Cardiology,* August 1993.

**McGill Cardiomyoplasty Group:** *Cardiothoracic Surgery:* Ray C.-J. Chiu, MD (Principal Investigator); Jonah N.K. Odim, MD (Coordinator); Peter E. Blundell, MD. *Cardiology:* John H. Burgess, MD; James A. Steward, MD (Echocardiography); Mark A. Rabinovitch, MD (Radionuclide Studies). *Plastic Surgery:* H. Bruce Williams, MD. *Anesthesiology:* Richard J.S. Robinson, MD; D.T. Truong, MD.

From Carpentier A, Chachques JC, Grandjean P: Cardiac Bioassist. © Futura Publishing Co, Inc, Armonk, NY, 1997.

# Methods

## Case Selection

Four patients with dilated cardiomyopathy were accepted for dynamic cardiomyoplasty after proper informed consent. All patients were deteriorating under intensive medical therapy, but were still New York Heart Association (NYHA) functional Class III. Terminal and refractory patients in NYHA functional Class IV were excluded because of the high operative mortality in this group of patients.[3] All four patients were initially referred for heart transplantation by their cardiologists, but were deemed unsuitable candidates: one patient for logistic reasons, and the rest because of age and other associated medical conditions. By echocardiography and radionuclide angiography, one patient had a preoperative ejection fraction of 17%, and the remainder had ejection fractions of less than 10%. All patients were free of significant coronary artery occlusive disease, and associated mitral insufficiency was mild to moderate. All had cardiac arrhythmias thought to be medically controllable. The type of preoperative studies carried out changed, reflecting our increasing understanding of the procedure. Routine hemodynamic studies alone were carried out for the first two cases. Cardiac catheterization and other noninvasive techniques emphasized ejection fraction and other parameters of systolic functions, in accordance with our earlier view that this operation simply provides systolic assist. In the latter two patients, the concept of gradual "myocardial sparing effect" was introduced, and additional investigations including exercise testing with spirometry, quality-of-life assessment, and neurohormone studies were carried out (Table 1).

## Operative Procedures

Details of the anesthetic technique and surgical procedure are already described elsewhere.[4,5] In brief, general anesthesia is employed and a double-lumen endotracheal tube is inserted to control breathing when the left lung is partially collapsed.[6] The patient is initially placed in the right lateral decubitus position. An incision is made from the axilla to the iliac crest along the lateral border of the latissimus dorsi muscle. This muscle is dissected out freely as a pedicle graft, detaching it from the iliac crest, the paravertebral fascia, and finally the humeral head. The thoracodorsal neurovascular bundle is carefully preserved. Bipolar neuromuscular electrodes are placed which depolarize the thoracodorsal nerve, thereby inducing contraction of the entire latissimus dorsi muscle. A segment of the third rib is then resected at the level of the anterior axillary line, and the distal portion of the muscle flap including the electrodes is transferred into the left pleural cavity. The divided tendon, originally attached to the humerus, is reattached by nonabsorbable sutures to the periosteum of the resected rib. The wounds are closed following the placement of closed subcutaneous suction drainage. A dressing is applied to the incision wound, and the patient turned to the supine position.

Although none of our patients to date have required cardiopulmonary bypass, the machine remains on standby during the operation. A guidewire is

**Table 1**
Preoperative Studies

| Case | % Wrap | LVEF (%) | | CI ($L/min/m^2$) | | LVEDV (cc) | | Stage I VeMax (L/min) | | Stage I $VO_2$Max (L/min) | | Follow-Up | Medications | | NYHA Class | | Clinical Status |
|---|---|---|---|---|---|---|---|---|---|---|---|---|---|---|---|---|---|
| | | Pre- | Post- | Pre- | Post- | Pre- | Post- | Pre- | Post- | Pre- | Post- | (months) | Pre- | Post- | Pre- | Post- | |
| #1<br>Male<br>40 yrs | 70 | 17 | 15.4 ± 0.82*<br>(14.3)** | 2.1 | 2.3 ± 0.14<br>(2.1) | 284 | 329 ± 7.2<br>(354) | NA | 56.7 ± 2.5*<br>(67 ± 3.2%)***<br>(52.3)**<br>(63%)*** | NA | 1.45 ± 0.17<br>(50 ± 5.4%)<br>(1.0)<br>(35%) | 36 | Captopril<br>Diltiazem<br>Digoxin<br>Lasix<br>Thiazide<br>Warfarin | Captopril<br>—<br>Digoxin<br>Lasix<br>Thiazide<br>Aldactone<br>Warfarin | III | I | Returned to clerical job |
| #2<br>Male<br>62 yrs | <60 | 8 | 8.12 ± .37<br>(8.8) | 1.3 | 1.2 ± 0.11<br>(1.6) | 358 | 361 ± 5.4<br>(352) | 54.7<br>(57%) | NA | 1.2<br>(52%) | NA | 7 | Captopril<br>Digoxin<br>Lasix<br>Warfarin | Captopril<br>Digoxin<br>Lasix<br>Warfarin<br>Amiodarone | III+ | IV | Died of heart failure |
| #3<br>Male<br>62 yrs | 100 | 9 | 19.68 ± 0.60<br>(21.6) | 1.4 | 2.5 ± 0.07<br>(2.6) | 304 | 301.5 ± 5.2<br>(291) | 28.8<br>(35%) | 48.2 ± 5.2<br>(58.5 ± 6.5%)<br>(43)<br>(52%) | 0.7<br>(30%) | 1.4 ± 0.1<br>(60 ± 2%)<br>1.3<br>(58%) | 24 | Lisinopril<br>Digoxin<br>Lasix<br>Warfarin<br>Tocanide | —<br>Digoxin<br>Lasix<br>Warfarin<br>Amiodarone | III | I | Retired<br>Active - swims, golfs, tennis |
| #4<br>Male<br>65 yrs | 100 | 8 | 15–20% | 1.6 | NA | NA | NA | 45.9<br>(49%) | 48.7<br>(58%) | 1.5<br>(56%) | 1.2<br>(44%) | 9 | Lisinopril<br>Digoxin<br>Lasix<br>Zaroxolvn | Lisinopril<br>Digoxin<br>Lasix<br>Amiodarone | III+ | II | Retired<br>Improving |

Pre = preoperative; Post = postoperative; NA = not available; % Wrap = estimated areas of ventricles covered by the muscle flap wrapping; LVEF = left ventricular ejection fraction; CI = cardiac index; LVEDV = left ventricular end-diastolic volume; VeMax = maximal ventilation (Jones protocol with bicycle ergometry); $VO_2$Max = maximal oxygen uptake (Jones protocol); NYHA = New York Heart Association functional class.

*Mean±SEM.

**Last follow-up data.

***% of predicted.

inserted percutaneously into the femoral artery for rapid insertion of an intra-aortic balloon if required, but this has not been necessary.

A sternotomy is carried out and a reversed C-shaped pericardial flap is made and reflected toward the right of the patient. Epicardial sensing electrodes are screwed into the myocardium. The muscle flap and accompanying electrodes are then retrieved from the left pleural cavity and wrapped around both ventricles in a clockwise manner. The pericardium is used to anchor this muscle wrap, without sutures placed directly in friable and diseased myocardium. Two key posterior stay sutures are placed. One is positioned in the posterior pericardial reflection just lateral to the pulmonary valve, and the other is placed on the posterior pericardium at the junction between the inferior vena cava and the right atrium. When the corresponding sites of the muscle flap are fixed to these points after slipping the bulk of the muscle behind the left ventricle, these two anchoring sutures fix the posterior border of the muscle flap to the posterior AV groove. The remaining muscle mass is turned over the right border of the heart as well as the apex and approximated in front of the heart. In the first two patients, only 60% and 70% of the biventricular mass was wrapped by the available muscle flap. In this instance, the pericardial flap previously constructed is used to cover the defect over the right ventricle. In the latter two cases, sufficient muscle flap was available to completely encircle both ventricles. Consequently, the pericardial flap was simply used to anchor the muscle wrap cephalad, leaving the pericardium lying over the right atrium and pulmonary artery.

Both the sensing and stimulating electrodes are then connected to a synchronizable burst stimulator (Medtronic® Cardiomyostimulator SP 1005), and placed within a subfascial pocket in the upper abdomen. The sternotomy is closed following the placement of mediastinal and pleural drainage tubes.

## Postoperative Management

All patients were extubated within 24 hours and their stay in the Intensive Care Unit ranged from 2 to 4 days during which period the patients were supported with inotropic and antiarrhythmic agents as indicated. Upon transfer to the ward, the cardiomyostimulator remained in the "off" status for 10 days to allow recovery of the vascular supply to the muscle flap and the formation of adhesions between the muscle and the epicardium. Following this period of "vascular delay," the cardiomyostimulator was turned on in a stepwise fashion, gradually increasing the number of pulses within the burst train delivered to the muscle flap, in order to transform it into fatigue-resistant type I fibers.[7] The adjustments in stimulation parameters were carried out at weekly intervals, and by 6 weeks postop, the patient received full burst stimulation (Table 2). Either 1:1 or 2:1 heart rate-to-burst stimuli ratio were used. Alternatively, the transformation of the muscle is carried out after the patient is discharged from the hospital, and programming of the cardiomyostimulator is conducted on an out-patient basis.

The patients returned regularly for clinical evaluation and follow-up studies according to protocol. Initially these studies centered on noninvasive he-

**Table 2**
Burst Stimulation Parameters

| | |
|---|---|
| Pulse amplitude | 5–8 V |
| Pulse width | 210 sec |
| Burst duration | 185 msec |
| Frequency | 30 Hz |
| Number of pulses/burst | 5–6 |
| Synchronization AV delay | 25–100 msec |
| *Synchronization ratio | 1:1 or 2:1 |

*Heart rate to pulse train (burst) ratio.

modynamic measurements. In later cases, additional exercise tolerance and neurohormonal studies were carried out (Table 1).

## Results

There has been no operative mortality, and the patients have been followed for 7 months to 4 years.

### Case #1 (JA)

This 40-year-old patient with dilated cardiomyopathy was admitted in NYHA functional Class III and was deteriorating despite maximal medical therapy. He was considered for heart transplantation, but post-transplant follow-up was deemed impractical since he lived in the Arctic on Baffin Island, nearly 2000 km away from a major medical center. His subsequent operation for cardiomyoplasty was uneventful. It is estimated that about 70% of his biventricular mass was wrapped with the muscle flap available. His preoperative ejection fraction of 17% has remained virtually unchanged in the postoperative period. Cardiac catheterization a year after operation revealed minimal hemodynamic improvement (Table 3). Nevertheless, at almost 4 years since operation, he is virtually asymptomatic, NYHA functional Class I, and has returned to his full-time clerical job. His medical regime, which consists of ACE inhibition, diuretics and digitalis, has remained essentially unchanged. He has been readmitted to the hospital, not for heart failure, but for management of choledocholithiasis and an inguinal hernia. He requires cardiac medications for predominant right heart failure which is now controlled.

### Case #2 (PG)

This 62-year-old patient with an ejection fraction of 8% and suffering from dilated cardiomyopathy was not accepted into the transplant program due to his age. He underwent dynamic cardiomyoplasty and his perioperative course

**Table 3**
Case #1 (JA): Right Heart Catheterization

| | *Preop* | *Postop (1 Year)* |
|---|---|---|
| RA (mm Hg) | (4) | (4) |
| RV (mm Hg) | 32/5 | 26/4 |
| PA (mm Hg) | 33/29 (22) | 26/16 (20) |
| PCW (mm Hg) | 13 | 13 |
| BP (mm Hg) | 94/64 (74) | 96/66 (80) |
| SVR (dynes.sec.cm$_{-5}$) | 1494 | 1543 |
| PVR (dynes.sec.cm$_{-5}$) | 192 | 142 |
| LVSWI (gm/m$^2$/beat) | 18.5 | 25.3 |
| RVSWI (gm/m$^2$/beat) | 5.5 | 6.1 |
| SV (mL/beat) | 41 | 53 |
| CI (L/min/m$^2$) | 2.1 | 2.1 |

RA = right atrial pressure; RV = right ventricular pressure; PA = pulmonary artery pressure; BP = aortic blood pressure; SVR = systemic vascular pressure; PVR = pulmonary vascular resistance; SV = stroke volume; PCW = pulmonary capillary wedge pressure; LVSWI = left ventricular stroke work index; RVSWI = right ventricular stroke work index; CI = cardiac index.

was uneventful. However, because of short stature and a very large heart, only less than the estimated 60% of the ventricular mass was covered with the muscle flap, with virtually all of the anterior surface of the heart draped with the pericardial flap. Postoperatively, his hemodynamic status remained unchanged and he gradually deteriorated clinically. Although he was eventually placed on the transplant waiting list, he never received a donor organ and died 7 months after cardiomyoplasty from heart failure.

## Case #3 (NW)

This 62-year-old man with dilated cardiomyopathy and an ejection fraction of 9% had been admitted to the hospital repeatedly for biventricular failure. He was also referred for but ultimately rejected from the heart transplant program because of his age. His postoperative course was uneventful. Although he too had a large heart, because of his larger body stature, he had sufficient latissimus dorsi muscle flap to achieve 100% complete biventricular wrap. Within 4 months after operation, his ejection fraction more than doubled to 22%, and his clinical condition improved to NYHA functional Class I. This patient was the first to undergo preop exercise tolerance studies. At 4 months postop and thereafter, both the maximum ventilation (Jones protocol) and the peak oxygen uptake doubled from the preop level of 30% predicted (Table 1). Cardiac catheterization 18 months postoperatively reflects an improved hemodynamic state (Table 4). Due to his dramatic clinical improvement, the ACE inhibitor was discontinued and his diuretic therapy reduced. He currently is maintained on amiodarone and digoxin for rhythm and rate control. This retired executive has had significant improvement in quality of life, and has returned to playing tennis and swimming without symptoms. It is now nearly 3 years postop, and he has not required rehospitalization for heart failure.

**Table 4**
Case #3 (NW): Right Heart Catheterization

| | *Preop* | *Postop (1.5 Years)* |
|---|---|---|
| RA | (14) | (2) |
| RV | 50/16 | 22/2 |
| PA | 50/32 (38) | 22/10 (14) |
| PCW | (30) | (4) |
| BP | 100/70 (80) | 95/60 (76) |
| SVR | 1913 | 1218 |
| PVR | 232 | 165 |
| LVSWI | 12 | 37 |
| RVSWI | 6 | 6 |
| SV | 31 | 70 |
| CI | 1.6 | 2.7 |

RA = right atrial pressure; RV = right ventricular pressure; PA = pulmonary artery pressure; BP = aortic blood pressure; SVR = systemic vascular pressure; PVR = pulmonary vascular pressure; PCW = pulmonary capillary wedge pressure; LVSWI = left ventricular stroke work index; RVSWI = right ventricular stroke work index; CI = cardiac index; SV = stroke volume.

## Case #4 (RE)

This 64-year-old retired dentist with dilated cardiomyopathy and an ejection fraction of 9%, was NYHA functional Class III-IV, and has been declined by several transplant programs because of his age and a remote history of ulcerative colitis. During surgery, this 6' tall gentleman had sufficient mass and length of latissimus dorsi muscle to completely encircle the markedly dilated ventricles. Although his perioperative course was uneventful, in the early postop period, he had a few episodes of sudden deterioration with the onset of transient atrial fibrillation. At 1 month postop, during a revisit for programming the cardiomyostimulator, he also had a episode of ventricular tachyarrhythmia which required defibrillation. He has showed gradual but steady improvement thereafter, and at 9 months postop, he shows clinical improvement (Class II). At 8 weeks postop, significant enhancement of blood flow velocity in the ascending aorta can already be demonstrated in the stimulated beats with Doppler echocardiographic recording. In this patient with intraventricular conduction block, ultrasound was used to time burst stimulation, delivered just after the closure of the mitral valve and opening of the aortic valve. At 6 months postop, the ejection fraction is between 15% and 20% by echocardiography and radionuclide angiography. Cardiac catheterization documented significant improvements in systolic functions (Table 5). Approximately 1½ years postop, he suddenly died during sleep, presumably from arrhythmias.

## Discussion

Although the concept of using native skeletal muscle for cardiac assistance had been proposed as early as the late 1950s,[8] this approach did not reach clinical fruition until two biological issues were addressed. The first constraint relates

**Table 5**
Case #4 (RE): Right Heart Catheterization

| | *Preop* | *Postop (1 Year)* |
|---|---|---|
| RA | 4 | 12 |
| RV | 28/4 | 44/12 |
| PA | 28/16 (20) | 44/22 (30) |
| PCW | 12 | 18 |
| BP | 85/50 (62) | 100/60 (73) |
| SVR | 1381 | 1036 |
| PVR | 191 | 204 |
| LVSWI | 20.9 | 23.2 |
| RVSWI | 6.7 | 7.6 |
| SV | 48 | 67 |
| CI | 1.56 | 2.16 |
| CPP | 38 | 42 |
| RPP | 5950 | 7000 |

RA = right atrial pressure; RV = left atrial pressure; PA = pulmonary artery pressure; BP = aortic blood pressure; SVR = systemic vascular resistance; PVR = pulmonary vascular resistance; SV = stroke volume; LVSWI = left ventricular stroke work index; RVSWI = right ventricular stroke work index; CI = cardiac index; CPP = cerebral perfusion pressure; RPP = rate-pressure product.

to the fatigue which sets into the skeletal muscle when it is stimulated to contract at the heart rate. The discovery of the phenomenon of skeletal muscle transformation in the late 1960s[9,10] and introduction of this technique into cardiac assist in the late 1970s[11] effectively solved the issue of muscle fatigue. It is now well established that low-frequency electrical stimulation of the skeletal muscle can modulate its gene phenotype expression and convert it into predominantly type I, highly fatigue resistant fibers. Accompanying these functional changes are many similarities to cardiac muscle at the molecular level, which range from myosin isoform expression to vastly increased aerobic capacity for energy production.[12,13] Our longest surviving patient (case #1) has had his latissimus dorsi muscle contract for over 3 years without signs of fatigue. This is confirmed by palpating the extrathoracic portion of the latissimus dorsi muscle flap, which was anchored to the periosteum of the resected rib in the left axilla.

The second constraint in assisting the failing heart with skeletal muscle relates to the inefficacy of an ordinary cardiac pacemaker to stimulate skeletal muscle and generate sufficient power for hemodynamic work. The difference in structure between cardiac and skeletal muscle forms the biological basis of this problem. Cardiac muscle is a synctium with each myocyte connected by an intercalated disk, thus a depolarizing impulse can spread and capture the whole organ. Therefore, once a threshold is attained, the myocardium will contract in an all-or-none fashion. In contrast, skeletal muscle consists of separate motor units, thereby increasing strength of depolarizing current recruits increasing numbers of motor units. A pulse train or burst electrical stimulation pattern, on the other hand, can summate the contractile force of skeletal muscle. To modulate the contractile pattern and force of skeletal muscle to resemble cardiac muscle, a synchronized burst stimulator was developed in the early 1980s.[14,15] Convergence of the capability for muscle transformation with synchronized burst stimulator technology made it possible to study, and eventually apply, the concept of muscle-powered cardiac assist to patients suffering from heart failure.

Our understanding of the mechanism underlying this procedure has continued to evolve over the past several years since its first clinical application in 1985.[16] Initially it was thought that skeletal muscle wrapped around the ventricles and stimulated during systole would improve the function of the heart immediately; consequently, many patients in terminal heart failure were operated upon. It soon became evident that any beneficial effect from cardiomyoplasty takes place gradually over weeks and months, and many patients who were moribund succumbed postoperatively. For end-stage heart failure patients in NYHA functional Class IV, who were operated on in the 1980s, the operative mortality exceeded 30%.[3] Thus, there is an emerging consensus that such patients are not appropriate candidates for dynamic cardiomyoplasty. Initially there was also considerable concern about the tightness of the muscle wrap around the ventricles. However, there have been no reports of constrictive pericarditis created by this maneuver. It would appear that the initial tension applied to the muscle wrap is not as crucial as originally thought in view of the "conformational change" that may occur gradually in the postoperative period.[17] Skeletal muscle appears able to delete or add sarcomeres to restore optimal length and recovery of its contractile functional capacity.[18,19] This adaptation may explain the gradual improvements seen in FDA phase I patients, and in our series, tending to reach a plateau at 6 months to a year postoperative.[3]

Several reports[20,21] have been published recently on the results of cardiomyoplasty, but many patients in these series underwent additional surgical procedures, such as coronary bypass, aneurysm resection, and valve replacement. It was therefore uncertain that the cardiomyoplasty procedure played a dominant role in any clinical improvement. In some, the technique of cardiomyoplasty had been altered during the study period. The early expectation was that when the cardiomyostimulator was turned on, there would be greater squeeze during cardiac systole to improve the ejection fraction and stroke volume. It is clear, based on experimental work and on the clinical results reported here, that such a systolic assist indeed can occur. By measuring the pressure volume loops, Lee et al. and others[22,23] have shown significant improvements in the stroke work index and ejection fraction in a number of experimental models. Our case #3 doubled the ejection fraction 4 months after operation. The flow velocity measured at the aortic root with Doppler ultrasound in case #4 showed a significant increase in flow velocity in stimulated beats, also supporting this view. Interestingly, in both experimental studies cited, as well as in these two patients (cases #3 and #4), both ventricles were wrapped completely by a thick latissimus dorsi muscle. It is postulated that under these conditions, clear systolic augmentation can indeed be documented. The improvements seen with cardiopulmonary exercise testing in case #3 provide objective data to support the notion that significant amelioration of the heart failure syndrome had occurred in this patient.

In contrast to such cases, our patient (case #1) showed no consistent improvement in ejection fraction and yet demonstrated considerable gradual improvement in his clinical functional status which appeared to remain stable for a prolonged period of time. In the worldwide phase I study for this procedure, of the 46 patients who were preoperative functional Class III and survived the operation, 41% attained functional Class I postoperatively, while another 44% improved to functional Class II. In spite of this, overall changes in ejection fraction did not achieve statistical significance.[3] These discrepancies could be interpreted in two ways. One is the possible placebo effect. This would be difficult to exclude since sham operations are not ethically acceptable for such patients. Another interpretation lies in the hypothesis of chronic "myocardial sparing effect" which we wish to postulate. In patients whose skeletal muscle wrap is less than ideal, such as a poor quality latissimus dorsi or insufficient muscle flap length to achieve a complete biventricular wrap, the immediate systolic functional improvements (e.g., left ventricular ejection fraction and cardiac output) may not be readily discernible. Nevertheless, by sharing the systolic workload with the underlying myocardium, it may spare and reduce myocardial stress which over time may result in stabilization and improvement in the functional status of these patients. An analogy may be drawn to the recent findings of improved survival in heart failure patients following the administration of ACE inhibitors. Even though important improvement in systolic function was not observed over the follow-up period by lowering the peripheral resistance with ACE inhibitors, reduction of the myocardial stress yielded improved survival.[24] Although clinical data indicating reduced myocardial stress following dynamic cardiomyoplasty are not yet available, experimental data supporting this hypothesis have been reported.[22] This hypothesis also explains the generally negative results obtained with acute stimulator "on"–"off" studies, whereas there have been anecdotal cases of patients who deteriorated following the prolonged absence of cardiomyostimulator function for 1 to 2 weeks.[25]

We postulate that a range of responses to dynamic cardiomyoplasty observed are, in some measure, related to the quality of muscle wrap achieved in each patient. This introduces a potential anatomical constraint in trying to match the autologous latissimus dorsi muscle to the native heart, which is grossly dilated. When the wrap is complete (e.g., cases #3 and #4 with 100% wrap), systolic hemodynamic improvements accompany clinical functional progress. When the wrap is inadequate (e.g., case #2 with less than 60% wrap), it may not be beneficial. In intermediate cases (e.g., case #1 with approximately 70% wrap), improvements in systolic hemodynamic parameters may not be readily measurable, but gradual clinical improvement may occur from the "myocardial sparing effect." In such cases, perhaps the end-point studied should be objective functional data rather than ejection fraction, which is known to correlate poorly with patients' exercise tolerance. Other plausible explanations for gradual improvements in these patients include prevention or delaying of further ventricular dilatation. Preliminary data on neurohormonal changes, such as the marked reduction in renin level seen in our case #3, also suggest possible extracardiac mechanisms.[26]

Thus, in our patients, as well as in those reported by others,[3] it appears that dynamic cardiomyoplasty improves the quality of life in many patients suffering from heart failure. Whether dynamic cardiomyoplasty will prolong the life of such patients[25] requires a prospective randomized control study to answer. However, preliminary data such as those reported here are required before undertaking such a study.

We conclude that this experimental procedure deserves further investigation for it improves the quality of life of many heart failure patients who continue to deteriorate under intensive medical therapy. We consider this procedure a pretransplant option, since truly terminal patients carry high operative mortality with this intervention. On the other hand, this operation does not preclude patients from receiving subsequent heart transplantation if their condition deteriorates. Follow-up after successful dynamic cardiomyoplasty has been highly cost-effective, since they need neither biopsies to detect rejection nor immunosuppression as in post-transplant patients.

## References


1. Chiu RCJ: Cardiomyoplasty: an overview. *PACE* 14:577–584, 1991.
2. Hill AB, Chiu RCJ: Dynamic cardiomyoplasty for treatment of heart failure. *Clin Cardiol* 12:681–688, 1989.
3. Grandjean PA, Austin L, Chan S, et al: Dynamic cardiomyoplasty: clinical follow-up results. *J Card Surg* 6:80–88, 1991.
4. Carpentier A, Chachques JC: Myocardial substitution with a stimulated skeletal muscle: first successful clinical case. *Lancet* 8440:1267, 1985.
5. Chiu RCJ, Odim JNK, Blundell PE, Williams HB: Dynamic cardiomyoplasty. In AS Kapoor (ed): *Atlas on Heart and Lung Transplantation,* NY, McGraw-Hill, 1992.
6. Robinson RJS, Truong DT, Odim JNK, et al: A 62-year-old man is scheduled for a new cardiac surgical procedure: dynamic cardiomyoplasty. *J Cardiovasc Anesth* 6:476–487, 1992.
7. Grandjean PA, Herpers L, Smits K, et al: Performance of the cardiomyostimulator and intramuscular leads in the cardiomyoplasty procedure. In Chiu RCJ (ed): *Transformed Muscle for Cardiac Assist and Repair.* Mount Kisco, NY, Futura Publishing Co Inc, 1990, pp 231–240.
8. Kantrowitz A, McKinnon WMP: The experimental use of the diaphragm as an auxiliary myocardium. *Surg Forum* 9:266, 1959.
9. Salmons S, Sreter FA: Significance of impulse activity in the transformation of skeletal muscle type. *Nature* 263:30–34, 1976.
10. Pette D, Simoneau JA: Chronic stimulation-induced alterations in phenotype expression and functional properties of skeletal muscle. In Chiu RCJ (ed): *Transformed Muscle for Cardiac Assist and Repair.* Mount Kisco, NY, Futura Publishing Co, Inc, 1990, pp 129–137.
11. Macoviak JA, Stephenson LW, Armenti F, Kelly AM, et al: Electrical conditioning of in situ skeletal muscle for replacement of myocardium. *J Surg Res* 32:429–439, 1982.
12. Ianuzzo CD, Hamilton N, O'Brien PJ, Desrosiers C, et al: Biochemical transformation of canine skeletal muscle for use in cardiac-assist devices. *J Appl Physiol* 68:1481–1485, 1990.
13. Acker MA, Anderson WA, Hammond RL, et al: Oxygen consumption of chronically stimulated skeletal muscle. *J Thorac Cardiovasc Surg* 94:702–709, 1987.
14. Drinkwater DC, Chiu RCJ, Modry D, et al: Cardiac assist and myocardial repair with synchronously stimulated skeletal muscle. *Surg Forum* 31:271–274, 1980.
15. Dewar ML, Chiu RCJ: Cardiomyoplasty and the pulse-train stimulator. In Chiu RCJ (ed): *Biomechanical Cardiac Assist: Cardiomyoplasty and Muscle-Powered Devices.* Mount Kisco, NY, Futura Publishing Co Inc, 1986, pp 43–58.
16. Chachques JC, Grandjean P, Carpentier A: Latissimus dorsi dynamic cardiomyoplasty. *Ann Thorac Surg* 47:600–604, 1989.

17. Odim JNK, Burgess JH, Williams BH, et al: Pathophysiology of dynamic cardiomyoplasty: a clinico-pathological case study. *J Card Surg* 5:336–346, 1990.
18. Herring SW, Grimm AF, Grimm BR: Regulation of sarcomere number in skeletal muscle: a comparison of hypotheses. *Muscle Nerve* 7:161–173, 1984.
19. Williams P, Watt P, Bicik V, Goldspink G: Effect of stretch combined with electrical stimulation on the type of sarcomeres produced at the ends of muscle fibers. *Exp Neurol* 93:500–509, 1986.
20. Magovern GJ, Kao RL, Christlieb IY, et al: Dynamic cardiomyoplasty in patients. *J Heart Transplant* 9:258–263, 1990.
21. Carpentier A, Chachques JC: Clinical dynamic cardiomyoplasty: method and outcome. *Semin Thorac Cardiovasc Surg* 3:136–139, 1991.
22. Lee KF, Dignan RJ, Parmar JM, et al: Effects of dynamic cardiomyoplasty on left ventricular performance and myocardial mechanics in dilated cardiomyopathy. *J Thorac Cardiovasc Surg* 102:124–131, 1991.
23. Molteni L, Almada H, Ferreira R: Synchronously stimulated skeletal muscle graft for left ventricular assistance. *J Thorac Cardiovasc Surg* 97:439–446, 1989.
24. The SOLVD Investigators: Effect of enalapril on survival in patients with reduced left ventricular ejection fractions and congestive heart failure. *N Engl J Med* 325:293–302, 1991.
25. Jatene AD, Moreira LFP, Stolf NAG, et al: Left ventricular function changes after cardiomyoplasty in patients with dilated cardiomyopathy. *J Thorac Cardiovasc Surg* 102:132–139, 1991.
26. Zelis R, Sinoway LI, Musch TI: Why do patients with congestive heart failure stop exercising? *J Am Coll Cardiol* 12:359–361, 1988.

Chapter 8

# *Discussion*

**Sir Magdi Yacoub (London):** The patients that you presented to us were in chronological order. Therefore, the 100% coverage came later. Are you sure that other factors and your expertise didn't change in the meantime? Do you think it was only the wrap or something else?

**Dr. Odim:** Our technique throughout the 3-year period was essentially the same. Perhaps our selection criteria changed because our very first case was a gentleman with an ischemic cardiomyopathy who actually developed arrhythmias 4 months later that we had not anticipated.

**Dr. Guiraudon (London, Ontario, Canada):** Was your estimation of the wrap accurate when you got the autopsy?

**Dr. Odim:** For the second patient, we were fortunate to get an autopsy. It showed viability of the muscle. There was indeed suboptimal muscular wrapping as estimated intraoperatively. There was some evidence of atrophy, particularly at the periphery, 1 to 2 mm fibers between the muscle and the epicardium. There was no evidence of any neovascularization at 7 months following surgery.

**Dr. Guiraudon:** So the question is: Was the extent of the wrap measured at the time of operation?

**Dr. Odim:** Yes.

**Dr. Guiraudon:** Does that correlate with what happens late? Did you attempt to measure it late?

**Dr. Odim:** We do not have a method of following the extent of wrapping in live patients.

**Unidentified:** The last patient you showed was interesting in the sense that the ejection fraction improved quite considerably, but the wedge pressure went up. I wonder whether in spite of the increase in improvement in systolic function, wrapping this muscle around the heart sometimes may not worsen the diastolic function of the heart?

**Dr. Odim:** In the postoperative course, the synchronization delay between sensing the R-wave and the burst stimulation to the muscle was set at 15 msec. However, on echocardiographic study and trying to time that burst with closure of the mitral valve, we discovered that there was some interference with the diastolic filling and we had to prolong this delay out to 100 msec to get optimal performance. But this gentleman, as seen from his cardiac lab data, had important right-sided problems with increased pulmonary vascular resistance. I am not sure, therefore, that we can definitely say that the wrap is bad for diastolic function.

Chapter 9

# Dynamic Cardiomyoplasty: La Pitie Experience

Valéria Bors, Richard Dorent, Guillaume Jondeau, Iradj Gandjbakhch

## Introduction

The management of chronic congestive heart failure patients remains a challenge. In recent years, pharmacological trials confirmed that vasodilator therapy is beneficial but demonstrated a deleterious effect of certain inotropic agents. At the same time, the increase in numbers of heart transplantation has not continued, probably a result of the limited number of available donor hearts. Furthermore, the improvement in early survival after cardiac transplantation has not been associated with an impact on rate of late deaths.[1]

Dynamic cardiomyoplasty, initially described by Carpentier and Chachques in 1985,[2] has been proposed as a method of ventricular assistance for patients with heart failure. We report our experience with cardiomyoplasty at La Pitie Hospital.

## Patients

From January 1992 to March 1996, 26 patients with moderate congestive heart failure underwent isolated cardiomyoplasty without cardiopulmonary bypass. All of them were referred to our center for cardiac transplantation. Four of them refused cardiac transplantation and two others preferred cardiomyoplasty. Nine patients were very stout with few chances to get an adequate donor heart in the following year.

There were 21 males and 5 females ranging in age from 34 to 62 years (mean, 49 years). The etiology of heart failure was idiopathic dilated cardiomyopathy in 20 patients and ischemic heart disease in six patients. Twenty-five had predominant or exclusive left heart failure. All patients were in sinus rhythm. The preoperative clinical and hemodynamic status of our patients is shown in Table 1.

From Carpentier A, Chachques JC, Grandjean P: Cardiac Bioassist. © Futura Publishing Co, Inc, Armonk, NY, 1997.

**Table 1**
Preoperative Status: 26 Patients

| | |
|---|---|
| LVEF (MUGA) | 22.3 ± 9.1% |
| CI | 2.6 ± 0.64 L/min/m$^2$ |
| $MVO_2$ | 17.6 ± 4.24 mL/kg/min |
| NYHA Class II | 2 patients |
| NYHA Class III | 24 patients |

LVEF = left ventricular ejection fraction; CI = cardiac index.

# Methods

## Surgical Procedure

Cardiomyoplasty was performed following the Carpentier and Chachques technique using the left latissimus dorsi muscle to reinforce the left ventricle, without cardiopulmonary bypass.[3] We implanted the Medtronic® intramuscular electrodes (Model SP 5528) and the Medtronic myocardial sensing lead (Model 5548) connected to the Medtronic cardiomyostimulator (Model SP 1005 and Model 4710, since January 94) located in the left upper abdominal wall. The wrapping was posterior (clockwise) with complete covering of the left ventricle. The covering of the right ventricle was complete in four cases, and more than 50% in the other cases.

## Electrostimulation Management

The muscle stimulation protocol was started usually 2 weeks after surgery and was progressive during 10 weeks. The heart/muscle contraction ratio was 2:1 and muscle contraction was effective in all patients. The skeletal muscle pulse amplitude used was 4.25 volts (range, 3.5 volts to 5 volts), 30 Hz burst, pulse width 210 μsec.

## Postoperative Follow-Up

Patients were preoperatively studied by Doppler echocardiography, 24-hour Holter recording, exercise stress testing, radionuclide left ventriculography, and right and left heart catheterization. All of these investigations except left heart catheterization were repeated at 6 months and at 1 and 2 years of follow-up. The follow-up period ranged from 2 to 50 months.

## Statistical Analysis

Student's paired test was used for comparison of preoperative and postoperative mean values. Chi square analysis was used when appropriate. Probability values less than 0.05 were considered statistically significant.

# Results

## Early Postoperative Complications

In our series of 26 patients, four postoperative deaths occurred. One patient died 4 hours after surgery of electromechanical dissociation. Three other patients developed a low cardiac output with final multiorgan failure and died on 7th, 10th, and 14th days after surgery. There were no postoperative complications in 10 patients. In 12 patients, postoperative management was difficult. Early complications are listed in Table 2.

## Late Results

The survival curve of our series is shown in Figure 1. Three late deaths occurred. Two patients died suddenly at 15 and 30 months after surgery and an-

**Table 2**
Postoperative Complications: 12 Patients

| | |
|---|---|
| Low cardiac output | n = 7 |
| Acute pulmonary edema | n = 2 |
| Atrial fibrillation | n = 1 |
| Mechanical ventilation longer than 2 days | n = 5 |
| Acute renal failure needing dialysis | n = 2 |
| Mediastinitis | n = 1 |

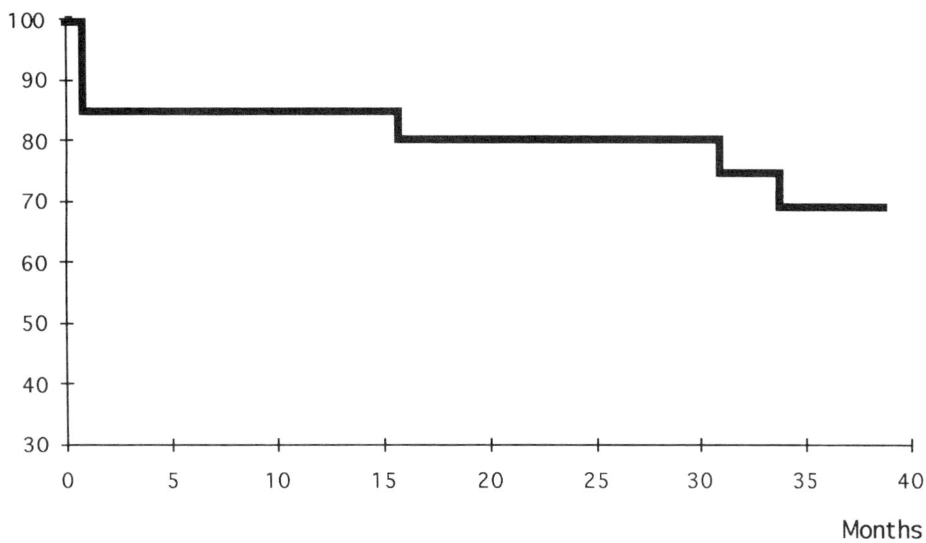


**Figure 1:** *Kaplan-Meier actuarial survival following cardiomyoplasty (26 patients).*

**Table 3**
Hemodynamic Data at 12 and 24 Months after Cardiomyoplasty

| | *Preoperative* | *12 Months* | *24 Months* |
|---|---|---|---|
| CI L/mn/m$^2$ | 2.5 ± .6<br>n = 16 | 2.52 ± .7<br>n = 16 | 2.36 ± .7<br>n = 13 |
| LVEF (MUGA) percent | 21.27 ± 6.83<br><br>n = 15 | 26.20 ± 8.69<br>p = 0.0275<br>n = 15 | 27.79 ± 9.74<br>p = 0.0077<br>n = 14 |

CI = cardiac index; LVEF = left ventricular ejection fraction.

other developed progressive biventricular heart failure and died 33 months after cardiomyoplasty. Another patient, after early functional improvement, developed congestive heart failure and underwent successful heart transplantation 15 months after cardiomyoplasty. Thus the 36-month actuarial survival for the 26 patients was 69%.

Hemodynamic data collected at 12 and 24 months after surgery, despite good clinical results and improvement in NYHA class in 16 patients, did not change significantly except for the increase of the radionuclide left ventricular ejection fraction (Table 3). Despite the mild change of hemodynamic parameters, the functional improvement was significant and began as early as 3 months after the procedure. Quality of life is much better for all of them except three patients. None of the patients complained of discomfort due to the contractions of the latissimus dorsi muscle and rotation into the chest.

## Conclusion

Our findings demonstrate that cardiomyoplasty produces short-term and long-term clinical benefits without significant hemodynamic effect. The symptomatic improvement is associated with high 36-month actuarial survival.

## References

1. Kaye MP: The registry of the international society for heart and lung transplantation: Ninth official report 1992. *J Heart Lung Transplant* 11:599, 1992.
2. Chachques JC, Grandjean PA, Carpentier A: Latissimus dorsi dynamic cardiomyoplasty. *Ann Thoracic Surgery* 47:600, 1989.
3. Chachques JC, Grandjean PA, Carpentier A: Patient management and clinical follow up after cardiomyoplasty. *J Cardiac Surg* 6(Suppl 1): 89-99, 1991.
4. Jondeau G, Dorent R, Bors V, Dib JC, et al: Dynamic cardiomyoplasty: Effect of discontinuing latissimus dorsi muscle stimulation on left ventricular systolic and diastolic performance and exercise capacity. *JACC* 26(1):129–134, 1995.

Chapter 10

# Cardiomyoplasty:

## The Russian Experience – Review of Early and Late Results

V. S. Chekanov, A. A. Krakovsky, V. V. Pekarsky*

### Introduction

The problem of congestive heart failure, from various causes, has been of particular interest and a challenge to practitioners for many decades. Its treatment remains one of the most difficult problems of cardiac surgery.[1,2] Congestion can be alleviated through aggressive management in many instances. However, when failure is due to irreversible myocardial pathology, the therapeutic effect is temporary and unstable, and progresses to an unmanageable stage.[3,4]

Cardiac transplantation is often the only treatment option available for these patients.[5,6] The mechanical artificial heart serves as a bridge to transplant. The limited availability of donor hearts as well as the numerous contraindications for cardiac transplantation are significant obstacles to widespread clinical implementation.[7,8] An alternative treatment option for these patients may be dynamic cardiomyoplasty: the use of stimulated skeletal muscle to support the weakened myocardium.[9–12]

Our experience with cardiomyoplasty in 25 patients follows. We have included early and late results, control of hemodynamic changes, and the description of the optimal regimen for the stimulation of the muscular graft.

### Methods and Materials

Twenty-five carefully selected patients underwent isolated cardiomyoplasty between October 1988 and March 1993. Operations were performed at two centers: Bakulev Institute for Cardiovascular Surgery in Moscow and

*With the cooperation of NS Buslenko, LG Riabinina, DB Andreev, and KV Shatalov.
From Carpentier A, Chachques JC, Grandjean P: Cardiac Bioassist. © Futura Publishing Co, Inc, Armonk, NY, 1997.

Siberian Scientific Institute of Cardiology in Tomsk. Twenty-one patients suffered from ischemic cardiomyopathy and four from dilated cardiomyopathy. All of the patients in this series were male. The age range was from 28 to 59 years, with a mean age of 45.7 years.

All patients with ischemic heart disease had a history of myocardial infarction. The mean was 1.7 occurrences. Four patients were in New York Heart Association (NYHA) Class III and 21 were in Class IV. Each patient in the series was on maximum medical therapy including long-acting nitrates, digitalis, and diuretics. There were 14 patients who had severe angina pectoris despite aggressive medical management, and who had to add an average of 15 tablets of sublingual nitroglycerin daily to the medical regimen. In the other patients, the clinical picture was characteristic for congestive heart failure (Table 1). Heart failure duration was an average of 18.1 months for these patients (from 2 to 36 months).

Exercise testing by means of bicycle ergometry in the sitting position was performed on 17 patients. The method of gradually increasing the load was used to determine the exercise threshold, which was expressed in watts. The exercise was stopped when ischemic changes appeared on the ECG and according to the WHO criteria established in 1969. Exercise thresholds ranged from 25 to 60 watts, with an average of 30.5 watts.

Left ventricular contractility was determined by two-dimensional echocardiography. End-systolic volume of the left ventricle (LVESV) varied from 128 to 293 mL with a mean of 228.2 (±3.8 mL). End-diastolic volume of the left ventricle (LVEDV) was from 264 to 420 mL with a mean of 310.2 (±0.6 mL). Left ventricular ejection fraction (LVEF) varied from 22% to 39% with a mean of 30.2% (±2.0%)

Radionuclide studies by myocardial scintigraphy with thallium-201 helped to determine the area of myocardial scarring. The area ranged from 15% to 50% with a mean of 38.1% (±1.6%). LVEF was measured by radionuclide ventriculography using technetium-99. The range was 21 to 29.2% with a mean of 24% (±1.4%) (Table 2).

All patients underwent selective coronary cineangiography by the Judkins technique. Those with greater than 75% luminal obstruction of the coronary arteries were classified as having severe atherosclerotic disease. Among the patients with severe coronary artery disease, six patients had occlusion of one vessel with no evidence of retrograde filling, six patients had two-vessel disease, and six patients had three-vessel disease. In 10 of these patients, there was diffuse distal disease.

Left ventriculography was performed in the right oblique view. Measurement of LVEF ranged from 12% to 32% with a mean of 25.2 (±1.4%). The range

**Table 1**

Characteristics of Patients Before the Operation of Cardiomyoplasty

| | |
|---|---|
| Mean age | 45.7 ± 2.4 |
| NYHA functional class | 3.8 ± 0.02 |
| Functional class of angina (n = 19) | 4.0 ± 0.02 |

**Table 2**
Two-Dimensional Echocardiography and Radionuclide Studies

| | | |
|---|---|---|
| End-systolic volume of the left ventricle (ESVLV) (mL) | 128–293 | (228.2 ± 3.8) |
| End-diastolic volume of the left ventricle (EDVLV) (mL) | 264–420 | (310.2 ± 4.6) |
| Left ventricle ejection fraction (LVEF) (%) | | |
| Echo | 22–39 | (30.2 ± 2.0) |
| Radioisotopic | 21–29.2 | (24.0 ± 1.4) |
| Area of myocardial scarring (%) | 15–50 | (38.1 ± 1.6) |

for left ventricular end-diastolic pressure (EDPLV) was from 16 to 32 mm Hg with a mean of 22.8 (±1.2 mm Hg).

A median sternotomy, in four patients, was used as the operative approach in the years between 1988 and 1990. Since 1990, the exposure of choice has been left anterolateral thoracotomy through the fourth intercostal space.

Thirteen patients received the first-generation neuromyostimulators (Stiminak 805, Russia). Since 1991, the second-generation neuromyostimulator (EKS 445, Russia) has been used. The advantages of Stiminak 805 and EKS 445 are not only the ability to change stimulation ratios from 1:1 to 1:8, but the capability to change the impulse voltage in the EKS 445 to the number of impulses in the burst. The EKS 445 can also be operated in the demand mode.

Preparative training by stimulation of the latissimus dorsi skeletal muscle was accomplished prior to the definitive operation in one patient. In the other patients, the operation was performed in one stage.

Two months following the operation, when the period of graft training was completed, postoperative studies were performed in 10 patients (all after left anterolateral thoracotomy). The hemodynamic state was measured at different stimulation parameters. The same patients were investigated in the follow-up period, which ranged from 6 months to 3.5 years.

To determine the optimal regimen of stimulation, a Swan-Ganz catheter was introduced into the pulmonary artery, and access to a central vein and peripheral artery was obtained. Then, successive changes of the myostimulation ratio from 1:1 to 1:8 were induced, and minute circulation volume was measured by thermodilution techniques.

## Mortality

Four patients died during the early postoperative period, within 7 days after the operation. Causes of death were coronary artery thromboembolism (1), progressive heart failure (2), and acute myocardial infarction (1). Two of the patients were in the group that underwent the operation through median sternotomy and two were in the group that had anterolateral thoracotomy. One patient died in the postoperative period of 8–30 days. Cause of death in this patient was cerebrovascular stroke, ischemia resulting from thrombosis of an atherosclerotic left middle cerebral artery. Anatomopathological examination showed that the left heart was free of thrombi which could serve as a source of embolism. Thus, the mortality rate was 16%.

In the late postoperative period, two patients died, one at 8 months following the operation and one at 1 year after the operation. One death was sudden and most probably heart-related, and the other death was due to myocardial infarction.

## Late Results

The follow-up period ranged from 6 months to 3.5 years, with a mean follow-up duration of 14.6 months. Fourteen patients were studied. Eleven patients had improved, and the status of three patients remained unchanged.

Improvement in clinical status consisted of a decrease in the signs of cardiac failure and a decrease in the NYHA functional class from a mean of 3.8 to a mean of 2.2. In patients with ischemic heart disease, a decrease in the functional angina class from a mean of 4.0 to a mean of 2.0 was noted.

Tolerance to physical exercise increased twofold from an average of 41.4 watts to 83.7 watts. The LVESV, as judged by echocardiographic data, decreased in average by 18%, from a mean of 228.2 mL (±3.8 mL) to 185.0 mL (±3.2 mL). The LVEDV decreased by an average of 21% from 310.2 mL (±4.6 mL) to 245.1 mL (±3.8 mL). The LVEF increased by an average of 10% from 30.2 (±2.6) to 41.2 (±1.6), which constituted 1/3 of the initial value (Table 3).

Ten patients were examined and selected to determine the optimal regimen of myostimulation. During this examination, a clear hemodynamic response to stimulation by the muscular graft was revealed. Mean value of the cardiac index (CI) without stimulation was 3.9 L/min/m$^2$ (±1.2). The extremes of these indices were fixed at different stimulation ratios and constituted an average of 5.1 L/min/m$^2$ (±1.2). The stroke index (SI) was subject to similar changes. At the start of stimulation, the mean value rose from 38.5 mL/m$^2$ (±3.2) to 51.0 mL/m$^2$ (±4.2).

As an average, cardiac output increased from 3.9 L/min without stimulation (±0.4 L/min) to 4.8 ± 0.5 L/min with stimulation. The most significant increase in CI, SI, and cardiac output (CO) was seen during stimulation regimen 1:4 or 1:6 (Table 4).

**Table 3**

Indices of Left Ventricular Myocardial Contractile Capacity Late After the Cardiomyoplasty Operation (as Judged by Echocardiography)

| | *Preoperative* | *Postoperative* |
|---|---|---|
| Left ventricular end-systolic volume (mL) | 228.2 ± 3.8 | 185.0 ± 3.2 |
| Left ventricular end-diastolic volume (mL) | 310.2 ± 4.6 | 245.1 ± 3.8 |
| Left ventricular ejection fraction (%) | 30.2 ± 2.6 | 41.2 ± 1.6 |

**Table 4**
Catheterization Results

| | *Without Stimulation* | *With Stimulation* | | | | | | | |
|---|---|---|---|---|---|---|---|---|---|
| | | *1:1* | *1:2* | *1:3* | *1:4* | *1:5* | *1:6* | *1:7* | *1:8* |
| CI (L/min/m$^2$) | 3.9 ± 1.2 | 4.1 ± 1.0 | 4.1 ± 0.9 | 4.4 ± 1.3 | 5.1 ± 1.2 | 4.9 ± 1.1 | 5.0 ± 1.2 | 4.8 ± 1.0 | 4.0 ± 1 |
| CO (L/min) | 3.9 ± 0.4 | 4.6 ± 0.3 | 4.5 ± 0.5 | 4.6 ± 0.4 | 4.7 ± 0.4 | 4.4 ± 0.5 | 4.8 ± 0.5 | 4.3 ± 0.6 | 4.2 ±0 |
| SI (mL/m$^2$) | 38.5 ± 3.2 | 48.1 ± 3.8 | 47.2 ± 3.5 | 48.0 ± 4.0 | 51.0 ± 4.2 | 50.1 ± 3.9 | 50.9 ± 4.1 | 49.1 ± 2.8 | 44.1 ± 3 |
| # of Patients | 10 | 10 | 8 | 8 | 10 | 8 | 10 | 10 | 6 |

CI = cardiac index; CO = cardiac output; SI = stroke index.

## Discussion

The prognosis for patients with ischemic heart disease who have extensive scarring of the left ventricular muscle and decreased contractility is unfavorable, especially in the presence of heart failure.[14–16] Recently, attempts have been made to treat these patients with new and powerful therapeutic agents.[17–19] The prognosis in dilated cardiomyopathy is also unfavorable.[20,21] Cardiac transplantation is a radical method of treatment, with an array of medical and social problems.[22,23] An alternative method of treatment for this group of patients may be cardiomyoplasty.

Functional coronary reserve is necessary to allow the patient to survive the operation and the difficult immediate postoperative period, and to allow the heart to adapt to the new conditions.

It has been the experience of all who perform cardiomyoplasty that the effect of the operation is not immediate and that it takes time for ventricular function to improve.[24–26]

Four patients died during the early postoperative period for an overall mortality rate of 16%. From 1988 to 1990, two of four patients who underwent the operation died. In the period from 1990 to 1992, mortality was 9.6%, 2/21 patients died. Increased experience, technical progress, and awareness of patient selection criteria are evident.

Early myostimulation was used in one patient to determine the possibility of arresting acute heart failure. Contraindications to early myostimulation are that it causes rapid fatigue of the unprepared muscle and there is a high probability of myocardial suture dehiscence during stimulation. These factors can be eliminated by preliminary training of the graft and fixation of the distal portion of the transplanted muscle to the pericardium, which was done in this patient.

In subsequent patients, the skeletal muscle was not pretrained. If the muscle is not stimulated during the first week after implant, the training is lost.[27] In performing subsequent operations, we considered the possibility of placing the intact muscle into the thoracic cavity, thus avoiding the duration of intervention. This is at the expense of scarring and adhesions forming in the zone of lead implantation.

Seven days after surgery, all patients were subjected to progressive stimulation aimed at assisting the new graft to adapt to its new conditions and transformation of fibers. The increase in impulse frequency was gradual, at week-long intervals, thus allowing good muscular adaptation to each new regimen. The risk of muscle damage when the stimulator was reprogrammed was eliminated by this gradual progression. The gradual increase of the ratio of work of the cardiosynchronized neuromyostimulator was 1:16, and after that, from 1:7 to 1:1.

After the period of skeletal muscle training was completed, 10 patients were examined to determine the optimal regimen of the neurostimulator's work. The term "optimal regimen" means the parameters of stimulation at which the complex "muscle-heart" produces an adequate minute circulation volume. In this investigation, we made an attempt to determine the influence of the synchronization ratio, as well as determine the impulse voltage and number of impulses in the burst with the EKS 445 implanted, on hemodynamic indices.

The investigation, which was done 1 month after surgery, consisted of calculation of the derivatives of the main hemodynamic parameters, fixed during successive changes of the myostimulator's work regimens at rather short intervals. The myostimulation ratio changed successively from 1:8 to 1:1.

When the study began, control measurements were done without stimulation and hypervolemic testing. The last was repeated at the end of the study with myostimulation at optimal levels. Control measurements showed improvement of the derivatives of the main hemodynamic indices as compared to preoperative values.

Neuromyostimulators which are generally available (Medtronic) can change the synchronization ratio from 1:1 to 1:3. The Russian stimulators have the advantage of changing the synchronization ratio from 1:1 to 1:7 and 1:16. In our experience, it is extremely important to have this flexibility. Our investigation, aimed at the choice of optimal regimen of myostimulation, showed the 1:4 and 1:6 ratios to be most advantageous. A positive hemodynamic response is obtained when a regimen of muscular graft rest is created.

Our data of results during the late postoperative period coincide with the data obtained at other centers following cardiomyoplasty. All investigators note improvement in the clinical status of the patients following surgery despite small changes in hemodynamic parameters.[28,29] Satisfactory results in our patients indicate correct patient selection criteria.

The majority of investigators assess the effectiveness of the operation by evaluation of clinical data as well as by the status of LV ejection fraction. The state of the formed "muscle-heart" complex and hemodynamic factors are not taken into account. There are two fallacies in this approach: (1) the improvement of hemodynamic parameters is the goal of this operation, and (2) it is possible that the investigation of the relationship between hemodynamic response and the type of operation and regimen of stimulation can reveal significant myocardial reserve and increase this intervention's effectiveness.

The data obtained in this study confirm that cardiomyoplasty has a significant positive effect on central hemodynamic indices. However, the mechanism of the muscular graft's influence appears to be more complex. At present, the following factors that influence hemodynamics are: mechanical compressive influence of the muscular graft during stimulation; improvement of myocardial metabolism as a result of indirect revascularization of ischemic muscle; changes in ventricular filling and changes in the relationship of compliance/compression after implantation of the graft and during stimulation. A mathematical model to study the effects of cardiomyoplasty should be completed for the follow-up of LV systolic and end-diastolic volume dynamics during both the intraoperative and postoperative phase.

## Conclusions

Based on our findings, we believe that cardiomyoplasty leads to clinical improvement in patients who have been followed up to 4 years, cardiomyoplasty has a positive effect on central hemodynamics, the myostimulation regimens of 1:4 and 1:6 are the most advantageous for graft stimulation and allow the most significant hemodynamic improvement, and skeletal muscle rest is an important factor in overall outcome.

## References


1. Messie BM, Conway M: Survival of patients with congestive heart failure: past, present and future prospects. *Circulation* 75(Suppl)IV-11–IV-19, 1987.
2. Bounous ED, Wark DB, Pollock BG, et al: Surgical survival benefits for coronary disease patient with left ventricular dysfunction. *Circulation* 78(Suppl) I-151–I-157, 1988.
3. The Consensus Trial Study Group: Effects of enalapril on mortality in severe congestive heart failure: results of the Cooperative North Scandinavian Study (CONSENSUS). *N Engl J Med* 316:1429–1435, 1987.
4. Likoff MJ, Chandler SL, Kay HR: Clinical determinants of mortality in chronic congestive heart failure secondary to idiopathic dilated or to ischemic cardiomyopathy. *Am J Cardiol* 59:634–638, 1987.
5. Hildebrandt A, Reichenspurner H, Reichbart B: Heart transplantation: the treatment of choice for patients with end-stage ischemic heart disease. *Thorac Cardiovasc Surg* 37:37–41, 1989.
6. Mohsin Hakim, Higenbottam T, Bethune D, Cory-Pearce R, et al: Selection and procurement of combined heart and lung grafts for transplantation. *J Thorac Cardiovasc Surg* 95:474–479, 1988.
7. Mannion JD, Stephenson LW: Potential uses of skeletal muscle for myocardial assistance. *Surg Clin North Am* 65:679–687, 1985.
8. Bodylak SF, Weiss R: Taking skeletal muscle to heart. *Science News* 134:334–335, 1988.
9. Carpentier A, Chachques JC: Myocardial substitution with a stimulated skeletal muscle: first successful clinical case. *Lancet* 1:1267, 1985.
10. Chekanov V, Krakowsky A: Possible use of skeletal muscle in various congenital and acquired cardiac pathology. In Chekanov V, Krakowsky A (eds): *Cardiomyoplasty.* Bombay, 1989, p 73–87.
11. Chachques JC, Grandjean PA, Vasseur B, et al: Preclinical research and first successful clinical myocardial substitution with a stimulated skeletal muscle. *Ann New Acad Sci* 494:445–448, 1987.
12. Dumcius AS, Sirvinskas EK, Skucas J, et al: A method of extended myoventriculoplasty with programmable cardiosynchronized electroneurostimulation: description and initial clinical results. *Cor et Vasa* 31:393–401, 1989.
13. Hamilton GW, Murray JA, Kennedy JW: Quantitative angiography in ischemic heart disease. *Circulation* 45:1065, 1972.
14. Califf RM, Horrell FE, Lee KL, et al: The prognosis in the presence of coronary artery disease. In Braunwald B, Mock MK, Watson J (eds): *Congestive Heart Failure.* New York, 1982, pp 31–35.
15. Balu V, Szmedra L, Dean D, Bhayama J: Long-term survival of patient with low ejection fraction. *Texas Heart Inst J* 15:44–48, 1988.
16. Faulkner SL, Honey WS, Alford WC, et al: Ischemic cardiomyopathy: medical versus surgical treatment. *J Thorac Cardiovasc Surg* 74:77–81, 1977.
17. Captopril Multicenter Research Group: A placebo controlled trial of captopril in congestive heart failure. *J Am Coll Cardiol* 2:755–763, 1983.
18. Chaterjee K, Warmley WW: The role of vasodilator therapy in heart failure. *Prog Cardiovasc Dis* 19:301–325, 1977.
19. Cody RJ: Do positive inotropic agents adversely affect the survival of patients with chronic congestive heart failure. *J Am Coll Cardiol* 12:559–561, 1988.
20. Fuster V, Gersch BJ, Giuliani ER, et al: Natural history of idiopathic dilated cardiomyopathy. *Am J Cardiol* 47:525–529, 1981.

21. Franciosa JA, Wilen M, Zieschle S: Survival in men with severe chronic left ventricular failure due to either coronary heart disease or idiopathic dilated cardiomyopathy. *Circulation* 75(Suppl)IV-1–IV-3, 1987.
22. Chekanov VS, Krakowsky AA, Pekarsky VV: Electrostimulated dynamic cardiomyoplasty: new trend in cardiac surgery for autotropic biomechanical cardiac support. In: Chekanov VS, Krakowsky AA, Pekarsky VV (eds): *Mechanical and Biomechanical Cardiac Support,* Tomsk, 1991, pp 9–27.
23. Walsh C, Chiu RC-J: Skeletal muscle for cardiac repair and assist: a historical overview. In: Chiu RC-J (ed): *Biomechanical Cardiac Assist.* Mt. Kisco, NY, Futura Publishing Co. Inc., 1986, pp 1–18.
24. Carpentier A: Hospital Broussais: Clinical experience from cardiomyoplasty. In: Carpentier A, Chachques JC, Grandjean P (eds): *Cardiomyoplasty.* Mt. Kisco, NY, Futura Publishing Co. Inc., 1991, pp 147–157.
25. Chachques JC, Grandjean P, Schwartz K, Mihaleanu S: Effect of latissimus dorsi dynamic cardiomyoplasty on ventricular function. *Circulation* 78(Suppl)III-203–III-216, 1988.
26. Chachques JC, Grandjean P, Carpentier A: Patient management and clinical follow-up after cardiomyoplasty. *J Cardiac Surg* 6:89–99, 1991.
27. Chekanov VS, Krakowsky AK: Cardiomyoplasty: a new approach to surgical treatment of heart failure. In: Lewis BS, Kimchi A (eds): *Heart Failure: Mechanisms and Management.* Springer-Verlag, Berlin Heidelberg, 1991, pp 425–433.
28. Magovern GJ, Park SB, Kao RL, et al: Dynamic cardiomyoplasty in patients. *Heart Transplant* 9:258, 1990.
29. Magovern GJ, Christlieb IV, Kao KL: The Allegeny Hospital experience. In: Carpentier A, Chachques JC, Grandjean PM (eds): *Cardiomyoplasty.* Mt. Kisco, NY, Futura Publishing Co., Inc., 1991, pp 159–170.

Chapter 11

# Clinical Results of Cardiomyoplasty

Shamil D. Akhmedov, Euvgenily V. Krivoschekov, Vikenty V. Pekarsky*

## Introduction

The aim of this chapter is to provide an overview of the clinical results in patients with ischemic and dilated cardiomyopathies following dynamic cardiomyoplasty performed at our institution.[1]

## Materials and Methods

### Patients

Between 1990 and 1994, 35 cardiomyoplasty procedures were performed in patients whose age ranged from 11 to 59 years. Five of these patients, including one child (11 years old), had dilated cardiomyopathy. Thirty patients had ischemic heart disease with a history of acute myocardial infarctions. Exertional angina was Canadian Heart Association Class III to IV, while functional status due to heart failure was New York Heart Association Class III to IV, with a maximum level of exercise at less than 25 W. Four patients had episodes of sudden cardiac arrest, but were successfully resuscitated. One patient had a complete atrioventricular (AV) block, and another had sick sinus syndrome. Fourteen patients were found to have ventricular extrasystoles (Lown III to IV) on Holter ECG monitor recordings.

### Surgical Techniques

In 21 patients, cardiomyoplasty was carried out as a one-step procedure; a two-step operation was performed in 14.

*With the cooperation of Mariana V. Pekarskaya, Alexander L. Krylov, Zhanna V. Vesnina, Vladimir I. Chernov, Alexander M. Chernyavskiy, Yuriy Y. Vechersky, Rostislav S. Karpov, and Edward A. Nechaev.

From Carpentier A, Chachques JC, Grandjean P: Cardiac Bioassist. © Futura Publishing Co, Inc, Armonk, NY, 1997.

During the preparation of the latissimus dorsi (LD) muscle, any curare-type drugs were avoided, since they may affect muscle contractility and interfere with testing of optimal electrode location placed on the thoracodorsal nerve. The second rib was resected and the LD muscle tendon was detached from the humerus bone and fixed to the third rib, followed by transferring the LD muscle flap into the left hemithorax. In the one-step procedure, a left thoracotomy was performed, and following pericardiotomy, the costal surface of the LD muscle flap was placed over the epicardium and wrapped around the ventricles in anteroposterior fashion. In the six patients who underwent the two-step procedure, coronary artery bypass was also carried out. In two patients, right and anterior descending coronary arteries were revascularized, while in four others, only the anterior descending coronary artery was bypassed. Because of the low ejection fraction (a mean of 15%), coronary artery bypass grafting (CABG) was performed without cardiopulmonary bypass. In the two-step operation, the second step—namely, a median sternotomy—facilitated the complete wrapping of the heart by the LD graft. Life-threatening cardiac rhythm disturbances were not seen during the procedures.

The CMS Stiminak-805 (Moscow Engineering Physics Institute, Moscow, Russia) was implanted in six patients, and CM-445 (Tochmash, Moscow, Russia) was used in 29 patients. Electrical stimulation of the LD flap was begun immediately after surgery with the ratio of 1:16, burst of four impulses, and an amplitude of 2.5 V. Synchronization ratio was reprogrammed to 1:7 in 10 days and to 1:3 in 3 weeks.

## Laboratory Studies

Preoperatively, all patients underwent left ventriculography and selective left and right coronary angiography. Akinetic and dyskinetic zones comprised 43.6% ± 2.3% of the left ventricular myocardial mass. The ejection fraction was 19% ± 2.6%, and the end-diastolic pressure was 23 ± 2.2 mm Hg. The contraindications for coronary artery bypass and resection of aneurysms in these patients included low left ventricular contractility, and multiple distal occlusions of the coronary arteries.

At 2 to 28 months after cardiomyoplasty procedures, repeated investigations were carried out. In eight patients, additional selective angiography of the left thoracodorsal artery supplying the LD graft was obtained (of those, seven patients suffered from ischemic cardiomyopathy and one patient had dilated cardiomyopathy) in order to visualize vascular anastomoses between the muscle wrap and the underlying myocardium. Radioisotopes (99m technetium pertechnetate with total activity of 185 mBk) were administered into the thoracodorsal artery of four patients to confirm that blood flow went from the LD muscle to the myocardium and not vice versa. The rate of isotope administration was 15 to 18 mL/sec using an automatic injector. Simultaneously, 18 blood samples were taken during 36 seconds via a catheter inserted into the coronary sinus, with subsequent determination of radioactivity using a Gamma-spectrometer (Tracor Analytic®, Boston, MA, USA). Similar studies were carried out in three patients as controls.

## Myocardial Scintigraphy

To objectively assess the degree of myocardial blood supply, tomoscintigraphic study of myocardial perfusion with dipyridamole (199 thallium-chloride, product of the Tomsk Institute of Nuclear Physics, Tomsk, Russia) was carried out before and 8 ± 3.8 months after the operation. Zones with stable and reversible myocardial perfusion defects were marked out by automatic processing of scintigrams. Relative volume of perfusion defect, expressed as percentage of left ventricular myocardial mass, was calculated. Scintigraphic studies were performed using the Gamma-camera "Omega-500" (Technicare, GE Medical Systems, Milwaukee, WI) supplied with a computer system Scintron MX (Matrix Computer AG, Miles Inc., Leverkusen, Germany).

# RESULTS

## Clinical and Hemodynamic Outcome

Out of 35 patients operated upon, six died in hospital (17%). Four patients died from acute heart failure, two from ischemic strokes 3 weeks after the operation although they were hemodynamically stable. In the follow-up period of 9 ± 2.1 months, seven patients died, four from sudden cardiac death and three from acute myocardial infarction. One patient developed sudden attacks of ventricular tachycardia and ventricular fibrillation 2 weeks after cardiomyoplasty, which were terminated by defibrillator discharges of 150 to 200 J. Amiodarone, with rhythmilen, lidocaine administered intravenously, neither terminated nor prevented these attacks. Resuscitation was carried out for 24 hours with more than 200 defibrillations and closed cardiac massage carried out. This patient recovered after reprogramming the CMS-445 stimulator to the overdrive ventricular stimulation with the rate of 110 beats/min, and intramuscular administration of eglonil (neuroleptic agent) in a dose of 400 mg/day. Resuscitation measures including defibrillations did not interfere with the function of the CMS-445 stimulator, and the stimulator was successfully reprogrammed to the usual regimen 3 days thereafter. The patient was discharged from the hospital in a satisfactory condition.

One of 28 patients discharged from the hospital died 2 months after operation with advanced cardiac failure. The remaining patients, at 1.5 to 2 months after cardiomyoplasty, showed signs of improvement, including the decrease in the dyspneic symptoms and improved of functional status to functional Class I to II.

Maximal level of exercise increased by 30 to 40 W (in four patients by 100 W). Ischemic heart disease patients showed decreased or disappearance of anginal attacks, and a decreased dose of antianginal and cardiotropic drugs required. Ejection fractions increased by an average of 12% as assessed by ultrasonography, and 14 of the 28 patients returned to their jobs. Four patients had episodes of decreased ventricular sensing by the CMS-445 stimulator 4 months after operation, resulting in asynchronous LD muscle and ventricular stimulation. This complication was overcome by reprogramming the sensitivity values of the CMS or additional implantation of endocardial electrodes into the right ventricle of two patients.

The results of contrast ventriculography in eight patients showed a tendency for improved hemodynamics, but were not consistent (Table 1). Pulmonary artery and right ventricular pressure tracings in three patients showed increased pressure by 5 to 7 mm Hg.

## Myocardial Scintigraphic Studies

Table 2 shows the dynamics of scintigraphic indices before and after cardiomyoplasty. The mean value at stable perfusion defect (SPD) zone did not change reliably, although in eight patients SPD volume decreased 2 to 3 weeks after operation; and in five patients SPD volume increased for more than 40%. In the follow-up period of 1 year, mean values of SPD did not change consistently, although individual analysis revealed decreased SPD values in four patients. Mean value of reversible perfusion defects (RPDs) was 11.4%. In the early postoperative period, RPD values consistently decreased (6.6%), and remained at this level during a long-term follow-up (Fig. 1). Myocardium/lung index remained stable with a tendency to increase.

**Table 1**
Hemodynamic Indices of LV Contractility in Patients Before and After CMP

| *No. Pts.* | *Follow-Up Period* | *EF* | *ESV** | *EDV*** | *EDP**** | *dP/dt* |
|---|---|---|---|---|---|---|
| 1 | 2 | 50/57 | 47/49 | 101/95 | 23/18 | 1700/1400 |
| 2 | 7 | 11/12 | 184/195 | 207/210 | 35/27 | 800/1100 |
| 3 | 12 | 62/65 | 39/31 | 107/89 | 11/11 | 1850/2000 |
| 4 | 12 | 13/24 | 191/187 | 220/215 | 31/22 | 700/900 |
| 5 | 18 | 40/44 | 87/105 | 150/161 | 30/33 | 1300/1000 |
| 6 | 18 | 12/13 | 121/118 | 138/136 | 35/24 | 1200/900 |
| 7 | 18 | 10/15 | 194/194 | 218/218 | 17/23 | 700/700 |
| 8 | 18 | 18/26 | 110/105 | 210/181 | 32/26 | 1000/900 |

*End-systolic volume (before and after CMP); **end-diastolic volume (before and after CMP); ***end-diastolic pressure (before and after CMP).

**Table 2**
Changes of Scintigraphic Indices Before and After CMP

| | *SPD%* | *RPD%* | *I M/L* |
|---|---|---|---|
| Before CMP | 31.3 ± 4.2 | 11.4 ± 2.6 | 1.58 ± 0.06 |
| After CMP | 28.0 ± 3.8 | 6.6 ± 1.8* | 1.72 ± 0.03* |
| 0.5–1 year after CMP | 26.1 ± 5.1 | 6.6 ± 1.6 | 1.81 ± 0.09 |

I M/L = index myocardium/lung; RPD = reversible perfusion defect; SPD = stable perfusion defect.
*$p < 0.05$ compared with preoperative indices.

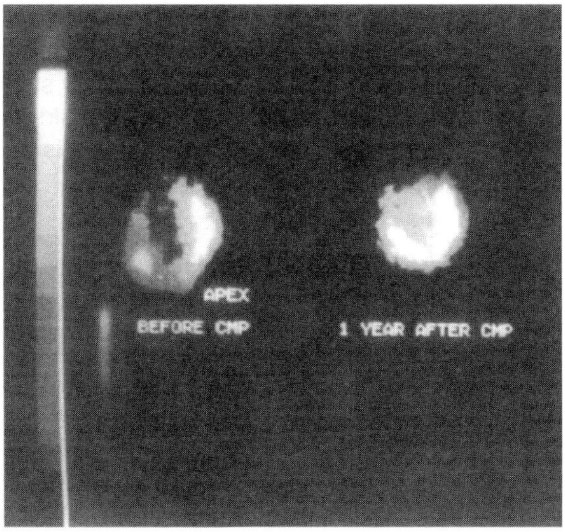


**Figure 1:** *Dynamic scintigraphy with T1-199 in a patient with dilated cardiomyopathy. One year after cardiomyoplasty, the volume of left ventricular cavity decreased and perfusion defects disappeared.*

We suspect that the decrease in the size of the myocardial perfusion defect zone could be due to the effect of indirect myocardial revascularization described below.

## Selective Angiography of the Thoracodorsal Artery

Selective angiograms of the left subclavian artery showed well-developed branches of thoracodorsal arteries that surround the contours of the heart in a circular manner. Twisted vessels 0.3 mm in diameter were seen in the region of muscle-to-myocardium interface and they were not the direct extension of thoracodorsal artery branches (Fig. 2A, B). Thus, selective arteriography demonstrated the formation of new vascular anastomoses between the thoracodorsal artery and the myocardial vessels. To confirm that myocardial perfusion came from the thoracodorsal artery, we injected radioisotopes into this artery and took blood samples from the coronary sinus for a 30-second period for radiometric studies. Two activity peaks were revealed (Fig. 3). The first peak was at 10 to 12 seconds, and the second at 22 to 24 seconds after injections. Three patients without cardiomyoplasty (controls) revealed only one activity peak at 20 seconds. Thus, the cardiomyoplasty patients demonstrated direct blood flow from the thoracodorsal artery into the myocardium.

## Removal of Cardiomyostimulators

We had to remove the CMS from five patients. Two had infectious complications after 6 and 11 months, respectively, and two had erosion of the CMS 8

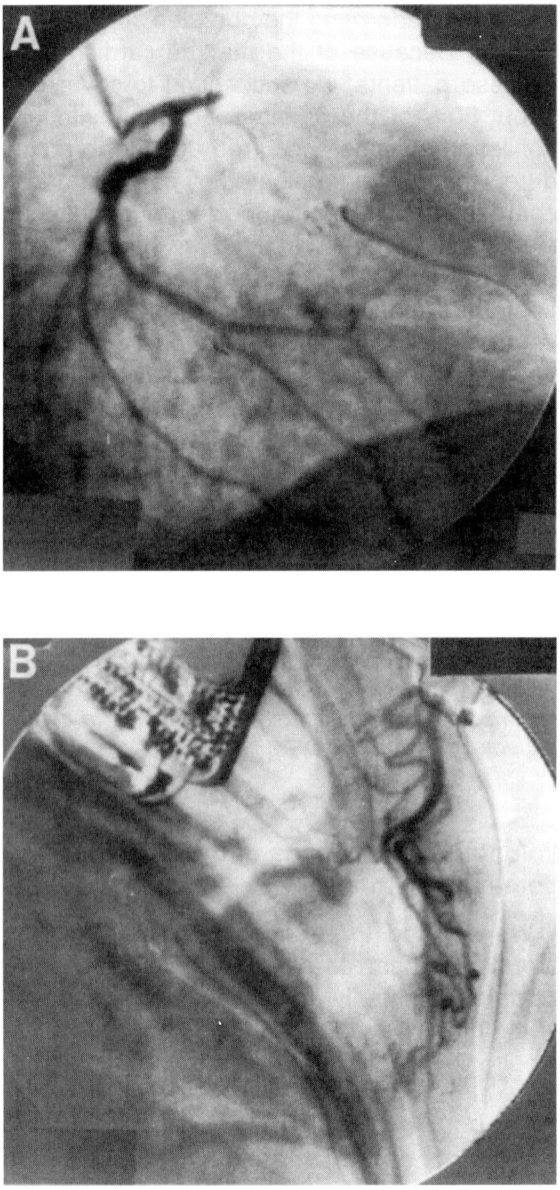

**Figure 2:** *Ischemic heart disease patient 1 year after cardiomyoplasty. (**A**) Occlusion of the anterior descending coronary artery seen on the coronarogram. A spiral myocardial electrode can be seen. (**B**) Thoracodorsal arterial angiogram revealed a broad vascular network, which covers the anterior wall and apex of the heart, while there is no visible blood flow in the anterior descending coronary artery.*

and 12 months postoperatively. Another patient had a breakage of a muscular electrode. We noted that all of these patients had deterioration of their clinical status after the removal of the CMS. Their dyspnea increased and angina pectoris reappeared. In these patients, the thoracodorsal artery was less developed in size than in those patients with a functioning CMS as assessed by ventricu-

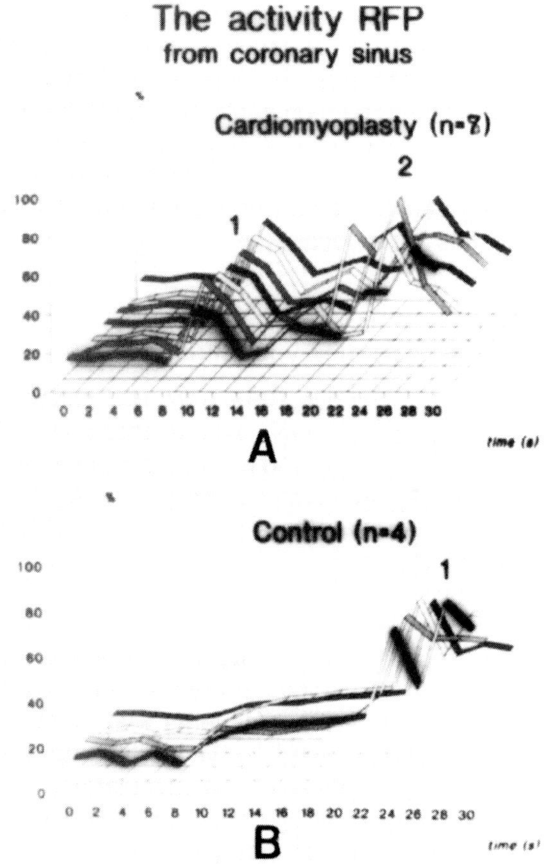


**Figure 3:** *Curves of isotope radioactivity in the blood obtained from the coronary sinus after the isotopes were injected into the thoracodorsal artery. (**A**) The first radioactive peak is recorded at 10 to 12 seconds after injection, and the second peak at 22 to 24 seconds in cardiomyoplasty patients. (**B**) In control patients, only the late peak is apparent.*

lography 6 months after removal of the stimulators and selective angiography of the thoracodorsal artery 1.5 years after cardiomyoplasty.

## Voluntary Contractions of the Latissimus Dorsi Muscle Graft

We decided to examine the LD muscle wrapped around the heart to see if it could be made to contract voluntarily, in response to commands of the brain. The LD muscle graft was punctured with monitoring electrodes, and rheomyosignals recorded using a technique described previously.[2] The patients were asked to initiate movements of the left hand and we were able to demonstrate that the LD muscle contracted not only in response to bursts of impulses originating from the stimulator, but to some active movements of the left hand as well. The amplitude and duration of the rheomyosignals recorded did not correspond to the strength and duration of the left hand movements.

Clearly, the possibility of voluntary contraction of such an innervated muscle pedicle graft should be taken into account even when the muscle is being stimulated by a CMS.

## Discussion

Our clinical experience with dynamic cardiomyoplasty is based on the treatment of 35 patients with ischemic and dilated cardiomyopathies who, according to our statistical data, are expected to live for about 1.5 to 2 years without operation. Based on our experience of 21 patients with the one-step and 14 patients with the two-step operations for cardiomyoplasty, we came to the conclusion that the two-step approach is more convenient for the surgeon. The latter allows the wrapping of the whole heart relatively easily and there is the possibility of carrying out concomitant coronary bypass surgery, as was done in six of our patients. Although three coronary bypass patients showed vein graft occlusion in the follow-up period, we suspect that these grafts played a positive role in decreasing the risk of acute myocardial infarction developing in the early postoperative period.

We were faced with certain technical difficulties while performing the one-step surgical procedure. Because of the marked cardiomegaly in these patients, we succeeded in covering only about 80% of the cardiac surface. Ventricular fibrillation episodes occurred during the procedure that were terminated by defibrillator discharges in six patients. Short-term manual cardiac massage was required in three patients because of the fall of arterial pressure. Two patients had marked adhesions between the left ventricle and the pericardium, and lysis of adhesions was technically more difficult. Nevertheless, postoperatively, the one-step procedure was better tolerated, which might be explained by less operative trauma. All four patients who died in the first 3 to 4 days after operation from acute myocardial infarction were operated on using the two-step approach. However, long-term clinical results were not different regardless of which surgical approach was used.

Cardiomyoplasty patients showed first clinical signs of improvement approximately 1.5 to 2 months after operation. Angina and dyspnea decreased and the level of exercise increased. Ejection fraction increased by a mean of 10% in the follow-up period as assessed by ventriculography, ultrasound, and radioactive scans. We also noted that positive hemodynamic contribution of LD muscle contraction was demonstrated mostly when the ejection fraction was less than 25%. In the long-term follow-up, when the ejection fraction increased and was more than 25%, LD muscle contraction did not appear to have positive influence on cardiac hemodynamics.

The question of indirect revascularization of ischemic myocardium by muscle wrap is of particular interest. Selective angiograms of the thoracodorsal artery revealed not only its well defined, broadened branches covering the contours of the heart, but a large number of twisted vessels 0.3 mm in diameter that were clearly not the natural extension of the thoracodorsal arterial branches. Significant decrease of perfusion defects in the myocardium and early detection of radioactivity in the coronary sinus following the injection of radioactive isotopes into the thoracodorsal artery not only confirmed the new vascularization across the skeletal muscle-myocardial interface, but also the direct blood flow from the muscle toward the myocardium. We suspect that electrical stimulation of the LD muscle which causes it to contract produces a positive pressure gradient, facilitating the blood flow from the muscle into the myocardium.

Cessation of electrical stimulation of the LD muscle led to gradual atrophy of the muscle and obliteration of newly formed vessels. We believe this is why such patients developed angina and dyspnea again after the removal of the CMS. The fact that myocardial indirect revascularization can be achieved with cardiomyoplasty should be taken into account when choosing surgical treatments for patients with ischemic heart disease, when there are distal coronary arterial occlusions and reasonable ejection fraction, which made the efficacy of routine coronary bypass surgery questionable.

Thus, dynamic cardiomyoplasty improves the clinical course of patients with ischemic and dilated cardiomyopathies, reverses heart failure symptoms, and is able to revascularize ischemic myocardium.[3–6]

## References

1. Akhmedov SD, Krivoschekov EV, Pekarskaya MV, Krylov AL, et al. Clinical results of dynamic cardiomyoplasty. *J Cardiac Surg* 10:573–579, 1995.
2. Pekarski VV, Akhmedov SD, Dubrovsky IA, et al: Optimal electrical stimulation for latissimus dorsi muscle after cardiomyoplasty. *J Cardiac Surg* 8:184, 1993.
3. Chiu RCJ, Bourgeois IM (eds): *Transformed Muscle for Cardiac Assist and Repair*. Mount Kisco, NY, Futura Publishing Co., 1990.
4. Carpentier A, Chachques JC, Grandjean P (eds): *Cardiomyoplasty*. Mount Kisco, NY, Futura Publishing Co., 1991.
5. Lorusso R, Zogno M, La Canna G, et al: Dynamic cardiomyoplasty as an effective therapy for dilated cardiomyopathy. *J Cardiac Surg* 8:177, 1993.
6. Stephenson L: Skeletal muscle ventricles in circulation. *Eur JCPE* 2:2, 1992.

Chapter 12

# Experience with Isolated Cardiomyoplasty in Patients with Contraindications for Heart Transplantation

Rüdiger Lange, Falk-Udo Sack, Siegfried Hagl*

## Introduction

The method of dynamic cardiomyoplasty was first applied clinically by Carpentier and Chachques in 1985. Since then, more than 400 cases have been performed worldwide. Some controlled clinical trials could show the efficacy of this procedure.[1,2] However, in all studies, a marked discrepancy between the subjective condition of the patient and the measurable hemodynamic improvement is evident. This discrepancy was also obvious when the data from the phase II multicenter clinical trial were analyzed.[3] Furthermore, the results of some studies were not conclusive because cardiomyoplasty was combined with reconstructing surgical procedures, such as left ventricular aneurysmectomy, valve replacement, or myocardial revascularization with the use of extracorporeal circulation. In those patients, it cannot be differentiated whether a postoperative hemodynamic improvement may be attributed to the latissimus dorsi contraction or to the surgical repair of the associated cardiac defect. Therefore, we intended to investigate the efficacy of dynamic cardiomyoplasty in a homogeneous group of patients with ischemic or dilated cardiomyopathy. All patients were required to have contraindications for heart transplantation. Until further experience has been gained about the hemodynamic efficacy and long-term outcome of cardiomyoplasty, this procedure cannot be considered an alternative to heart transplantation.

*With the cooperation of Werner Saggau, Raffaele De Simone, Angelique Nair, Manfred Heinen, Martin Grunze, Johannes Brachmann, Ranier Haussmann, and Franz Fleischer.

From Carpentier A, Chachques JC, Grandjean P: Cardiac Bioassist. © Futura Publishing Co, Inc, Armonk, NY, 1997.

## Material and Methods

Between August 1990 and July 1992, six patients suffering from end-stage cardiomyopathy were operated on. All patients were in NYHA Class III prior to the operation and had suffered from one or more periods of cardiac decompensation. The diagnosis was dilated cardiomyopathy in three and ischemic cardiomyopathy in three patients. The operation date, age, diagnosis, NYHA status, and preoperative ejection fraction (angio) are shown in Table 1. All patients had contraindications for heart transplantation (Table 2). These consisted of chronic infections, severe sequelae of diabetes mellitus, or alcohol abuse. Before the operation, the following examinations were performed:

- Pulmonary function test (forced vital capacity = FVC [L], forced expiratory volume in 1 s = $FEV_1$ [L/sec], $FEV_1$/FVC, airway resistance = $R_{tot}$ [L/kpa × sec]);
- Treadmill-exercise test with a modified Naughton-protocol[4] (max. exercise capacity [watt], max. oxygen consumption [mL/min × kg]);
- Transthoracic Doppler-echocardiography (fractional shortening, peak aortic flow) (Aloka SSD 870 color-Doppler, Hellige, Freiburg, Germany, 2.5 MHz probe, Aloka UST-5226-2.5/2). End-diastolic (EDD, mm) and end-systolic (ESD, mm) ventricular dimensions were assessed with M-mode echocardiography at the level of the cordae tendineae at the parasternal position. Fractional shortening of the LV (FS, %) was calculated with the following formula:

$$FS\% = \frac{EDD - ESD}{EDD} \times 100$$

Blood flow velocity in the left ventricular outflow tract (Vmax aorta, m/sec) was determined using continuous wave (CW) and pulsed wave (PW) Doppler. Isovolumetric relaxation time (IRT, msec) was measured by positioning the CW Doppler between the outflow and the inflow tract of the mitral valve. The time between the end of the outflow curve and the onset of the inflow curve was defined as isovolumetric relaxation time.

- Right heart catheterization with supine bicycle exercise (cardiac index by thermodilution, pulmonary artery pressure). Values shown for "exercise" are the last determination before exercise was stopped because of exhaustion.

**Table 1**
Operation Date, Age, Diagnosis, and NYHA Status

| *Patient* | *Op* | *Age* | *Diagnosis* | *NYHA Class* |
|---|---|---|---|---|
| M.H. | 8/90 | 60 | Dil.CMP | III–(IV) |
| N.L. | 3/91 | 56 | Isch.CMP | III–(IV) |
| Mö.H. | 3/91 | 36 | Dil.CMP | III–(IV) |
| G.H. | 4/91 | 52 | Dil.CMP | III–(IV) |
| K.H. | 1/92 | 67 | Isch.CMP | III–(IV) |
| W.N. | 7/92 | 56 | Isch.CMP | III–(IV) |

Dil.CMP = dilated cardiomyopathy; Isch.CMP = ischemic cardiomyopathy.

**Table 2**
Contraindications for Heart Transplantation

| *Patient* | *Contraindications for Heart Transplantation* |
|---|---|
| M.H. | IDDM, chronic diabetic gangrene, diabetic late complications |
| N.L. | IDDM, diabetic late complications, cerebral infarction, alcohol abuse |
| G.H. | chronic bronchitis, recurrent putride exacerbations |
| Mö.H. | IDDM, chronic osteomyelitis, pulmonary hypertension |
| K.H. | chronic osteomyelitis |
| W.N. | IDDM, peripheral occlusive disease, small vessel disease |

IDDM = insulin-dependent diabetes mellitus.

• Left heart catheterization (EF%). Determination of the EF was obtained using the RAO projection.

In principle, the operative technique was the one described by Carpentier and Chachques.[5] A posterior cardiocostal wrapping procedure was performed without the use of extracorporeal circulation in all cases.[6] As a minor modification of the Carpentier technique, we used 4-5 single, pledged 3-0 Prolene sutures to fix the latissimus dorsi muscle to the posterior wall of the left ventricle, which made repeated lifting of the heart necessary. A remaining part of the right anterior wall, which could not be covered by muscle tissue in some cases, was bridged with a pericardial flap in continuity with the right pericardium. The Cardiomyostimulator™ (Medtronic® SP 1005/1005 A) was implanted under the left M. rectus abdominis. For the postoperative stimulation protocol, we followed the guidelines by Carpentier and Chachques.[7] Three months after the operation, the latissimus dorsi was stimulated in all patients with a 185 ms, 30–33 Hz burst impulse in a 1:1 mode. The delay was set according to the echocardiographically determined closure of the mitral valve at 50 ms.

Every 6 months, the following examinations were repeated: lung function test, exercise test, right heart catheterization, left heart catheterization.

## Results

According to a surgical learning curve, the operative time (skin-to-skin) decreased with each procedure from an initial 420 min to 290 min. The time in the ICU and the time for required ventilatory support varied from 3 to 10 days and from 10 to 44 hours, respectively (Table 3). In-hospital stay varied from 16 to 27 days. One patient exhibited ventricular fibrillation early after the operation, which was successfully converted by electrical defibrillation and IV amiodarone. The same patient had been on mexiletine therapy prior to the operation. Two patients with ventricular ectopies were temporarily treated with IV xylocaine. All patients received inotropic support with dobutamine; in two patients low-dose norepinephrine was temporarily added. None of the patients exhibited a significant increase in the CK level. Immediately before the initiation of electrical muscle stimulation, all patients were fully mobilized and in relatively good condition. Six to 24 months following the operation, 2/6 patients

**Table 3**
Operative Time (skin-to-skin), Time Required for Ventilatory Support, and Time in ICU

| *Patient* | *Op (min)* | *Intubation (hr)* | *ICU (days)* | *Complications* |
|---|---|---|---|---|
| 1 | 420 | 22 | 7 | VT/Amiodarone |
| 2 | 400 | 10 | 3 | — |
| 3 | 360 | 44 | 3 | — |
| 4 | 315 | 14 | 3 | VES/Xylocaine |
| 5 | 315 | 11 | 3 | — |
| 6 | 290 | 23 | 10 | VES/Xylocaine |

One patient exhibited ventricular fibrillation early after the operation that was successfully converted by electrical defibrillation and IV amiodarone. Two patients with ventricular ectopies were temporarily treated with IV xylocaine. Op = operative time; VT = ventricular tachycardia; VES = ventricular extrasystoles.

were in NYHA Class I, 3/6 in Class II, and 1/6 in Class III. Three of six patients went back to work, 2/6 had already retired prior to the operation but would have been able to work, and 1/6 remained disabled (Table 4).

In one patient, pulmonary function at rest showed a decrease of FVC from 4.5 L prior to the operation to 3.5 L after the operation and in another patient, an increase in $FEV_1$ from 1.4 L/sec to 2.6 L/sec, and a decrease in $R_{tot}$ from 0.4 L/kpa × s to 0.2 L/kpa × s, respectively. In all other patients, FVC, $FEV_1$, $FEV_1$/FVC, and $R_{tot}$ did not change. The maximal exercise level (Watt) increased in all but one patient (Fig. 1), while the maximal $O_2$ consumption increased in only 4/6 patients (Fig. 2).

Right heart catheterization revealed no consistent change of cardiac index (CI) neither at rest nor during exercise when the preoperative values were compared with the postoperative values. Before the operation, the mean (±SD) CI was 2.5 ± 0.4 L/min/m$^2$ (at rest) and 3.6 ± 0.8 L/min/m$^2$ (during exercise) ($p<0.015$ rest vs. exercise). After the operation, the CI was 2.7 ± 0.5 L/min/m$^2$ (at rest) and 3.9 ± 1.4 L/min/m$^2$ (during exercise) ($p<0.015$), respectively. The values after the operation are the mean calculated from all 6-month interval determinations. They are not significantly different from the values before the operation, neither at rest nor during exercise. In contrast, resting systolic pulmonary artery pressure tended to decrease after the operation in four of six patients (Fig. 3). However, the mean decreased not significantly from 43.5 ± 25.2 mm Hg to 37.3 ± 22.4 mm Hg. The increase in pulmonary artery pressure during exercise remained pathological after the operation but peak values were lower than before the operation.

Left ventricular ejection fraction increased considerably in one of six patients from a preoperative value of 29.9% to a postoperative value of 69.3% (last determination). This striking increase was not found in the other patients. However, except for one, all other patients exhibited a moderate increase in left ventricular ejection fraction (LVEF) (Fig. 4). The mean for all six patients increased from 20.5 ± 5.3% to 37.9 ± 17.1% (mean value of all postoperative measurements, $p<0.03$). Since the increase to almost normal values in one patient is not typical for cardiomyoplasty, we calculated the mean change in LVEF again based on the other five patients. For these five patients, LVEF increased

**Table 4**
Patient Status*

| Patient | NYHA Class pre | | NYHA Class post | State of Employment pre | | State of Employment post |
|---|---|---|---|---|---|---|
| M.H. | III | → | I | disabled | → | housekeeper |
| N.L. | III | → | II | " | → | secretary |
| Mö.H. | III | → | III | " | → | disabled |
| G.H. | III | → | I | " | → | truck driver |
| K.H. | III | → | II | " | → | retired |
| W.N. | III | → | II | " | → | retired |

*6–24 months following the operation, 2/6 patients are in NYHA Class I, 3/6 in Class II, and 1/6 in Class III. 3/6 patients went back to work, 2/6 had retired prior to the operation, but would have been able to work, and 1/6 continued to be disabled.

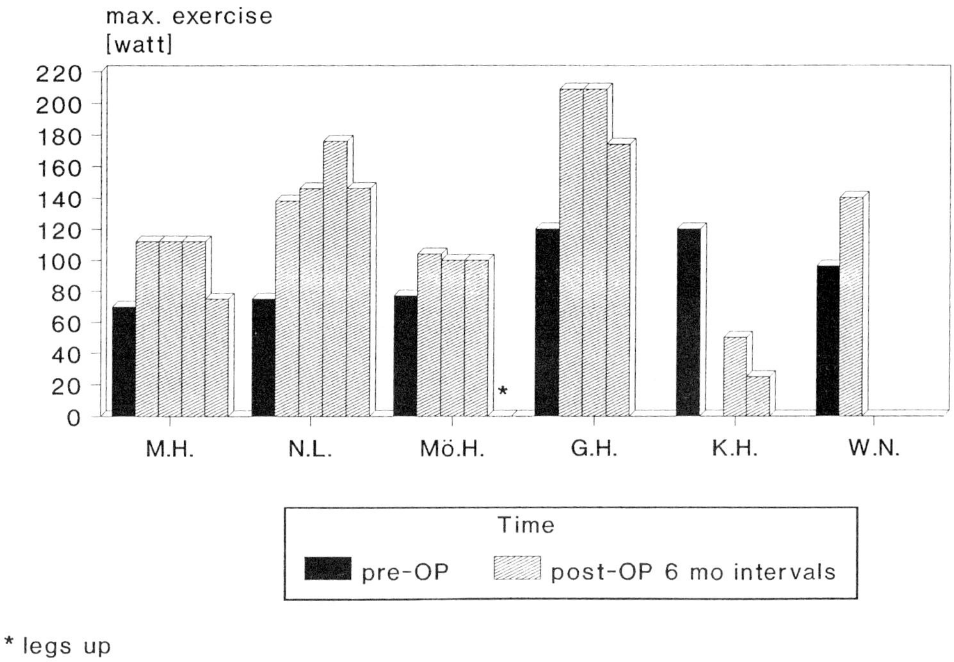


**Figure 1:** *Maximal exercise level (Watt).*

from 18.6 ± 2.8% to 33.0 ± 10.5% ($p$<0.02). A typical example of a postoperative angiogram with the stimulator turned off and on is shown in Figure 5. In this example, ventricular wall motion is enhanced by skeletal muscle contraction primarily at the antero- and posterobasal, as well as at the diaphragmatic level of the left ventricle. The contribution to the anterolateral and apical wall motion is only small. In this example EF increased from 13% to 39%.

The echocardiographically determined end-diastolic diameter showed no change when values before the operation and after 1 year were compared

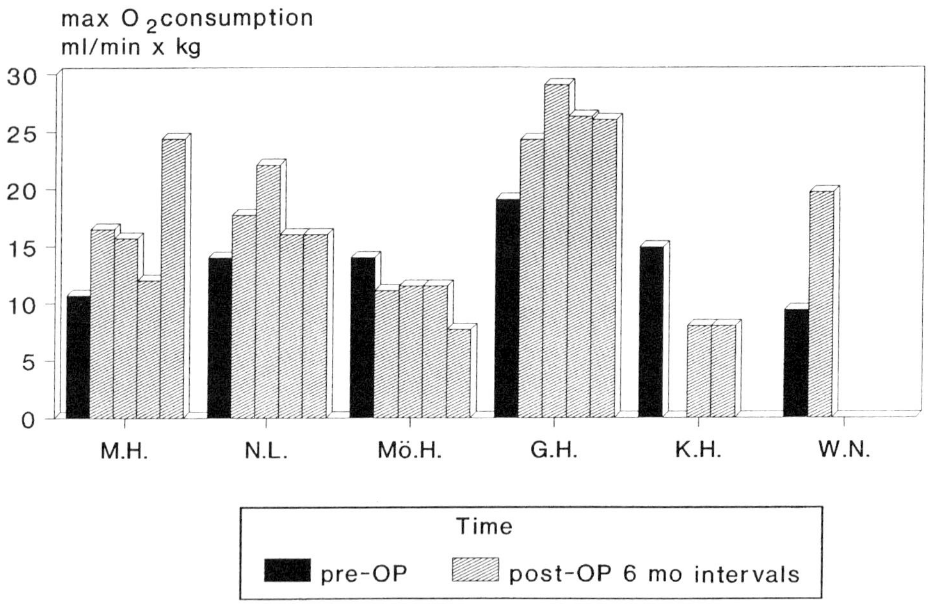


**Figure 2:** *Maximal $O_2$ consumption.*

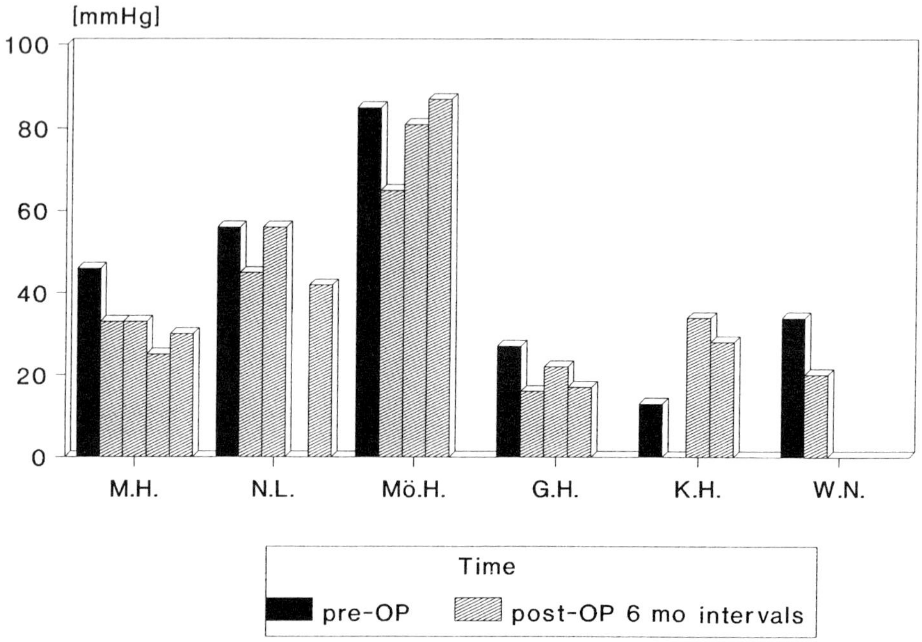


**Figure 3:** *Systolic pulmonary artery pressure.*

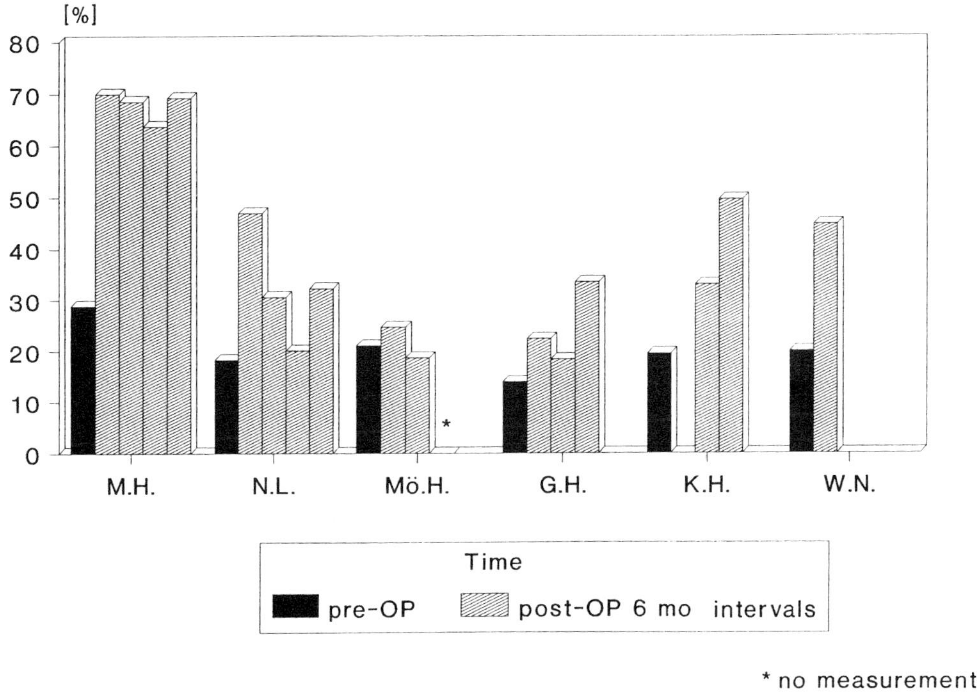


**Figure 4:** *EF (LV angiography).*

(Table 5). However, end-systolic diameter decreased in all patients and fractional shortening increased. The isovolumic relaxation time did not change.

All patients could be stimulated according to the protocol. An increase of the burst amplitude was necessary in all patients during the first months after the operation. In addition, the sensitivity of the Cardiomyostimulator™ had to be adjusted in some patients when the postoperative ECG showed that either ectopic beats were incorrectly accompanied by a burst or that burst impulses occurred in the ECG without a triggering QRS complex. Beyond 3 months after the operation, all patients were stimulated in a 1:1 mode, with a burst frequency of 30 or 33 Hz (according to six impulses in the burst), respectively, with a delay time of 50 ms and an amplitude ranging from 3.5 to 7.0 V.

## Discussion

Cardiomyoplasty was conceived as a new surgical method to treat end-stage heart failure. In the presence of increasing donor organ shortage and still unsolved problems with the long-term application of mechanical assist devices, there would be a place for cardiomyoplasty as an additional treatment option. However, even 8 years after its first introduction, it remains difficult to yield objective and consistent evidence of the efficacy of this method in regard to improved performance of the heart/skeletal muscle complex.[8] One reason for this lack of convincing hemodynamic data might be the nonhomogeneous patient

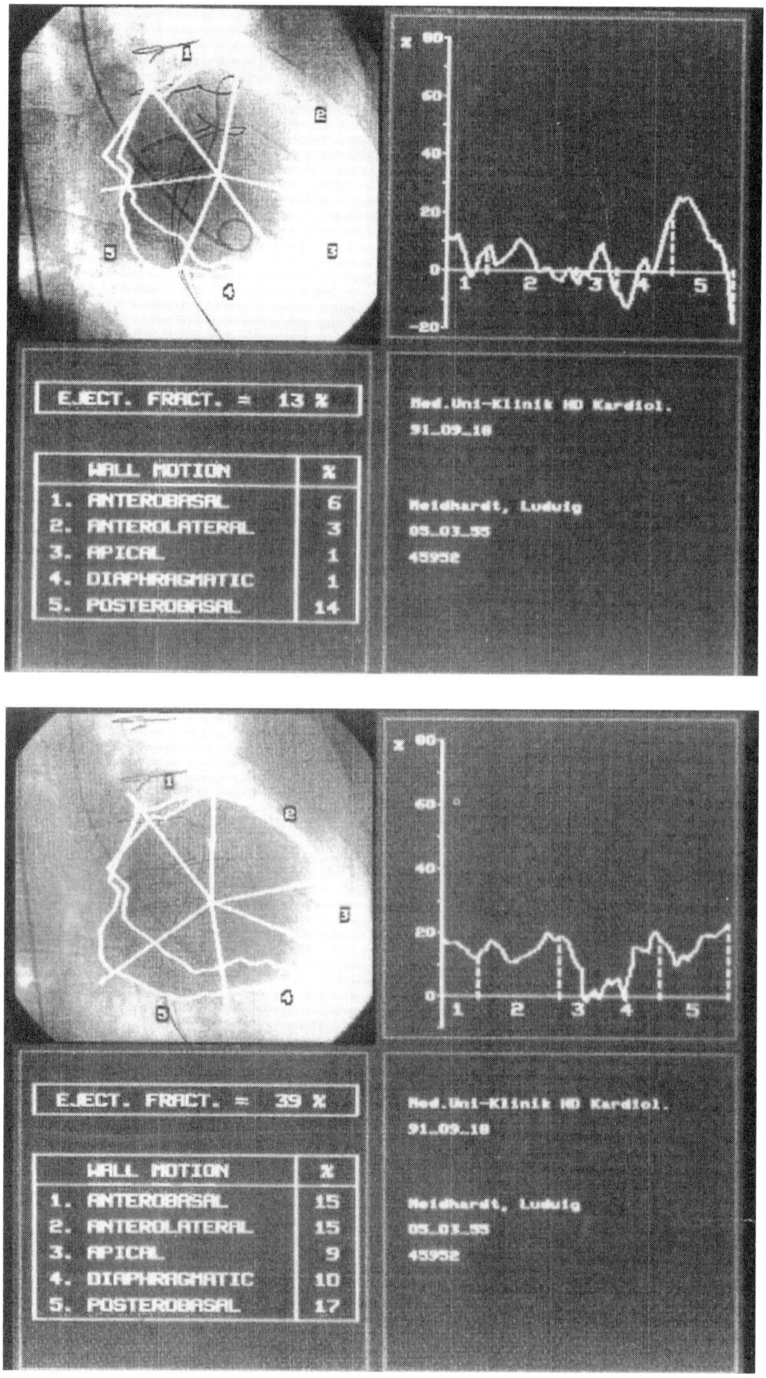


**Figure 5:** *Example of a postoperative angiogram with the stimulator turned off and on. Ventricular wall motion is enhanced by skeletal muscle contraction primarily at the antero- and posterobasal, as well as the diaphragmatic level of the left ventricle. The contribution to the anterolateral and apical wall motion is only small. In this example, EF increased from 13% to 39%.*

**Table 5**
Echocardiographically Determined End-Diastolic and End-Systolic Diameter and Fractional Shortening

| | | M-Mode | | |
|---|---|---|---|---|
| | | *EDD mm* | *ESD mm* | *FS %* |
| M.H. | pre | 65 | 55 | 15 |
| | post | 63 | 48 | 32 |
| N.L. | pre | 76 | 66 | 13 |
| | post | 77 | 56 | 27 |
| Mö.H. | pre | 69 | 59 | 14 |
| | post | 67 | 50 | 25 |
| G.H. | pre | 73 | 64 | 12 |
| | post | 74 | 58 | 22 |
| W.N. | pre | 64 | 50 | 21 |
| | post | 66 | 49 | 25 |
| K.H. | pre | 65 | 50 | 15 |
| | post | 64 | 45 | 29 |

EDD = end-diastolic dimension; ESD = end-systolic dimension; FS = fractional shortening.

populations receiving cardiomyoplasty: patients in different preoperative conditions presenting with a variety of heart diseases were operated on in various centers by different surgeons with probable modifications of the technique. More than 20% of the patients even underwent associated reconstructive cardiac procedures, such as valve replacement or aneurysmectomy, requiring cardiopulmonary bypass.[2,9,10] This makes the differentiation between the hemodynamic effect of cardiomyoplasty and the associated cardiac repair impossible. Some centers used single impulse stimulation instead of burst stimulation for the skeletal muscle,[11,12] although experimental studies by Dewar and Chiu had shown as early as 1984 that a significant augmentation of left ventricular function is achieved only by burst stimulation of the skeletal muscle.[13] Furthermore, the hemodynamic results of patients with complete muscle wrap were analyzed together with those who had only a partial "substitution cardiomyoplasty"[7] following left ventricular aneurysmectomy.[14]

Another reason why cardiomyoplasty is only hesitatingly accepted might be the high operative and long-term mortality that was reported in the beginning of the clinical experience.[2] More recently, the operative mortality lies between 0% and 23%.[15–21] The operative mortality is reported to be due to myocardial failure, hemorrhage, sepsis, pulmonary infection, multiorgan failure, or arrhythmia.[8,22] The strongest determinant for the postoperative mortality is the proper patient selection.[21] Factors such as the surgical technique and/or the adequacy of perioperative management[23–25] might also play a role. At our center, extensive animal studies had been performed before the clinical series was begun.[26–31] This deepened the pathophysiological understanding of the procedure and improved the technique of wrapping and harvesting the muscle. Postoperatively, the patients are closely followed and treated by a highly dedicated team of surgeons and anesthesiologists. Although our series of six patients is small, we think that these factors might have contributed to the primary success.

After a mean follow-up period of 26.7 ± 8.2 months, the midterm survival in our series is also 100%. Overlooking a much larger patient population of 28 patients, the Sao Paulo group reported most recently about an excellent 1-year survival of 80%.[16] Carpentier reported that long-term survival of 59 patients was 74% after a mean follow-up period of 26 months (2 months to 8 years).[32] Others report about a 1-year actuarial survival of 58% (n = 45)[32] and 68% (n = 13).[22] The 4-year actuarial survival in the Brazil study group was 40.8%. In order to establish cardiomyoplasty as a treatment option for end-stage heart failure, survival following cardiomyoplasty should be regarded in respect to already established treatment methods for end-stage heart failure, such as heart transplantation and medical therapy. At our institution, patients who undergo cardiomyoplasty fulfill all criteria of the indication for heart transplantation, except for the fact that they present with extracardiac contraindications that preclude transplantation. Survival after heart transplantation, according to the 1992 registry report by the International Society for Heart and Lung Transplantation, is 79.1% at 1 year, 67.8% at 5 years, and 55.8% at 10 years[33] and thus considerably better than following cardiomyoplasty. In the Consensus study, the mortality of patients with congestive heart failure was compared in a double-blind trial.[34] One group received a placebo with conventional treatment and the other group received enalapril beyond conventional treatment. One-year survival was 48% in the placebo group and 64% in the enalapril group, respectively. No measurements of cardiac function were reported for the Consensus study patients, who were required to be in NYHA Class IV, defined as having symptoms of dyspnea, fatigue, or fluid retention. However, since ACE inhibitors are regarded as the current "gold-standard" in the medical treatment of congestive heart failure, it may still be concluded that survival following cardiomyoplasty is considerably better, at least in the hands of experienced centers. Furthermore, quality of life is reported to be noticeably improved after cardiomyoplasty, whereas no mention is found in the Consensus study about this issue.

To date, the cardiomyoplasty procedure is performed in many different centers, most of which perform only very few operations. Therefore, the results are significantly affected by differences in preoperative patient condition, indication, surgical technique, postoperative care, and experience. The survival data from the Sao Paulo group and from Carpentier in Paris suggest that the best results may be achieved when a large group of patients is treated at one center. Otherwise, the operative success is strongly affected by few unfavorable outcomes. Some preoperative risk factors associated with increased operative and midterm mortality have been identified.[21,32] These include atrial fibrillation, severely increased pulmonary artery pressure, very low ejection fraction of the right ventricle, left ventricular ejection fraction below 15%, and preoperative functional Class IV. Avoiding these risk factors may help in the future to decrease mortality of the cardiomyoplasty procedure. In our series there were no cases with atrial fibrillation or preoperative Class IV. All patients had predominant left ventricular failure, except one patient with consecutive right ventricular failure whose systolic pulmonary artery pressure was 85 mm Hg before the operation. This patient did not improve after cardiomyoplasty. This one case may support the suggestion by Carpentier to consider severe right ventricular compromise and severely increased pulmonary artery pressure as a risk factor. A recent analysis of the phase II study patients by the Dynamic Cardiomyoplasty Study Group also emphasizes the importance of the proper indication for this procedure.[3] Following cardiomyoplasty, 47 patients were divided into two groups according to score. One group of patients had less advanced disease with a lower incidence of symptomatic arrhythmia and better aerobic capacity prior to the operation than the other group. Analysis of the results showed that the patients with less advanced cardiac symptoms benefited more from cardiomyoplasty. This group of patients exhibited an increase of left ventricular ejection fraction from 23% to 30%, of left ventricular stroke work index from 28.7 gm/m$^2$/beat to 37.6 gm/m$^2$/beat and of peak oxygen uptake from 17.6 mL/min/kg to 20.5 mL/min/kg, respectively. The mean NYHA functional class improved in this group from 3.0 before the operation to 1.6 after the procedure. In the other group, left ventricular ejection fraction and left ventricular stroke work index did not change significantly; NYHA class changed from 3.1 prior to the operation to 2.0 after the procedure. Hence, these data suggest that there may be a meaningful clinical improvement following cardiomyoplasty, if the indication is carefully selected.

The expectations of the cardiologists and surgeons regarding the hemodynamic improvement following cardiomyoplasty might have been influenced by the hemodynamic results following heart transplantation. However, it is well known that patients may be functionally well compensated with an ejection fraction of just over 30%. However, their condition may rapidly deteriorate when the ejection fraction reaches values of around 20% or less. Therefore, the increase in ejection fraction in our series (from 18.6 $\pm$ 2.8% to 33.0 $\pm$ 10.5%) and in the Brazil study patients (from 20 $\pm$ 2% to 25 $\pm$ 5% at 1 year)[16] may explain the improvement in NYHA class functional status and maximal exercise capacity. Furthermore, we observed a trend for the systolic pulmonary artery pressure to fall after cardiomyoplasty. In the Brazil study patients, there was a significant fall in the pulmonary capillary wedge pressure from 26 $\pm$ 5 mm Hg to 16 $\pm$ 4 mm Hg at 1 year.[16] The heart may work at a reduced preload following cardiomyoplasty, suggesting improved contractility in spite of no concomitant change in cardiac index.

Although only moderate hemodynamic changes are observed following cardiomyoplasty, there is a significant and consistently reported improvement in quality of life. However, patients remain on their cardiac medication and their exercise capacity is reduced. Following heart transplantation, quality of life is reported to be excellent and exercise capacity dramatically improved.[35] However, the resources for transplantation are limited and no improvement is invisible. In Germany, approximately 30% of the patients on the waiting list die before a proper donor organ is found.[36] Hence, by direct comparison, cardiomyoplasty is not an alternative treatment to heart transplantation but may become an option in patients with contraindication for transplantation or as a "bridge to transplantation." Because of the need for an additional surgical method to treat end-stage heart failure and in light of favorable recent results with cardiomyoplasty at some centers, the question arises of which factors prevent a more widespread application of cardiomyoplasty. One limiting factor might be the lack of information about this procedure among cardiologists and surgeons. Others might be confused by controversial data or even advised that cardiomyoplasty is hemodynamically ineffective,[37] impairs ventricular filling,[38,39] or must fail because of progressive skeletal muscle structural decay.[40] However, these are results of experimental studies that, to our knowledge, could never be reproduced in patients. We could show in our experimental laboratory that chronic electrical stimulation of a skeletal muscle with burst impulses per se does not lead to structural damage.[41] Clinically, a structurally well-preserved and functioning latissimus dorsi was found in a patient who underwent heart transplantation 9 months after cardiomyoplasty.[42] Furthermore, impaired diastolic ventricular function has never been shown in patients. Based on the limited experience, one might summarize that cardiomyoplasty has been shown to improve quality of life, survival, and hemodynamic function, although the latter is less pronounced than initially expected. In the hands of experienced surgeons, cardiomyoplasty is performed with a low mortality rate. A clear definition of the indication and the risk factors for this procedure is mandatory. A constructive discussion about this important issue has been initiated by Carpentier and Magovern[10,19,32] and may help to further improve the results. In addition, we believe that more emphasis should focus on the surgical technique and the perioperative management, especially when new centers start their initial experience. In order to achieve more consistent results, it would be preferable to have fewer experienced centers perform more operations instead of the current trend that more surgeons start a procedure in a state when the efficacy of the method has yet to be proven.

## References

1. Moreira LF, Bocchi EA, Stolf NA, et al: Current expectations in dynamic cardiomyoplasty. *Ann Thorac Surg* 55:299–303, 1993.
2. Carpentier A, Chachques JC: Clinical dynamic cardiomyoplasty: Method and outcome. In Loop FD, Magovern GJ (eds): *Seminars in Thoracic and Cardiovascular Surgery,* Vol. 3, No. 2., Philadelphia, W. B. Saunders, 1991, p 136.
3. Medtronic Inc: Phase II Clinical Results. 1993.
4. Naughton J: *Exercise Testing: Physiological, Biochemical and Clinical Principles.* Mount Kisco, NY, Futura Publishing Co, 1988.
5. Carpentier A, Chachques JC: The use of stimulated skeletal muscle to replace diseased human heart muscle. In Chiu RC-J (ed): *Biomechanical Cardiac Assist.* Mount Kisco, NY, Futura Publishing Co, 1986, p 85.
6. Furnary AP, Christlieb IY, Magovern JA, et al: A standardized nomenclature for latissimus dorsi cardiomyoplasty. *J Card Surg* 6(Suppl):74, 1991.
7. Chachques JC, Grandjean PA, Carpentier A: Latissimus dorsi dynamic cardiomyoplasty. *Ann Thorac Surg* 47:600, 1989.
8. Medtronic Inc: Phase I Clinical Results: Dynamic Cardiomyoplasty System: SP1005 Cardiomyostimulator(TM) Pulse Generator; SP5528 Intramuscular Lead. 1992.
9. Chachques JC, Grandjean PA, Nataf P, et al: Dynamic cardiomyoplasty: A surgical approach for ventricular assistance. *Int J Artif Organs* 11:469, 1988.
10. Magovern JA, Furnary AP, Christlieb IY, Kao RL, et al: Indications and risk analysis for clinical cardiomyoplasty. In Loop FD, Magovern GJ (eds): *Seminars in Thoracic and Cardiovascular Surgery,* Vol. 3, No. 2., Philadelphia, W.B. Saunders, 1991, p 145.
11. Almada H, Molteni L, Ferreira R, et al: Clinical experience with dynamic cardiomyoplasty. *J Cardiac Surg* 5:193, 1990.

12. Magovern GJ, Heckler FR, Park SB, et al: Paced latissimus dorsi used for dynamic cardiomyoplasty of left ventricular aneurysms. *Ann Thorac Surg* 44:379, 1987.
13. Dewar M, Drinkwater DC, Wittnich C, et al: Synchronously stimulated skeletal muscle graft for myocardial repair. *J Thorac Cardiovasc Surg* 87:325, 1984.
14. Magovern GJ, Park SB, Kao RL, et al: Dynamic cardiomyoplasty in patients. *J Heart Transplant* 9:258, 1990.
15. Odim JNK, Burgess JH, Chiu RC-J: Dynamic cardiomyoplasty: The extent of biventricular coverage on outcome. *World Symposium on Cardiomyoplasty, Biomechanical Assist and Artificial Heart,* Paris, France, May 24–26, p 42, 1993 (abstract).
16. Moreira LF, Bocchi EA, Stolf NA, et al: Long-term clinical and hemodynamic improvement after cardiomyoplasty in patients with dilated cardiomyopathies. *World Symposium on Cardiomyoplasty, Biomechanical Assist and Artificial Heart,* Paris, France, May 24–26, p 46, 1993 (abstract).
17. Lorusso R, Sandrelli L, Borghetti V, et al: Long-term myocardial assistance by a wrapped skeletal muscle: A clinical experience. *World Symposium on Cardiomyoplasty, Biomechanical Assist and Artificial Heart,* Paris, France, May 24–26, p 30, 1993 (abstract).
18. Lange R, Saggau W, Sack F-U, et al: Dynamische Kardiomyoplastie: Untersuchungen zur Hämodynamik und Lungenfunktion. Jahrestagung der Deutschen Gesellschaft für Thorax-, Herz-und Gefäßchirurgie Bonn, 1992 (abstract).
19. Furnary A, Magovern JA, Swanson J, et al: Preoperative risk factors affecting survival after cardiomyoplasty: A multivariate analysis. *World Symposium on Cardiomyoplasty, Biomechanical Assist and Artificial Heart,* Paris, France, May 24–26, p 54, 1993 (abstract).
20. Bors V, Dorent R, Jault F, et al: Dynamic cardiomyoplasty: One year experience. *World Symposium on Cardiomyoplasty, Biomechanical Assist and Artificial Heart,* Paris, France, May 24–26, p 34, 1993 (abstract).
21. Furnary AP, Magovern JA, Christlieb IY, et al: Clinical cardiomyoplasty: Preoperative factors associated with outcome. *Ann Thorac Surg* 54:1139, 1992.
22. Trehan H, Swanson J, Furnary A, et al: Clinical cardiomyoplasty: Analysis of results. *World Symposium on Cardiomyoplasty, Biomechanical Assist and Artificial Heart,* Paris, France, May 24–26, p 48, 1993 (abstract).
23. Chachques JC, Grandjean PA, Carpentier A: Patient management and clinical follow-up after cardiomyoplasty. *J Cardiac Surg* 6(Suppl):89, 1991.
24. Blanc P, Girard C, Vedrinne C, et al: Latissimus dorsi cardiomyoplasty: Perioperative management and postoperative evolution. *Chest* 103:214, 1993.
25. Auler JOC, Moreira LF, de Carvalho MJ, et al: Anesthetic management of patients undergoing cardiomyoplasty. *Anesthesiology* 77:379, 1992.
26. Lange R, Sack F-U, Saggau W, De Simone R, et al: Influence of cardiac function on the performance of the heart/skeletal muscle complex in dynamic cardiomyoplasty. In D'Alessandro LC (ed): *Heart Surgery 1991.* Rome, Casa Editrice Scientifica Internationale, 1991, p 559.
27. Lange R, Sack F-U, Saggau W, et al: Influence of cardiac function on the performance of the heart/skeletal muscle complex in dynamic cardiomyoplasty. *4th International Symposium on Cardiac Surgery,* Rome, Italy, May 28–31, 1991 (abstract).
28. Lange R, Sack F-U, Saggau W, et al: Effektivität der dynamischen Kardiomyoplastie in Abhängigkeit von Funktionszustand des unterstützten Herzens. Jahrestagung der Deutschen Gesellschaft für Thorax-, Herz- und Gefäßchirurgie Bonn 1991 (abstract).
29. Lange R, Sack F-U, Saggau W, et al: Performance of dynamic cardiomyoplasty related to the functional state of the heart. *J Cardiac Surg* 6(Suppl):225, 1991.
30. Lange R, Sack F-U, Saggau W, et al: Ventricular function and contraction pattern of cardiomyoplasty in canine hearts with left ventricular wall defects. *4th World Symposium on Transformed Skeletal Muscle for Cardiac Assist,* Oct 3–6 Palm Springs, CA, 1990 (abstract).
31. Sack F-U, Lange R, Saggau W, et al: Hemodynamic performance of cardiomyoplasty in the sufficient canine heart. *4th World Symposium on Transformed Skeletal Muscle for Cardiac Assist,* Oct 3–6 Palm Springs, CA, 1990 (abstract).

32. Carpentier A, Chachques JC, Acar C, et al: Dynamic cardiomyoplasty at eight years. *World Symposium on Cardiomyoplasty, Biomechanical Assist and Artificial Heart,* Paris, France, May 24–26, p 52, 1993 (abstract).
33. Kaye MP: The registry of the international society for heart and lung transplantation: Tenth official report, 1993. *J Heart Lung Transplant* 4:541, 1993.
34. Consensus Trial Study-Group: Effects of enalapril on mortality in severe congestive heart failure. *N Engl J Med* 316:1429, 1987.
35. Bunzel B, Grundböck A, Laczkovics A, et al: Quality of life after orthotopic heart transplantation. *J Heart Transplant* 10:455, 1991.
36. Schüler S, Warnecke H, Loebe M, et al: Extended donor age in cardiac transplantation. *Circulation* 80(Suppl III):III–133, 1989.
37. Anderson WA, Andersen JS, Acker MA, et al: Skeletal muscle grafts applied to the heart: A word of caution. *Circulation* 78(Suppl III):III–180, 1988.
38. Cheng W, Sobermann MS, Justica AG, et al: Dynamic cardiomyoplasty on left ventricular systolic and diastolic functions in a canine model of chronic heart failure. *Surg Forum* 41:260, 1990.
39. Corin WJ, George DT, Sink JD, et al: Dynamic cardiomyoplasty acutely impairs left ventricular diastolic function. *J Thorac Cardiovasc Surg* 104:1662, 1992.
40. Lucas CM, van der Veen E, Cheriex EC, et al: Long-term follow-up (12 to 35 weeks) after dynamic cardiomyoplasty. *J Am Coll Cardiol* 22:758, 1993.
41. Lange R, Nair A, Sack F-U, et al: Biomechanical support of the heart: Does chronic electrical stimulation damage the skeletal muscle? *23rd Annual Meeting of the German Society for Thoracic and Cardiovascular Surgery,* Bonn, February 16–19, 1994 (abstract).
42. Jegaden O, Delahaye F, Montagna P, et al: Cardiomyoplasty does not preclude heart transplantation. *Ann Thorac Surg* 53:875, 1992.

# Chapter 12

# *Discussion*

**Dr. El Kaim (Los Angeles):** As a cardiologist, I have been listening to these presentations. This is the first time that I have been exposed to this technique. It sounds exciting but it all comes across as quite confusing. The results are variable: some patients do better, some do worse, some die. Also, nobody took the time and the effort to have a control group, and I wonder why it is not possible to compare this technique to either medical therapy, if you consider this as an alternative to medical therapy, or to transplantation. Dr. Carpentier said that this technique may be indicated for patients who are awaiting cardiac transplantation.

**Dr. Stolf:** Randomization is one way to approach the answer for the definitive benefits of cardiomyoplasty. The other way is to have large series compared with medical therapy. What is controversial, from the presentation, is the objective demonstration of ventricular function improvement. So these issues have to be addressed.

**Dr. Lange:** To answer your question: I think that, so far, we have dealt with an experimental technique. It may be the point of this meeting to establish the state of the art and perhaps to compare it to other techniques. But thus far, for ethical reasons, it was not possible to do a randomized trial against transplantation or against established methods of medical treatment.

**Dr. Carpentier:** Dr. Stolf, I know that you have made a sort of randomized study in your group. Can you talk about it?

**Dr. Stolf:** We compared two series of patients; from clinical and all the other parameters, they were comparable. They were not randomized but were comparable. In these two groups, medical therapy versus cardiomyoplasty, the survival rate was 100% better in the cardiomyoplasty group than in the medical therapy group. So I think there are two things to consider: one is the functional benefit of cardiomyoplasty compared to medical therapy, the other is influence on survival. The controversial point remains the objective demonstration of benefit on ventricular function.

**Dr. Mikaeloff (Lyon):** I think that from the learning curve we have had in the last 3 years and from the experience of Alain Carpentier, we have learned to have better indications, in order to decrease perioperative mortality and not lose too many patients in the first 2 years after surgery. Now, the indications are selective and unless we group together many centers, we will not be able to randomize, in a single city, two series of patients in a short time period. Do you agree, Dr. Carpentier?

**Dr. Carpentier:** This question has two answers, depending on the type of patients dealt with. There are patients in whom cardiomyoplasty is an alternative to cardiac transplantation or left ventricular assist devices and there are patients in whom cardiomyoplasty is the only surgical treatment because of contraindications to these two other procedures. Randomization is ethically correct for patients belonging to the first group but incorrect for patients belonging to the second group. I have heard all my professional life people advising randomized studies. It is not that simple in practice. Patients belonging to the second group are sent to us by their cardiologists because medical treatment has become inefficient with repeated bouts of pulmonary edema and so forth. Dr. El Kaim, you are a cardiologist, let us assume that you have such a patient whom you sent to me because you have exhausted all medical means. What would you think if I replied: "Your patient has been included in a randomized trial, I am sorry he did not get the right number." And what is your patient going to say? Most probably: "I will just go and see other specialists who are not ' "randomizers.' "

**Dr. Rebecca:** Just two more comments. If the patients who had the elevations of norepinephrine postprocedure were the ones who had been withdrawn from the ACE inhibitors, that would be encouraging. Also ACE inhibitors cause plasmarenin activity to be elevated, so if your plasmarenin activity went down, it could be explained by the negative feedback. The other comment I want to make is that since all of these studies have begun, there have been several major heart failure trials that have come out showing the benefits of using ACE inhibitors in asymptomatic LV dysfunction, so I would strongly encourage everyone to continue to use all of those medications with or without the procedure. Probably digitalis is very important because of its effect on hormones as well.

**Dr. Lorusso:** This is an outstanding experience and I will make a very brief comment: I saw the German experience and they have a patient who improved from a 30% ejection fraction to an almost 68% ejection fraction. I don't think such a result can be achieved with any kind of left ventricular assist device. Like Dr. Carpentier, we have patients who do not improve but we have patients who improve so much that we can't understand why. Since the technique improves some patients, this is the future direction of the technique. In the future, we should be able to understand why some muscles in some patients react in a way that they can do a lot of work and why in other patients they do almost nothing. This is something that is seen in athletic games. Only a few athletes perform in an outstanding way and I think this is the same in our field.

We have some muscles that react in a proper way to the stimulation protocol. The future direction will be to understand more of skeletal muscle physiology. If we improve skeletal muscle performance, we will have a better outcome.

**Dr. Carpentier:** The Olympic games for stimulated muscle are open and this session is closed. Thank you.

# Part II

## Ventricular Function

Chapter 13

# Beat-to-Beat Analysis of Left Ventricular PV Loops in Nine Cardiomyoplasty Patients

J. J. Schreuder, F. Delahaye, O. Jegaden, F.H. van der Veen

## Introduction

Since the introduction of cardiomyoplasty,[1] a discrepancy has been observed between improvements in clinical condition, on the one hand, judged by the New York Heart Association (NYHA) criteria and unchanged hemodynamic measurements in the same patient on the other. The absence of significant changes in cardiac output or ejection fraction in patients that show clinical improvement[2] may have several causes. First, inappropriate cardiomyostimulator settings can have a negative effect on cardiac function.[3] Second, cardiovascular compensatory mechanisms may counteract or mask effects of latissimus dorsi (LD) stimulation; when the heart as a pump is not the limiting factor in providing adequate organ perfusion, an increase in contractility will not result in an increase in cardiac output. Third, the resolution of the applied evaluation techniques may have been too small to observe changes of the measured variables.[4] Finally, it has been suggested by Chachques et al.[5] that active prevention of ventricular dilatation may be a major factor in clinical improvement.

## Methods

To evaluate these possibilities, the acute hemodynamic effects of LD muscle stimulation were studied in nine patients several months after the operation on a beat-to-beat basis. The conductance catheter technique, as introduced by Baan and co-workers,[6] was used to measure left ventricular pressure-volume (PV) relationships. Therefore, a conductance catheter and a catheter with two solid-state pressure transducers were introduced into the left ventricle. To validate conductance stroke volume (SV), SV was also estimated using the aortic

From Carpentier A, Chachques JC, Grandjean P: Cardiac Bioassist. © Futura Publishing Co, Inc, Armonk, NY, 1997.

model flow method according to Wesseling and co-workers.[7] This method computes SV from aortic pressure by a nonlinear time-varying three-element model of aortic impedance.

The study was performed in nine male patients, 53–69 years old, who had undergone dynamic cardiomyoplasty (CMP). All patients had dilated cardiomyopathy related to ischemia or to an idiopathic origin. At the time of the CMP, all patients were in NYHA Class III with a mean ejection fraction (EF) of 22%. Every individual stimulator setting was examined during 15-second sample periods with breath-holding in order to prevent respiration-related changes in venous return and to exclude cardiovascular compensatory reflexes. The LD muscle was stimulated at a 1:2 ratio for 10 seconds followed by a nonpaced period of 5 seconds. Two variables of the stimulator were changed: the synchronization delay was changed from 4 up to 125 ms, with increments of 25 ms. The stimulus strength was set at the patient's own clinical amplitude and at a maximal amplitude.

## Results

Figure 1 shows an example of a 15-second sample period with a 1:2 stimulated 10-second period at the patient's best stimulator setting, followed by a nonpaced 5-second period. The left ventricular volume tracing indicates an increased SV and an increased EF during the LD-stimulated beats.

In Figure 2 the PV relationships of the first two beats of the same recording are shown. The dotted line represents the unstimulated beat. Systolic

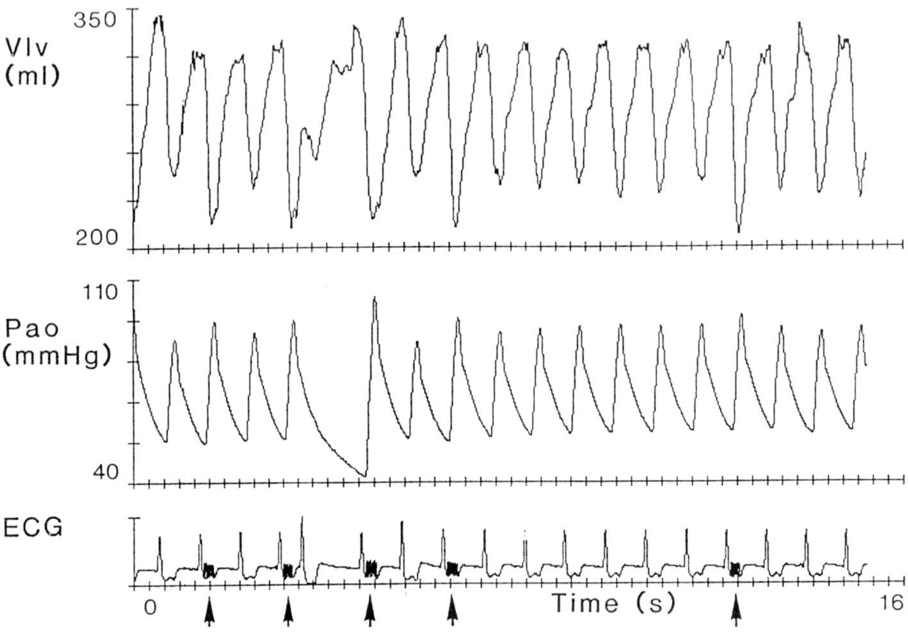


**Figure 1:** *See text for explanation.*

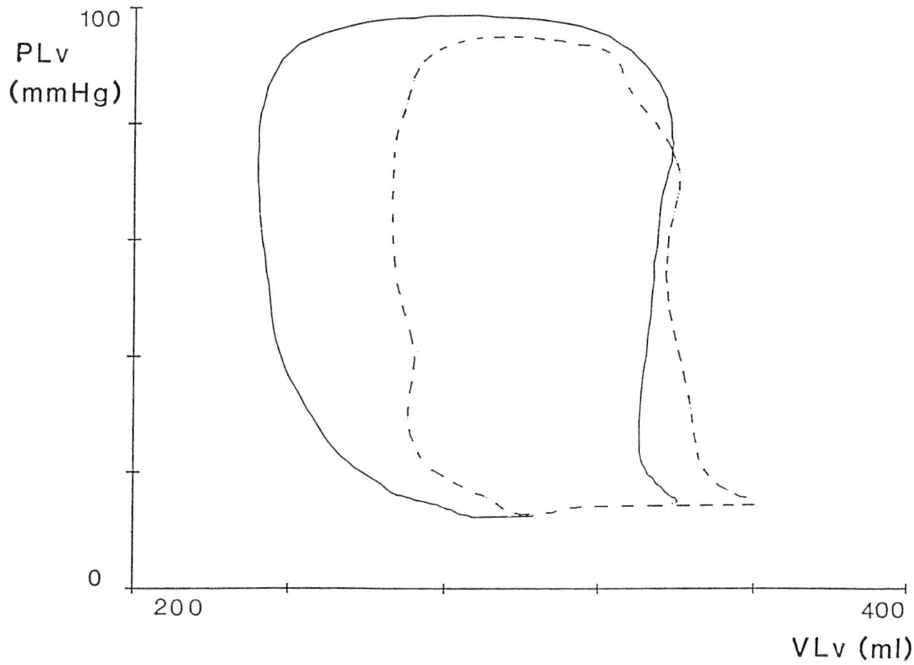


**Figure 2:** *Pressure volume loops. Dashed line represents the unassisted beat. Solid line is the LD assisted beat.*

pressure SV and therefore SW increased during the stimulated beat. The end-diastolic PV relationships of the stimulated and unstimulated beats are similar.

Table 1 presents hemodynamic results of the nine patients at the clinical setting. "Stim" and "unstim" refer to the stimulated and unstimulated beats of the assisted first 10-second period. "Post" refers to the beats of the subsequent unstimulated 5-second period.

Comparisons in % SV were made between stimulated and unstimulated beats of the assisted period and the postassisted period. Although a slight increase in SV of the stimulated beats was observed during the 10-second assisted period, no significant change in SV was found when the postassisted "post" period was compared with the stimulated period.

Systolic aortic pressure (Pao) was not changed significantly between stimulated and unstimulated beats. Left ventricular end-diastolic pressure (PLVED) was unchanged during the stimulated period but increased significantly ($p<0.05$) during the nonpaced period. Peak negative dP/dt was unchanged. Peak ejection rate (PER, -dV/dt) increased significantly ($p<0.01$) with a mean of 30% during the stimulated beats.

## Patients' Individual Best Setting

The best settings were selected as the settings with the largest increases in SV resulting from LD stimulation at the maximal applied amplitude (Table 2). In all patients, the best setting was observed at the maximal applied stimulus

**Table 1**
Clinical Setting

| | *Stim* | *Unstim* | *Post* |
|---|---|---|---|
| SV (%) | +3 ± 2 | −3 ± 2 | −1.8 ± 3 |
| Pao (mm Hg) | 120 ± 23 | 119 ± 23 | 120 ± 22 |
| PLVED (mm Hg) | 15 ± 7 | 15 ± 6 | 16 ± 8 |
| −dP/dt (mm Hg/sec) | 972 ± 160 | 952 ± 153 | 956 ± 160 |
| PER (mL/sec) | 643 ± 253 | 534 ± 248 | 511 ± 225 |

See text for abbreviations.

**Table 2**
Best Setting

| | *Stim* | *Unstim* | *Post* |
|---|---|---|---|
| SV (%) | +20 ± 15 | −20 ± 15 | −8 ± 5 |
| Pao (mm Hg) | 117 ± 16 | 110 ± 17 | 112 ± 15 |
| PLVED (mm Hg) | 12 ± 5 | 11.6 ± 4 | 13.6 ± 5 |
| −dP/dt (mm Hg/sec) | 983 ± 155 | 934 ± 148 | 953 ± 150 |
| PER (mL/sec) | 796 ± 308 | 492 ± 224 | 530 ± 232 |

See text for abbreviations.

strength between 7 and 10 volts, and the delays ranged from 25 to 125 ms. There was a significant ($p<0.01$) increase in SV with a mean of 20% during LD stimulation. During the nonpaced 5-second period, SV was significantly ($p<0.01$) lower with a mean of 8% compared with all the beats of the preceding stimulated period.

Systolic aortic pressure increased significantly ($p<0.01$) with a mean of 7 mm Hg. PLVED did not change during the stimulated period but increased significantly ($p<0.05$) during the 5-second nonpaced period. Peak negative dP/dt was slightly but significantly ($p<0.05$) higher during the stimulated beats. PER increased significantly ($p<0.01$) during the stimulated beats with a mean of 70% compared with the unstimulated beats of the stimulated period.

The worst setting is the setting with the smallest increase in SV due to LD stimulation at the maximum applied stimulus strength (Table 3). The worst settings were observed for early delays in four patients and a very late delay in the remaining five patients. Mean SV during LD stimulation was negative compared with the unstimulated beats of the stimulated period. Systolic aortic pressure did not change significantly. PLVED increased ($p<0.05$) during the nonpaced period. Maximum negative dP/dt remained unchanged, whereas PER increased significantly ($p<0.01$) by a mean of 30% during stimulated beats.

## Conclusions

The findings from the present study demonstrate that the settings of the cardiomyostimulator are critical if increases in SV and ejection fraction are to be achieved after a CMP procedure.

**Table 3**
Worst Setting

| | *Stim* | *Unstim* | *Post* |
|---|---|---|---|
| SV (%) | −0.5 ± 4 | +0.5 ± 4 | +0.2 ± 5 |
| Pao (mm Hg) | 115 ± 21 | 112 ± 20 | 114 ± 19 |
| PLVED (mm Hg) | 12.3 ± 4 | 12.7 ± 5 | 13.5 ± 5 |
| −dP/dt (mm Hg/sec) | 885 ± 203 | 911 ± 167 | 902 ± 160 |
| PER (mL/sec) | 656 ± 220 | 544 ± 253 | 518 ± 217 |

See text for abbreviations.

The evidence points to an increased contractile state of the left ventricle-LD muscle combination during the stimulated beats at the best settings, based on: (a) increased PER, increased max negative dP/dt and increased SV; (b) decreased PLVED during the stimulated periods; (c) leftward shifts of the ESPV points. All of these changes during LD stimulation were observed under preload and afterload conditions similar to the unstimulated beats in between.

The positive effect of CMP at the clinical setting may be largely due to active prevention of ventricular dilatation. This is suggested by the direct significant rise in end-diastolic pressure after the stimulated period. However, the increase of about 30% in PER is suggestive of a decreased workload of the heart muscle itself during LD stimulation.

## References


1. Carpentier A, Chachques JC: Myocardial substitution with a stimulated skeletal muscle: first successful clinical case. *Lancet* 1:1267 (letter), 1985.
2. Delahaye F, Jegaden O, Montagna P, Desseigne P, et al: Latissimus dorsi cardiomyoplasty in severe congestive heart failure: The Lyon experience. *J Cardiac Surg* 6:106–112, 1991.
3. Geddes LA, Janas W, Bourland JD, Cook J, et al: The importance of timing muscle contraction in dynamic cardiomyoplasty. *PACE* 16:2255–2265, 1993.
4. Lee KF, Dignan RJ, Parmar JM, Dyke CM, et al: Effects of dynamic cardiomyoplasty on left ventricular performance and myocardial mechanics in dilated cardiomyopathy. *J Thorac Cardiovasc Surg* 102:124–131, 1991.
5. Chachques JC, Acar C, Tapia M, Guibourt P, et al: Résultats à moyen terme de la cardiomyoplasty. *Arch Mal Coeur* 87:49–56, 1994.
6. Baan J, van der Velde ET, De Bruin HG, Smeenk GJ, et al: Continuous measurement of left ventricular volume in animals and humans by conductance catheter. *Circulation* 70:812–823, 1984.
7. Wesseling KH, Janssen JRC, Settels JJ, Schreuder JJ: Computation of aortic flow from pressure in humans using a nonlinear, three-element model. *J Appl Physiol* 74:2566–2573, 1993.

Chapter 13

# *Discussion*

**Dr. Carpentier:** Pressure-volume loops studies are indeed important in assessing not only results but also the mechanism of function. Dr. David Kass has experience in this field. How do the changes we see involve the volumes, the pressures, and the contractility?

**Dr. Kass (Baltimore):** I don't think one can separate these variables. I don't know that any of these relations tell me what the contractility is and I would warn people in interpreting parameters such as Vmax stroke work. In contractility, we are looking at a change that is very complex: it is a remodeling type of change. I think we are showing that systolic function, which is a less loaded way of saying contractility, is increased. There is no question that the heart starts at virtually the same diastolic curve, and when it ends, it ends at a systolic curve that is further away from the diastolic curve than the one that we had originally. So this kind of a leftward shift increases the range in which the heart can function.

**Dr. Chachques:** But don't you get the same thing as a change of volume?

**Dr. Kass:** We do not care whether it is a slope change or a shift in volume. It was shown what the data look like; either change, whether it is a slope change or a volume change is going to represent a substantial increase in the contractile systolic performance of the heart.

**Dr. Lorusso (Italy):** I would like to comment that we have been doing the same study with PV loops in Brescia and in Lyon. We now have studied 11 patients with PV loops and we have the same results. But I did not get the point concerning 1:1 mode. In our patients with a 1:1 mode, we saw a dramatic reduction in stroke volume and as soon as we restored the 1:2 mode, the volume increased dramatically. We even tried to see, with PV loops, differentiation in AV delay. I would like to know if you saw the same thing.

**Dr. Kass:** You have studied patients and you should be commended. I would love to do more. It is going to vary from patient to patient. There is no question that it could have significant constraining effect of how much net filling you get with that kind of stimulation.

**Dr. Salmons:** In the nonpaced situation, the PV loop improved. We are definitely not talking about beat-to-beat assistance.

**Dr. Kass:** The quest for worrying about acute effects of pacing on/off is misguided. They are just like other forms of therapy. This is a chronic intervention that leads to chronic changes in the chambers and that is the kind of improvement we are going to see.

**Dr. Lazzara (Allegheny General Hospital):** Did you use single or dual-held conductances? Since cardiomyoplasty changes the geometry of the ventricle and the heart in general, then it must change conductance. How does this affect these results or the results from other people? Is there any doubt about supporting the longitudinal use of conductance catheters in this type of situation?

**Dr. Kass:** We use two different actual boxes: in one box, it is a dual field and in the other it is a CPI box. We have looked at parallel conductance, at least in some dogs, and it does not change very significantly. Most of it is coming from the muscle itself, which moves entirely with the catheter and surrounding it at all times. The other thing that should be noted is that most of the data I have shown you are with the stimulator off, so there is really very little change in parallel conductance. The last thing is that in the longitudinal studies, we are calibrating to independent external measures of LV function, using ejection fraction and cardiac output as the two parameters, which provide us with our reference volumes. So there are no assumptions made in terms of parallel conductance. I don't care what it does; if it changes, it changes and I will get that from my continuously repeated external calibration.

**Dr. Moreira (Sao Paulo):** Your study is in agreement with what we observed with angiography and pressure volume loop determinations. I would like to ask you if the stimulator is turned off for 24 hours or more, are there real significant changes as we observed?

**Dr. Kass:** I would love to believe that but I am not all that optimistic. I don't know how long one would have to do it; but it is the same question that cardiologists could raise: if they take a patient who is doing well and stop three verapamil how long does one have to wait before one would see some reduction of LV function? I don't know if 24 hours would be enough.

**Unidentified (Sydney):** How much of the effect is due to the rotational changes? This is directed to Dr. Cho. You showed a big improvement in rotation of the left ventricle with the flap. Is that important?

**Dr. P. Cho (John Hopkins Hospital, Baltimore):** We feel that if one looks at the actual axis dimensions in three dimensions, the long axis appears to account for most of the volume changes.

**Unidentified (Sydney):** That's long axis shortening, but also the twist?

**Dr. Cho:** Insofar as any twist would contribute to ejection fraction, it would also show up as a shortening of the short axis. I believe that it is mostly the long axis shortening.

**Dr. Kass:** As a reminder, the data that I have are with the pacer off, whereas Dr. Cho's data would be important for evaluating the acute stimulation effects. They are not applicable to the kind of chronic changes we are seeing here.

**Dr. Furnary:** Have you looked at the left cardiomyoplasty because it is hypothesized that the left anterior or posterior cardiomyoplasty will contract in a radial direction whereas the right contracts longitudinally as you have shown? How did you get the dog and the stimulator into the MRI room?

**Dr. Cho:** We did a preliminary study on one dog with a left posterior wrap and we had almost identical findings. There is virtually no radial compression augmentation. As far as getting the animal into the MRI lab, we have people working in biomechanical engineering who have designed special filters and isolators that allow us to take the dog into the chamber. The myostimulator is explanted and we hook the dog up to stimulator cables.

**Dr. Furnary:** So you have to explant it. We cannot do this to a patient.

**Dr. Cho:** One possibility: They are also working on MRI-compatible electronic instruments. However, one could conceivably do this sort of study on humans when changing the pacemaker for battery power failure.

**Dr. Salmons:** We are beginning to get some hard data on the modus operandi and I think few people now would argue that this technique is not effective but there has been a great deal of argument about the mechanism.

Chapter 14

# Correlation between Echocardiographic and Isotopic Studies after Clinical Cardiomyoplasty

Jesús Herreros, Ignacio Iglesias, Joaquín Barba*

## Introduction

Congestive heart failure (CHF), regardless of its etiology, is an important cause of morbidity and mortality in the Western world.[1] The present treatment alternatives for patients with congestive heart failure refractory to medical treatment are cardiac transplantation and mechanical ventricular assistance. Nevertheless, these two methods have their limitations.[2,3] For this reason, other treatment modalities are currently being studied for patients with CHF refractory to medical treatment. One of them is mechanical support to the heart with a skeletal muscle, generally the latissimus dorsi (LD). The muscle is electrically stimulated synchronically with the heart using an apparatus that is a hybrid between a dual chamber pacemaker and a muscle stimulator (dynamic cardiomyoplasty or DC). Despite its theoretical advantage and the initially promising results, the clinical experience is still limited.[4] It is thus premature to make definite conclusions about its efficacy since a different stimulation protocol and surgical techniques have been used.

The aim of this study is to evaluate any change in systolic and diastolic function after DC, stimulating the muscle and without stimulating, by means of echocardiography and isotopic ventriculography, and to find new parameters of systolic function more sensitive to these changes and independent of volumetric calculations.

*With the cooperation of Martín Salvador Zabala, Javier Arbizu, Maria José García, and José Richter.

From Carpentier A, Chachques JC, Grandjean P: Cardiac Bioassist. © Futura Publishing Co, Inc, Armonk, NY, 1997.

## Patients, Material, and Methods

Since February 1991 we have done eight dynamic cardiomyoplasties at our institution. The clinical features of our patients are summarized in Table 1. All patients were male, 57.9 ± 11.4 years of age, and they had a formal contraindication to cardiac transplantation (active infectious disease or marked elevation in vascular pulmonary artery resistance).

Surgery was indicated in two cases for a left ventricular aneurysm and systolic dysfunction of the remaining ventricular segments without any possibility of coronary revascularization, or a small left ventricular cavity of the nonaneurysmatic segments. We trained the latissimus dorsi (LD) 6 weeks before the procedure with a temporal pacemaker and a percutaneous electrode in its pedicle, increasing the pulse amplitude and rate to 5 V and 60 ppm by 4 weeks.

Surgery was done according to Broussais Hospital and Allegheny Hospital protocols,[5,6] wrapping the muscle graft in a clockwise manner. Three patients underwent cardiopulmonary bypass (Table 1).

In three patients, we implanted a conventional dual chamber pacemaker (single pulse) to stimulate the LD. In the remaining five, a cardiomyostimulator (CMS) was used (Biotronik Myos) with a bipolar lead, placing the anodic electrode in the muscle pedicle 5–6 cm distally. In all cases, we sensed the heart placing one lead in the anterior wall of the right ventricle.

The post-DC protocol of stimulation for the CMS is summarized in Table 2. The main parameters of the CMS and dual chamber pacemaker are: CMS: pacing mode: $DDD_c$, lower rate: 60 ppm, upper rate limit: 160 ppm; AV delay (sensed or paced): 105 ms; pulse amplitude: 4.8 V; pulse width: 0.5 ms; dual chamber pacemaker: pacing mode: DDD, lower rate: 60, upper rate limit: 160; AV delay: 150 ms; pulse amplitude: 5 V; pulse width: 0.5 ms. We programmed these parameters synchronizing contraction and left ventricular outflow tract maximum velocity (LVOTv) using Doppler echocardiography.

The echocardiographic studies were done with a Hewlett-Packard Sonos 1500 echocardiograph and a 2.5 MHz probe. Volumes were measured according to the Teicholz formula[7] in the parasternal short-axis view (papillary muscles

**Table 1**
Clinical Features

| *Patient* | *Disease* | *Surgery* | *Device* | *NYHA* |
|---|---|---|---|---|
| 1 | IM | C | Single pulse | IV |
| 2 | LVA | A+C | Single pulse | III |
| 3 | LVA | A+C | Single pulse | III |
| 4 | IM | C | CMS | IV |
| 5 | DiC | C | CMS | IV |
| 6 | IM | A+MVR+CABG+C | CMS | IV |
| 7 | DiC | C | CMS | IV |
| 8 | IM | C | CMS | IV |

IM = ischemic cardiomyopathy; LVA = left ventricular aneurysm; DiC = dilated cardiomyopathy; A = aneursymectomy; C = cardiomyoplasty; MVR = mitral valve replacement; CABG = coronary artery bypass graft; CMS = cardiomyostimulator.

**Table 2**
Protocol of Stimulation (Cardiomyostimulator)

| *Days after Surgery* | *Cadence* | *Spikes/Burst* |
|---|---|---|
| 10 | 4:1 | 1 |
| 17 | 3:1 | 1 |
| 32 | 3:1 | 2 |
| 47 | 3:1 | 4 |
| 62 | 2:1 | 2 |
| 77 | 2:1 | 4 |
| 92 | 2:1 | 6 or 8 |

level), using M-mode, and ejection fraction (EF) was calculated, following the recommendations of the American Society of Echocardiography.[8] Pulsed-wave Doppler was used to evaluate left ventricular filling parameters, E-wave and deceleration time (DT), from the apical four-chamber view 1 cm away from the mitral annulus, and continuous-wave Doppler signal from mitral regurgitation was used to calculate dP/dt (Chung's method).[9] Left ventricular outflow tract maximum velocity was measured with pulsed-wave Doppler in this position, from the apical four-chamber view. Isotopic ventriculography was done with $^{99}{}_{m}$Tc labeled red blood cells obtaining images in left anterior oblique (LAO) projection, 16 frames, measuring EF. All studies were done with the CMS turned off and on.

We compared the results with a paired *t* test and $p<0.05$ was considered statistically significant.

## Results

### Clinical Results

The mean follow-up of our patients was 9.1 ± 5.8 months. There were no operative deaths. One patient died 3 months after DC of a brain stroke. Another patient died 11 months after DC after a palliative coronary angioplasty. There was marked improvement in functional class (Fig. 1). Nearly all patients were in Class I or II (except one) in the midterm follow-up.

### Echocardiographic Studies

*Systolic Function*

The preoperative and postoperative results are shown in Figures 2 and 3. We show the postoperative results with the CMS on (see protocol, Table 2). A significant increase in EF and LVOTv between preoperative data and 1 month/ 6 months after surgery was noted.

With the CMS off, there is also a significant increase in EF comparing preoperative data and data after 6 months (24.9 ± 5.8 vs. 26.8 ± 8.6, $p<0.05$) and 1 and 6 months (26.8 ± 8.6 vs. 34.0 ± 11.0, $p<0.01$). No significant change

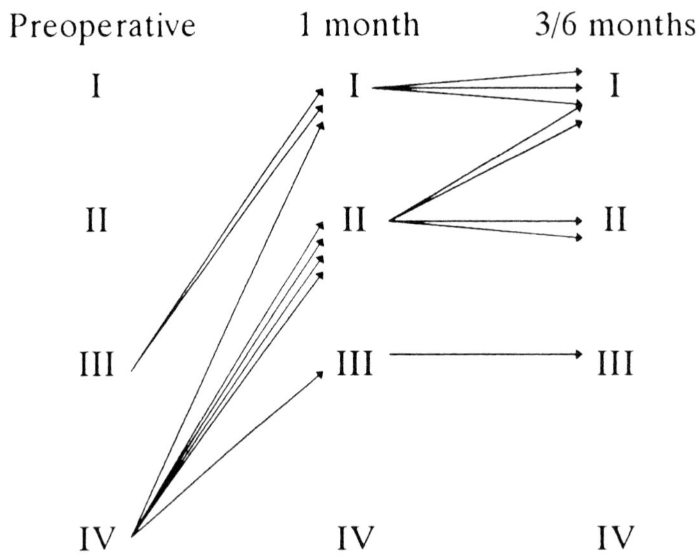


**Figure 1:** *Functional class.*

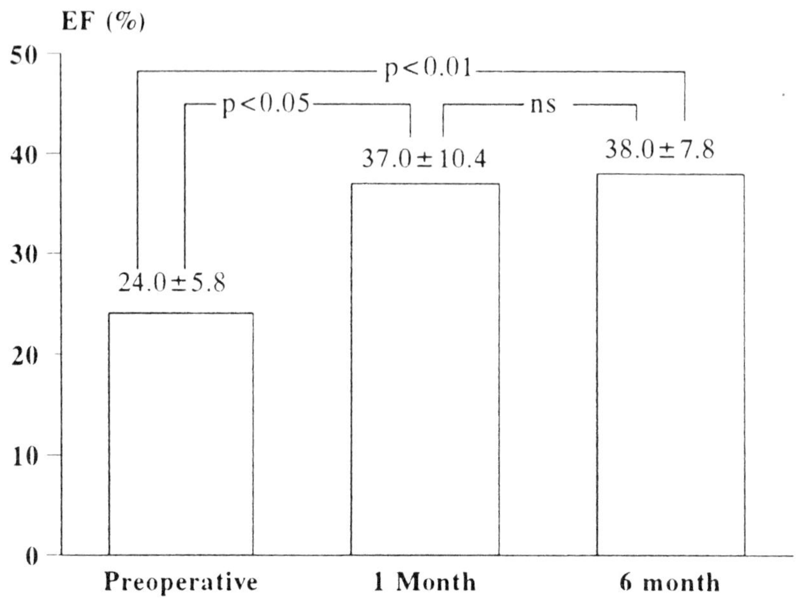


**Figure 2:** *Echocardiographic ejection fraction.*

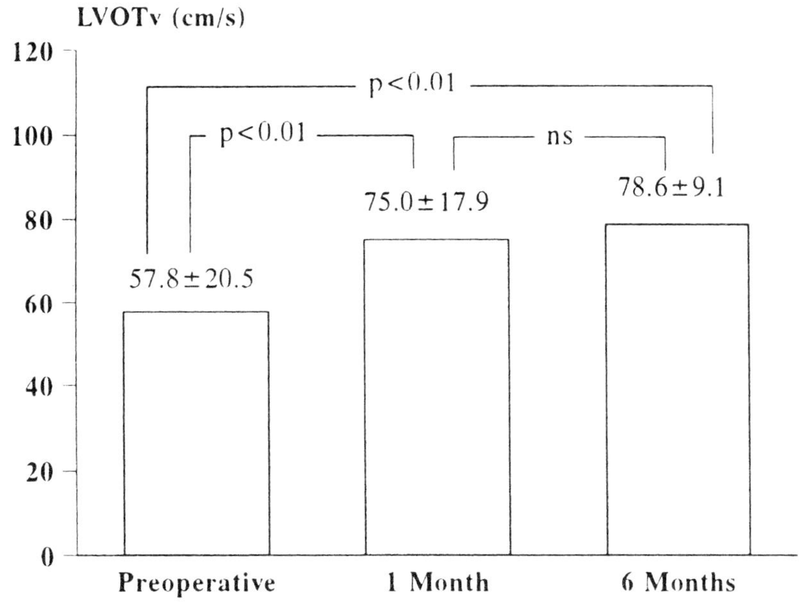


**Figure 3:** *Left ventricular outflow tract maximum velocity (pulsed-wave Doppler).*

exists comparing preoperative EF and 1 month EF (24.9 ± 5.8 vs. 26.8 ± 8.6, ns) with CMS off. There is also a significant increase in LVOTv between 1 month and 6 months (56.9 ± 20.4 vs. 68.0 ± 19.5 cm/s, $p<0.05$) with the CMS off but there is no difference between preoperative LVOTv and 1 month (57.8 ± 20.5 vs. 56.9 ± 20.4 cm/s, ns) or 6 months (68.0 ± 19.5 cm/s, ns). We noted, when comparing data derived with the CMS off and on, that a significant increase in echocardiographic EF occurs 1 month after DC (26.8 ± 8.6 vs. 37.0 ± 10.4, $p<0.05$) and this comparison is nonsignificant in the 6 months study (34.0 ± 11.0 vs. 38.0 ± 7.8, ns). One month after surgery, there is also a significant difference turning on and off the CMS in the LVOTv (56.9 ± 20.4 vs. 75.0 ± 17.9, $p<0.05$), but this difference is less evident in the 6 months study (68.0 ± 19.5 vs. 78.6 ± 9.1, ns). The evolution in echocardiographic EF and LVOTv is shown in Figure 4. The mechanical effect of the muscle seems to be less important at 6 months than at 1 month postoperatively. As a noneffective phase index of left ventricular performance, dp/dt was measured in patients with mitral regurgitation. We found a significant difference with the CMS off and on in this parameter (592.6 ± 181.6 vs. 706.3 ± 291.5 mm Hg/s, $p<0.05$) 1 month after surgery.

### *Diastolic Function*

We did not find a significant change in E-wave (early left ventricular filling) over time or with the CMS off and on. Preoperative: 80.9 ± 9.3 cm/s; 1 month (CMS off/on) 83.3 ± 14.4/80.3 ± 20.3 cm/s; 6 months (CMS off/on) 82.7 ± 15.3/80.1 ± 17.5 cm/s. The results of the determination of DT are: preoperative: 125.1 ± 40.0 ms; 1 month (CMS off/on): 123.1 ± 41.5/129.6 ± 31.1 ms; 6 months:

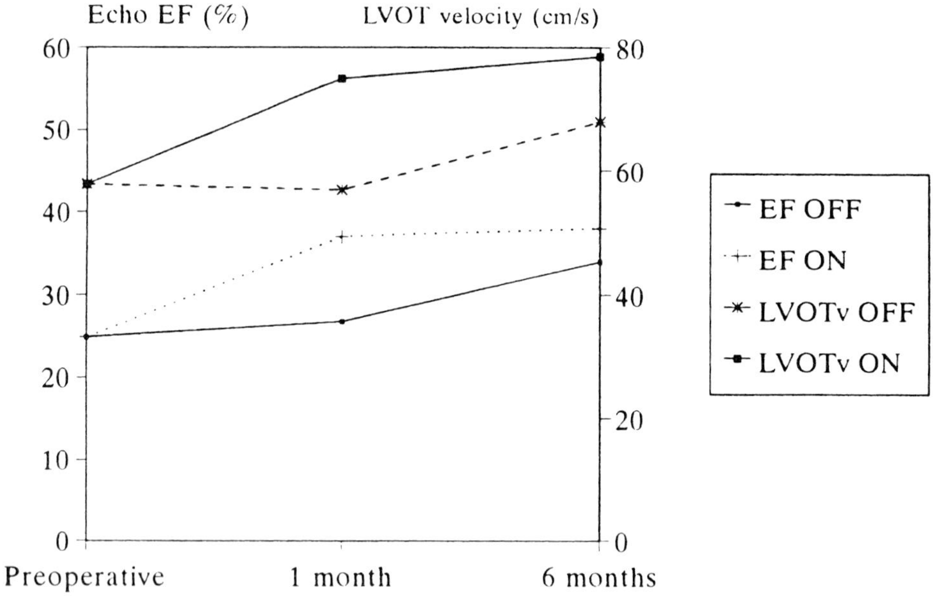


**Figure 4:** *Evolution in echocardiographic ejection fraction and left ventricular outflow tract maximum velocity.*

98.9 ± 12.4/106.3 ± 9.5 ms. A significant difference was found comparing deceleration time 1 month and 6 months after the DC with the CMS on (129.6 ± 31.1 vs. 106.3 ± 9.5 ms, $p<0.05$).

## Isotopic Ventriculography

The preoperative and postoperative results with the CMS on are shown in Figures 5 and 6. The results are very similar to the echo studies. A significant difference exists in EF preoperatively and 1 or 6 months after DC, with the CMS on (Fig. 5). Comparing the results, with the CMS off we have found a significant difference in EF presurgery and 6 months after surgery (20.3 ± 8.3 vs. 28.1 ± 11.7, $p<0.05$), but no difference is noted comparing preoperative data and 1-month studies (20.3 ± 8.3 vs. 24.4 ± 10.3, ns) or 1-month and 6-month studies (24.4 ± 10.3 vs. 28.1 ± 11.7, ns). When we studied the effect of the stimulation, we found a significant difference one month after DC with the CMS off and on (24.5 ± 9.5 vs. 33.4 ± 12.3, $p<0.05$) and 6 months after surgery (27.4 ± 11.1 vs. 32.9 ± 12.3, $p<0.05$). The evolution in isotopic EF is shown in Figure 6. The mechanical effect of the muscle seems to be less important over time.

## Conclusions

There is general agreement that DC improves symptoms in patients with heart failure, Class III–IV NYHA, with a contraindication to cardiac trans-

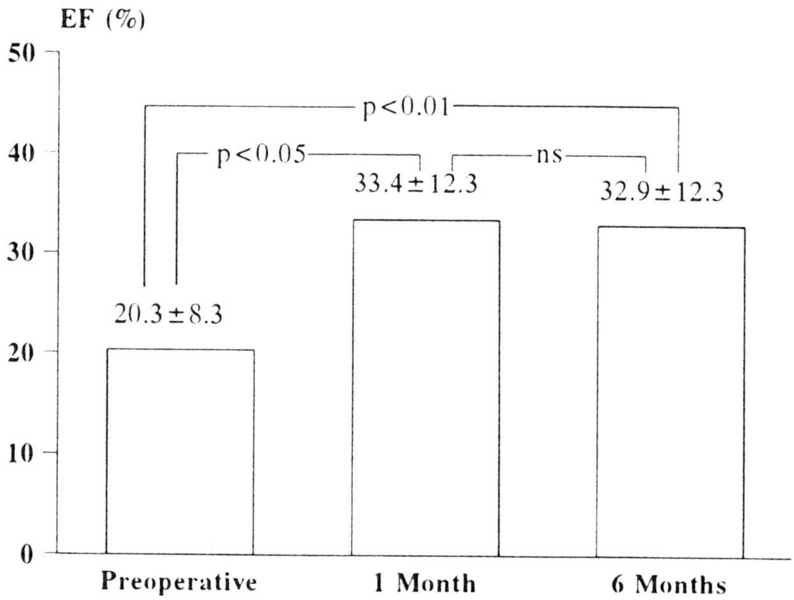


**Figure 5:** *Isotopic ejection fraction.*

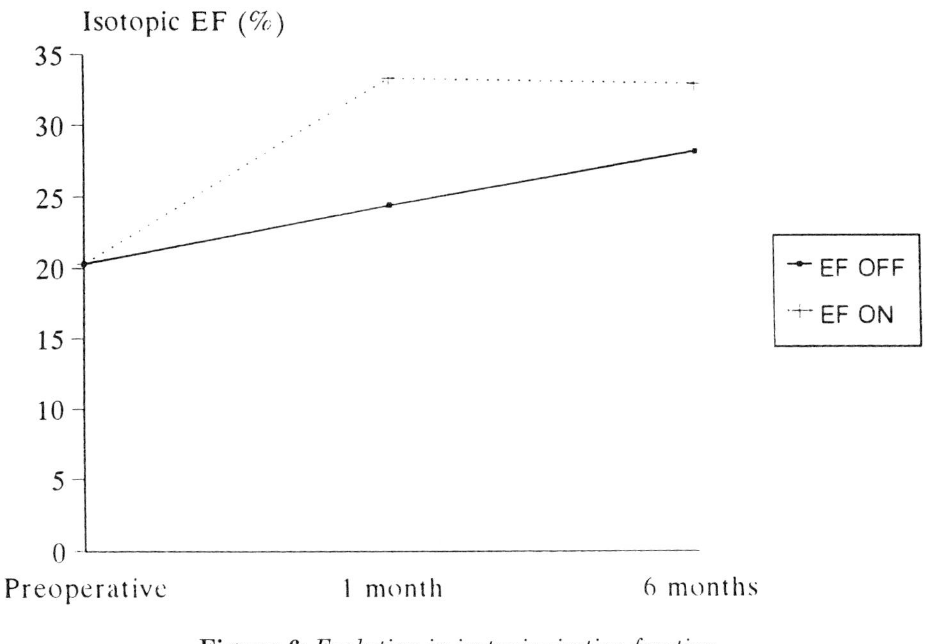


**Figure 6:** *Evolution in isotopic ejection fraction.*

plantation, but studies differ as to when this occurs. Franquiz et al.[10] note a symptomatic improvement 8 months after surgery, whereas Magovern et al.[11] found an earlier improvement. In our study we found an improvement in functional class 1 month after DC that persists in the midterm follow-up, but the mechanism seems to be different, as we will discuss later. The discrepancies in these studies could be related to the different clinical features of the patients included. In our initial experience, three patients have been operated on for left ventricular aneurysm, and this can induce per se an early improvement in functional class.

Several studies have been reported focusing on systolic function.[12–14] There is also general agreement that DC improves systolic function measuring echocardiographic and isotopic parameters. Nearly all of these parameters are derived from calculation of left ventricular volumes, and are an expression of the systolic ejection phase. For this reason we have studied the maximum velocity in left ventricular outflow tract and noninvasive dp/dt with Doppler echocardiography as a nonejective phase index. In our study we noted a significant improvement in systolic parameters over time, with the CMS off and on. In the 1-month study, there is a significant improvement in echocardiographic and isotopic ejection fraction and echocardiographic left ventricular outflow tract maximum velocity with the stimulator off and on. This improvement is also demonstrated in the 6-month study, but only in isotopic ejection fraction. With the CMS turned on, there is a sharp increase in dp/dt 1 month after surgery. We think that the stimulator improves systolic function early after surgery by its mechanical force, but several months later other mechanisms could play a role, and that the stimulation induces a sharp increase in the nonejection systolic index, the first phase of left ventricular contraction. This index could be used as a measure of the mechanical force of the latissimus dorsi, and of its influence on systolic function. Among the mechanisms that could play a role several months after surgery, two are important: neovascularization of the myocardium,[15] and a muscle barrier for the progressive dilation of the left ventricle.

Diastolic function does not seem to deteriorate over time. A significant difference was found in deceleration time 1 month and 6 months after DC, without any change in peak E-wave. We hypothesize that this could be related to progressive hypertrophy of the muscle that restricts the filling of the left ventricle, but more studies are necessary to demonstrate this.

We conclude that dynamic cardiomyoplasty is an alternative, although still under study, for treatment of end-stage congestive heart failure refractory to medical treatment. The clinical experience is still very limited but it seems that the symptomatic improvement, as demonstrated by a lower NYHA functional class, has a relation to the parameters of ventricular function. However, there are also contradictory data. New parameters of systolic and diastolic function (echocardiographic and isotopic), more sensitive to the mechanical action of the muscle are necessary, and new mechanisms of action could play a role in the symptomatic improvement. Until then, echocardiographic studies and isotopic studies are very useful to determine the global left ventricular function after this new surgical procedure.

## References


1. Parmley WW: Pathophysiology and current therapy of congestive heart failure. *J Am Coll Cardiol* 13:771, 1989.
2. Heck CF, Shumway SJ, Kaye MP: The registry of International Society for Heart Transplantation: Sixth official report, 1989. *J Heart Transplant* 8:271, 1989.
3. Pae WE, Miller CA, Pierce WS: Combined registry for the clinical use of mechanical ventricular assist pumps and the total artificial heart: Third official report, 1988. *J Heart Transplant* 8:277, 1989.
4. Moreira LFP, Stolf NAG, Bocchi EA, et al: Latissimus dorsi cardiomyoplasty in the treatment of patients with dilated cardiomyopathy. *Circulation* 82:257, 1990.
5. Chachques JC, Grandjean PA, Pfeffer TA, et al: Cardiac assistance by atrial or ventricular cardiomyoplasty. *J Heart Transplant* 9:239, 1990.
6. Chachques JC, Grandjean PA, Carpentier A: Latissimus dorsi dynamic cardiomyoplasty. *Ann Thorac Surg* 47:600, 1989.
7. Teicholz LE, Kreulen T, Herman MV, et al: Problems in echocardiographic volume determinations: Echocardiographic-angiographic correlations in the presence or absence of asynergy. *Am J Cardiol* 37:7, 1976.
8. Schiller ND, Shah PM, Crawford M, et al: Recommendations for quantitation of the left ventricle by two dimensional echocardiography: Committee on standards. Subcommittee on quantitation of two dimensional echocardiograms. *J Am Soc Echocardiogr* 26:358, 1989.
9. Chung N, Nishimura RA, Holmes DR, et al: Measurement of left ventricular dp/dt by simultaneous Doppler echocardiography and cardiac catheterization. *J Am Soc Echocardiogr* 5:147, 1992.
10. Franquiz García JM, Carrera Alonso C, Dortiods Balea F, et al: Valor de la ventriculografía isotópica en el pronóstico y seguimiento de los pacientes sometidos a cardiomioplastia dinámica. *Rev Esp Cardiol* 45:381, 1992.
11. Furnary AP, Magovern JA, Christlieb IY, et al: Clinical cardiomyoplasty: preoperative factors associated with outcome. *Ann Thorac Surg* 50:1139, 1992.
12. Jatene AD, Moreira LF, Stolf NA, et al: Left ventricular function after cardiomyoplasty in patients with dilated cardiomyopathy. *J Thorac Cardiovasc Surg* 102:132, 1991.
13. Moreira LF, Stolf NA, Bocchi EA, et al: Latissimus dorsi cardiomyoplasty in the treatment of patients with dilated cardiomyopathy. *Circulation* 82(Suppl IV):257, 1990.
14. Moreira LF, Seferian P, Bocchi EA, et al: Survival improvement with dynamic cardiomyoplasty in patients with dilated cardiomyopathy. *Circulation* 84(Suppl III):296, 1991.
15. Beyer M, Hoffer H, Eggeling T, et al: Cardiomyoplasty to improve myocardial collateral blood supply as an alternative to transplantation in intractable angina. *J Heart Lung Transplant* 11:189, 1992.

Chapter 14

# Discussion

**Dr. Carpentier:** We have the opportunity to discuss the much debated question of the value of the different noninvasive investigations we have at our disposal to assess the results of cardiomyoplasty. May I ask Dr. Gottlieb, a specialist in echocardiography, to join us for the discussion?

**Dr. Chekanov:** Skeletal muscle wrapping may change the configuration of the heart and the echocardiographic picture may also change. Perhaps it is difficult to compare the echo data before and after cardiomyoplasty. What is your opinion?

**Dr. Gottlieb (Philadelphia):** I think what you see is the decrease in end-diastolic volume, which changes the heart's position on the Starling curve and it is not unreasonable to use the echo to look at these parameters. The shape does change but perhaps that shape change is important for the outcome.

**Dr. Plehn (from Lebanon in New Hampshire):** There may be another possibility for diastolic improvement, as has been suggested by a number of other reports. What may be happening is either restrictive cardiomyopathy or constrictive pericarditis. E/A ratio is very problematic and when you increase your E and decrease your A over time, you may be increasing atrial pressure. We have previously shown that atrial naturetic factor increases caused by atrial stretch, which is what you get in constrictive pericarditis and restricted cardiomyopathy. You get big atria, stretched atria, and the ANP can go up. I would like to suggest that in fact what is happening here is that the ventricles are getting smaller because you have a restrictive or constrictive physiology and the ratio is changing because the atrial pressure is high, which is actually a bad thing to happen. How would you respond to that?

**Dr. Gottlieb:** I think it is clearly a possibility. My opinion is, without much data to back it up, that perhaps part of the mechanism and the success of cardiomyoplasty is that it is buttressing the heart and changing its geometry and volume so that it is working on a different part of the Starling curve. As to whether the E/A ratio really means improvement in diastolic function or is it due to a pseudonormalization you have alluded to, I can't answer that. It is the early peak filling velocity that has increased. It is not decreasing, which is what you might expect to some degree in the scenario.

From Carpentier A, Chachques JC, Grandjean P: Cardiac Bioassist. © Futura Publishing Co, Inc, Armonk, NY, 1997.

**Sir Magdi Yacoub (London):** You should not use the word "restrictive" in a ventricle that is huge. It is a contradiction in terms.

**Dr. Gottlieb:** Pressure volume loops show that it may be somewhat restrictive. At the end of diastole, you have a very dilated ventricle but restrictive patterns with the very steep pressure volume curve at the end of the curve but not in the middle part of the curve during normal volumes. So, in a sense, it is a type of restrictive cardiomyopathy. You don't have the typical square root sign on pressure tracings, but you do get a restrictive pattern with a steep curve.

**Sir Magdi Yacoub:** So a useful thing rather than a primary bad thing could explain the A/E ratio, but it is still not a restrictive cardiomyopathy.

**Dr. Plehn:** We are talking about a filling pattern that is bad for the heart where you have a very steep pressure volume slope, which is not something we want to happen in this situation. It is quite possible that is what you are causing by wrapping the heart.

**Dr. Acker (Johns Hopkins):** We have shown at Hopkins using three-dimensional tagged MRI imaging techniques, that there is a change in heart motion with skeletal muscle wrap contraction. Are even sophisticated 2D echo techniques applicable in a heart that is moving dramatically in three dimensions, and what artifacts might be introduced when one is looking at a cross-sectional ejection fraction?

**Dr. Gottlieb:** It might not be the most optimal technique to use long term. However, it is a simple noninvasive technique with which one can follow these patients very easily longitudinally. The fact that one is doing it on the same patient and the technique is reasonably reproducible makes it worthwhile. There are other techniques that will certainly surpass it in the future.

Chapter 15

# Heart Failure Model for Evaluation of Skeletal Muscle Cardiac Assist

E. Christopher Orton, Eric Monnet, June Boon*

## Introduction

Considerable physiological evidence now supports the feasibility of using skeletal muscle to assist the failing myocardium. Skeletal muscle cardiac assist has appeal over cardiac transplantation because the problems of tissue rejection and limited donor supply are avoided. Dynamic cardiomyoplasty shows promise for treatment of chronic progressive heart failure, by optimization of the procedure probably has not yet been achieved. New methods of skeletal muscle cardiac assist such as aortomyoplasty and skeletal muscle ventricles are emerging and soon may be ready for clinical evaluation. The goals of further evaluating and optimizing cardiomyoplasty and of comparing cardiomyoplasty with new methods of skeletal muscle cardiac assist would be advanced by a clinically realistic animal model of progressive heart failure.

Naturally occurring idiopathic dilated cardiomyopathy of large-breed dogs has clinical, pathological, ultrastructural, and biochemical findings that are similar to human idiopathic dilated cardiomyopathy.[1–9] The progressive nature of canine dilated cardiomyopathy makes it a potentially realistic model for evaluating the long-term effects of skeletal muscle cardiac assist on cardiac function. The clinical course for dilated cardiomyopathy is reported to be rapid, although actuarial survival analysis for dogs with dilated cardiomyopathy has not been reported. Development of canine dilated cardiomyopathy as a clinically realistic model might allow evaluation and optimization of skeletal muscle cardiac assist before procedures are performed in humans.

To further define the clinical course for dogs with idiopathic dilated cardiomyopathy, retrospective actuarial survival analysis on 20 dogs presented for dilated cardiomyopathy and treated with standard medical therapy was performed. To test the feasibility of canine dilated cardiomyopathy as a model for skeletal muscle cardiac assist, dynamic cardiomyoplasty was performed on three dogs with advanced dilated cardiomyopathy.

*With the cooperation of Gordon B. Jacobs, Phillip Steyn, and Mark Guadagnoli.

From Carpentier A, Chachques JC, Grandjean P: Cardiac Bioassist. © Futura Publishing Co, Inc, Armonk, NY, 1997.

## Material and Methods

### Retrospective Survival Analysis

Medical records of dogs diagnosed with idiopathic dilated cardiomyopathy at Colorado State University Veterinary Teaching Hospital were evaluated retrospectively. Criteria for diagnosis of dilated cardiomyopathy were: (1) evidence of left ventricular heart enlargement on echocardiography (left ventricular end-diastolic dimension >44 mm/$M^2$), (2) decreased fractional shortening of the left ventricle (<25%), (3) lack of hypertrophy of the left ventricular wall, and (4) no evidence of primary valvular disease. Entry time was established as the time of the first echocardiogram confirming the diagnosis of dilated cardiomyopathy. The product limit method of Kaplan-Meier was used to construct a survival curve. Survival rates at 1 and 2 years were determined from the survival curve.

### Cardiomyoplasty Surgery and Protocol

Three dogs with advanced dilated cardiomyopathy underwent dynamic cardiomyoplasty surgery. Monitoring during surgery included electrocardiogram, direct arterial pressure, central venous pressure, end tidal $CO_2$, oxygen saturation, and arterial blood gases. Pre-anesthetic medications were oxymorphone (0.1 mg/kg) and diazepam (0.2 mg/kg). Anesthetic induction was by intravenous injection of propofol (5 mg/kg). Dogs were intubated, and balanced anesthesia was maintained by inhalation of isoflurane, and intravenous injections of fentanyl (0.01 mg/kg) and atracurium (0.1 mg/kg). Soon after induction of anesthesia, a Swan-Ganz catheter was placed via a jugular vein to monitor pulmonary artery pressure, pulmonary wedge pressure, and cardiac output during and after surgery.

Dogs were placed in left lateral recumbency for surgery. A diagonal incision across the lateral thorax was made in the skin, subcutaneous tissues, and cutaneous trunci muscle. The right latissimus dorsi muscle was exposed and isolated on its neurovascular pedicle. Two myostimulator electrodes were placed on either side of the insertion end of the muscle flap 2 cm distal to the bifurcation of the thoracodorsal nerve. The second rib was resected and a fifth intercostal thoracotomy performed. The muscle flap was transferred into the thoracic cavity via the rib resection. The insertion end of the muscle flap was included in the closure of the rib resection incision. The pericardium was opened with an L-shaped incision along the apex and cranial aspects of the heart. Two screw-in epicardial leads were placed in the ventricular myocardium for R-wave sensing. An anterior cardiosubcutaneous wrap was formed by suturing the muscle flap to the left lateral and caudal aspects of the pericardium at the level of the atrioventricular groove. The remaining flap was sutured back to itself to cover the right ventricle. The myostimulator and epicardial electrodes were connected to a teleprogrammable cardiosynchronous myostimulator made by Telectronics Pacing Systems. The myostimulator generator unit was implanted in the lateral abdominal wall medial to the external abdominal oblique muscle. The intercostal thoracotomy and lateral thoracic wound were closed in routine fashion. Oxymorphone (0.1 mg/kg) was administered for 24 hours to control postoperative pain.

The skeletal muscle flap was rested for 14 days to allow for revascularization of the flap and adhesion of the flap to the epicardium. Thereafter, the skeletal muscle flap was conditioned with 6-V pulses of 0.1 ms duration according to the schedule in Table 1. Pulses were delivered in a 35-Hz burst with a 23-ms delay after the R-wave was sensed. The heart:myostimulator synchronization ratio was 2:1 for heart rates <130 bpm and 3:1 for heart rates >130 bpm. Pulse voltage and duration were adjusted to achieve maximal skeletal muscle contraction assessed by palpation of the thoracic wall and echocardiography.

## Echocardiography

Echocardiographic examinations were obtained with a Hewlett Packard Sonos 1000 machine and a 3.5- or 5-mHz transducer. Dogs were placed in right lateral recumbency on a raised table with windows for obtaining right paracostal scans. Measurements of left ventricular dimension, septal wall thickness, and posterior wall thickness during systole and diastole were obtained from M-mode echocardiography and normalized to 1 $M^2$ by linear regression. Shortening fraction, septal thickening fraction, and posterior wall thickening fraction were calculated. Left ventricular end-diastolic volume, end-systolic volume, ejection fraction, and stroke volume were calculated from two-dimensional echocardiography using the modified method of Simpson.[10] Aortic ejection velocities were measured by Doppler echocardiography. Peak velocity, velocity flow integral, mean velocity, mean acceleration, acceleration time, ejection time, and pre-ejection period were determined as measures of systolic function. Indices were determined for both skeletal muscle-assisted and -unassisted systoles (n=5). Indices also were obtained with the myostimulator off for 20 minutes.

## MUGA Scan

Red blood cells were labeled in vivo with Tc-99m. MUGA scans were acquired on a Technicare Omega 500 SPECT system with dogs lying quietly in right lateral recumbency. A left ventral oblique view was adjusted to show the

**Table 1**
Schedule for Progressive Burst Stimulation after Cardiomyoplasty Surgery

| *Postoperative Period* | *Number of Pulses/Burst* |
|---|---|
| 14 days | 1 pulse |
| 24 days | 2 pulses |
| 34 days | 3 pulses |
| 44 days | 4 pulses |
| 55 days | 5 pulses |

interventricular septum. Data acquisition was obtained over a 10-minute period at 16 frames per cardiac cycle. A region of interest was drawn around the left ventricle and a time activity curve for the left ventricle was generated. NucLear MAC clinical software was used to determine the left ventricular ejection fraction. Scans were obtained with the myostimulator on and off.

## Results

### Retrospective Study

Twenty dogs met the diagnostic criteria for dilated cardiomyopathy during the time period of this study. The 50% probability of survival for dogs with dilated cardiomyopathy occurred at 6.9 months (Fig. 1). Probability of survival at 1 year was 48% and at 2 years was 16%. The frequency of clinical findings from the cardiac history, physical examination, electrocardiogram, and thoracic radiographs are listed in Table 2. The means ±SD for echocardiographic indices are reported in Table 3.

### Cardiomyoplasty Surgery

Three dogs with advanced dilated cardiomyopathy underwent dynamic cardiomyoplasty surgery. Dog 1 was a 3-year-old flat-coated retriever presented

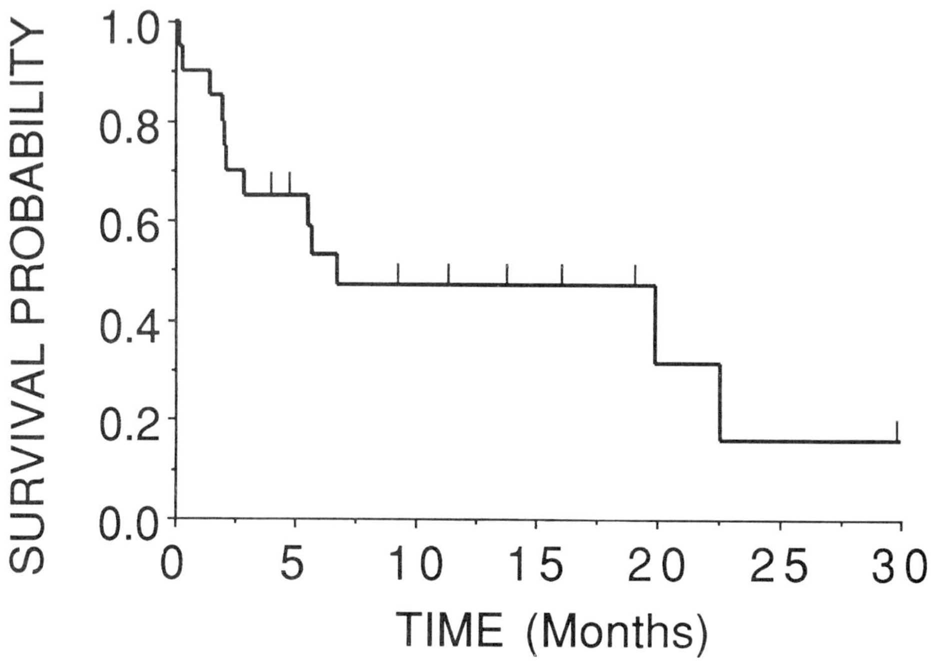


**Figure 1:** *Actuarial survival of 20 dogs with idiopathic dilated cardiomyopathy.*

for syncope and collapse during exercise. Left ventricular end-diastolic diameter was 62 mm (normal left ventricular diameter, 41.5 to 45.1 mm), left ventricular fractional shortening was 11.7%, and left ventricular ejection fraction was 24.8%. Holter examination revealed ventricular ectopy, including 189 nonsustained runs of ventricular tachycardia in a 24-hour period. Ventricular ectopy was controlled incompletely by oral mexiletine therapy. Additional therapies included digoxin and enalapril. Dynamic cardiomyoplasty surgery was performed without complication. Six hours after surgery, the dog experienced a witnessed cardiac arrest due to ventricular fibrillation. Attempts at electroconversion were unsuccessful.

**Table 2**

Frequency of Clinical Findings from Cardiac History, Physical Examination, Electrocardiogram, and Thoracic Radiographs in 20 Dogs with Dilated Cardiomyopathy

| *Clinical Finding* | *Number of Dogs* | *Frequency (%)* |
|---|---|---|
| Weight loss | 7 | 35 |
| Syncope | 7 | 35 |
| Exercise intolerance | 7 | 35 |
| Ascites | 4 | 20 |
| Atrial fibrillation | 2 | 10 |
| Ventricular ectopy | 4 | 20 |
| Left ventricular enlargement | 3 | 8 |
| Biventricular enlargement | 12 | 60 |
| Pulmonary venous congestion | 11 | 55 |
| Pulmonary edema | 16 | 80 |
| Pleural effusion | 5 | 20 |
| Class of heart failure | | |
| I | 3 | 15 |
| II | 5 | 25 |
| III | 10 | 50 |
| VI | 2 | 10 |

**Table 3**

Mean ± Standard Deviation (SD) for Echocardiographic Indices from 20 Dogs with Dilated Cardiomyopathy*

| *Index* | *Mean ± SD* | *Normal Dog 95% CI* |
|---|---|---|
| Left ventricular diastolic diameter (mm/M$^2$) | 55.9 ± 10 | 40.9–44.4 |
| Left ventricular systolic diameter (mm/M$^2$) | 49.2 ± 8.6 | 25.4–27.9 |
| Shortening fraction (%) | 14.6 ± 3.8 | 33.7–45.9 |
| Ejection fraction (%) | 30.5 ± 6.9 | 63.2–78.0 |
| Left ventricular diastolic wall thickness (mm/M$^2$) | 7.3 ± 1.4 | 8.3–9.3 |
| Left ventricular systolic wall thickness (mm/M$^2$) | 8.9 ± 2.5 | 13.4–14.6 |
| Thickening fraction (%) | 30.8 ± 23.5 | 45.7–75.9 |

*Confidence interval (95% C.I.) from 70 normal dogs are listed for comparison. Ventricular dimensions normalized by linear regression to 1 M$^2$ body surface area.

Dog 2 was an 11-year-old Doberman pinscher presented for collapse, coughing, and shortness of breath. On presentation, the dog had pulmonary edema and was in modified NYHA Class IV heart failure. Initial therapy consisted of intravenous furosemide and dobutamine. Subsequently, the dog was placed on oral digoxin, furosemide, and enalapril therapy. Left ventricular end-diastolic dimension was 59 mm and left ventricular fractional shortening was 4%. Left ventricular ejection fraction was 25.7% by echocardiography and 28% by MUGA scan. Dynamic cardiomyoplasty surgery was performed 3 weeks after initial presentation. Medically refractory pleural effusion and ascites developed 26 days after surgery. The dog died from progressive cardiac and multiorgan failure 44 days after surgery before latissimus dorsi muscle conditioning was completed.

Dog 3 was a 5-year-old Rhodesian ridgeback dog presented for exercise intolerance, collapse, and shortness of breath. Cardiac workup confirmed a diagnosis of advanced idiopathic dilated cardiomyopathy. Medical therapy included furosemide, digoxin, and enalapril. Dynamic cardiomyoplasty was performed without complication. Six months after surgery, dog 3 was alive and clinically improved. Echocardiography derived left ventricular fractional shortening and ejection fraction improved after surgery for both skeletal muscle-assisted and -unassisted systoles (Figs. 2 and 3). Six months after surgery, MUGA-derived and echocardiography-derived ejection fractions were higher with myostimulation on than with myostimulation off (Figs. 3 and 4). Other indices of left ventricular function were either improved or not different 3 and 6 months after surgery compared to values obtained before surgery (Table 4).

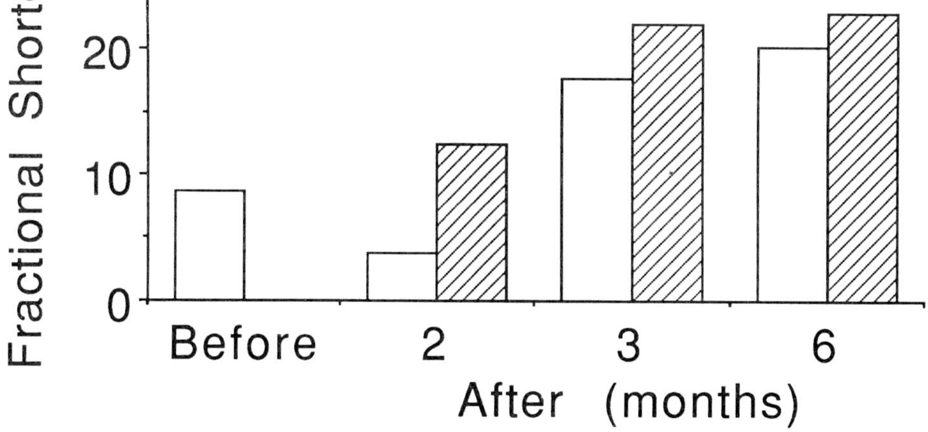


**Figure 2:** *M-mode echocardiography-derived left ventricular fractional shortening (%) for skeletal muscle-assisted and -unassisted systoles from dog 3 before and after dynamic cardiomyoplasty.*

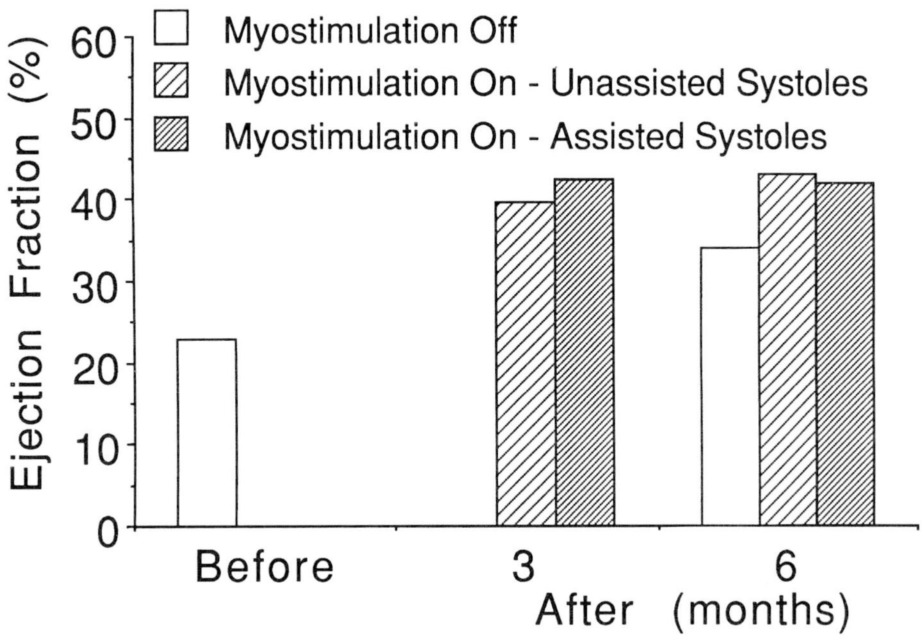


**Figure 3:** *Two-dimensional echocardiography-derived left ventricular ejection fraction (%) from dog 3 before and after dynamic cardiomyoplasty with myostimulation off and on. Ejection fractions with myostimulation on determined for both skeletal muscle-assisted and -unassisted systoles.*

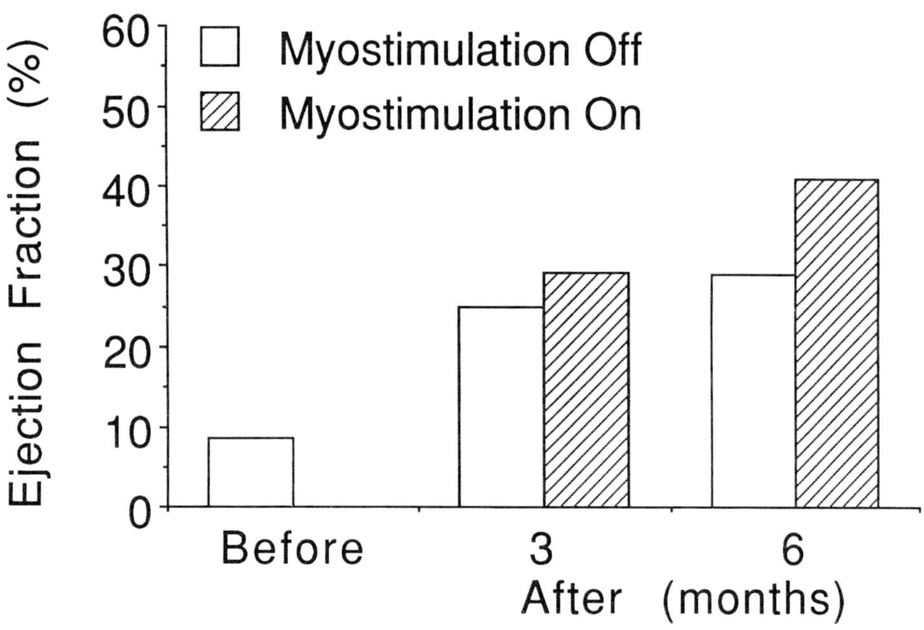


**Figure 4:** *MUGA-derived left ventricular ejection fraction (%) from dog 3 before and after dynamic cardiomyoplasty with myostimulation off and on.*

**Table 4**
M-Mode, Two-dimensional, and Doppler Echocardiographic Indices of Left Ventricular Function from Dog 3 Before and After Dynamic Cardiomyoplasty for Skeletal Muscle Assisted- and Unassisted Systoles*

| | | *3 months* | | *6 months* | |
|---|---|---|---|---|---|
| | Before | Unassisted | Assisted | Unassisted | Assisted |
| M-Mode | | | | | |
| Diastolic diameter (mm) | 50.8 | 48.7 | 50.0 | 48.5 | 48.2 |
| Systolic diameter (mm) | 46.4 | 40.1 | 39 | 38.7 | 37.2 |
| Fractional shortening (%) | 8.6 | 17.6 | 22 | 20.2 | 22.9 |
| Two-Dimensional | | | | | |
| End-diastolic volume (mL) | 139 | 133 | 142 | 140 | 135 |
| End-systolic volume (mL) | 107 | 80.3 | 81.8 | 79.1 | 79.8 |
| Stroke volume (mL) | 32 | 52.7 | 60.2 | 60.9 | 55.2 |
| Ejection fraction (%) | 23 | 39.6 | 42.4 | 43.5 | 40.9 |
| Doppler | | | | | |
| Max velocity (cm/s) | 141 | 155 | 158 | 136 | 139 |
| Flow integral (cm) | 16.0 | 14.4 | 14.8 | 13.4 | 13.0 |
| Mean velocity (cm/s) | 99.5 | 104 | 107 | 92.2 | 91.6 |
| Mean acceleration ($cm/s^2$) | 2326 | 2896 | 2939 | 2826 | 2805 |
| Acceleration time (s) | .061 | .054 | .055 | .051 | .053 |
| Ejection time (s) | .161 | .138 | .138 | .146 | .142 |
| Pre-ejection period (s) | .100 | .089 | .085 | .094 | .098 |

*Cardiosynchronous stimulation ratio was 3:1.

Left ventricular dimensions were not substantially different after cardiomyoplasty surgery (Table 4).

## Discussion

Idiopathic dilated cardiomyopathy occurs naturally in large and giant-breed dogs. The etiology of dilated cardiomyopathy in dogs is unknown but is likely multifactorial.[1] There is a familial component to the disease in Doberman pinschers.[2] Although the incidence of dilated cardiomyopathy is unknown, the disease is considered common in large-breed dogs, especially Doberman pinschers.[1,2] The most common clinical presentations for dogs with dilated cardiomyopathy are left-sided congestive heart failure or syncope.[1–4] Signs of right heart failure are unusual except in advanced cases. Survival analysis for cardiomyopathic dogs has not been reported previously, but it is suggested that 50% of affected dogs die within 6 months of onset of signs.[1–4] Kaplan-Meier analysis of 20 dogs with dilated cardiomyopathy in this report confirms the rapidly progressive course of this disease. Most dogs with dilated cardiomyopathy die from progressive heart failure, although approximately 20% of affected dogs experience a sudden death probably from malignant ventricular tachycardia.[1–3] Echocardiographic findings associated with dilated cardiomyopathy in dogs include left ventricular dilation, left atrial enlargement, decreased left ventricular fractional shortening, decreased septal and free wall thickening fractions, and increased E-point septal separation.[1–5] Echocardiographic indices from dogs in this report were consistent with previous reports. Pathological, histologic, ultrastructural, and biochemical findings in dogs with dilated cardiomyopathy are reported to be similar to findings in humans with idiopathic dilated cardiomyopathy.[6–8] Together, these findings suggest that idiopathic dilated cardiomyopathy in dogs is rapidly progressive and clinically similar to idiopathic dilated cardiomyopathy in humans, and as such could be a clinically realistic model of chronic heart failure. Experimental end-points using this model could include invasive and noninvasive indices of cardiac function as well as survival. A randomized trial of cardiomyopathic dogs could provide early information on potential survival benefits associated with different strategies for skeletal muscle cardiac assist.

Dogs have been the most common animal model used to study dynamic cardiomyoplasty, although goats and sheep also have been used.[11–28] Glantz et al.[29] have shown that dogs and goats are physiologically and biochemically different in the way their skeletal muscle adapts to chronic electrical stimulation. It is unclear which physiological pattern more closely resembles human skeletal muscle adaptation. Although useful information about dynamic cardiomyoplasty has been gained by studying animals with normal hearts, investigators recently have focused on evaluating cardiomyoplasty under more realistic circumstances by studying animals with experimentally induced cardiac compromise. Experimental models of cardiac compromise have included rapid ventricular pacing,[17,18] acute intravenous propranolol,[12,14,16] coronary ligation,[15,27] ventricular wall replacement,[13,23,26] and Adriamycin toxicity.[20,24,28] These studies have provided useful information about cardiomyoplasty, although each of these models has limitations as a model of chronic heart failure. Rapid pacing and propranolol are limited to studying acute effects of cardiomyoplasty during heart failure. Coronary ligation results in a more regional rather than global ventricular dysfunction that may be less amenable to assist by cardiomyoplasty. Adriamycin toxicity is perhaps the best model of chronic heart failure; however, toxic effects of this drug may not be limited to cardiac muscle. Injury to skeletal muscle may make this model less appropriate for study of skeletal muscle cardiac assist. Canine idiopathic cardiomyopathy could be an ideal model for study of cardiomyoplasty and other skeletal muscle assist strategies. Although dogs are not anatomically or physiologically identical to humans, it seems likely that cardiac assist strategies that work in such a severe and progressive model would hold promise for human patients.

Risk factor analysis of human patients who have undergone cardiomyoplasty has begun to clarify indications and contraindications for this procedure. Biventricular failure and pulmonary hypertension clearly have emerged as relative contraindications for cardiomyoplasty.[30–32] Persistent Class IV heart failure or a left ventricular ejection fraction $<15\%$ are also contraindications because patients must have some cardiac reserve to survive surgery and the postoperative conditioning period.[30,33] Excessive left ventricular dilation, atrial fibrillation, and complex ventricular arrhythmias have emerged as further absolute or relative contraindications for this procedure.[30,31] If cardiomyoplasty is performed on cardiomyopathic dogs, it is likely that similar contraindications for the surgery will emerge. Dog 1 in this report had medically refractory ventricular tachycardia and experienced sudden death soon after surgery. As is the current practice in human patients, dogs with complex ventricular arrhythmias should not undergo cardiomyoplasty surgery. Dog 2 in this report was in Class IV heart failure that required intravenous inotropic support prior to surgery. This dog's condition was likely too advanced to benefit from cardiomyoplasty and died 6 weeks after surgery despite evidence that cardiomyoplasty was beginning to improve systolic function. Unfortunately, some dogs will not be presented for medical attention until cardiac failure is quite advanced and this may decrease the number of suitable candidates for surgery.

Results from dog 3 demonstrate that cardiomyoplasty can be successfully performed on a dog with advanced dilated cardiomyopathy. Left ventricular ejection fraction, measured by two methods, increased substantially in this dog after cardiomyoplasty surgery. Most patient series report modest but significant improvement in left ventricular ejection fraction after cardiomyoplasty.[31,32,34–38] One report of seven patients showed no improvement in left ventricular ejection fraction 6 months after surgery.[39] It is unclear why the magnitude of improvement in ejection fraction was greater in dog 3 than generally has been observed in humans. One explanation is that results achieved in this one dog are not representative of what would be achieved if more cardiomyopathic dogs were to undergo cardiomyoplasty. Anatomic and physiological differences between humans and dogs also could account for the results observed in this dog. Finally, most studies report results from human patients who have undergone left latissimus dorsi cardiomyoplasty whereas the dogs in this report underwent right latissimus dorsi cardiomyoplasty. Furnary et al.[19] have shown in acute studies of normal dogs that greater enhancement of left ventricular flow and pressure can be achieved from the right latissimus dorsi muscle when compared to the left muscle.

An interesting observation in dog 3 is that cardiac function was improved for both skeletal muscle-assisted and -unassisted systoles. One explanation is that myocardial function spontaneously improved in this dog independent of cardiomyoplasty. While spontaneous improvement in cardiac function in this dog cannot be absolutely excluded, it is unlikely, given the invariably progressive nature of idiopathic dilated cardiomyopathy in dogs.[1–9] An alternative explanation is that benefits from cardiomyoplasty go beyond simple direct cardiac assist. Lee et al.[40] have proposed that cardiomyoplasty augments cardiac output by increasing wall thickness, decreasing wall stress, and normalizing afterload mismatch. These effects could provide benefits that go beyond simple augmentation of stroke volume by contracting skeletal muscle, including improvement in the myocardial oxygen supply-demand relationship. It is tempting to suggest from the above observations that benefits from cardiomyoplasty may be more passive than active. However, it is worth noting that ejection fraction decreased substantially when myostimulation was turned off, even for a short period.

In summary, idiopathic dilated cardiomyopathy in dogs is rapidly progressive and clinically similar to idiopathic cardiomyopathy in humans. Dynamic cardiomyoplasty can be successfully performed and results in improved systolic function in cardiomyopathic dogs. Thus, canine idiopathic dilated cardiomyopathy could be an ideal and realistic model of chronic progressive heart failure. This model could be used to evaluate survival benefits associated with cardiomyoplasty, to investigate mechanisms of altered systolic and diastolic function after cardiomyoplasty, and to test new strategies of skeletal muscle cardiac assist.

## References


1. Calvert CA: Update: Canine dilated cardiomyopathy. In Kirk RW, Bonagura JD (eds): *Current Veterinary Therapy XI: Small Animal Practice.* Philadelphia, W.B. Saunders Co., 1992, pp 773–779.
2. Calvert CA, Chapman WL, Toal RL: Congestive cardiomyopathy in Doberman pinscher dogs. *J Am Vet Med Assoc* 181:598–602, 1982.
3. Thomas RE: Congestive cardiac failure in young cocker spaniels: Details of eight cases. *J Small Anim Pract* 28:265–279, 1987.
4. Lombard CW: Echocardiographic and clinical signs of canine dilated cardiomyopathy. *J Small Anim Pract* 25:59–70, 1984.
5. Gooding JP, Robinson WF, Mews GC: Echocardiographic characterization of dilatation cardiomyopathy in the English cocker spaniel. *Am J Vet Res* 47:1978–1983, 1986.
6. Calvert CA, Brown J: Use of M-mode echocardiography in the diagnosis of congestive cardiomyopathy in Doberman pinschers. *J Am Vet Med Assoc* 189:293–297, 1986.
7. Van Vleet JF, Ferrans VJ, Weirich WE: Pathologic alterations in congestive cardiomyopathy of dogs. *Am J Vet Res* 42:416–424, 1981.
8. Bishop L: Ultrastructural investigations of cardiomyopathy in the dog. *J Comp Pathol* 96:685–698, 1986.
9. Bishop L: Biomechanical investigations of cardiomyopathy in the dog. *Res Vet Science* 43:1–6, 1987.
10. Schiller NB, Shah PM, Crawford M: Recommendations for quantitation of the left ventricle by two-dimensional echocardiography. *J Am Soc Echo* 2:358–367, 1989.
11. Andersen WA, Andersen JS, Acker MA, et al: Skeletal muscle grafts applied to the heart. *Circulation* 78:III/180–III/190, 1988.
12. Chagas ACP, Moreira LFP, Da Luz PL, et al: Stimulated preconditioned skeletal muscle cardiomyoplasty. *Circulation* 80:III/202–III/208, 1989.
13. Soberman MS, Wornom IL, Justicz AG, et al: Latissimus dorsi dynamic cardiomyoplasty of the right ventricle. *J Thorac Cardiovasc Surg* 99:817–827, 1990.
14. Kao RL, Christlieb IY, Magovern GJ, et al: The importance of skeletal muscle fiber orientation for dynamic cardiomyoplasty. *J Thorac Cardiovasc Surg* 99:134–140, 1990.
15. Takemura H, Watanabe G, Sakakibara N, et al: Ventricular assistance by right free wall dynamic cardiomyoplasty following acute right heart failure in canines. *J Cardiac Surg* 6:1:132–136, 1991.
16. Niihami H, Pochettino A, Ruggiero R, et al: Canine latissimus dorsi cardio-double myoplasty: acute feasibility study. *J Cardiac Surg* 6(1):124–131, 1991.
17. Lee KF, Dyke CM, Dignan RJ, et al: Effects of dynamic cardiomyoplasty on left ventricular dynamic geometry in a canine model of dilated cardiomyopathy. *Surg Forum* 42:263–265, 1991.
18. Lee KF, Dignan RJ, Parmar JM, et al: Effects of dynamic cardiomyoplasty on left ventricular performance and myocardial mechanics in dilated cardiomyopathy. *J Thorac Cardiovasc Surg* 102:124–131, 1991.
19. Furnary AP, Magovern JA, Christlieb IY, et al: Improved ventricular augmentation with right latissimus dorsi cardiomyoplasty. *Surg Forum* 42:307–309, 1991.
20. Cheng W, Soberman MS, Justicz AG, et al. Dynamic cardiomyoplasty on left ventricular systolic and diastolic functions in a canine model of chronic heart failure. *Surg Forum* 42:260–263, 1991.

21. Magovern JA, Furnary AP, Christlieb IY, et al: Bilateral latissimus dorsi cardiomyoplasty. *Ann Thorac Surg* 52:1259–1265, 1991.
22. Kawaguchi O, Goto Y, Futaki S, et al: Mechanical enhancement and myocardial oxygen saving by synchronized dynamic left ventricular compression. *J Thorac Cardiovasc Surg* 103:573–581, 1992.
23. Morita K, Koyanagi K, Sakamoto Y, et al: Full-thickness dynamic cardiomyoplasty of the left ventricle with free revascularized latissimus dorsi myografts. *J Thorac Cardiovasc Surg* 104:1125–1134, 1992.
24. Cheng W, Justicz AG, Soberman MS, et al: Effects of dynamic cardiomyoplasty on indices of left ventricular systolic and diastolic function in a canine model of chronic heart failure. *J Thorac Cardiovasc Surg* 103:1207–1213, 1992.
25. Corin WJ, George DT, Sink JD, et al: Dynamic cardiomyoplasty acutely impairs left ventricular diastolic function. *J Thorac Cardiovasc Surg* 104:1662–1671, 1992.
26. Chachques JC, Grandjean PA, Tommasi JJ, et al: Dynamic cardiomyoplasty: A new approach to assist chronic myocardial failure. *Life Support Systems* 5:323–327, 1987.
27. Millner RWJ, Burrows M, Pearson I, et al: Dynamic cardiomyoplasty in chronic left ventricular failure: an experimental model. *Ann Thorac Surg* 55:493–501, 1993.
28. Cheng W, Michele JJ, Spinale FG, et al: Effects of cardiomyoplasty on biventricular function in canine chronic heart failure. *Ann Thorac Surg* 55:893–901, 1993.
29. Glantz JFC, De Jong YF, Coumans WA, et al: Differences in metabolic response of dog and goat latissimus dorsi muscle to chronic stimulation. *J Appl Physiol* 73:806–811, 1992.
30. Chachques JC, Acar C, Carpentier A, et al: Dynamic cardiomyoplasty for long-term cardiac assist. *Eur J Cardiothorac Surg* 6:642–648, 1992.
31. Magovern JA, Furnary AP, Christlieb IY, et al: Indications and risk analysis for clinical cardiomyoplasty. *Semin Thorac Cardiovasc Surg* 3:2:145–148, 1991.
32. Furnary AP, Magovern JA, Christlieb IY, et al: Clinical cardiomyoplasty: Preoperative factors associated with outcome. *Ann Thorac Surg* 54:1139–1143, 1992.
33. Grandjean PA, Austin L, Chan S, et al: Dynamic cardiomyoplasty: Clinical follow-up results. *J Cardiac Surg* 6:80–88, 1991.
34. Carpentier A, Chachques JC: Clinical dynamic cardiomyoplasty: Method and outcome. *Semin Thorac Cardiovasc Surg* 3:136–139, 1991.
35. Jatene AD, Moreira LFP, Stolf NAG, et al: Left ventricular function changes after cardiomyoplasty in patients with dilated cardiomyopathy. *J Thorac Cardiovasc Surg* 102:132–139, 1991.
36. Moreira LFP, Stolf NAG, Jatene AD: Benefits of cardiomyoplasty for dilated cardiomyopathy. *Semin Thorac Cardiovasc Surg* 3:2:140–144, 1991.
37. Bocchi EA, Moreira LFP, De Moraes AV, et al: Effects of dynamic cardiomyoplasty on regional wall motion, ejection fraction, and geometry of left ventricle. *Circulation* 86:II/231-II235, 1992.
38. Moreira LFP, Bocchi EA, Stolf NAG, et al: Current expectations in dynamic cardiomyoplasty. *Ann Thorac Surg* 55:299–303, 1993.
39. Delahaye F, Jegaden O, Montagna, et al: Latissimus dorsi cardiomyoplasty in severe congestive heart failure: The Lyon experience. *J Cardiac Surg* 6:106–112, 1991.
40. Lee KF, Dyke CM, Wechsler AS: Theoretical considerations in the use of dynamic cardiomyoplasty to treat dilated cardiomyopathy. *J Cardiac Surg* 6:119–123, 1991.

Chapter 15

# *Discussion*

**Dr. Salmons:** How do you decide whether or not a dog has pain in the chest at rest?

**Dr. Orton:** We have a modified class system that is based on the NYHA for veterinary patients and it is probably more subjective than yours, but basically, a dog in Class IV is a dog that is restricted to a cage, and cannot go out and move around for any substantial period of time. So we don't know if they have pain. We think they do, but we don't know.

**Dr. Salmons:** Most of these dogs are actually people's pets, aren't they?

**Dr. Orton:** Yes. These dogs were catheterized and had everything done that you would do clinically in humans. The same restrictions would apply. But if you were to set up a study, unless a breeding colony of these dogs was established, you would have to work with owners and the study would have to have some hope of improving the dogs.

**Dr. Starr:** This is very important research. It may be that our surgical advances will have to be confined to another species, at least for the time being. Every large city has a significant reservoir of Dobermans and other large dogs that have cardiomyopathy and we can probably learn a lot from them.

**Dr. Carpentier:** We have not talked about our Russian colleagues' statement that the 1:4 mode or 1:5 mode works better than the 1:2 mode. Do you have the impression that when you go from the 1:2 or 1:3 mode, you get progressively better efficiency of the cardiomyoplasty?

**Dr. Orton:** The way it works with this myostimulator is that the synchonization ratio is dependent on the rate and the way this is set is that when the rate goes above 130 (and the rates in dogs are relatively high compared to humans) it automatically goes to 1:3. When the rate is less than 130, it is set at 1:2. We have no idea what is really optimal. Generally, when we have studied this dog, it is with a little apprehension, and all of these data were derived at 1:3 ratios. We have no idea what is the best way to stimulate a dog.

**Dr. Carpentier:** You have been using the right LD and there has been some concern for possible adhesions between the sternum and the right LD when crossing the midline. I have been told that there have been some early excellent results with progressive deterioration of the results after a few months as a result of these adhesions. This is something that should be investigated in the future. Have you seen any impairment of the function as a result of adhesions?

**Dr. Orton:** We have done this surgery in several normal dogs and after a year, there are a lot of adhesions. We are very curious as to whether these results will last; we have no idea if they will. I am not sure that in a dog where the shoulders are so close together and the chest is narrow that there is a big difference between a right anterior wrap and a left posterior wrap even though data in dogs would suggest otherwise. It does not seem to me that the angle would change that much.

**Unidentified (Lasalle University):** Although the cardiomyopathy seems similar to those in humans, have you any information on the skeletal muscle characteristics of the dog since we know that the metabolic profiles are quite different from those of humans.

**Dr. Orton:** I do not have the expertise to say how close a dog compares to a human and I am very curious to hear that as well. Apparently the circulation is similar and it is a good model from that standpoint, but physiologically I cannot say.

**Dr. Salmons:** It is fair to say that a dog has a much more oxydated LD, so you began with an advantage in that species.

**Dr. Kass (Baltimore):** Could you get dogs in a less severe class of heart failure? Do their owners bring them in only when they are in Class IV?

**Dr. Orton:** Unfortunately, they are often quite advanced and we have lost out doing this surgery on several dogs because they presented in a too advanced state. For some reason, this syndrome sneaks up on people and their dogs and they don't see it as a common disease. How many dogs are going to present that would have a good indication for the surgery? We concluded that we would have to include cases from several centers in order to do a study on a significant number of dogs.

**Dr. Kass:** How well has neurohumoral status been worked out in the spontaneous heart failure in the dog?

**Dr. Orton:** It has been worked out incompletely. The assays exist and we know that elevated norepinephrine levels in dogs with heart failure correlate with poor survival. We know that much but we have not done any further studies.

**Dr. Cheng (New York):** Perhaps we have a wrong idea that the LD wraps around the heart. Where did you get this idea? Surgeons practicing manual massage of the heart know that this is totally different from wrapping the heart with a muscle. When you use manual massage, the hand is free from the ventricle when the heart contracts. The hand may or may not contract. If the hand does not contract, it won't influence the ventricle. On the other hand, you wrap the LD muscle around the ventricle; they adhere together. When the ventricle contracts and the muscle does not contract, the ventricle has to pull this muscle with it. This may decrease the cardiac function.

**Dr. J. Magovern:** These discussions point out that there really is an art to surgery in constructing these wraps. There is no question that cardiomyoplasty can depress cardiac function but it is not necessarily an inherent property of cardiomyoplasty. Dr. Cheng must be congratulated because if you are going to talk about depression of cardiac function you really need to measure load-independent indices of ventricular function. It is clear that cardiomyoplasty affects ventricular geometry and volume probably more than it affects contractility. If you are going to change ventricular volume, you then have to use volume or load-independent measures of contractility.

Chapter 16

# Static Cardiomyoplasty Effects on Load-Dependent and Load-Independent Left Ventricular Systolic Function

David T. George, William J. Corin, James D. Sink, William P. Santamore

## Introduction

Cardiomyoplasty is a new alternative approach under investigation for the treatment of congestive heart failure.[1–4] This surgical procedure uses the patient's latissimus dorsi muscle (LDM) to provide direct cardiac assistance. In this procedure, the LDM is isolated, positioned in the chest, and wrapped around the heart. In current clinical practice, the muscle is not stimulated for the first 2 weeks following the wrapping procedure.[2] Thus, in the early postoperative period, the effects of cardiomyoplasty are due primarily to the application of passive muscle to the epicardium (static cardiomyoplasty).

Due to the risk and difficulty in assessing a patient's hemodynamic state early after a surgical procedure, there are no reports of hemodynamic measurements either immediately after or in the first 2 weeks following the cardiomyoplasty procedure. It has been suggested, however, that because of delay between surgery and the beginning of cardiac augmentation, patients should have sufficient preoperative cardiac reserve to survive this period.[1,4,5] Despite this caution, there is little documentation of left ventricular function in the early postoperative period. Most clinical and experimental studies have emphasized left ventricular functional measurements with and without muscle stimulation[2,4,6] or compared stimulated beats with unstimulated beats[7,8] or compared late postoperative (3–6 months) hemodynamics with preoperative function.[2,4,9] Several experimental studies comparing pre-and postwrap hemodynamics suggest that the application of the muscle wrap to a normal heart depresses left ventricular function.[10–12] However, these studies did not measure preload-independent indices of left ventricular function.

From Carpentier A, Chachques JC, Grandjean P: Cardiac Bioassist. © Futura Publishing Co, Inc, Armonk, NY, 1997.

To better understand left ventricular function during the immediate postoperative period, we measured the effect of static cardiomyoplasty in dogs. We used preload-independent indices of left ventricular systolic function, including maximum systolic elastance and preload recruitable stroke work. Data were taken before and after wrapping the β-adrenergic blocked heart with the LDM.

## Methods

### Overview

We analyzed the acute effects of cardiomyoplasty on left ventricular (LV) systolic function in a canine preparation. The LV pressure–short axis area relationship was obtained using micromanometry and sonomicrometry over a wide range of systolic pressures, produced by occluding the inferior and superior venae cavae. Data were analyzed to obtain the maximum elastance and recruitable stroke work.

### Animals

Six mongrel dogs (20–30 kg) were used in this study. All animals were cared for a humane fashion, in accordance with guidelines published by the National Institutes of Health (*Guide for Care and Use of Laboratory Animals*, NIH Publication 85-23, revised 1985). This animal investigation was approved by the Institutional Animal Care and Use Committee of the Presbyterian Medical Center.

### Experimental Preparation

The surgical protocol used to isolate the LDM and create the cardiomyoplasty was similar to that previously described from this laboratory.[2,9,10] General anesthesia was induced using intravenous sodium pentobarbital (25 mg/kg) and the dogs were intubated. Ventilation was maintained using a Harvard Respirator and volume ventilator with 100% oxygen. Anesthesia was supplemented as needed with sodium pentobarbital (100 mg IV). A limb lead electrocardiogram (ECG) was monitored throughout the experiment. After adequate anesthesia was confirmed, the left LDM was exposed via a transverse left axillary skin incision, and skin flaps developed. Dissection of the LDM was carried out carefully to preserve the thoracodorsal pedicle. A 5-cm arc of the lateral portion of the second rib was resected and the LDM was then positioned in the chest via the defect in the second rib. The thorax was opened by a median sternotomy and the heart suspended in a pericardial cradle.

### Instrumentation

Piezo crystals (ID3, 4 mm diameter, 3 MHz, Triton Technology, San Diego, CA) were introduced into the LV cavity via a small puncture in the apex of the heart. To ensure correct positioning of the crystals, a needle was inserted sequentially across the anterior-posterior and septal free wall diameters at the base of the heart. The piezo crystal wires were retracted from the ventricular cavity through these small holes and positioned on the endocardial surface of the anterior, posterior, septal, and lateral walls (Fig. 1). LV short axis area was calculated from the dimensional data obtained by sonomicrometry. At the completion of each experiment, proper piezo crystal placement was confirmed by visual inspection.

A 5F micromanometer (Millar Instruments, Houston, TX) was inserted via the LV apex and a 7F fluid-filled catheter was inserted into the LV via the carotid artery. The fluid-filled catheter was connected to a pressure transducer (Transpac II, Abbott Laboratories, Salt Lake City, UT) and was balanced to zero at the level of the LV and to 100 mm Hg using a physiological monitor (VR-12, PPG Biomedical, Pleasantville, NY). Using the same monitor, the micromanometry catheter was calibrated to zero and to the mean pressure of the fluid-filled catheter. Pressure and dimension data were digitally converted at 200 Hz (MacAdios II, GW Laboratories, Somerville, MA) and stored on computer disc (MAC IIcx, Apple Computers, Cupertino, CA) for analysis after completion of the study. Finally, the azygos vein was tied off and snare occluders were placed around the superior and inferior venae cavae. Lidocaine (50 mg IV) was given as needed to abolish arrhythmias.

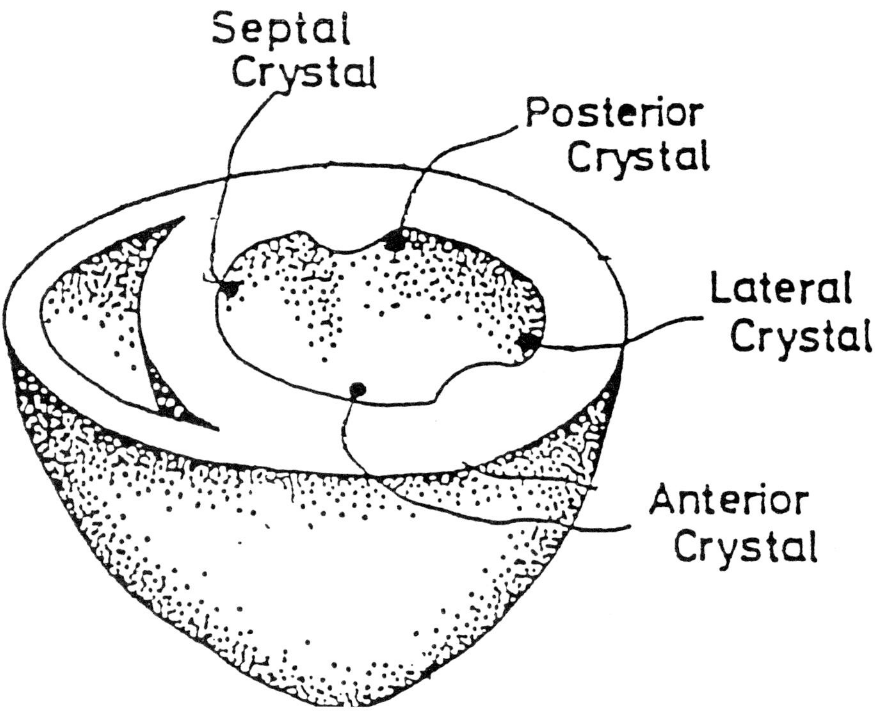


**Figure 1:** *A schematic drawing illustrating sonomicrometry crystal placement on the endocardial surface to measure the anterior-posterior and septal free wall dimensions. Crystals were inserted into the left ventricle via the apex and positioned on the endocardial surface at the base of the heart.*

## Experimental Protocol

After confirming satisfactory signals, baseline systolic function was evaluated. The respirator was turned off at end-expiration and LV pressure and dimensions were measured during vena caval occlusion. Contractile function data were determined from pressure and short axis area measurements from beats occurring during vena caval occlusion. β-adrenergic receptors were blocked using intravenous propranolol (1 mg/kg) and systolic function was again evaluated using LV preload reduction.

A left posterior cardiocostal LDM wrap was then done.[13] The most proximal portion of the muscle that reached the heart was applied just below the atrial ventricular groove under the left atrial appendage. The costal aspect of the LDM was placed on the epicardium, with the spinal aspect closest to the atrioventricular groove. In this way, the LDM was wrapped posteriorly around the heart, encompassing the entire left and right ventricles (Fig. 2). The tightness of the muscle wrap was adjusted so that there was no change

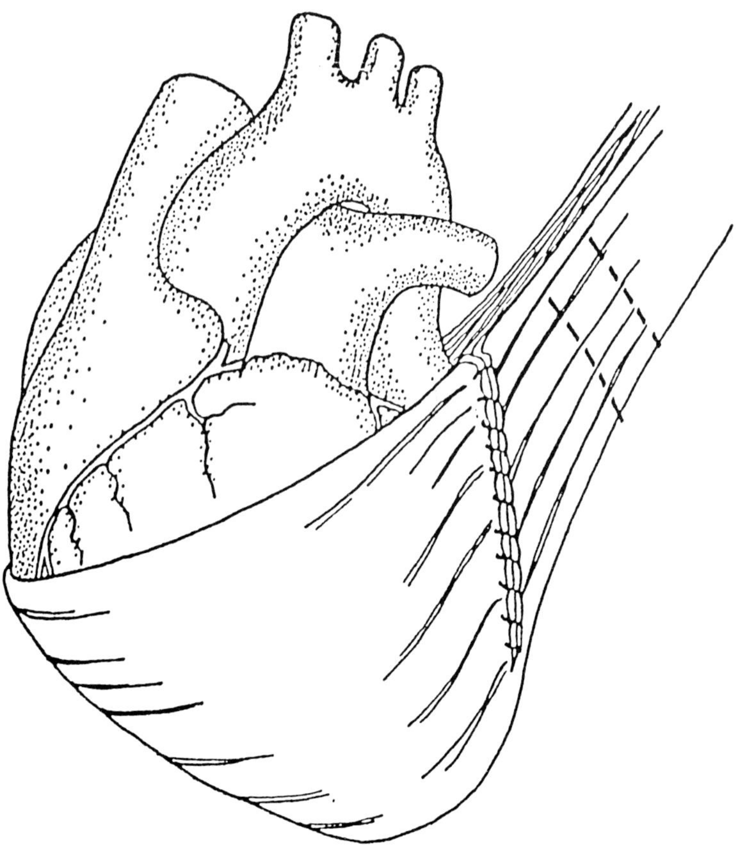

**Figure 2:** *A biventricular wrap was done using the left latissimus dorsi muscle. The latissimus muscle was wrapped posteriorly around the two ventricles.*

in end-diastolic short axis area, as determined by the real-time signals from the piezo crystals. This is comparable to the technique of Morwick and colleagues,[14] who used intraoperative echocardiography to prevent constrictive pathophysiology.

After completion of the wrap, LV systolic function was reevaluated at steady state and during preload reduction. At completion of the study, the animal was euthanized, the heart removed, and positioning of the crystals was confirmed by visual inspection.

## Data Analysis

Using data analysis software developed in our laboratory (ASYST, Keithly-Metrabyte, Taunton, MA), we extracted hemodynamic variables from the digitally stored data to create LV pressure–short axis area loops. After excluding irregular beats, hemodynamic data from the remaining beats were used to evaluate LV contractile function.

Left ventricular area (A, $cm^2$) was calculated using Eq. 1:

$$A = \pi D_{fw\text{-}sep} D_{a\text{-}p}/4 \quad [1]$$

where $D_{fw\text{-}sep}$ and $D_{a\text{-}p}$ were the LV free wall septum and anterior-posterior diameters (cm), respectively.

The first time derivative of ventricular pressure, dP/dt, was calculated by numeric differentiation of the Millar pressure signal. Differentiation was accomplished using a second-order interpolating polynomial fit algorithm (ASYST). End-systole and end-diastole were determined using differential analysis of instantaneous LV pressure (dP/dt).[6,15]

An area stroke work analog (SW, mm Hg-$cm^2$) was calculated from the integral of ventricular pressure (P, mm Hg) and cavitary area over each cardiac cycle, using Eq. 2:

$$SW = \int (PdA) \quad [2]$$

Preload recruitable stroke work (RSW) was calculated by linear regression analysis of the SW and end-diastolic area (EDA, $cm^2$) data, using Eq. 3[16]:

$$SW = RSW\,(EDA - A_w). \quad [3]$$

Preload recruitable stroke work was defined as the slope of the relationship between stroke work and end-diastolic area, with $A_w$ as the x-intercept.

Left ventricular systolic function was also evaluated from the slope of the end-systolic pressure (ESP, mm Hg) end-systolic area (ESA, $cm^2$) relationship[17] shown in Eq. 4:

$$ESP = Emax\,(ESA - Ao) \quad [4]$$

## Statistical Analysis

Hemodynamic and contractility data at baseline, after propranolol, and after the muscle wrap were compared by repeated-measures one-way analysis of variance. When this analysis indicated a significant difference among the three conditions, Scheffe's test was used to compare the conditions. Differences with a statistical probability less than 0.05 were considered significant. All data are presented as the mean and the standard error of the mean.

## Results

Figure 3 shows an example of left ventricular pressure and area before and after the muscle wrap in the β-adrenergic blocked heart. The beats are time-matched to the ECG. In this record, the static muscle wrap decreased peak LVP by about 12 mm Hg. Left ventricular end-diastolic and end-systolic areas were decreased slightly by the wrap.

Left ventricular hemodynamic data at baseline, after propranolol administration, and after the LDM wrap are summarized in Table 1. β-adrenergic blockade decreased heart rate ($p<0.05$). End-diastolic area and pressures were increased by propranolol ($p<0.05$). After propranolol, peak systolic LVP decreased and peak positive LV dP/dt decreased ($p<0.05$), while area stroke work increased. The wrap did not affect heart rate. The wrap tended to decrease end-diastolic area and end-diastolic pressure (Fig. 4), but these changes did not reach statistical significance. Peak left ventricular systolic pressure was decreased by the muscle wrap. Peak positive dP/dt was reduced 19% ($p<0.05$) and area stroke work by 40% ($p<0.05$) after the LDM wrap.

Figure 5 shows left ventricular pressure and short axis area from one experiment during a vena caval occlusion, immediately before the wrap procedure. Peak left ventricular pressure was near 100 mm Hg before the occlusion. As the venae cavae were occluded, systolic pressure decreased rapidly and then more gradually, approaching about 60 mm Hg after 20 seconds of preload reduction. Similarly, short axis area decreased during the occlusion maneuver. Figure 6 shows left ventricular pressure-area loops and the calculated end-systolic pressure-area relation (ESPAR) as measured immediately before (left panel) and then after wrapping the heart (right panel), from the same experiment as in Figure 5. In this study, the slope of the ESPAR (Emax) was slightly increased after the muscle wrap; the x-intercept was shifted slightly to the right.

Preload-independent measures of left ventricular systolic function are presented in Table 2 and Figure 7. β-adrenergic block reduced maximum systolic elastance ($p<0.05$) but the x-intercept of the ESPAR was unaffected. After propranolol, preload recruitable stroke work tended to decrease while the x-intercept of the stroke work–end-diastolic area relation was unchanged. The muscle wrap had no effect on Emax or the x-intercept of the ESPAR. Preload recruitable stroke work tended to decrease with the LDM wrap, but this change was not statistically significant. The muscle wrap did not affect the x-intercept of the stroke work-end-diastolic area relation.

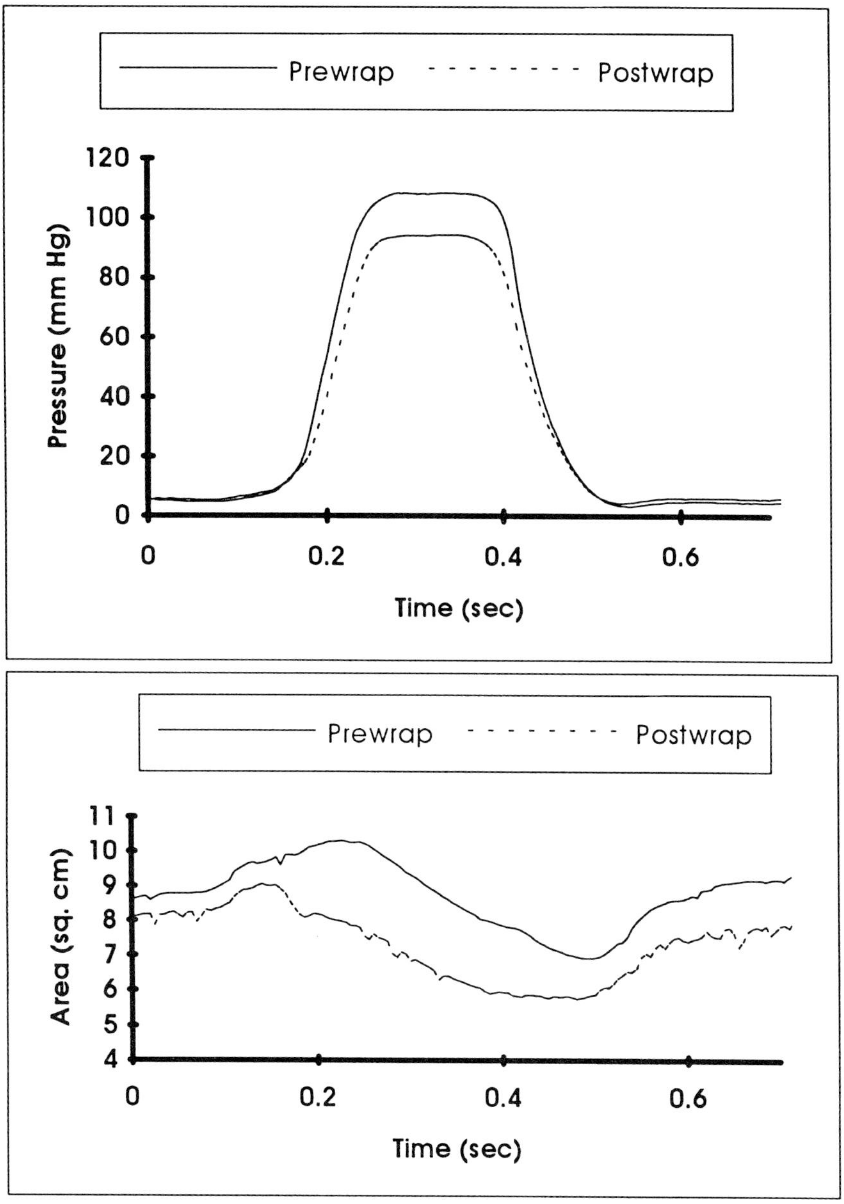


**Figure 3:** *Experimental record of left ventricular pressure and area from before and immediately after the muscle wrap. The signals are time-matched to the ECG.*

**Table 1**
Hemodynamic Effects of Muscle Wrap

| *Variable* | *Baseline* | *Prewrap* | *Postwrap* |
|---|---|---|---|
| HR (bpm) | 136 ± 12 | 94 ± 9* | 102 ± 8 |
| EDA ($cm^2$) | 5.7 ± 0.9 | 6.9 ± 1.2* | 6.3 ± 1.3 |
| EDP (mm Hg) | 5.8 ± 0.4 | 7.8 ± 0.8* | 6.7 ± 0.7 |
| LVP (mm Hg) | 100 ± 7 | 89 ± 7 | 79 ± 8 |
| LV dP/dt (mm Hg/sec) | 1540 ± 129 | 1159 ± 94* | 934 ± 115** |
| SW (mm Hg*$cm^2$) | 139 ± 17 | 162 ± 26 | 99 ± 24** |

HR = heart rate; EDA = end-diastolic area; EDP = end-diastolic pressure; LVP = left ventricular pressure; LV dP/dt = time derivative of LV pressure; SW = area stroke work.

Data are reported as mean ± the standard error of the mean.

*$p<0.05$ compared with baseline.

**$p<0.05$ compared with prewrap.

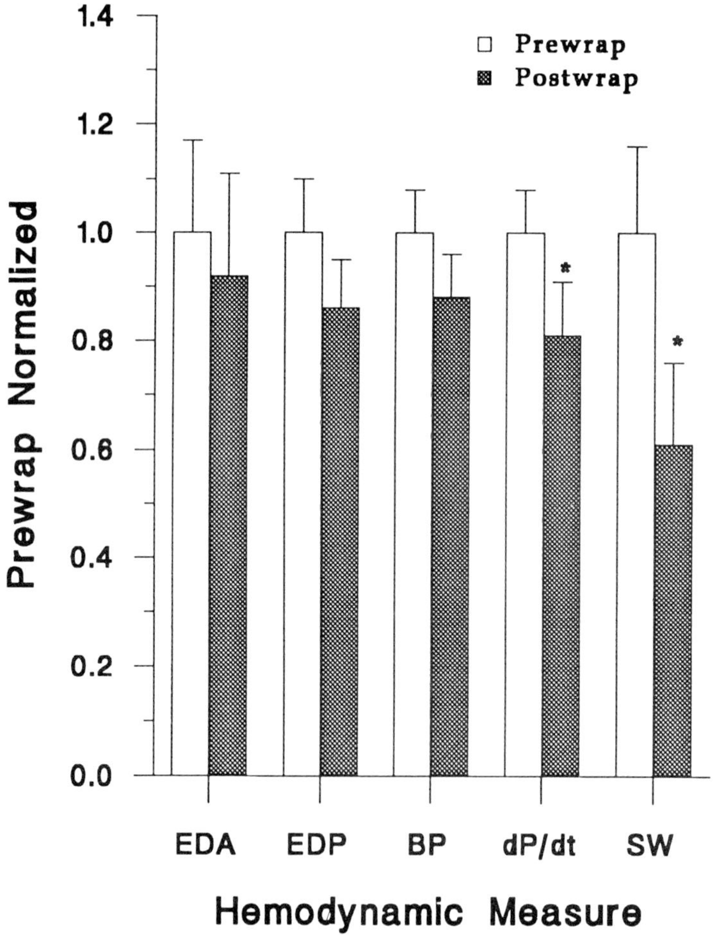


**Figure 4:** *Prewrap-normalized hemodynamic measures. End-diastolic area (EDA) and end-diastolic pressure (EDP) were unchanged by the muscle wrap. Peak left ventricular systolic pressure (BP), peak positive dP/dt (dP/dt), and area stroke work (SW) decreased with the muscle wrap. *p<0.05 compared with prewrap.*

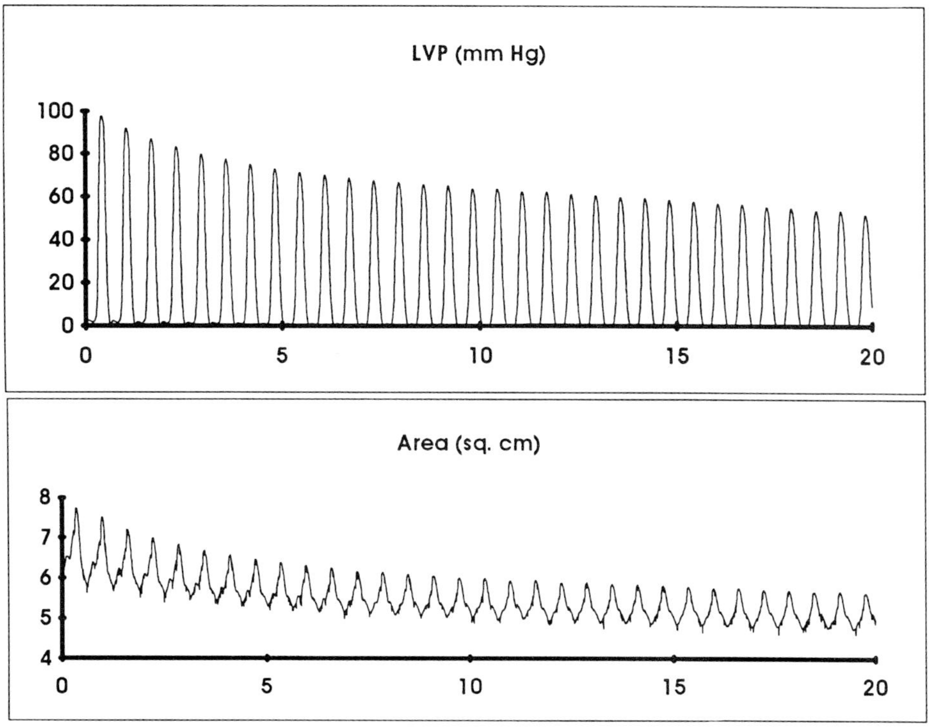


**Figure 5:** *Left ventricular pressure and short axis area as measured during a vena caval occlusion of the β-adrenergic blocked heart. Peak left ventricular pressure decreased from about 100 mm Hg to 60 mm Hg during the occlusion.*

## Discussion

The effect of cardiomyoplasty on LV function in the early postoperative period is an important determinant of the success of the procedure. In current practice, the muscle is not stimulated during the first 2 postoperative weeks. During this period, the muscle adheres to the epicardium and revascularizes after isolation of its collateral blood flow. Therefore, the primary effect of the muscle wrap is due to the application of the passive LDM (static cardiomyoplasty). Earlier work suggested that static cardiomyoplasty caused depression of preload-dependent measures of LV systolic[11,12] and diastolic[10] function in normal hearts. Our results show that in a β-adrenergic blocked heart, some preload-dependent measures of LV systolic function are impaired with the passive wrap, but that preload-independent measures of contractility are unchanged. The passive wrap decreased peak LV dP/dt and stroke work (Table 1); however, the wrap did not change maximum systolic elastance, preload recruitable stroke work, or their intercepts (Table 2).

Because of the risk and difficulty in assessing a patient's hemodynamic state early after a surgical procedure, there are no reports of hemodynamic measurements in the first 2 weeks following the cardiomyoplasty procedure. However, it has been observed that New York Heart Association (NYHA) Class IV patients have a poorer prognosis following the cardiomyoplasty procedure

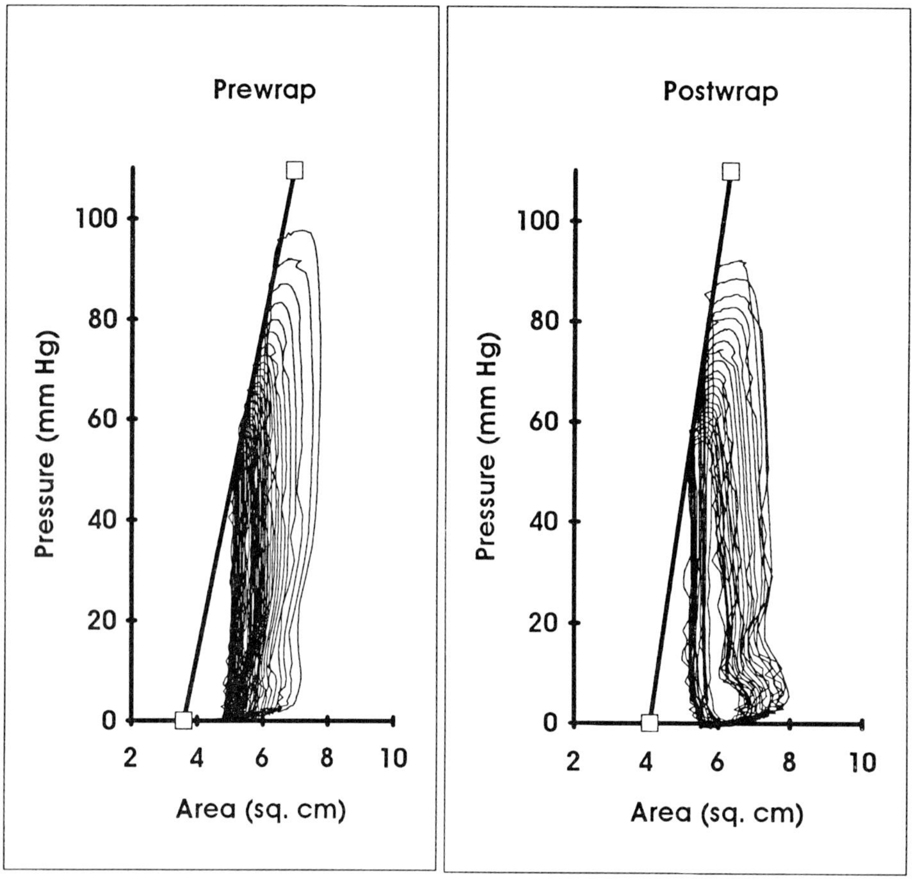


**Figure 6:** *Pressure-area loops during vena caval occlusion as calculated from data obtained before and after static cardiomyoplasty. Left panel shows loops from before the muscle wrap and the right panel shows loops immediately after the muscle wrap. The end-systolic–pressure area relations are shown.*

**Table 2**
Contractility Measures

| *Variable* | *Baseline* | *Prewrap* | *Postwrap* |
|---|---|---|---|
| Emax (mm Hg/cm$^2$) | 96 ± 5 | 59 ± 8* | 65 ± 15 |
| Ao (cm$^2$) | 3.4 ± 0.9 | 3.2 ± 1.0 | 3.4 ± 1.0 |
| RSW (mm Hg) | 80 ± 18 | 70 ± 16 | 57 ± 15 |
| Aw (cm$^2$) | 4.0 ± 0.8 | 4.2 ± 0.9 | 4.4 ± 1.1 |

Emax-maximum systolic elastance; Ao = x-intercept of the end-systolic pressure-area relation; RSW = preload recruitable stroke work; Aw = x-intercept of the stroke work-EDA relation.

Data reported as mean ± the standard error of the mean.

**p*<0.05 compared with baseline.

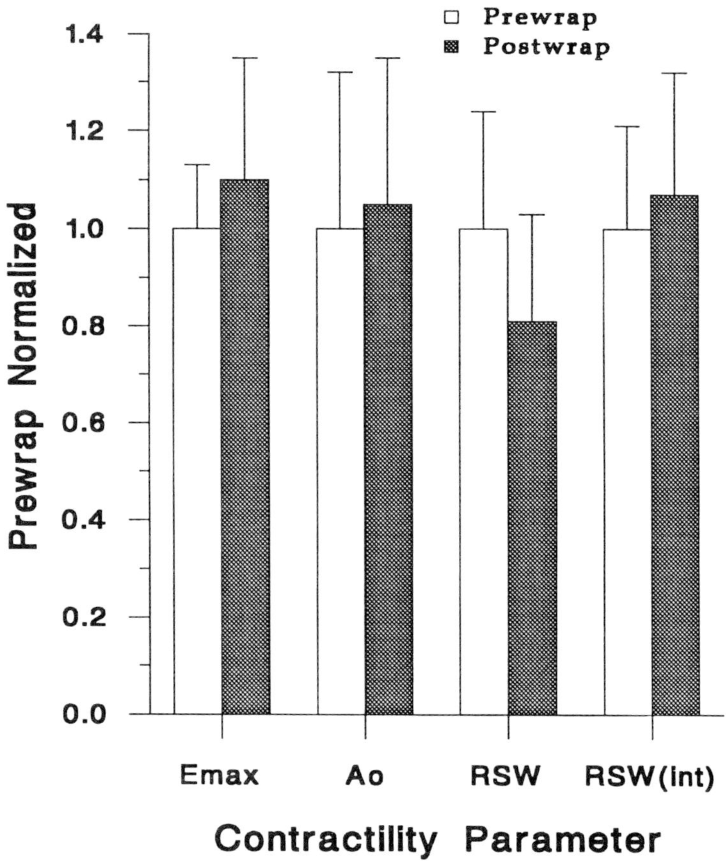


**Figure 7:** *Prewrap-normalized contractility measures. Maximum systolic elastance (Emax) and its x-intercept (Ao) were increased slightly by the wrap. Preload recruitable stroke work (RSW) decreased and its x-intercept (RSW(int)) increased after the muscle wrap.*

than NYHA Class III patients.[18] In a review of 78 clinical cardiomyoplasty procedures, early deaths, defined as those that occur prior to discharge, were significantly higher in preoperative Class IV patients (33%) than in class III patients (12%). Of the 29 deaths occurring in the study group, the most common cause was given as perioperative complications (13 deaths). Perioperative depression of LV function may contribute to the high early mortality of the NYHA Class IV patients. This is also consistent with the suggestion that patients have sufficient cardiac reserve to overcome the delay between the surgical procedure and initiation of muscle contraction.[1,3,5]

These observations have led to proposed modifications in the cardiomyoplasty procedure, with the goal of using the muscle sooner after surgery. Fibrin glue has been proposed to fix the skeletal muscle to the heart epicardium more rapidly.[19] Pharmacological and electrical means of improving skeletal muscle performance have been proposed.[20,21] Preconditioning of the skeletal muscle prior to cardiomyoplasty has also been reported.[3,22–24]

## Comparison with Literature

In recent experimental studies, hemodynamic function was measured immediately following the cardiomyoplasty surgery.[10–12] Earlier work from our laboratory suggested that static cardiomyoplasty caused mild LV diastolic dysfunction in the normal heart.[10] Comparison of pre- and postwrap diastolic function showed that although end-diastolic area and end-diastolic pressure were unchanged by the static wrap, more sensitive indices suggested the presence of diastolic dysfunction. The static wrap reduced peak negative left ventricular dP/dt by 20%, caused an eightfold increase in the constant of passive stiffness, and increased the time constant of diastolic relaxation ($\tau$) by 40%.

Magovern's group performed left, right, and bilateral LDM cardiomyoplasty in dogs and measured depressed ventricular function immediately following each procedure.[11,12] They reported significant decreases in peak right ventricular systolic pressure, peak positive right ventricular dP/dt, peak LV pressure, and peak aortic pressure and flow. Peak LV systolic pressure decreased 19% with the left wrap and 27% with the bilateral wrap. Similarly, left and bilateral wraps decreased peak dP/dt by 26% and 39%, respectively.[12]

To this first manuscript, they added data from right LDM cardiomyoplasty and compared pre- and postwrap hemodynamic function.[11] As with the left wrap, application of the passive right muscle decreased peak positive right ventricular dP/dt, peak left ventricular systolic pressure, peak left ventricular dP/dt, peak aortic flow, and aortic pressure. The severity of depression was similar to the left wrap. They report that, in general, bilateral cardiomyoplasty caused a more severe depression of LV function than did cardiomyoplasty using solely the left or the right LDM. They did not measure left ventricular dimensions in these studies.

Our results demonstrated a less severe depression in systolic function than measured by the Pittsburgh group.[11,12] It is possible that the effects of static cardiomyoplasty differ in pericardium-intact, normal hearts compared to pericardectized, β-adrenergic blocked hearts. In addition, they did not report end-diastolic area, so constrictive pathophysiology following the muscle wrap cannot be ruled out. Finally, Magovern and colleagues used a two-stage procedure wherein the LDM was first isolated and 7 to 10 days later the muscle wrap was done. For this study, we isolated the muscle and measured LV hemodynamics on the same day. We have also performed the two-stage procedure and found that a preisolated LDM has greater passive stiffness than a freshly isolated muscle. A stiffer LDM has the potential to cause more severe dysfunction. Both the single[3,25] and multiple surgery procedures[3,22] have been reported clinically. It is thought that the two-stage procedure may be better for patients who cannot tolerate long surgical procedures.[26,27] However, a comparison of the single-day versus multiple-day cardiomyoplasty procedures has not been made.

## Mechanism

Our laboratory measured impairment of preload-dependent measures of LV systolic function with the muscle wrap, but we did not find greatly decreased end-diastolic area or elevated end-diastolic pressure. Potential mechanisms leading to LV systolic dysfunction include reduced myocardial contractility, preload or afterload changes, and changes in diastolic chamber properties. The small change in end-diastolic area (Table 1) suggests that preload may have been reduced slightly after the wrap; however, this change was not statistically significant. Direct measurement of contractility showed unchanged myocardial contractility (Table 2). Similarly, previous work from our laboratory suggests that sensitive indices of diastolic function show a decline in the rate of diastolic pressure decay and a prolongation of the pressure relaxation constant, without evidence of constrictive pathophysiology after the LDM wrap.[10] The likeliest mechanism of depression is due to the increased heart mass caused by the addition of the passive muscle. The mass of the LDM applied to the heart is comparable to the mass of the heart. If intrinsic myocardial force does not change with the muscle wrap, increased inertial effects will lead to decreased wall motion.

It is difficult to interpret the findings of Magovern and colleagues[11,12] with regard to potential mechanisms of impaired LV hemodynamics because they did not report end-diastolic area or end-diastolic pressure. As a result, constrictive pathophysiology following the muscle wrap cannot be excluded. In addition to reduced LV preload, observations of reduced peak positive LV dP/dt are consistent with the ventricular wall carrying along the additional mass of the passive LDM. It is interesting that Magovern's group measured greater decreases in LV systolic performance in the bilateral wrap which has, presumably, about twice the muscle mass applied to the heart as with the left. This is comparable to hypertrophic hearts where decreased dP/dt has been observed.[28] A potential mechanism is that increased muscle mass caused increased inertial effects. It is reasonable that a similar mechanism is at least partly responsible for the acute LV depression seen after cardiomyoplasty in the study presented here and in the previous works.[10–12] The greater impairment of LV function with the bilateral wrap, without any evidence to suggest constrictive pathophysiology, is a potential indication of the significance of the additional mass. In the acute setting, this is difficult to measure, because the muscle is not yet adhered to the epicardium. In our studies, however, we did not observe loss of contact between the epicardium and the LDM. We believe that the decreases in preload-dependent measures of left ventricular function following cardiomyoplasty are due to the combination of mild reduction in left ventricular preload and increased inertial effects.

An important but difficult-to-quantify aspect of the muscle wrap procedure is the "tightness" of the muscle wrap. It is generally agreed that the muscle should be wrapped as tightly as possible but not so tight as to impair ventricular filling.[6] We followed this heuristic rule by using the crystal and pressure signals to monitor end-diastolic area and pressure during the wrapping procedure. Other investigators report using echocardiography to insure no constrictive pathophysiology following the muscle wrap.[14]

The use of sonomicrometry has allowed us to do advanced analysis on cardiac function. In particular, we can calculate preload-independent measures of systolic function by taking pressure and dimension measurements during preload reduction. Two previous studies reported using sonomicrometry to measure LV dimensions during cardiomyoplasty,[6,10] and one study measured LV dimensions during extra-aortic counterpulsation.[29]

Wechsler's group[6] used sonomicrometry to measure one minor axis dimension, wall thickness, and, in some studies, the long axis dimension in a pacing-induced dilated cardiomyopathy model in the dog. Dimensions were measured immediately after the LDM wrap, both with and without LDM stimulation. Their results suggested that LDM stimulation augmented systolic shortening in the minor axis. Their data cannot be compared with our study, however, because they did not measure LV function before the LDM wrap. Our laboratory has also used sonomicrometry to measure ventricular dimensions during cardiomyoplasty.[10] We measured diastolic dysfunction in normal dog hearts after static cardiomyoplasty.

Wechsler's group[29] used micromanometry and sonomicrometry to measure the effects of skeletal muscle extra-aortic counterpulsation on left ventricular unloading and functional mechanics. They measured ventricular short axis dimension and wall thickness and found that counterpulsation decreased left ventricular minor axis diameter and increased wall thickness. In addition, left ventricular work loops calculated from wall stress and minor axis dimension shifted downward and to the left with skeletal muscle counterpulsation.

## Limitations

This study measured the perioperative effects of static cardiomyoplasty in a β-adrenergic blocked heart. The effects of the static wrap may differ in a setting of congestive heart failure where chronic cardiac dilatation and more severely compromised cardiac function are present. Comparison of pre- and postwrap hemodynamics will be a valuable component of any chronic study.

It has been suggested that one cannot augment function of a normal heart subjected to dynamic cardiomyoplasty, and that some cardiac dysfunction must be present.[30,31] This point is unclear, however, because augmentation of normal hearts has also been reported.[7,8,10–12] Analogously, it is possible that the perioperative effects of static cardiomyoplasty may be related to the severity of prewrap cardiac dysfunction. This study observed dysfunction following static cardiomyoplasty in the β-adrenergic blocked heart whereas earlier works also reported dysfunction in normal hearts.[10–12]

## Conclusion

We used well-established measures of LV function to assess LV function before and after wrapping the heart with the left LDM. After static cardiomyoplasty, we observed decreases in preload-dependent measures of LV hemodynamics (dP/dt and stroke work), while preload-independent measures remained unchanged. These results suggest that static cardiomyoplasty causes mild LV systolic dysfunction in this model. Likely mechanisms leading to depression are slight preload reduction and increased inertial effects. A "loose" muscle wrap configuration that does not affect preload will minimize the potential dangers of constrictive pathophysiology; however, inertial effects will be difficult to avoid. Future studies involving a chronic heart failure model should include careful measurement of pre- and postwrap function.

*Acknowledgment:* We acknowledge the superb technical support of Gioia V. Di Loreto-Sharp and John J. Michele.

## References


1. Carpentier A, Chachques JC: Clinical dynamic cardiomyoplasty: Method and outcome. *Semin Thorac Cardiovasc Surg* 3(2):135–139, 1991.
2. Cheng W, Justicz AG, Soberman MS, et al: The effect of dynamic cardiomyoplasty on indices of left ventricular systolic and diastolic function in a canine model of chronic heart failure. *J Thorac Cardiovasc Surg* 103:1207–1213, 1992.
3. Magovern JA, Furnary AP, Christlieb IY, et al: Indications and risk analysis for clinical cardiomyoplasty. *Semin Thorac Cardiovasc Surg* 3(2):145–148, 1991.
4. Moreira LFP, Bocchi EA, Noedir AG, et al: Current expectations in dynamic cardiomyoplasty. *Ann Thorac Surg* 55:299–303, 1993.
5. Orie JE: Dynamic cardiomyoplasty: A possible alternative treatment of congestive heart failure. *Semin Thorac Cardiovasc Surg* 3(2):98–100, 1991.
6. Lee KF, Dignan RJ, Parmar JM, et al: Effects of dynamic cardiomyoplasty on left ventricular performance and myocardial mechanics in dilated cardiomyoplasty. *J Thorac Cardiovasc Surg* 102:124–131, 1991.
7. Chachques JC, Grandjean MS, Schwartz K, et al: Effect of latissimus dorsi dynamic cardiomyoplasty on ventricular function. *Circulation* 78(Suppl III):203–206, 1988.
8. Fischer EIC, Chachques JC, Garcia A, et al: Effect of cardiomyoplasty on left ventricular diastolic function. *BAM* 1(3):253–258, 1991.
9. Cheng W, Michele JJ, Spinale FG, Sink JD, et al: Effects of cardiomyoplasty on biventricular function in canine chronic heart failure. *Ann Thorac Surg* 55(4):893–901, 1993.
10. Corin WJ, George DT, Sink JD, et al: Dynamic cardiomyoplasty acutely impairs left ventricular diastolic function. *J Thorac Cardiovasc Surg* 104:1662–1671, 1992.
11. Furnary AP, Magovern JA, Christlieb IY, et al: Component analysis of bilateral anterior cardiomyoplasty. *Ann Thorac Surg* 55:72–77, 1993.
12. Magovern JA, Furnary AP, Christlieb IY, et al: Bilateral latissiumus dorsi cardiomyoplasty. *Ann Thorac Surg* 52:1259–1265, 1991.
13. Furnary AP, Christlieb IY, Magovern JA, et al: A standardized nomenclature for latissimus dorsi cardiomyoplasty. *J Cardiac Surg* 6:74–79, 1991.
14. Morwick TH, Novoa R, Salsaidu EE, et al: Influence of latissimus dorsi cardiomyoplasty on left ventricular filling. *RBM* 13(2):106–108, 1991.
15. Lew WYW, LeWinter MM: Regional comparison of midwall segment and area shortening in the canine left ventricle. *Circ Res* 56:31–39, 1985.
16. Glower DD, Spratt JA, Snow ND, et al: Linearity of the Frank-Starling relationship in the intact heart: the concept of preload recruitable stroke work. *Circulation* 71:994–1009, 1985.
17. Sagawa K, Suga H, Shoukas AA, et al: End-systolic pressure/volume ratio: a new index of ventricular contractility. *Am J Cardiol* 40:748, 1977.
18. Grandjean PA, Austin L, Chan S, et al: Dynamic cardiomyoplasty: clinical follow-up results. *J Cardiac Surg* 6(1 Suppl):80–88, 1991.
19. Lorusso R, Lucas C, van der Veen F, et al: Early latissimus dorsi stimulation after cardiomyoplasty procedure: a preliminary study. *BAM* 1(1):83–87, 1991.
20. Dubelaar ML, Lucas CMBH, Hulsmann WC: The effect of L-carnitine on force development of the latissimus dorsi muscle in dogs. *J Cardiac Surg* 6(1):270–275, 1991.
21. Delosso TN, George DT, Cruz MP, et al: Variable frequency stimulation of latissimus dorsi muscle for cardiomyoplasty. In Li JKJ, Reisman SS (eds): *Proceedings of the Nineteenth Annual Northeast Bioengineering Conference.* IEEE Publishing, Inc., 1993, pp. 154–155.
22. Almada H, Molteni L, Ferreira R, et al: Clinical experience with dynamic cardiomyoplasty. *J Cardiac Surg* 5(3):193–198, 1990.

23. Chagas ACP, Moreira LFP, da Luz PL, et al: Stimulated preconditioned skeletal muscle cardiomyoplasty. An effective means of cardiac assist. *Circulation* 80(Suppl III):202–208, 1989.
24. Soberman MS, Wornom IL, Justicz AG, et al: Latissimus dorsi dynamic cardiomyoplasty of the right ventricle. *J Thorac Cardiovasc Surg* 99:817–827, 1990.
25. Jatene AD, Moreira LFP, Stolf NAG, et al: Left ventricular function changes after cardiomyoplasty in patients with dilated cardiomyopathy. *J Thorac Cardiovasc Surg* 102:132–139, 1991.
26. Magovern GJ, Heckler FR, Park SB: Paced skeletal muscle for dynamic cardiomyoplasty. *Ann Thorac Surg* 45:614, 1988.
27. Chachques JC, Grandjean PA, Carpentier A: Patient management and clinical followup after cardiomyoplasty. *J Cardiac Surg* 6:89–99, 1991.
28. Lorell BH, Grossman W: Cardiac hypertrophy: The consequences for diastole. *J Am Coll Cardiol* 9:1189–1193, 1987.
29. Lee KF, Hanan SA, Tuchy GE, et al: Skeletal muscle extraaortic counterpulsation: A true arterial counterpulsation. *J Thorac Cardiovasc Surg* 102:757–765, 1991.
30. Anderson WA, Anderson JS, Acker MA, et al: Skeletal muscle grafts applied to the heart: A word of caution. *Circulation* 78(Suppl 3):180–190, 1988.
31. Hill A, Li C, Tchervenkov C, et al: Dynamic cardiomyoplasty for hemodynamic support during acute pulmonary hypertension. An experimental study. *J Thorac Cardiovasc Surg* 103:1200–1206, 1992.

Chapter 16

# Discussion

**Dr. Salmons:** The inertial effects should increase as adhesions developed between the wrap and the heart. That would be difficult in your model to emulate.

**Dr. Sink:** The model was designed to look at the acute and static effects prior to the beginning of stimulation. Some of these patients have a difficult time immediately following the operation and we wanted to investigate that.

**Dr. Salmons:** It is interesting that you see changes in speed of development of tension rather than in some of the more static parameters. When you do a statistical test, you can't induce whether it is an increase or a decrease if it is not statistically different.

**Dr. Chachques:** Regarding the conclusion that preload recruitable stroke work is impaired, if I understand it correctly, you based that on a situation in which the end-diastolic pressure was decreased. I believe that your end-diastolic diameter or area as measured by the crystals was decreased significantly not only because of the pressure decrease but because of the lesser compliance induced by the wrap. If you had filled the ventricle to the same diameter prior to systole, would you have achieved the same amount of preload recruitable stroke work?

**Dr. Sink:** The end-systolic area and end-systolic pressure were not significantly decreased. I believe I said they tended to decrease but not significantly.

From Carpentier A, Chachques JC, Grandjean P: Cardiac Bioassist. © Futura Publishing Co, Inc, Armonk, NY, 1997.

Chapter 17

# Can Time-Varying Interpulse Intervals in the Stimulation Burst Improve Cardiac Function in Dynamic Cardiomyoplasty?

Tuan Bui, Gordon B. Jacobs, Todd Nixon, John A. Spratt, Vince Doerr

## Introduction

Heart failure (HF) is a prevalent disease affecting at least 2 million people in the United States alone.[1] The prognosis is poor with a mortality from all causes of 52% at 1 year.

Medical therapy and cardiac transplantation are the conventional treatments for HF. However, the mortality rate of HF patients with these treatments is still high and the limited availability of donor hearts severely limits the number of patients able to receive heart transplants. Dynamic cardiomyoplasty may provide an alternative treatment for cardiomyopathic patients and has been shown to improve survival and functional status in uncontrolled studies using carefully selected patients.[2] Cardiomyoplasty is a surgical procedure that requires mobilization of the latissimus dorsi muscle (LDM), keeping the neurovascular pedicle intact, then wrapping the LDM around the ventricular portion of the heart. The LDM is electrically stimulated by bursts of pulses to contract synchronously with the heart and thereby to augment cardiac function. Prior to its use for cardiac assistance, the LDM is trained in order to improve resistance to fatigue. This is done with a gradually increasing number of stimulating pulses during the first 6–8 weeks after surgery.

Since skeletal muscle is not a syncytium, tetany can only be achieved with a series of stimulation pulses delivered in the vicinity of the thoracodorsal nerve. A number of studies have been conducted to determine the ideal electrical pulse burst for stimulating skeletal muscle. Lucas et al.[3] investigated the effect of variations in the frequency of the stimulating burst on contractile force

From Carpentier A, Chachques JC, Grandjean P: Cardiac Bioassist. © Futura Publishing Co, Inc, Armonk, NY, 1997.

in untrained and trained LDM. Contractile force was measured with a force displacement transducer connected to the dog's left front leg. It was found that for trained muscle, contractile force increased progressively with a stimulus frequency of five pulses per second (pps) to reach a maximum at a stimulus rate of 30 pps. For untrained muscle, near maximal force was obtained at a stimulation frequency of 65 pps.

Delosso et al.[4] compared the contractile performance of untrained canine LDM during constant frequency bursts (CFB) to that with variable frequency bursts (VFB); the CFB was a six-pulse burst at 30 pps while the VFB was a five-pulse burst starting with a 100 pps triplet followed by a 24 pps doublet. Contractile force was again measured with a force transducer connected to the left forefoot of the dog. Contractile performance was better with VFB than CFB in the nonfatigued state with the difference becoming even greater during muscle fatigue.

Shea et al.[5] evaluated the contraction time and time to peak shortening of untrained LDM stimulated with the same CFB and VFB stimulus regimens. Contraction time was found to be 18% shorter with VFB than CFB and they noted that this observation may have implications for diastolic function.

Since the burst length of the VFB was shorter than that of the CFB in these studies, it is not clear whether the reduction in contraction time was caused by the VFB or by a shorter burst length. Also, since the studies by Delosso and Shea were done with unconditioned muscles, their observations are not directly applicable to the conditioned LDM used in cardiomyoplasty.

The effects of variable frequency bursts on trained LDM wrapped around the heart were evaluated in the present study. We hypothesized that muscle relaxation would be faster with no reduction in maximum contractile force or systolic cardiac augmentation if a VFB stimulus regimen was used in contrast to a CFB regimen. The burst length was kept constant to eliminate its effect on contraction time. Muscle mechanics was evaluated by measuring contraction time and fractional shortening while the hemodynamic parameter used was left ventricular (LV) pressure. Measurements were made at constant interpulse intervals and at a range of increasing interpulse intervals.

## Materials and Methods

### Surgical Procedure

Four mongrel dogs (20–25 kg) were used in this study, which was approved by the Institutional Animal Care and Use Committee. All animals were cared for in a humane fashion in accordance with guidelines published by the National Institutes of Health (*Guide for the Care and Use of Laboratory Animals,* NIH publication 85-23, revised 1985).

Anesthesia was induced with sodium thiopental (25 mg/kg IV), and the animals were intubated. The animals were then shaved, placed on the operating room table, and sterility prepped. Anesthesia was maintained with isoflurane (0.5% to 3.0%) via an anesthesia machine and a volume ventilator. Prophylactic antibiotics (penicillin G; 25,000 U/kg) were administered 30 minutes before the skin incision and daily for 7 days after initial surgical procedure. A transverse left axillary skin incision was made and the left LDM was dissected free from all attachments except the thoracodorsal neurovascular pedicle. Two intramuscular leads (Telectronics IML-03U) were then placed 5 cm apart across the width of the muscle with the proximal cathode lead placed within the LDM on the costal side at the region of the thoracodorsal nerve trifurcation. A 3-cm segment of the second rib was resected, allowing the LDM to be passed into the thoracic cavity. The humeral insertion of the muscle was then divided and sutured to the periostium of the third rib.

A thoracotomy was then performed through the fifth intercostal space and the heart was exposed. After placement of an epicardial pace/sense lead (Telectronics Model 033-572) near the apex of the right ventricle, a biventricular anterior cardiocostal cardiomyoplasty wrap[6] was then performed. The LDM was then sutured to the epicardium and the leads were exteriorized and connected to the myostimulation device (Telectronics MyoStim 7220). The myostimulator was placed in a subcutaneous pocket, and all wounds were closed in layers. The animals were then allowed to recover from anesthesia.

## LDM Training

A 2-week vascular delay period was used prior to starting the conditioning regimen. The conditioning protocol used is shown in Table 1. The burst synchronization ratio (heart beat: myostimulation rate) was 2:1 for heart rates below 130 bpm and 3:1 for rates above this level.

## In Vivo Measurements

A terminal study was performed at 13 weeks after implantation. The animals were anesthetized with thiamylal sodium (25 mg/kg), intubated, and secured on the operating room table in the supine position. A median sternotomy was performed to expose the heart and cardiomyoplasty wrap. Micromanometer-tipped catheters (Millar Instruments, Houston, TX) were inserted through the apex of the LV and through the femoral artery to measure intracavitary LV and distal aortic pressures, respectively. A pair of ultrasonic transducers were placed in the body of the latissimus muscle 2–3 cm apart and in the region of the distal intramuscular stimulating lead in order to measure LDM shortening. Electrocardiogram lead II was continuously monitored.

The LDM was then stimulated using three CFB and two VFB regimens. The stimulus modes were changed in random fashion, and 5–10 minutes were allowed before data collection and between different interventions. The five stimulating conditions used are described in Table 2 and shown graphically in Figure 1. Condition 1 was the chronic programmed burst, a CFB of six pulses at 25 pps, with a burst length of 200 ms. In condition 2, a CFB of eight pulses at 35 pps (28.5-ms interval) was used with the same burst length of 200 ms. In condition 3, a variable frequency burst of 35 pps was used. The interval between the first two pulses was 28.5 ms (35 pps), while each subsequent interpulse interval

**Table 1**
LDM Training Regime

| | *Vascular Delay Period* | *Conditioning Period* | *Conditioning Period* | *Conditioning Period* | *Chronic Programmed Parameters* |
|---|---|---|---|---|---|
| Week | 1–2 | 3–4 | 5–6 | 7–8 | 9–12 |
| Burst Frequency | | 25 pps | 25 pps | 25 pps | 25 pps |
| Pulses per Burst | 0 | 1 | 2 | 4 | 6 |
| Burst Duration | | 0.1 ms | 40 ms | 120 ms | 200 ms |
| Sync Ratio* | | 2:1 | 2:1 | 2:1 | 2:1 |
| Stimulus Amplitude | | 5 volts | 5 volts | 5 volts | 5 volts |
| Burst Pulse Width | | 0.10 ms | 0.10 ms | 0.10 ms | 0.10 ms |

*The sync ratio was 2:1 for heart rates below 130 bpm and 3:1 for higher heart rates.

**Table 2**
Stimulation Conditions

| *Condition* | *Number of Pulses* | *Frequency (pps)* | *Increment (ms)* | *Burst Length (ms)* |
|---|---|---|---|---|
| 1 | 6 | 25 | 0 | 200 |
| 2 | 8 | 35 | 0 | 200 |
| 3 | 6 | 35 | +5.9 | 202 |
| 4 | 18 | 85 | 0 | 200 |
| 5 | 6 | 85 | +13.7 | 195.5 |

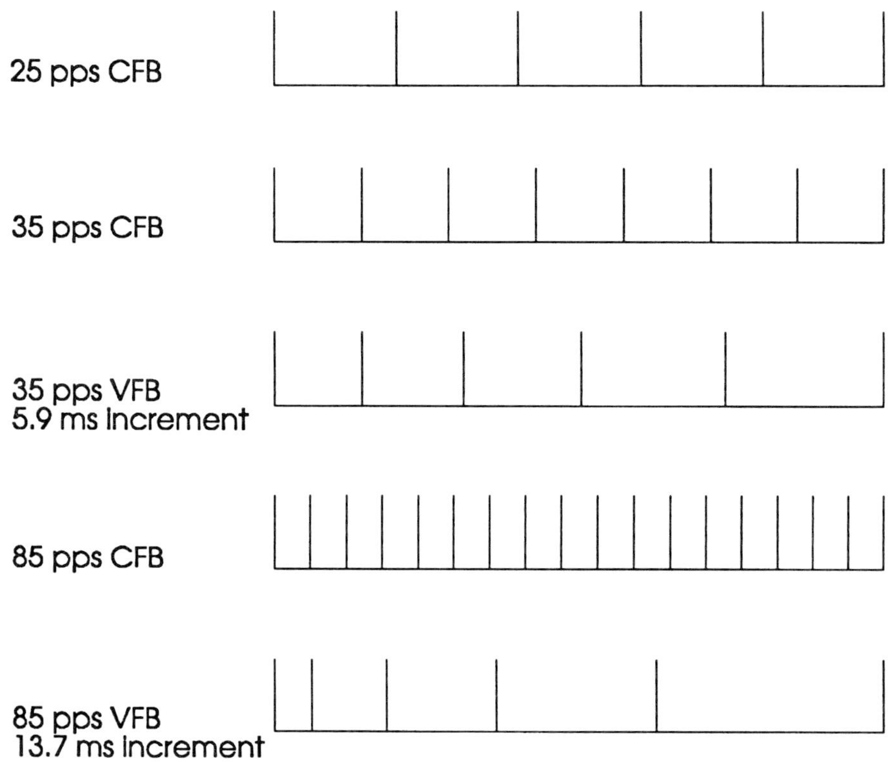


**Figure 1:** *Burst of stimulating pulses.*

was progressively increased by 5.9 ms. In condition 4, a CFB of 18 pulses of 85 pps (11.7-ms interval) was used. In condition 5, a VFB of 85 pps was used with a larger increment between the interpulse intervals. The interval between the first two pulses was 11.7 ms (85 pps), while each subsequent interpulse interval was progressively incremented by 13.7 ms. The total burst lengths of each of the five conditions was kept close to 200 ms.

During each stimulus regimen, data were digitally recorded at 200 Hz and stored for subsequent analysis. The muscle shortening and aortic pressure were later analyzed using custom designed programs available in our laboratory.

## Results

Muscle shortening, reported as percentage shortening from the unstimulated length, ranged from 23.2 ± 9.5% to 31.4 ± 7.6%. It was greatest during the 85 pps CFB regimen (condition 4) as shown in Table 3.

Contraction time was defined as the time from the first stimulation pulse to the onset of muscle relaxation. Figure 2 shows a typical contraction time for condition 4 (85 pps CFB) and condition 5 (85 pps VFB). One observes from this figure that the degree and rate of muscle shortening is nearly identical to the two stimulus regimens. However, the VFB regimen shows earlier relaxation. Contraction times were shorter for both VFB regimens compared to the CFB conditions. When the increment in the interpulse interval was small (5.9 ms), the reduction was not significant (e.g., between conditions 2 and 3). However, when a large increment (13.7 ms) in the interpulse interval was used, the contraction time decreased from 298 ± 12 to 179 ± 48 ms as shown in Table 3 (conditions 4 and 5).

The LV pulse pressure of the stimulated beats was found to be highest with condition 4 (85 pps CFB) and lowest for conditions 5 (85 pps VFB) and 1 (25 pps CFB) as shown in Table 4. There was no statistically significant difference in LV pulse pressure between CFB and VFB.

The percentage change in LV pulse pressure from unstimulated beats to stimulated beats is another way to measure the effectiveness of myostimulation (Fig. 3). The percentage improvements are shown in Table 4. The highest was 7.9% for 85 pps CFB (condition 4). In general, CFB stimulus regimens produced greater improvement than VFB.

There were no noticeable differences in the maximum dP/dt between CFB and VFB stimulus regimens. There was no consistent relationship between maximum dP/dt and increasing stimulus frequency (conditions 1, 2, and 4). In the VFB regimens, maximum dP/dt decreased slightly with an increase in the interpulse interval (condition 5).

Maximum negative dP/dt, calculated from the LV pressure curve, was used as an index of diastolic function. The absolute values of -dP/dt were within the range of normal values reported by Corin et al.[7] (typically 1,400 mm Hg/sec at 80 mm Hg and 1,790 mm Hg/sec at 110 mm Hg). There was a consistent trend of an increasing slope when the stimulating bursts were changed from CFB to VFB. At 35 pps, the increase was 2.6 ± 0.5% while the increase was 3.5 ± 2.8% for 86 pps bursts.

Table 3

Muscle Mechanics Results

| *Condition* | *Muscle Shortening (%)* | *Contraction Time (ms)* |
|---|---|---|
| 1 | 23.2 ± 9.5 | 262 ± 35 |
| 2 | 28.2 ± 6.1 | 263 ± 30 |
| 3 | 24.3 ± 8.4 | 258 ± 15 |
| 4 | 31.4 ± 7.6 | 298 ± 12 |
| 5 | 23.5 ± 8.2 | 179 ± 48 |

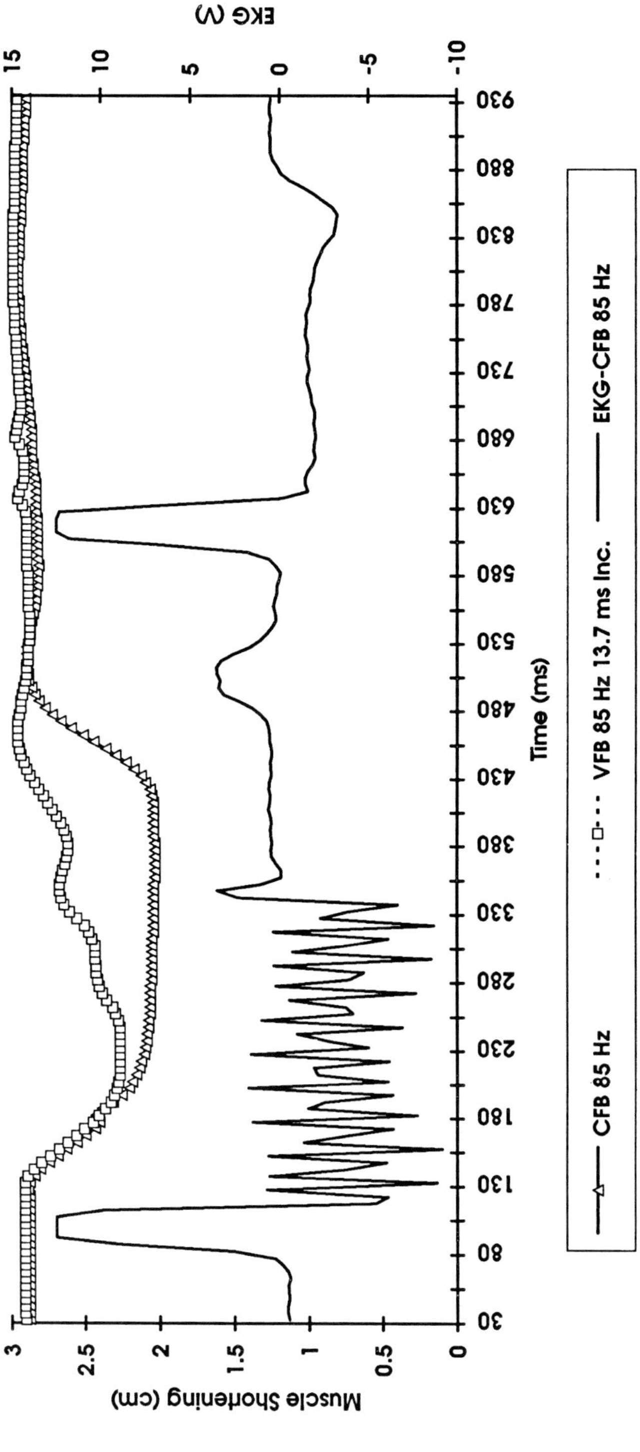


Figure 2: *Muscle shortening.*

**Table 4**
Systolic Parameters

| *Condition* | *LV Pulse Pressure (mmHg)* | *Improvement in LV Pulse Pressure (%)* | *Max. dP/dt (mm Hg/sec)* |
|---|---|---|---|
| 1 | 86.5 ± 17.2 | 4.3 ± 3.0 | 1642.4 ± 20.7 |
| 2 | 87.5 ± 15.5 | 5.7 ± 2.8 | 1682.5 ± 30.4 |
| 3 | 87.7 ± 14.3 | 5.1 ± 3.2 | 1665.0 ± 28.6 |
| 4 | 92.1 ± 22.1 | 7.9 ± 4.0 | 1672.5 ± 50.3 |
| 5 | 84.9 ± 12.0 | 5.8 ± 3.8 | 1642.5 ± 35.2 |

## Discussion

When a skeletal muscle is conditioned for fatigue resistance, the physiology is straightforward and has been increasingly well defined over the last 10 years. With cardiomyoplasty, however, the situation is more complicated in that the conditioned muscle has been mobilized from much of its vascular supply and its physical configuration has been changed. Muscle length and tension are therefore more difficult to measure and vary with position throughout the muscle. Measurements are made more difficult due to the confounding effects of cardiac activity. One of the ongoing concerns with using trained LDM for cardiac assist is the significant increase in both contraction and relaxation times[8] after training. This increase may result in a loss of power available for systolic augmentation,[9–11] while the slower relaxation speeds may not allow the LDM sufficient time to relax and consequently inhibit diastolic filling. In clinical cardiomyoplasty, device-related considerations such as battery life span and the electronics to control the stimulus regimens are also additional factors. The problem can be reduced to the following question: Given a period of time in the cardiac cycle (up to approximately 200 ms), what is the best way to stimulate the cardiomyoplasty wrap to augment cardiac performance? The term "best" involves considerations of muscle conditioning and physiology, the stimulus regimen used, and myostimulator limitations. In the present study, we investigated the effects of CFB and VFB stimulus patterns in a chronically conditioned LDM cardiomyoplasty preparation.

The trained LDM in a myoplasty configuration provides a realistic model for studying the effect of time-varying interpulse intervals on muscle mechanics and on cardiac hemodynamics. The percentages of muscle shortening were in the range of 23.2 ± 9.5% to 31.4 ± 7.6%. Since the muscles were wrapped around the heart, load could not be accurately measured, but the amount of contraction was comparable to that reported by Chachques and Carpentier[12] (19% at a 1,000-g load to 46% at a 200-g load).

For CFB, the results from Table 3 showed that muscle contraction tended to be stronger with increasing myostimulation frequencies. The percentage muscle shortening at 85 pps CFB was 36% higher than that at 25 pps CFB (31.4% vs. 23.2%). Muscle shortening decreased slightly with VFB. However,

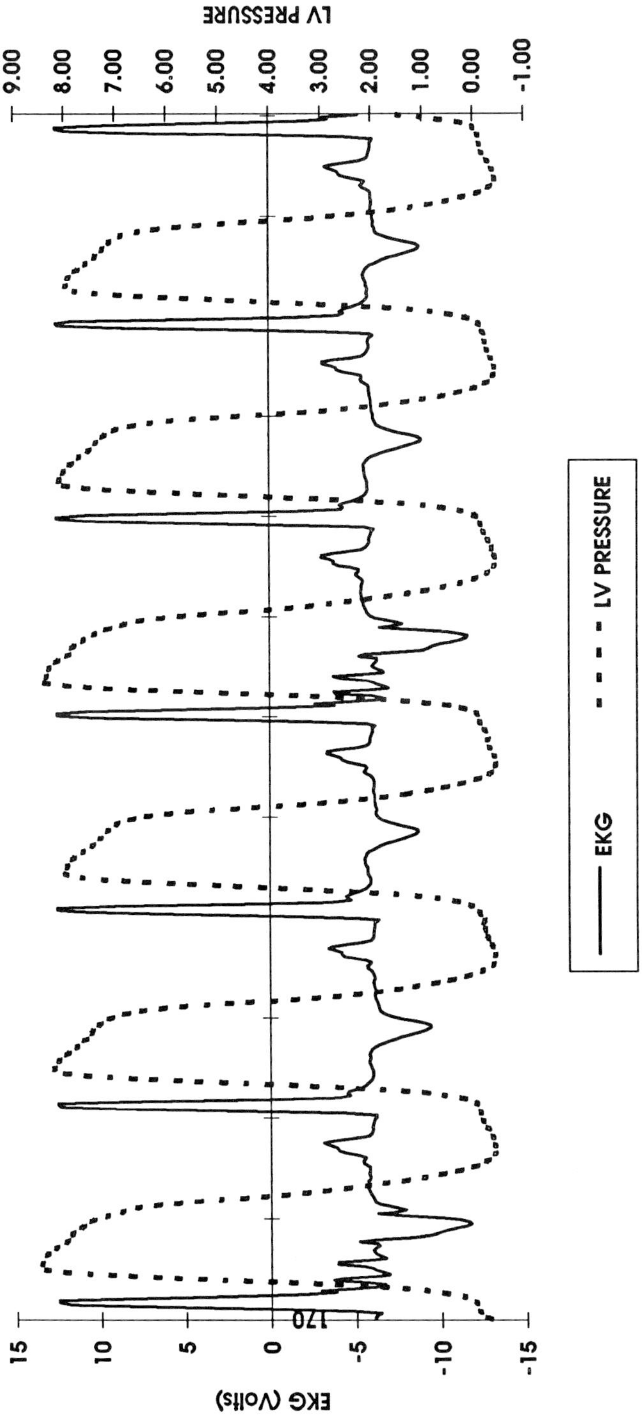


**Figure 3:** *Left ventricular pressure.*

when evaluated on a per pulse basis, the normalized shortening was higher for VFB than CFB. At 85 pps, the shortening was 3.91% (23.5/6 pulses) per pulse for VFB and 1.74% (31.5/18 pulses) for CFB. This indicates that the VFB is more efficient at causing muscle contraction than CFB.

Contraction time was found to be relatively constant for CFB at 25, 35, and 85 pps. This agrees with Neilson and Chiu[13] who found that the contraction time increased with stimulation frequency from 10 pps to 20 pps, then remained constant. Contraction times decreased, however, when the VFB stimulation was used. This reduction was not significant with the 5.9 ms increment, but was significantly reduced by 66% with the 13.7 ms increment, from 298 ms at 85 pps CFB to 179 ms at 85 pps VFB. The reduction was higher than that measured by Shea at al.[5] in which the total contraction decreased by 15% with their VFB. It is difficult to directly compare the two experimental results because the contraction time in our experiment was calculated from the time of first stimulation pulse to the onset of relaxation, while Shea et al. measured from the beginning of contraction to return to baseline.

The reasons for a decrease in contraction time in condition 5 are twofold. First, only six stimulus pulses were used in contrast to 8 or 18 in conditions 2 and 4. Second, the degree of muscle tetany was less as expressed by slight decreases in both muscle shortening and LV pulse pressure. Since less tetany was achieved, contraction time also decreased.

Muscle shortening, shown in Figure 2, sometimes showed stepwise changes in contraction. This may mean that the muscle reached full tetanic contraction only at the beginning of the cycle and reverted to twitching at the end of the cycle. However, the frequency used in the experiment was higher than the fusion frequency of 12 ± 3 pps for trained muscle as reported by Chachques and Carpentier.[12] Quite possibly, this LDM was not completely transformed. The waveforms in this figure suggest a future area of research in which the time-varying interpulse interval feature is used to optimize training, similar to the approach attempted by Badylak et al.[14]

A reduction in contraction time is of benefit only if the hemodynamic gains are not decreased. These benefits were analyzed by examining the changes in systolic function, such as the LV pulse pressure and maximum dP/dt. The LV pulse pressure difference between the assisted and nonassisted beats ranged from 4.3 ± 3.1% to 7.9 ± 4.2%. This is within the range of differences seen by Lucas et al.[15,16] who found an 11% acute improvement in the assisted beats for normal goats and a 2% improvement after 12 weeks of stimulation. This indicates that the improvements observed here with VFB are within the normal range of augmentation expected in cardiomyoplasty. Systolic function did not seem to change significantly when the CFB was changed to VFB. The LV pulse pressures were found to decrease by about 10% for bursts of 85 pps and there were no noticeable changes for bursts of 35 pps. Minimal changes in maximum dP/dt were observed when the CFB was changed to VFB.

Diastolic function, which was measured indirectly by the changes in maximum negative dP/dt, increased when the stimulating bursts were changed from CFB to VFB. This faster negative dP/dt would suggest a more compliant isovolumic relaxation phase, and hence an overall improvement in ventricular filling.

Levin, Tsitlik, and Halperin[17] developed a mathematical model to study the importance of timing between the natural heart and LDM. They found that residual LDM tension early in diastole would limit rapid filling and significantly reduce the benefits of cardiomyoplasty. Lucas et al.[18] analyzed the effect of muscle relaxation during dynamic cardiomyoplasty and also argued that diastolic filling of the heart may be impaired by a prolonged contraction of the LDM and furthermore that insufficient relaxation may inhibit coronary blood flow, possibly causing myocardial ischemia. Davies et al.[19] demonstrated in goats that at heart rates above 87 bpm, the total cycle time was extended to 460 ms and prevented the muscle from achieving maximal fractional shortening. In our experiments, the significant reduction in contraction time for the 85 pps VFB has the potential to improve diastolic function.

There are two major limitations to this study. The first is that only four animals were used. As a result, the statistical power to test the significance of our observations was low. The second is that although the LDM was conditioned, cardiac function was normal. This undoubtedly decreased the magnitude of the changes in systolic and diastolic function that we observed.

## Conclusion

In this study, we examined the effects of CFB and VFB stimulus regimens in a conditioned LDM cardiomyoplasty model. We observed that the VFB mode produced nearly comparable systolic cardiac augmentation to that obtained with CFB stimulation. Additionally, however, VFB stimulation produced a shorter contraction time that may improve diastolic performance and consequently extend the battery life of the myostimulator. These data, therefore, suggest that cardiomyoplasty stimulus regimens that employ VFB pacing may have advantages over ones that employ only CFB stimulation. These observations need to be verified in a larger number of animals, preferably with induced or natural heart failure. Finally, the approach of using a smaller number of pulses but at CFB should be examined as a reasonable alternative.

*Acknowledgment:* The authors acknowledge valued comments and contributions by Dr. Jonathan Jarvis.

## References

1. SOLVD Investigators: SOLVD Rationale, Design and Methods: Two trials that evaluate the effect of enalapril in patients with reduced ejection fraction. *Am J Cardiol* 66:315–322, 1990.
2. Moreira LFP, Seferian P, Bocchie EA, et al: Survival improvement with dynamic cardiomyoplasty in patients with dilated cardiomyopathy. *Circulation* 84:(III) 296–302, 1991.
3. Lucas CMHB, Van Der Veen F, Grandjean PA, et al: What is the ideal pulse frequency for skeletal muscle stimulation after cardiomyoplasty? *PACE* 14:778–782, 1991.
4. Delosso TN, George DT, Cruz MP, et al: Variable frequency stimulation of latissimus dorsi muscle for cardiomyoplasty. In Li JKJ, Relsman SS (eds): *Proc Nineteenth Annual Northeast Bioengineering Conference.* IEEE Publishing, Inc., 1993, pp 154–155.

5. Shea JS, Cruz MP, Delosso TN, et al: Comparison of cardiac and skeletal muscle contraction times: Relevance to cardiomyoplasty. In Li JKJ, Relsman SS (eds): *Proc Nineteenth Annual Northeast Bioengineering Conference.* IEEE Publishing, Inc., 1993, 19–20.
6. Furnary AP, Christlieb IY, Magovern JA, et al: A standardized nomenclature for latissimus dorsi cardiomyoplasty. *J Cardiac Surg* 6(Suppl):74–79, 1991.
7. Corin WJ, George DT, Sink JD, et al: Dynamic cardiomyoplasty acutely impairs left ventricular diastolic function. *J Thorac Cardiovasc Surg* 104:1662–1671, 1992.
8. Salmons S, Henriksson J: The adaptive response of skeletal muscle to increased use. *Muscle Nerve* 4:94–105, 1981.
9. Salmons S, Jarvis JC: Cardiomyoplasty: A look at the fundamentals. In Carpentier A, Chachques JC, Grandjean PA (eds): *Cardiomyoplasty.* Mount Kisco, NY, Futura Publishing Co., 1991, pp 3–17.
10. Salmons S, Jarvis JC: The working capacity of skeletal muscle transformed for use in a cardiac assist role. In Chiu RCJ, Bourgeois IM (eds): *Transformed Muscle for Cardiac Assist and Repair.* Mount Kisco, NY, Futura Publishing Co., 1990, pp 89–104.
11. Salmons S, Jarvis JC: Cardiac assistance from skeletal muscle: A critical appraisal of the various approaches. *Br Heart J* 68:333–338, 1992.
12. Chachques JC, Carpentier A: Experimental basis of cardiomyoplasty. In Carpentier A, Chachques JC, Grandjean PA (eds): *Cardiomyoplasty.* Mount Kisco, NY, Futura Publishing Co., 1991, pp 77–96.
13. Neilson IR, Chiu RCJ: Skeletal muscle-powered cardiac assist using an extra-aortic balloon pump. In Chiu RCJ (ed): *Biomechanical Cardiac Assist: Cardiomyoplasty and Muscle-Powered Devices.* Mount Kisco, NY. Futura Publishing Co., 1986, pp 141–150.
14. Badylak SF, Hinds M, Geddes LA: Comparison of three methods of electrical stimulation for converting skeletal muscle to a fatigue resistance power source suitable for cardiac assist. *Ann Biomed Eng* 18:239–250, 1990.
15. Lucas CMHB, Kloosterman-Castro-Ravelo EN, Van Der Veen FH, et al: Long-term follow-up after cardiomyoplasty in goats. In Lucas CMHB (ed): *The Use of the LDM for Cardiac Assist.* Maastrict, UPM, 1992, pp 99–121.
16. Lucas CMHB, Lorusso RC, Dubelaar ML, et al: Hemodynamic study following cardiomyoplasty: Comparison of different stimulation protocols. In Lucas CMHB (ed): *The Use of the LDM for Cardiac Assist.* Maastrict, UPM, 1992, pp 79–97.
17. Levin HR, Tsitlik JE, Halperin HR: Optimization of the timing of skeletal to cardiac muscle contraction during dynamic cardiomyoplasty: Analysis using a mathematical model. *J Cardiac Surg* 6:236–244, 1991.
18. Lucas CMHB, van der Veen FH, Cheriex EC, et al: The importance of muscle relaxation in cardiomyoplasty. *PACE* 5:1430–1436, 1992.
19. Davies CR, Novoa RM, Jacobs GB, et al: Optimization of pacing parameters for conditioned LDM in cardiomyoplasty. *ASAIO Trans* 37(3):163–164, 1991.

# Chapter 17

# *Discussion*

**Sir Magdi Yacoub:** Have you looked at the influence of your protocols on either fatigue or damage?

**Dr. Bui:** No, we have not looked at the effects of fatigue or damage to LD muscle using conventional training techniques such as 25 pulses per second, one pulse in the first 2 weeks, and then increasing the number of pulses to six pulses at the end.

**Dr. Jarvis:** You have not taken into account the fact that the variable frequency bursts have a smaller number of impulses than the constant frequency trainings.

**Dr. Bui:** Exactly. The reason that we want to maintain a constant burst length which was maintained around 200 msec is that we believe that the change in burst length probably has more effect than the number of pulses.

**Dr. Jarvis:** You would have seen exactly the same thing if you had just shortened the burst length of the constant frequency training. If you are going to look at nonconstant frequency trains, you need to express your results as whatever per impulse. Otherwise you never see a benefit. There is a potential benefit of optimized patterns but you have not shown them in this way.

**Dr. Bui:** Maybe the future area of study should be comparing short bursts with variable frequency bursts.

**Dr. Jarvis:** If you just express things as "per impulse," you'll do better.

**Sir Magdi Yacoub:** What benefit do you expect? Could you express your views a bit more clearly?

**Dr. Jarvis:** It certainly is possible, using fewer impulses to produce the same force from a skeletal muscle, for example by using a high frequency at the start of the burst with the force maintained by a lower frequency. That has been documented.

**Sir Magdi Yacoub:** That is for producing more power?

From Carpentier A, Chachques JC, Grandjean P: Cardiac Bioassist. © Futura Publishing Co, Inc, Armonk, NY, 1997.

**Dr. Jarvis:** Yes, you can do the same with fewer impulses. So in terms of the undesirable transformation that I have talked about, you should be able to avoid some of that undesirable reduction in power and still obtain forceful contractions.

**Sir Magdi Yacoub:** What about fatigue and/or damage?

**Dr. Jarvis:** If you use smaller impulses, you should cause less damage and less fatigue.

**Dr. Bui:** We also suspect that by loosing a number of pulses, you may have a shorter contraction time and that is what we want to do in the future. However, if you compare the results, in the conditioning of a fiber, you use six pulses, and this is probably equivalent to the 25 pulses per second constant frequency burst.

**Dr. Jarvis:** The contraction time has nothing to do with the pattern of impulses. It is the time between your first and last impulse. That is what you have measured as contraction time.

**Dr. Bui:** That is quite true. However, if you look at the way the muscle relaxes, you can see that the muscle tends to contract, and maintains the contraction for a long time before relaxing for constant frequency burst. However, when you have variable frequency, the muscle starts to relax earlier than the constant frequency.

**Dr. Salmons:** There is a lot of fundamental physiology, which I think you are missing. There is a thing called a force/frequency curve, which has been established for over 50 years, that can explain a lot of the observations you have seen. Dr. Jarvis is being excessively modest. He actually studied these so-called optimized variable frequency bursts in great detail and showed that you can get a similar force, a similar work and similar force time interval with a constant frequency pattern and with a variable burst which has far fewer impulses. Is that good in terms of fatigue? Yes, it is, because each impulse has a cost in terms of energy; you release calcium and you have to get the calcium back. So, the fewer impulses, the less the energy cost of contraction. And the less the energy cost of contraction, the sooner you can have the muscle fully working. We now have a stimulator that delivers variable pulses and we will be using it for chronic use. You definitely need to express your results per impulse if you have different lengths of burst as well as different frequencies.

**Dr. Bui:** We did not have different lengths of bursts. We had constant lengths of bursts. They all maintain 200 msec.

**Sir Magdi Yacoub:** They are very similar ideas anyway. You are on the same track, but it is how you analyze the results. What about relaxation? That is a very important parameter. That seems to be quite a useful thing to have a higher dp/dt/min.

**Dr. Salmons:** Again there is a frequency effect there, and since relaxation depends on calcium release, the more calcium that is released, the longer the relaxation. But I don't think that is a major effect. What we are talking about has been established for years. It is sometimes referred to as the catch property of skeletal muscle. Our muscles don't burst at constant frequency. There is an initial high frequency burst lasting 2 or 3 msec that quickly develops tension. That can be maintained with a lower frequency. We should certainly be looking at the possibility of using it instead of our rather old-fashioned constant frequency bursts.

**Sir Magdi Yacoub:** We need to know more about the catch properties.

**Dr. Carpentier:** It is a Catch 22 situation!

Chapter 18

# Left Ventricular Diastolic Compliance at Different Skeletal Muscle Tensions in Dynamic Cardiomyoplasty

Wang Cheng, Rafael A. Avila, Bobby S. David
Joseph N. Cunningham, Jr., Israel J. Jacobowitz

## Introduction

Dynamic cardiomyoplasty has been evaluated in the laboratory setting for more than 10 years and has been used clinically for the past 10 years.[1,2] Despite the absence of widely corroborated laboratory data in the chronic animal model, surgeons in Europe, South America, Canada, and the United States have used the latissimus dorsi muscle (LDM) cardiomyoplasty as a new form of cardiocirculatory support in patients with end-stage cardiac failure.[2–10] At the time of this writing, approximately 300 patients have undergone this procedure worldwide.[11]

Early preliminary reports on cardiomyoplasty in the clinical arena appeared to indicate that patients treated with cardiomyoplasty were experiencing significant improvement in their functional status; however, objective evidence of improved hemodynamics has not been consistent in those clinical trials that have shown improved clinical performance of patients.[12] These favorable reports have led to the use of this new modality by several centers worldwide despite the absence of objective laboratory data that showed improvement of quantitative parameters such as end-diastolic volume, pressure-volume loops, dP/dT, and ejection fraction.

More recently, however, the clinical use of the LDM cardiomyoplasty has been associated with unexpectedly high mortality (40%) and morbidity rates.[12] Additionally, laboratory studies have identified significant limitations of this technique, including a *girdling* effect, which may compromise cardiac function,

With the cooperation of Robert Robertazzi, Ira Nathan, and Corrado P. Marini.
Supported in part by the Maimonides Research and Development Foundation.

and a decrease of as much as 40% in cardiac output due to compromised diastolic function following LDM cardiomyoplasty.[13] The detrimental effects of skeletal muscle cardiomyoplasty on the diastolic component of cardiac function is of major concern to those clinicians willing to use this modality, since a significantly reduced preload (from impaired diastolic function) will consequently offset any beneficial effect of the procedure on the augmentation of systolic function.[14]

Because LDM cardiomyoplasty can affect ventricular compliance, we designed a study to evaluate the acute effects of LDM cardiomyoplasty on left ventricular (LV) compliance at three different skeletal muscle tensions in a normal canine heart, and after propranolol-induced acute LV failure.

## Materials and Methods

Ten dogs were used in this study. The animals were anesthetized with intravenous sodium pentobarbital (30 mg/kg) and fentanyl (4μg/kg). After endotracheal intubation, they were ventilated with a volume-controlled ventilator. Respiratory parameters included a tidal volume of 12 mL/kg, a respiratory rate to maintain the $pCO_2$ between 25 and 35 mm Hg, 5 cm PEEP, and an $FiO_2$ of 100%. Animals were monitored with a cardiac monitor. Arterial blood pressure was monitored with a catheter placed in the femoral artery. Lactated Ringer's solution was administered at the rate of 3–5 mL/kg/hr, and blood loss was replaced with lactated Ringer's solution. A left sagittal thoracic skin incision was made at the posterior axillary line. Dissection of the left LDM was carried out with care to preserve the thoracodorsal pedicle (nerve and vessels). After isolation, the LDM was restored to its original anatomic location, and the tension was measured by a strain transducer. This tension was designated as the original or optimal preload of the LDM. A biventricular LDM wrap was performed on 10 dogs.

A 5-cm arc of the lateral portion of the left second rib was resected. The LDM was then inserted into the chest through the wall defect. A median sternotomy and pericardiotomy provided anterior exposure of the heart. For sonomicrometric study, two pairs of hemispherical crystals were positioned on the endocardium to measure LV anterior-to-posterior and septal-to-free-wall dimensions. A micromanometer tip catheter (Millar Instruments, Houston, TX) was placed through the stab wound at the apex into the LV in order to record the LV pressure.

The LDM was extended by suturing a synthetic patch at the free end. The muscle was wrapped around the heart, forming a loop to encompass both the LV and the right ventricle (RV). The patch extension was channeled through the ipsilateral chest wall at the fourth intercostal space. This end was then attached to a force transducer. Once each of the three preloads (tensions) were set, the extension was fixed to the chest wall. This LDM wrap was perpendicular to the interventricular septal axis. The LDM was wrapped around both ventricles at three different tensions (preloads): original (optimal), double the original, and triple the original tension. LV pressure and two minor axis dimensions were measured at the different wrapping tensions before and after wrapping, and at 0, 5, and 10 volts LDM stimulation, respectively. After these measurements, propranolol 11.6 mg/kg was administered and all parameters were recorded again. The data were acquired by on-line computer. Computer-acquired two minor axis dimensions were converted into a volume value by the formula for a prolate ellipsoid model: volume $= 4/3 \times a/2 \times b/2 \times (a+b)/2$ ($a$ and $b$ are two minor axis dimensions.[15] LV pressure and volume loops were constructed by the computer program Excel (Microsoft Corporation, Redmond, WA). The segments, so-called passive pressure-volume curve, from onset to the end-diastole in the PV loops were rebuilt and their slopes calculated. These slopes represented wall stiffness and their reciprocals represented LV diastolic compliance. Compliance was defined as dV/dP (delta volume over delta pressure).

## Statistics

Data were analyzed by ANOVA for repeated measures. In the event of a significant F value, differences were localized by the method of Newman and Keuls. Statistical significance was accepted to correspond to a $p$ value less than 0.05.

## Results

Left ventricular pressure-volume curves for the latissimus dorsi muscle at its original tension and at the protocol's stipulated double and triple muscle tension cardiomyoplasty configuration for both the normal and propranolol-induced heart failure models were compared to the pre-wrap baseline (Table 1). Compliance of the pre-wrap left ventricular pressure-volume system was calculated at 1.79 $cm^3$/mm Hg. Post-wrap LV compliances exhibited by the incremental muscle tensions during the passive (0 volt) state and at 5- and 10-volt stimulation, respectively, decreased significantly, ranging from 0.61 to 0.99 $cm^3$/mm Hg.

**Table 1**
Left Ventricular Diastolic Compliance (dV/dP, $mm^3$/mm Hg)
Before (pre) Wrap and After (post) Wrap

| | | | |
|---|---|---|---|
| Pre-wrap | 1.79 ± 0.11 | | |
| Post-wrap with LDM* | *0 volt* | *5 volt* | *10 volt* |
| Orig tension | 0.99 ± 0.24 | 0.76 ± 0.08 | 0.70 ± 0.12 |
| 2X Orig tension | 0.77 ± 0.09 | 0.74 ± 0.14 | 0.61 ± 0.06 |
| 3X Orig tension | 0.69 ± 0.07 | 0.75 ± 0.09 | 0.78 ± 0.19 |
| Post-propranolol* | *0 volt* | *5 volt* | *10 volt* |
| Orig tension | 0.74 ± 0.06 | 0.72 ± 0.13 | 0.77 ± 0.15 |
| 2X Orig tension | 0.67 ± 0.07 | 0.69 ± 0.14 | 0.82 ± 0.15 |
| 3X Orig tension | 0.81 ± 0.13 | 0.93 ± 0.17 | 0.80 ± 0.16 |

0, 5, and 10 volt = LDM stimulation with 0, 5, or 10 volts, respectively; orig = original.
* = $p<0.05$ when compared to pre-wrap.

Compliances among the various muscle tensions and voltage stimuli were not found to be significant. Similar (post-wrap) results were observed for the propranolol-treated group. Left ventricular compliance was not altered by the introduction of propranolol. As in the normal heart model group, compliances among the distinct tension and voltage stimuli subgroups were not significantly different after propranolol infusion.

## Discussion

Diastolic compliance is an appropriate system property to evaluate ventricular relaxation in a cardiomyoplasty model. As the left ventricle fills progressively, a passive relationship develops between each increment of volume and the steady rise in pressure. For elastomeric tissue elements, the ensuing pressure-volume curve or loop is generally sigmoidal in character (denoting its elastic properties), and its slope, dP/dV, defines the system's volume-storage capability. This change in volume per unit change in pressure ($cm^3$/mm Hg) describes the ventricular compliance. As a measure of the myocardium's distensibility or ease with which the ventricle can be filled or stretched, it follows that any decline in LV compliance reduces the degree of ventricular relaxation, preload, and subsequently, end-diastolic volume.

In our series, all subgroup post-wrap LV compliances, determined from their individual pressure-volume profiles, were significantly decreased from their original pre-wrap status and as a result, the ventricular relaxation was compromised by the wrap. In addition, the LV compliance was not significantly changed by the degree of LDM wrap tension or voltage stimuli in either normal or failing heart groups, suggesting that mere modification of technical parameters would do little to nullify this deleterious effect.

Actually, previous studies have shown similar outcomes of post-wrap declines in cardiac function. In a chronic canine model, we induced heart failure with adriamycin.[18] After an initial 30% drop in LV ejection fraction (LVEF), an LDM wrap cardiomyoplasty was performed. The wrapping caused a further 40% drop in LVEF from 30% to 18%. In an acute canine study evaluating LDM wrap cardiomyoplasty techniques, Magovern's group noted an average 41% decrease in the peak aortic flow.[19]

Most investigators have concentrated their efforts on evaluating the effects of the stimulation of the LDM on cardiac functions, but have failed to evaluate the influence of the unstimulated wrap on systolic and diastolic function. This approach has led to rather inaccurate statements about the efficacy of the LDM cardiomyoplasty. In question is whether the stimulation of the wrap increases cardiac function to the degree necessary to offset the loss in stroke volume caused by the reduction in preload. To address this question, one should consider that the passive LDM wrap and the stimulated LDM wrap each act during distinct transient phases (Fig. 1). The unstimulated wrap alone acts "upstream" (diastole) to restrict filling, while LDM stimulation acts "downstream" (systole) to increase force of ejection. Intuitively, it is doubtful that LDM stimulation could increase ejection volume from a ventricular chamber that has not filled completely.

Since LDM cardiomyoplasty compromises not only the systolic function but also the diastolic filling function, it is arguable that the most frequently re-

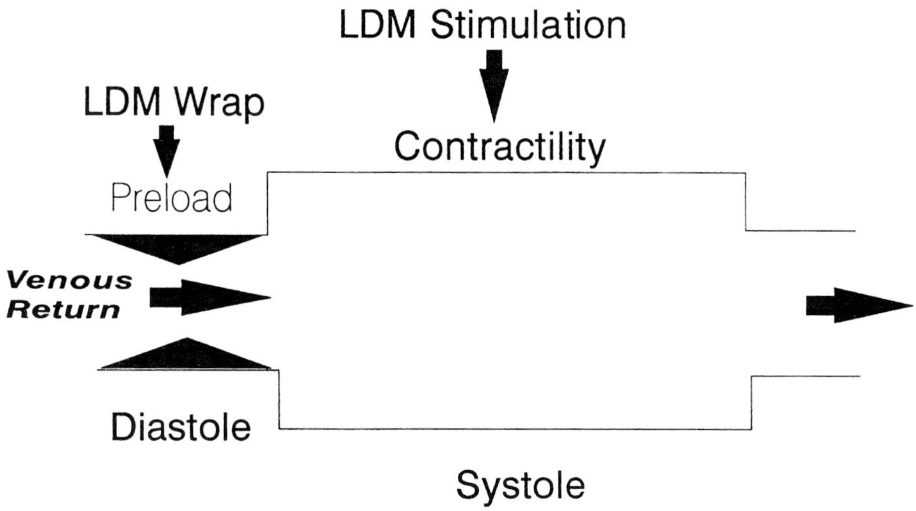


**Figure 1:** *Schematic representation of a two-component effect of the LDM wrap.*

ported evaluation parameter, the MUGA scan ejection fraction, can accurately appraise the results of cardiomyoplasty. The rationale for this is that the ejection fraction is an expression of a ratio, which in itself does not measure absolute volume. Hypothetically, an end-diastolic volume of 100 mL and an end-systolic volume of 70 mL would result in a stroke volume of 30 mL or an ejection fraction of 30%. Following cardiomyoplasty, the end-diastolic volume could conceivably be reduced to 75 mL. In this scenario, an end-systolic volume of 50 mL would result in stroke volume of 25 mL, an actual reduction of 5 mL. The reported ejection fraction, however, would indicate an increase from 30% to 33%, a net gain of 3%.

This study was related exclusively to the limitation of diastolic ventricular relaxation by the LDM wrap as represented by the LV compliance. Any comprehensive evaluation of the influence of the LDM wrap on cardiac function should also include a conscientious analysis of heart organ motion, the skeletal muscle inertia opposing the myocardium, muscular force and direction analysis during systole, and LDM flap occlusion on both pulmonary venous return to the left atrium and the superior and inferior vena cava blood flow to the right atrium.

While this study has certain limitations in its extrapolation to the clinical setting, specifically, it does not take into consideration either the conformation of the LDM or the conditioning of the LDM. Furthermore, the propranolol-induced heart failure model may not be a satisfactory representation of dilated cardiomyopathy. Nevertheless, it may explain the high *early* mortality, particularly in patients with Class IV heart failure.[12]

The data in this study suggest that the prevailing cardiomyoplasty methodology may, in fact, impair LV compliance to the extent that it limits the skeletal muscle's augmentation of cardiac function. We believe that this conclusion may explain some of the recently reported unexpected experimental and clinical results.[20] In light of these findings, it is conceivable that investigators may be compelled to contemplate a change in direction in the use of skeletal muscle for cardiac assistance. The new starting point should commence from a design, method, or model that does not significantly impede heart function first.

*Acknowledgments:* The authors would like to express their thanks to Anthony P. Siconolfi for technical assistance and Mary Ann Bottali for manuscript preparation.

## References

1. Carpentier A, Chachques JC: Myocardial substitution with a stimulated skeletal muscle. First successful clinical case (letter). *Lancet* 8840:1267, 1985.
2. Chachques JC, Grandjean PA, Pfeffer TA, et al: Cardiac assistance by atrial or ventricular cardiomyoplasty. *J Heart Transplant* 9:239, 1990.
3. Moreira LF, Seferian R Jr., Bocchi EA, et al: Survival improvement with dynamic cardiomyoplasty in patients with dilated cardiomyopathy. *Circulation* 82(Suppl III):III–713, 1990.
4. Magovern GJ, Park SB, Kao RL, et al: Dynamic cardiomyoplasty in patients. *J Heart Transplant* 9:258, 1990.
5. Jatene AD, Moreira LFP, Stolf NAG, et al: Left ventricular function changes after cardiomyoplasty in patients with dilated cardiomyopathy. *J Thorac Cardiovasc Surg* 102:131, 1991.
6. Delahaye F, Jegaden O, Montagna P, et al: Latissimus dorsi cardiomyoplasty in severe congestive heart failure: The Lyon experience. *J Cardiac Surg* 6:106, 1991.
7. Chachques JC, Grandjean PA, Carpentier A, et al: Patient management and clinical follow-up after cardiomyoplasty. *J Cardiac Surg* 6:89, 1991.
8. Furnary AP, Magovern JA, Christlieb IY, et al: Clinical cardiomyoplasty: Preoperative factors associated with outcome. *Ann Thorac Surg* 54:1139, 1992.
9. Odim JNK, Burgess JH, Williams BH, et al: Pathophysiology of dynamic cardiomyoplasty: A clinico-pathologic case study. *J Cardiac Surg* 5:336, 1990.
10. Magovern JA, Furnary AP, Christlieb IY, et al: Right latissimus dorsi cardiomyoplasty for left ventricular failure. *Ann Thorac Surg* 53:1120, 1992.
11. Chiu R C-J: Dynamic cardiomyoplasty: efficacy and mechanisms. *Cardiac Chronicle* 6:1, 1992.
12. Grandjean PA, Austin L, Chan S, et al: Dynamic cardiomyoplasty: Clinical follow-up results. *J Cardiac Surg* 6:80, 1991.
13. Cheng W, David BS, Avila RA, et al: Cardiomyoplasty: Unstimulated latissimus dorsi muscle wrap reduces cardiac output. *Surg Forum* 43:228, 1992.
14. Silverman NA: Invited letter concerning: Left ventricular function changes after cardiomyoplasty in patients with dilated cardiomyopathy (letter). *J Thorac Cardiovasc Surg* 102:156, 1991.
15. Weyman AE: *Cross-sectional Echocardiography.* Philadelphia, PA, Lea & Febiger, 1982, p 283.
16. West JB: *Best and Taylor's Physiological Basis of Medical Practice.* Baltimore, MD, Williams & Wilkins, 1991, p 224.
17. Corin WJ, George DT, Sink JD, et al: Dynamic cardiomyoplasty acutely impairs left ventricular diastolic function. *J Thorac Cardiovasc Surg* 104:1662, 1992.
18. Cheng W, Justicz AG, Soberman MS, et al: Effects of dynamic cardiomyoplasty on indices of left ventricular systolic and diastolic function in a canine model of chronic heart failure. *J Thorac Cardiovasc Surg* 103:1207, 1992.
19. Magovern JA, Furnary AP, Christlieb IY, et al: Bilateral latissimus dorsi cardiomyoplasty. *Ann Thorac Surg* 52:1259, 1991.
20. Magovern JA: Left ventricular function changes after cardiomyoplasty in patients with dilated cardiomyopathy (discussion). *J Thorac Cardiovasc Surg* 102:131, 1991.

Chapter 18

# Discussion

**Dr. Salmons:** Do you think you have been entirely fair by using the original in situ tension of the muscle when you did the wrap? It strikes me that that is fairly high compared to what the average surgeon uses in cardiomyoplasty.

**Dr. Jacobowitz:** I think it is very difficult to tell what the tension is at cardiomyoplasty; it is very subjective.

**Dr. Acker:** That is exactly what I want to comment on. If in the OR, one tightens that muscle to the original tension, signs and symptoms of tamponade will develop. We apply the wrap loosely as done Dr. Carpentier. In 3 months, it will no longer be loose since there is a gradual reduction in the size of the fibers and in the weight of the muscle as it becomes more aerobic and fatigue resistant.

**Dr. Jacobowitz:** This was measured with the muscle detached distally and not with the muscle in situ. It was left without putting any tension on it.

**Dr. Acker:** So you are saying that if you wrap the muscle without tension, you have this reduction in function?

**Dr. Jacobowitz:** Correct.

**Dr. Starr:** Reduction in function was only a derived pressure volume loop. We don't know whether the magnitude of that decrease in compliance would have any clinical relevance whatsoever. It would produce increased wedge pressures that a patient would feel uncomfortable with which we don't see clinically.

**Dr. Jacobowitz:** I suspect that clinically much of this is overcome by volume loading. This is a lot like a ventricular aneurysmectomy where one has to keep a certain amount of volume to improve the cardiac output. Insufficient volume will cause constriction and a low-output state; excessive volume will create a heart failure situation.

**Dr. Moreira (Sao Paulo):** We also did not observe any kind of clinical impairment in our patients. Using pressure volume loop studies, we observed a great change regarding compliance when we stimulated the muscle in long-term

From Carpentier A, Chachques JC, Grandjean P: Cardiac Bioassist. © Futura Publishing Co, Inc, Armonk, NY, 1997.

follow-up. Comparing data preoperatively and postoperatively, we showed benefits in compliance rather than impairing the compliance of the left ventricle.

**Dr. Chachques:** I would like to make a comment and ask a question. On your compliance curve, you measured elastance as a measure of compliance, since there was a shift in the curve as well as a change in its slope. I think you might have cheated yourself! Do you think it is fair to say that ventricular properties are altered by this? Aren't you after all measuring the properties of a neocomposite structure which consists of a ventricle and a muscle? As a neocomposite structure, it has a different compliance. I don't think that it implies that the ventricular compliance or ventricular performance itself is altered.

**Dr. Jacobowitz:** That may be correct. On the other hand, the clinical situation is one of a complete structure and not two individual ones: the heart muscle and the cardiomyoplasty. If they work in unison, this may in fact be what is being seen.

**Dr. Chachques:** I guess an altered characteristic curve does not necessarily reflect an impairment but reflects a different structure consisting of two thicknesses instead of one.

**Dr. Odim (Boston):** Have you looked at the static wrap in the chronic setting? I do agree that acutely you will get changes in compliance, but I suspect that if you looked at those same animals after 3 months, you would have adjustments and I just want to reemphasize Michael Acker's point that you have to distinguish between acute versus chronic tamponade.

**Dr. Jacobowitz:** This was an acute study and no consideration was given to accommodation and time. A chronic study might in fact reveal differences.

**Dr. David Kass (Johns Hopkins):** Your volume data are based on two presumably orthogonal short-access dimensions and so you have made an assumption by converting that to some form of chamber volume. What we see with clinical imaging is that cardiomyoplasty changes cardiac shape dramatically. I would guess that the relationship between your derived equations based on these dimensions before the wrap and after the wrap may change. It may change differently in different animals, but it is likely to have changed. This could critically change your coordinates for any of those compared diastolic pressure volume curves. I would be interested to know if you have tested to see if this change exists. One way would be to compare a stroke volume derived before wrap and after wrap based on your critical data, to that from some independent measure such as an ultrasonic flow probe that could clearly determine whether or not the relationship that you are assuming between these dimensions and real chamber volume in fact changes because of the shape change induced by cardiomyoplasty. Have you done that?

**Dr. Jacobowitz:** No, we have not. Your point is well taken with regard to the change in configuration.

**Dr. Kass:** Particularly the long access, which you left out of your calculations.

**Dr. Jacobowitz:** That was taken into consideration with the formula that we corrected. Whether or not that formula is in fact true when there are some changes in configuration, I can't tell you, but it holds true for the normal state and shape of the ventricle. I think that the emphasis for this was to try to determine what the early mortality in this operation was due to and to see whether we could find any way to confirm the rationale and how best to correct it.

Chapter 19

# Does Skeletal Muscle Steal Blood from the Heart Following a Latissimus Dorsi Cardiomyoplasty?

William F. Bailey Jr., John D. Mannion, Michael G. Magno*

## Introduction

Cardiomyoplasty is currently undergoing worldwide clinical evaluation as a biological left ventricular assist device. We have investigated using cardiomyoplasty to indirectly revascularize ischemic myocardium in patients with presently inoperable distal vessel disease. We have recently shown that following a latissimus dorsi (LD) cardiomyoplasty, collaterals develop between the skeletal muscle and chronic ischemic myocardium.[1] Furthermore, chronic electrical stimulation of the latissimus dorsi results in a sustained increase in skeletal muscle-derived collateral blood flow to the heart.[2] If these newly formed collaterals allow for bidirectional flow as was reported for intracoronary collaterals,[3] then the latissimus dorsi could steal blood flow from the coronary circulation and could further compromise the failing heart. The purpose of this preliminary study is to determine if the transposed latissimus dorsi might steal blood from the coronary circulation following a latissimus dorsi cardiomyoplasty.

## Material and Methods

### Overview of Experimental Design

Eleven adult, castrated male goats were studied. The animals were cared for according to the *Principles of Laboratory Animal Care* prepared by the National

*With the cooperation of Peter D. Buckman, Vincent Blood, and Fred DiMeo.

Supported by NHLBI R01 HL41918-04.
From Carpentier A, Chachques JC, Grandjean P: Cardiac Bioassist. © Futura Publishing Co, Inc, Armonk, NY, 1997.

Society for Medical Research and the *Guide for the Care and Use of Laboratory Animals* prepared by the National Academy of Science (NIH Publication No. 86-23, revised 1985). The latissimus dorsi received chronic electrical stimulation via an implanted pulse generator starting on postoperative day 10. After 6 weeks of continuous electrical stimulation, we measured the flow from the latissimus dorsi muscle to the heart and from the coronary circulation to the transposed latissimus dorsi muscle.

## Latissimus Dorsi Cardiomyoplasty (Fig. 1)

The details of the LD cardiomyoplasty and ameroid placement have been previously described.[1] All animals were anesthetized with 2% isoflurane solution after premedication with ketamine (500 mg IM) and thiopental (25 mg/kg IV). Prophylactic antibiotics (1 gm cefazolin IV) were administered. The rumen of each animal was decompressed with an oral-gastric plastic tube (0.5 inch ID). Using sterile surgical technique, the left latissimus dorsi was mobilized, while preserving its neurovascular pedicle.

A fourth interspace, lateral thoracotomy incision was performed, and the circumflex coronary artery, or a moderate-sized branch, was isolated. A permanent, indwelling, silastic catheter was placed in the left atrium through the left atrial appendage.

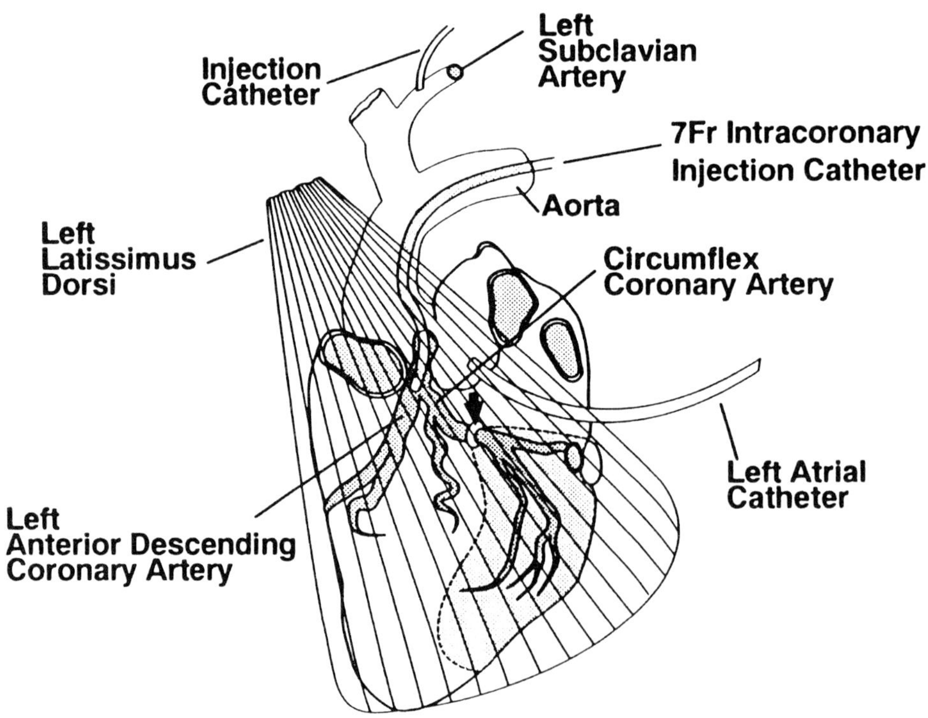


**Figure 1:** *Left lateral view of the goat heart instrument with catheters and ameroid constrictor, showing the placement of the left latissimus dorsi muscle.*

An ameroid constrictor was placed around the dissected coronary artery. The latissimus dorsi was then delivered into the chest through the bed of the resected second left rib, and was sutured to the inner surface of the pericardium. The configuration of the cardiomyoplasty was left anterior cardiocostal. There was no attempt to remove the epicardium or the fascia of the LD muscle. A nerve cuff electrode (Medtronic, Minneapolis, MN) was placed around the thoracodorsal nerve and attached to an electrical pulse generator (Medtronic) implanted within the rectus sheath. The left atrial catheter was implanted into a subcutaneous pouch, the chest closed, and the animals permitted to recover. The animals resumed normal activity within the university's animal facility.

A neurostimulator (Itrel, model no. 7421, Medtronic) was used for thoracodorsal nerve stimulation in eight of the animals that survived the 7.5-week protocol. In three other animals, an SP 1005 cardiomyostimulator was substituted. The pulse generators were turned on after 9.8 ± 1.2 postoperative days. The initial voltage was set at that voltage which resulted in distinct muscle twitching, as determined by palpation. The initial mean voltage was 2.4 ± 0.6 volts. During the course of the study, the voltage had to be increased to 3.4 ± 0.8 volts to maintain a palpable twitch as determined by physical examination. The stimuli were single and were delivered at 2 Hz for 6 weeks prior to the final study. After 6 weeks of stimulation, anesthesia was induced as above and maintained with sodium pentobarbital infusion (1.0 mg/kg/min, IV) and the regional blood flow determinations performed.

## Regional Blood Flow Measurements

Regional blood flows were measured with the reference organ method of Rudolph and Heymann[4] or by the reference withdrawal modification of this method. Table 1 summarizes the details of the various injections and the formulas used to calculate the different regional flows. The determinations of coronary flow, the LD muscle flow, and the latissimus-derived collateral flow were made by two simultaneous injections. The animals were then moved to the fluoroscopic unit for the intracoronary injections.

Since virtually all of the microspheres are trapped by systemic or pulmonary capillaries, they do not recirculate. Hence, any microspheres found in the latissimus dorsi that were injected into the coronary circulation had to be delivered by collaterals originating from the coronary circulation. Similarly, any microspheres trapped by the heart that were injected into the latissimus arterial supply had to be delivered by collaterals originating in the latissimus dorsi.

## Definition and Characterization of Risk Area

The animals were sacrificed with an overdose of anesthetic and saturated KCl. The coronary artery was cannulated just distal to the ameroid constrictor and injected with 10 mL of brilliant green dye. The heart and attached latissimus were then divided into four rings. Each ring was further divided into normal zone and risk area, based on the brilliant green dye staining. Myocardium

**Table 1**
Blood Flow Measurements

| To measure: | | |
|---|---|---|
| CBF | Injected 15 UN microspheres into: left atrium (red, 15 million) | |
| LD flow | Injected 15 UN microspheres into: left atrium (red, 15 million) | |
| LDCBF | Thoracodorsal artery (blue, 1.5 million) Subclavian artery (7.5 million) | |
| LD steal | Coronary artery (green, 1.5 million) | |

*Calculations*

| *blood flow –* | *tissue count ×* | *reference flow ×* | *reference count*[1] |
|---|---|---|---|
| CBF | red count in myocardium | syringe withdrawal rate[1] | red count in syringe blood |
| LD flow | red count in latissimus | syringe withdrawal rate | red count in syringe blood |
| LDCBF | blue count in myocardium | LD muscle blood flow | blue count in latissimus |
| LD steal | green count in latissimus | coronary blood flow | green count in myocardium |

[1]For these two determinations, a syringe withdrawing blood at a known, constant rate is substituted for an organ with a known blood flow. CBF = coronary blood flow; LD flow = latissimus muscle flow; LD steal = latissimus steal from the heart; LDCBF = latissimus-derived collateral blood flow.

not stained with brilliant green dye was labeled as normal. Myocardium stained with the dye was labeled as chronically ischemic, or infarcted based on blood flow characteristics. The criteria used to label each myocardial sample has been previously described.[5]

## Statistical Analysis

All data are presented as means ± standard errors and ranges. Paired *t*-tests were conducted on the data and the Bonferroni correction was applied where multiple comparisons were made. A probability of less than 0.05 was used to declare statistical significance.

## Results

In four animals, the intracoronary catheter delivered many of the microspheres into the aorta as indicated by high counts (more than 400/gram) in the kidneys. These animals were excluded because the collaterals originating in the heart were not the only pathway for these microspheres to enter the latissimus dorsi. Two more animals were excluded because collaterals did not form between the heart and the latissimus dorsi muscle.

In the five remaining animals, the mass of the chronically ischemic myocardium was 20.7 ± 2.8 grams. Left ventricular weight was 97.5 ± 10.2 grams.

## Hemodynamic Data

Table 2 summarizes the hemodynamic data. There are no cardiac output data for the LD steal measurements because there were no simultaneous left atrial injections. Due to equipment failure, the hemodynamic data for one animal during the intracoronary injection was lost. The data in this table show that blood pressure, heart, and cardiac output are within normal limits for pentobarbital anesthetized small ruminants. There is no difference between the time-tension index for the two sets of measurements, verifying that myocardial oxygen consumption was unchanged.

## Blood Flow Data

Figure 2 shows the comparison of the LD steal with the latissimus-derived collateral blood flow (LDCBF). As can be seen, the LD steal is virtually nonexistent in three of the five goats. In the other two, the LD steal is small.

Table 3 summarizes the regional blood flows for these animals. The LD steal is significantly less ($p<0.05$) than the LDCBF. The data in this table also show that the latissimus contributes about 20 times more to the nutrient flow of the heart than it takes from the heart.

Virtually all of the intracoronary injected microspheres were recovered from the distal portion of the latissimus that was in contact with the heart. There were no intracoronary injected microspheres recovered from the proximal latissimus in three animals. In the other two animals, less than 5% of the intracoronary injected microspheres recovered from the whole latissimus dorsi were recovered from the proximal latissimus dorsi.

The latissimus-derived collateral flow is modest, about 6% of the total coronary flow to the left ventricle. However, the latissimus-derived collateral flow to the chronically ischemic zone was delivered almost exclusively to the viable myocardium within the area at risk (flow to the ischemic area was significantly

**Table 2**
Hemodynamic Data

| | *BP* *mm Hg* | *HR* *Beat/min* | *TTI* *BP × HR* | *CO* *1/min* |
|---|---|---|---|---|
| LDCBF[1] | | | | |
| Mean | 71 | 85 | 8029 | 2.9 |
| SE | 4 | 5 | 724 | 0.2 |
| n | 5 | 5 | 5 | 5 |
| LD Steal[2] | | | | |
| Mean | 64 | 91 | 8198 | — |
| SE | 6 | 4 | 893 | — |
| n | 4 | 4 | 4 | — |

[1]Parameters measured during the determination of latissimus-derived collateral blood flow (LDCBF).
[2]Parameters measured during the determination of latissimus dorsi steal from the heart.
BP = arterial blood pressure; HR = heart rate; TTI = time-tension index; CO = cardiac output.

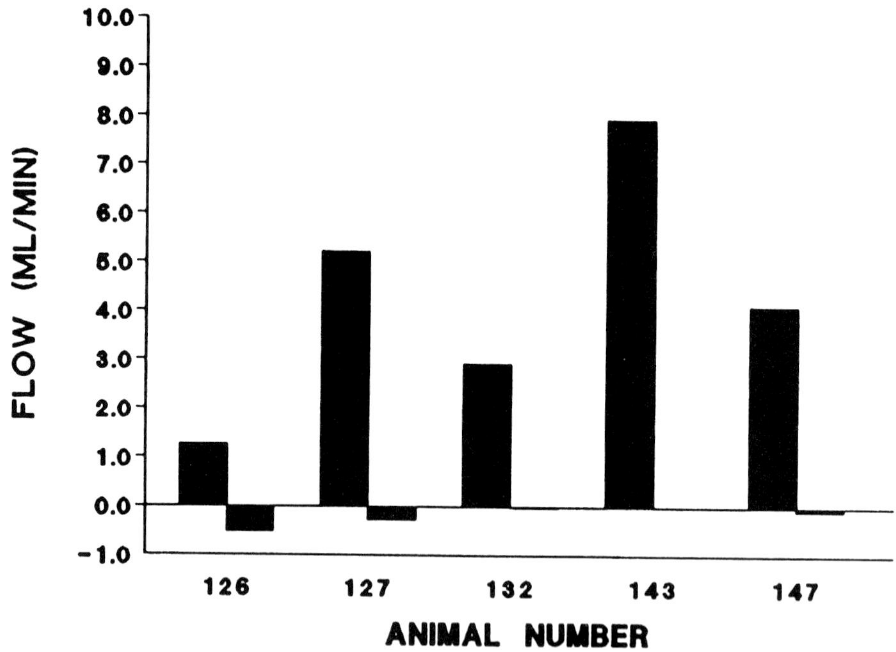


**Figure 2:** *Comparison of latissimus-derived collateral blood flow (positive values) with the latissimus dorsi steal (negative values) for each animal.*

**Table 3**
Summary of Regional Blood Flows (mL/min)

| | *CBF* | *LDCBF* | *LD Steal* |
|---|---|---|---|
| Mean | 70 | 4.29 | 0.18 |
| SE | 14 | 1.12 | 0.10 |
| n | 5 | 5 | 5 |

CBF = coronary blood flow; LDCBF = latissimus-derived collateral blood flow; LD Steal = latissimus dorsi steal.

greater than to the infarcted or normal myocardium $p<0.05$). These data are presented in Figure 3. In this figure, the latissimus-derived collateral flow per gram of tissue is presented as a percentage of the coronary flow per gram of healthy myocardium. Approximately one-fifth of the total flow needed by normal myocardium is delivered to the risk area by the latissimus. Thus, the latissimus-derived collateral flow is not trivial.

## Mixing Index

The use of intra-arterial injections carries with it the risk that the microspheres may not be uniformly mixed and therefore their distribution may not be identical with that of regional blood flow. This possibility was assessed

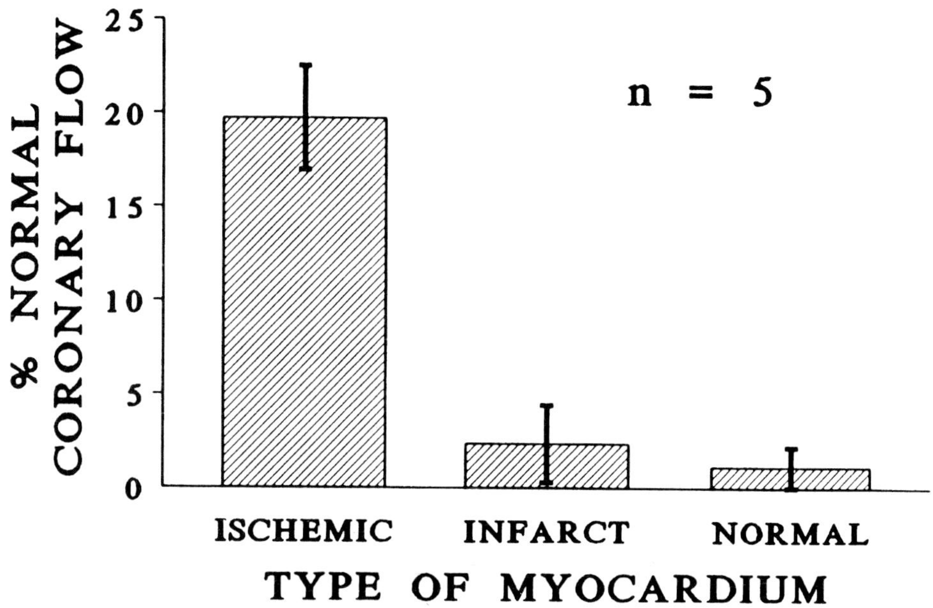


**Figure 3:** *Distribution of the latissimus-derived collateral blood flow (LDCBF) to the risk area, which is composed of chronic ischemic and infarcted myocardium and to the normal myocardium. The LDCBF is expressed as a percentage of the coronary flow to the normal myocardium measured by the left atrial microsphere injection. The vertical bars show ±1 SE.*

by comparing the distribution of the intra-arterially injected microspheres with that of the left atrial injected microspheres. The latter are considered to be well mixed by virtue of the turbulence in the left ventricle.

To make this comparison, a mixing index was calculated. The mixing index is the ratio of the distribution of the intra-arterial injection divided by that of the left atrial injection. The distribution of the microspheres in a specimen was calculated as the percentage of the total number of microspheres found in the whole organ.

For the injections into the latissimus arterial supply, there were 92 specimens from all the animals; for the intracoronary injections, there were 255 specimens. Figure 4A shows the distribution of the logarithm of mixing index for the thoracodorsal (or subclavian injections); Figure 4B shows the distribution for the intracoronary injections. A logarithmic transformation was used to correct for the non-Gaussian distribution of ratios.

If the distribution of the intra-arterially injected microspheres perfectly matched the distribution of the microspheres injected into the left atrium, then there would be a single column at zero, the log of 1.0. The distribution for the injections into the latissimus arterial supply is more or less symmetrical about 0, (the log of 1). Figure 4A shows that 74.4% of the latissimus mass had a mixing index within ± 0.2 log units of zero (arithmetic range 0.6 to 1.6). Thus, the microspheres injected into the latissimus arterial supply appear to be uniformly distributed and the error introduced is small.

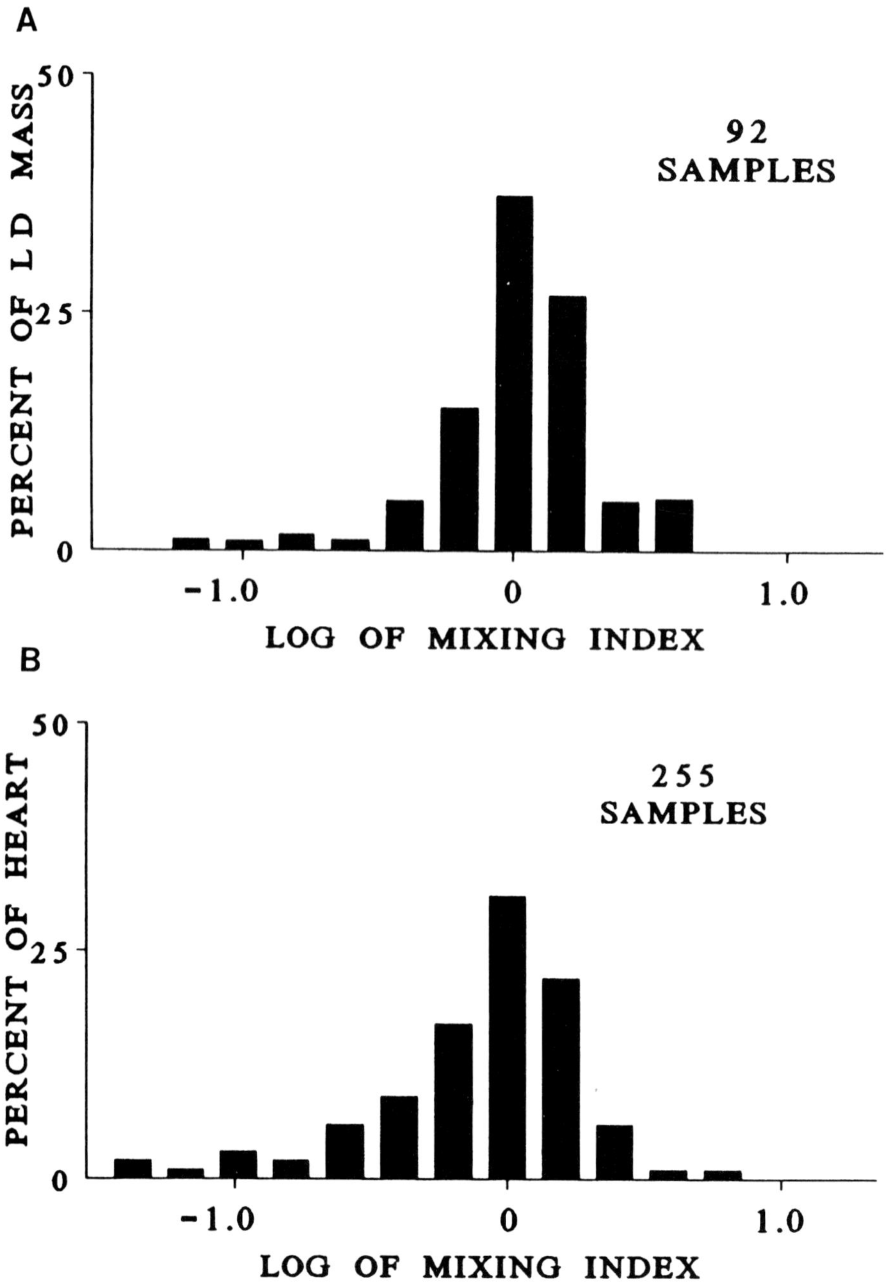


**Figure 4:** *Histograms showing the distribution of the logarithm of the mixing index for: A: the microspheres injected into the arterial supply of the latissimus dorsi; and B: for the microspheres injected into the coronary artery.*

The data in Figure 4B show that the distribution of the mixing index of the microspheres injected into the coronary artery is skewed slightly to the left and only 66.5% of the heart mass were within ± 0.2 log units of zero. The skew to the left would result in a slight overestimate of the LD steal because the reference count would be low (refer to Table 1, calculation of LD steal, green count in myocardium).

## Discussion

We have been investigating the use of skeletal muscle to indirectly revascularize ischemic myocardium for patients with inoperable distal coronary disease.[1,2,5] Because cardiomyoplasty is presently performed most commonly in patients with ischemic cardiomyopathy, we have speculated that in some patients, improvement in symptoms and ventricular function may be due, in part, to indirect revascularization. However, coronary collateral flow can be bidirectional.[3] Placement of an actively contracting skeletal muscle next to ischemic myocardium raises the possibility of a steal syndrome.

Another factor to consider regarding latissimus steal is the status of the vascular supply to the mobilized distal latissimus. The distal half of the latissimus receives its blood supply from intercostal vessels from the chest wall, and these are interrupted during mobilization. While initially the blood supply to the distal muscle through intramuscular collaterals is sufficient to support noncontracting muscle, it is clearly insufficient if the muscle immediately resumes contractile activity.[6] A collateral delay was developed to permit maturing of intramuscular collaterals. However, it is also possible that collaterals can form from the surrounding environment, which, after a cardiomyoplasty, would include the heart and the visceral pleura.

*Under the conditions of this experiment,* collateral flow was predominantly directed from the skeletal muscle to ischemic myocardium. There are several possible reasons for the apparent lack of a latissimus steal. First, unidirectional collateral blood flow has been noted before. In a canine ameroid constrictor model, Scheel et al.[7] noted that collateral flow between the right coronary artery and the left-sided coronary circulation occurred predominantly from right to left. Collateral flow between different areas of the left coronary circulation was bidirectional. Scheel et al.[7] speculated that there might be anatomic differences between the two collateral circulations to account for the directional nature of the flow.

A factor favoring the direction of collateral flow from the latissimus dorsi to the heart is the difference in metabolic activity between skeletal muscle and myocardium. In this experiment, the LD muscles were electrically conditioned at 2 Hz for 6 weeks. Prolonged, continuous electrical stimulation with this pattern induces a transformation of the skeletal muscle, which in the goat and canine species also significantly lowers muscle blood flow. In this experiment, the average LD blood flow per gram in the stimulated muscles was less than one-tenth of the regional myocardial blood flow. Such a large difference in blood flow requirements between skeletal muscle and the heart favors flow to the heart.

It might be argued that one of the purposes of the avascular pericardium is to limit the cross circulation between the heart and other organs. Therefore, we do not contend that the collateral blood flow between skeletal muscle and myocardium will favor the myocardial circulation in all circumstances. What factors would favor an LD steal are not known. However, the preliminary information presented here finds no evidence of a significant steal. Rather, the latissimus dorsi appears to contribute to the nutrient flow to the myocardium.

## References

1. Buckman P, Mannion JD, Magno M, DiMeo F, et al: After a cardiomyoplasty collaterals from skeletal muscle form to chronic ischemic myocardium. *Artificial Organs* 16:273–280; 1992.
2. Bailey WF Jr, Magno MG, Buckman PD, DiMeo F, et al: Chronic stimulation enhances extramyocardial collateral blood flow after a cardiomyoplasty. *Ann Thorac Surg* 56:1045–1052, 1993.
3. Fujita M, McKown DP, McKown MD, Franklin D: Bi-directional function of coronary collateral channels in conscious dogs. *Cardiovasc Res* 25:58–67, 1991.
4. Rudolph AM, Heymann MA: The circulation of the fetus in utero. *Circ Res* 21:163–184; 1967.
5. Mannion JD, Magno M, Buckman P, et al: Acute stimulation increases extramyocardial collateral blood flow after a cardiomyoplasty. *Ann Thorac Surg* 56: 1351–1358, 1993.
6. Mannion JD, Velchik M, Hammond R, et al: Effects of collateral blood vessel ligation and electrical conditioning on blood flow in dog latissimus dorsi muscle. *J Surg Res* 47:332–340; 1989.
7. Scheel KW, Rodriguez RJ, Ingram LA: Directional coronary collateral growth with chronic circumflex occlusion in the dog. *Circ Res* 40:384–390, 1977.

Chapter 20

# Cardiomyoplasty to Improve Myocardial Perfusion:

## Long-Term Results

M. Beyer, H. Hoffer, M. Lass, W. Fleischmann, A. Hannekum

## Introduction

Prior to the advent of direct coronary artery surgery, several methods were attempted to revascularize the ischemic myocardium. They basically all had the same purpose: to provide the heart with an extra-anatomical collateral circulation. Only the Vineberg operation, i.e., the implantation of the internal mammary artery directly into the myocardium, found a greater acceptance than the others. When the direct aortocoronary bypass technique was introduced by Favaloro in the late 1960s, indirect myocardial revascularization procedures were ultimately abandoned.

Some patients, however, are not suitable for direct coronary artery surgery. For those groups of patients, we developed a new surgical approach of myocardial revascularization based on observations after cardiomyoplastic interventions. These investigators described the development of vascular connections between the graft and the heart after cardiomyoplastic interventions performed for augmenting the pump performance of the failing heart.[1–3] Only very recently, Mannion[4] studied the significance of these neovessels for augmentation of myocardial perfusion. He found that the flow was insufficient, in case of acute myocardial ischemia, after grafting a neurovascular pedicle muscle flap onto the heart of a sheep. A few weeks after the intervention, he concluded that the collateral blood flow from the muscle flap may be augmented by establishing more favorable conditions to angiogenesis.

In order to find optimal conditions for angiogenesis after grafting a skeletal muscle flap onto the heart, the most important principle (in our opinion) of angiogenesis was applied to a new model of indirect myocardial perfusion, adopting a skeletal muscle; this is because skeletal muscle is, due to its high

From Carpentier A, Chachques JC, Grandjean P: Cardiac Bioassist. © Futura Publishing Co, Inc, Armonk, NY, 1997.

energy demand, very rich in capillaries. Therefore, a skeletal muscle flap was transplanted onto the heart. In order to avoid twitching of muscle fibers that might interfere with adherence of the graft to the heart, and thus sprouting of neovessels, the graft was denervated. Therefore, instead of the pedicled neurovascular flap, a free flap was adopted. Furthermore, due to neurogenic atrophy of the muscle fibers, the capillary network of the muscle flap may be stimulated to expand because the muscle itself no longer has an energy demand. Thus, the most important stimulus for neoangiogenesis was to bring an overproportional blood supply to the graft. The historical observations of Thoma[5] of the importance of a high perfusion pressure for the maintenance of angiogenesis recently confirmed by others[6] is, in our opinion, the most important influence for successful outcome of this grafting intervention for myocardial revascularization. Therefore, the graft was anastomosed to the internal mammary artery (IMA) and venous flow was drained into the right atrium. In order to study the vascular development, vascular corrosion casts were performed. Thereafter, at the time of grafting the free flap onto the anterior wall of the heart, an ameroid constrictor was implanted into the left anterior descending coronary (LAD). Thus, we established a condition of an "overperfused" muscle grafted onto an "underperfused (ischemic)" heart.

The animals were studied angiographically 4 weeks after the operation in vivo, and postmortem about 12 months afterwards.

The first clinical application is very briefly presented here, although the operation was only very recently done.

## Materials and Methods

Mongrel dogs, age 8 to 12 years, weighing 28 to 32 kg (FBI, Fa. Dr. Karl Thomae GmbH, Biberach/Riss, Germany), were adopted for the experiments. The surgical intervention is described in detail elsewhere.[7] After intubation and anesthesia with pentobarbital sodium, the musculus pectoralis, pars obliqua, was harvested as a free flap with its vascular pedicle. A median sternotomy was then performed in order to gain access to the heart. In the first series of experiments, the flap was grafted onto the heart of the dog, which had previously undergone induced myocardial infarction by means of selective injection of microspheres into the LAD.[8] The animals were studied about 20 weeks after the grafting operation with a microcorrosion cast preparation, as described in detail elsewhere.[9] A blue-colored casting material was injected into the stump of the IMA after isolation of the heart. A red one was injected into the coronaries. After maceration of the tissue, the casts were studied for vascular development.

In another series, the muscle flap was grafted together with an ameroid constrictor implantation into the LAD (the ameroid constrictors, a gift from Dr. W. Schaper, Director of the Max-Planck Institute for Circulation Research, Bad Nauheim, Germany). The occlusion of the LAD was documented angiographically about 3 weeks after implantation of the constrictor. Thereafter, some animals were again studied with a vascular cast about 20 weeks later, whereas others were left for long-term survival (12 months) and then studied with postmortem angiography. Flow determinations (regional myocardial blood flow) with the radioactive microsphere technique were performed as well. This technique is described in detail elsewhere.[10]

## Results

All animals tolerated the surgical intervention well. When the animals were sacrificed 20 weeks from the intervention, the muscle flap was transformed into a white fibrotic tissue that adhered firmly to the underlying heart (Fig. 1). When the blue casting material was injected by slight manual pressure, the blue color appeared readily in the underlying heart. After maceration of the tissue was achieved, the flap still adhered to the heart. After careful removal of some lateral parts of the heart, a prominent blue vascular network was evident that deeply ramified in the myocardium (Fig. 2). In some preparations, an admixture of the blue and red casting material was evident as a sign of communication between the two vascular networks. This was found in the animals with the multiple microinfarctions as well as in the animals with the ameroid constrictor. The ameroid constrictor completely occluded the LAD. This was evident from in vivo coronary angiographies. Postmortem studies 12 months after the grafting operation indicated that a significant amount of neovessels had again penetrated into the underlying heart. These neovessels established anastomosis with the coronary artery system (Fig. 3). Furthermore, the LAD, completely occluded by the ameroid constrictor, was retrogradely filled by these neovessels originating from the skeletal muscle flap.

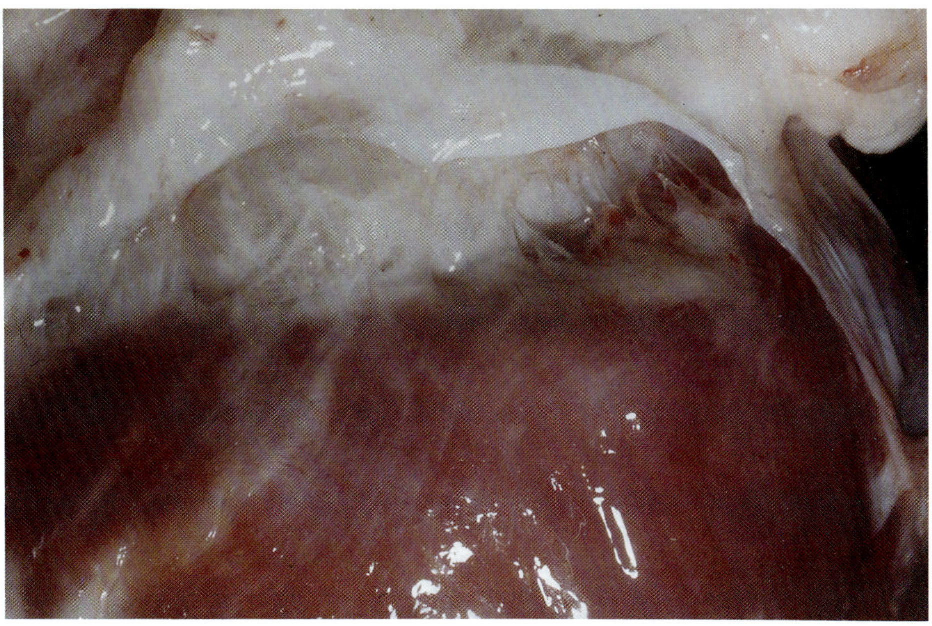

**Figure 1:** *The heart with the skeletal muscle flap 20 weeks after the grafting intervention. The flap is fibrotic, but adheres firmly to the heart.*

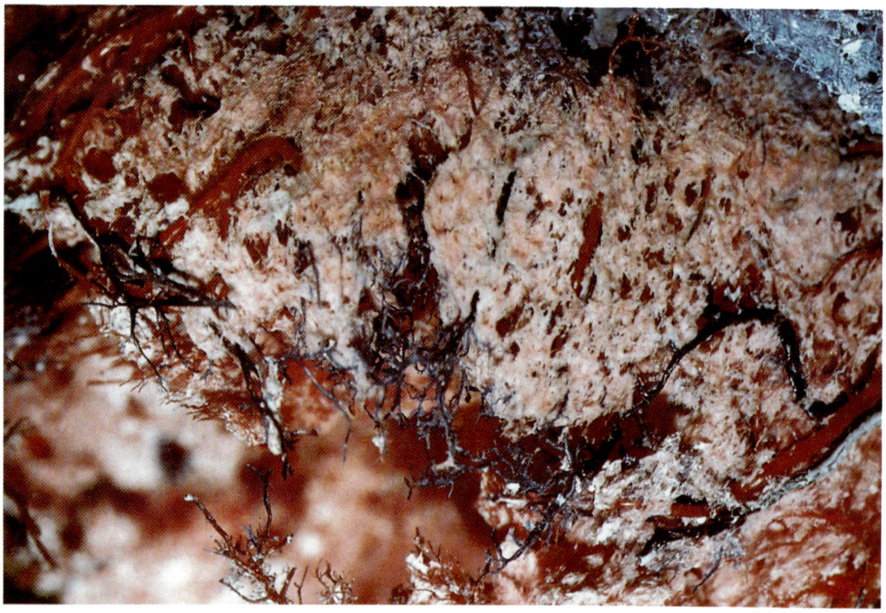

**Figure 2:** *Corrosion cast preparation of the heart with the graft. Vessels of the same color of casting material injected into the graft were found to form a large network in the myocardium.*

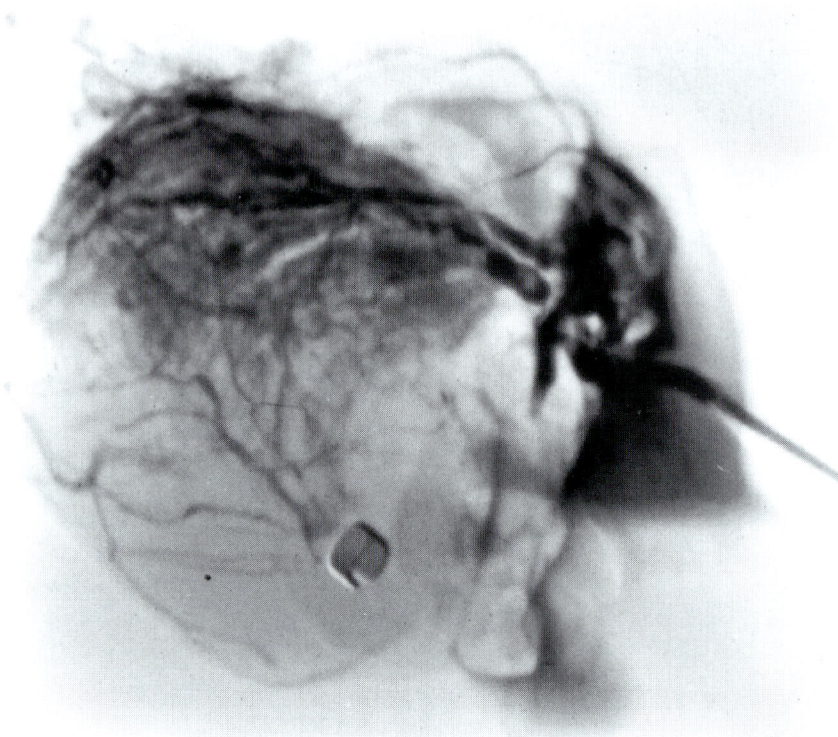

**Figure 3:** *Postmortem angiography 12 months after the intervention showed retrograde filling of the LAD from vascular anastomosis originating from the skeletal muscle graft.*

The flow determinations, adopting the radioactive microsphere technique, showed that an almost normal flow was evident in the myocardium perfused by the occluded LAD. This flow, therefore, was entirely dependent on the neovessels originating from the muscle flap. The flow in these anterolateral parts of the heart was from 0.46 to 1.0 mL/min/gram.

## Discussion

The results of our experimental study clearly indicated that a significant myocardial neovascularization is induced by grafting a free skeletal muscle flap onto the heart. In fact, in the vascular casts, it was evident that optimal adherence, as well as vascular development, is induced after such an intervention. These vessels clearly originated from the skeletal graft, as was shown by the fact that they had the same color of casting material that was injected into the IMA muscle flap. On the other hand, postmortem angiography confirmed that these neovessels persist even 12 months after the grafting operation. Furthermore, they establish anastomosis with the coronaries and are able to compensate for the occlusion of a major coronary artery as shown by retrograde filling of the LAD. The functional aspect of these neovessels was definitively confirmed by the flow measurements. This demonstrated that flow in the myocardium supplied by the IMA graft was the same as in the myocardium supplied by a normal coronary. Therefore, at least in the dog, coronary occlusion can be completely compensated by grafting a free skeletal muscle flap.

Indirect myocardial revascularization procedures have been performed since the 1930s. Many investigators aimed to augment myocardial perfusion by creating an extra-anatomic collateral circulation.[11–15] None of these operations gained general acceptance. Although the principal ideas that were the basis for these studies may have been of a theoretical clinical value, they could never be truly successful. This is due to the following factors:

1. Selective coronary angiography has been possible only since 1960 when Sones introduced this technique. Therefore, all patients who underwent these operations were selected basically for subjective symptoms and electrocardiographic findings.
2. Follow-up angiographic studies were impossible for the same reason mentioned above. Therefore, only subjective improvement could be assessed.
3. Only since 1960[16] has it been possible to perform microvascular anastomosis. Therefore, optimal perfusion of any graft could never be guaranteed in these early attempts.

Optimal perfusion, though, is in our opinion the most important stimulus for neoangiogenic activity. The historical indirect myocardial revascularization attempts probably produced only the formation of a granulation tissue due to wound healing. In order to stimulate these capillaries to further growth, and, most important, prevent regression of these newly formed vessels, a good perfusion pressure as postulated by Thoma is essential. We therefore conclude that grafting of a free skeletal muscle flap can induce a myocardial revascularization when a good perfusion pressure of the graft is surgically produced.

In our first clinical case, we adopted the latissimus dorsi muscle. The patient was suffering from small vessel coronary artery disease and unstable angina and therefore not suitable for bypass surgery. The skeletal muscle was grafted as a free flap onto the anterior lateral wall of the patient's heart. The vascular pedicle was directly anastomosed to the aorta, thus providing strong, good perfusion pressure. Venous flow was drained into the right atrium. The patient tolerated this surgical intervention well.

*Acknowledgments:* We greatly acknowledge the help of the Dr. Karl Thomae Company, Biberach a.d. Riss, where this study was conducted. The study was supported by a grant from the Deutsche Herzhilfe, e.V., Germany.

## References

1. Goldberg N, Gaynes M, McLaughlin I, Houlton F: Microvascular myocardioplasty. In Chiu RCJ (ed): *Biomechanical Cardiac Assist: Cardiomyoplasty and Muscle Powered Devices.* Mount Kisco, NY, Futura Publishing Company, 1991.
2. Mannion I, Stephenson L: Potential uses of skeletal muscle for myocardial assistance. *Surg Clin N Am* 65:679, 1983.
3. Christ IE, Spira M: Application of latissimus dorsi muscle to the heart. *Ann Plast Surg* 8:118, 1982.
4. Mannion JD, Buckman PD, Magno MG, DiMeo F: Collateral blood flow from skeletal muscle to normal myocardium. *J Surg Res* 53:578, 1992.
5. Thoma R: Über die Histomechanik des Gefäsystems und die Pathogenese der Angiosklerose. *Virch Arch Pathol Anat* 204:1, 1911.
6. Ziada AM, Hudlicka O, Tyler KR, Wright AI: The effect of long-term vasodilatation on capillary growth and performance in rabbit heart and skeletal muscle. *Cardiovasc Res* 18:724, 1984.
7. Beyer M, Hoffer H, Eggeling T, Matt O, et al: Free skeletal muscle transplantation to an infarction area: An experimental study in the dog. *Microsurgery* 14:125, 1993.
8. Beyer M, Eggeling T, Hoffer H, Mierdl S, et al: Experimental selective myocardial infarction in the dog without open chest surgery. *Res Exp Med* 192:169, 1992.
9. Beyer M, Hoffer H, Mierdl S, Beyer U, et al: Neoangiogenese nach Transplantation eines freien Skelettmuskellappens auf das Myokard des Hundes. *Vasa* 21:132, 1992.
10. Bartrum R, Berkowitz D, Hollenberg N: A simple radioactive microsphere method for measuring regional flow and cardiac output. *Invest Radiol* 9:126, 1974.
11. O'Shaugnessy L: An experimental method of providing a collateral circulation to the heart. *Br J Surg* 23:665, 1936.
12. Beck C, Tichy VL: The production of a collateral circulation to the heart. *Am Heart J* 10:849, 1935.
13. Carter RN, Gall SA, Wadsworth CL: An experimental study of collateral coronary circulation produced by cardiopneumoplexy. *Surgery* 25:489, 1949.
14. Lezius A: Die künstliche Blutversorgung des Herzmuskels. *Arch Klin Chir* 189:342, 1937.
15. Moran RE: Revascularization of the heart by tubed pedicle graft of skin and subcutaneous tissue. *Plast Reconstr Surg* 10:295, 1952.
16. Tamai S, Komatsu S, Sakamoto H: Free muscle transplants in dogs with microsurgical neurovascular anastomosis. *Plast Reconstr Surg* 46:219, 1970.

Chapter 20

# Discussion

**Dr. Mannion:** This is quite an exciting study. I wonder if you could speculate on the relationship between denervation and an increase in angiogenesis.

**Dr. Beyer:** I have the feeling that denervation may be important for collateralization. We have relatively high arterial inflow in the muscle flap and a relatively low energy demand on the part of the muscle flap. So we have a fit capillary network and no energy demand on the part of the muscle. Perhaps this may favor the formation of collaterals.

**Sir Magdi Yacoub:** I would also like to congratulate you; this is a brilliant study. The Vineberg experience taught us that you cannot evaluate postmortem angiographic studies with flow during life. You have done your microsphere measurement flow not in the internal mammary artery but in the circumflex artery. Can you indicate the relationship between the cast of the postmortem studies to flow in the internal mammary to the anterior surface of the heart?

**Dr. Beyer:** We have not measured flow in the internal mammary artery because it is not significant. We cannot say if the flow from the mammary artery is going directly into the right atrium or directly into the myocardium. What we have done is the original blood flow determination of postmortem heart tissue and this was done with radioactive microspheres to have milliliter heart tissue flow per gram per minute.

**Sir Magdi Yacoub:** But the flow in the anterior surface is very low. Isn't that right, or am I wrong?

**Dr. Beyer:** No, we have a high flow there!

**Sir Magdi Yacoub:** Is it normal?

**Dr. Beyer:** Yes.

# Part III

## Muscle Function

Chapter 21

# Tissue Velocity Imaging in Cardiomyoplasty

Neil R. Grubb, George R. Sutherland,
Ciro Campanella, Keith A. A. Fox

## Introduction

Optimization of skeletal muscle training and muscle stimulation parameters is of key importance in maximizing functional benefit after cardiomyoplasty. In the first 10 years of its clinical application, several methods have been used to monitor latissimus dorsi (LD) graft function. Palpation of the LD impulse in the axilla is often used to identify muscle contraction,[1] but this clinical assessment can be rendered insensitive by the patient's build and by the amount of muscle stump remaining outside the thoracic cavity. Furthermore, clinical examination can only assess the function of the most proximal portion of the graft. An alternative approach involves the use of fluoroscopy to measure shortening between the two intramuscular electrodes. Although this is likely to be more sensitive than the palpation method, it provides only information about function within a localized portion of the muscle. The use of ionizing radiation limits its use to comparatively brief assessments. An experimental approach to enhance this technique has used placement of metal clips at intervals along the LD graft during surgery, allowing fluoroscopic measurement of contraction throughout the muscle. This interesting technique is still under appraisal, but even using digital image acquisition and measurement methods, it provides only a limited, semiquantitative assessment. Left ventricular angiography provides accurate assessment of left ventricular ejection fraction, and provides an assessment of regional ventricular distortion.[2] This technique has high precision and has provided a useful insight into left ventricular mechanics in cardiomyoplasty, but does not lend itself to repeated assessments in the clinical setting.

From Carpentier A, Chachques JC, Grandjean P: Cardiac Bioassist. © Futura Publishing Co, Inc, Armonk, NY, 1997.

## Ultrasound Assessment

M-mode, Doppler, and two-dimensional B-mode echocardiography have been widely used in an attempt to optimize graft function after cardiomyoplasty. The currently accepted and widely applied method of setting the ventricle-muscle synchronization delay involves M-mode echocardiography of the mitral valve using a synchronized electrocardiogram to program initiation of the burst stimulus after closure of the mitral valve. Several centers have demonstrated that initiation of LD muscle contraction prior to mitral valve closure can have deleterious effects on hemodynamics and on subjective well-being.[3,4] M-mode echocardiography of the left ventricle has also been used to identify beat-to-beat variation in ventricular wall motion resulting from myograft contraction.[5] This provides useful information about whether latissimus dorsi force is transmitted to the heart. However, conventional ultrasound is limited in its application for several reasons. First, it depends on good image quality to demonstrate differences in ventricular wall motion induced by graft contraction. Second, it is prone to artifact effects caused by motion of the heart along the axis perpendicular to the ultrasound plane. This is a potential limitation in all echocardiographic assessments of ventricular function but is particularly relevant after cardiomyoplasty, where whole heart displacement is most marked during assisted cycles. Finally, the technique is at best semiquantitative and is not capable of providing information about proximal latissimus dorsi contraction (the portion of the muscle not wrapped around the ventricles). Information can only indirectly be inferred about wall motion velocity, and latissimus dorsi dynamics cannot be assessed.

## Tissue Velocity Imaging

Tissue velocity imaging (TVI) is a novel ultrasound technique that can provide quantitative information about motion in solid tissues.[6,7] The technique is based on the principle of color Doppler imaging of blood flow, which is now a standard component of the echocardiographic repertoire. Filtering hardware is modified to exclude relatively high blood pool velocities (usually greater than 25 cm/second), and to encompass slower solid tissue velocities. Post-processing is also modified to eliminate blood pool information. Tissue velocity information is displayed either as a two-dimensional color map, or with greater temporal resolution as a color M-mode plot. The color map provides information about *direction* and *speed* of tissue movement. In the examples shown in this chapter, tissue motion toward the ultrasound transducer is encoded red/yellow, and motion in the opposite direction is encoded green/blue (Fig. 1). Limited on-line analysis software is available on current systems, and to obtain useful quantitative information, an image acquisition system should be used to store images on optical media or high quality (super VHS) video tape. It is beyond the scope of this chapter to provide a detailed account of off-line analysis of TVI images; the details of this technique are previously reported.[8,9] In brief, off-line analysis of color M-mode traces involves marking a region of interest, normally within the myocardium or a layer of skeletal muscle. The mean velocity across this thickness of tissue is calculated for each point in time. These data can be used to generate tissue velocity-time plots.

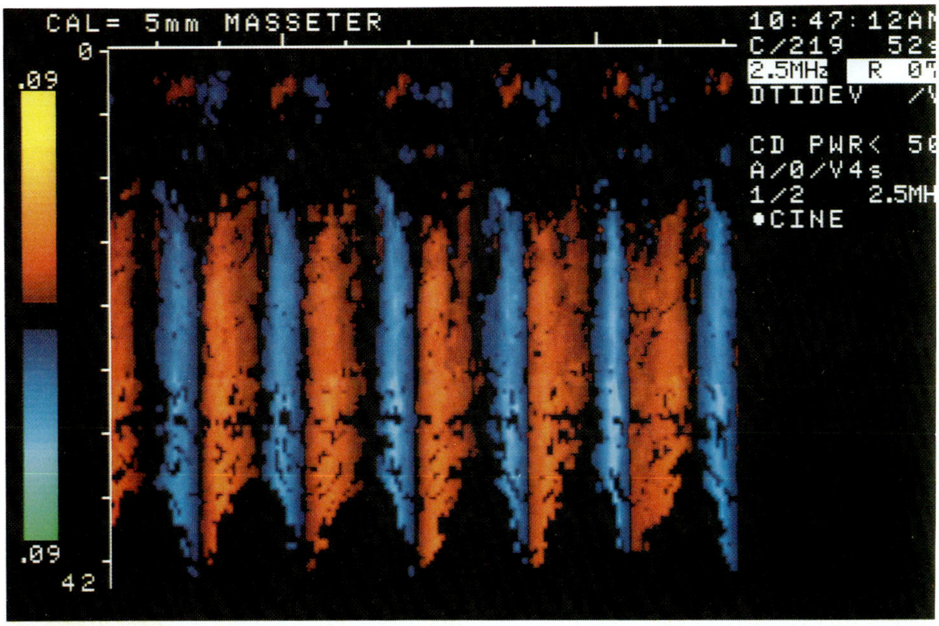


**Figure 1:** *TVI M-mode image of skeletal muscle contraction. The muscle group shown here is masseter; the subject is chewing. The horizontal axis represents time (one tick = 200 ms), the vertical axis tissue depth (one tick = 5 mm). Cyclic changes in muscle velocity can clearly be seen. The color scale is shown on the left in meters per second. Motion towards the transducer encodes red/yellow, motion in the opposite direction encodes green/blue.*

## Validation Studies

Initial studies validated the velocity and spatial resolution of TVI using a series of test phantoms.[8] Velocity resolution was found to be precise in the upper 90% of a selected velocity range, comparing TVI measured velocities with the actual velocity of a rotating foam phantom. Spatial resolution was validated using moving blocks of gel into which grooves were cut. Using a standard 2.5 MHz ultrasound transducer, spatial resolution is 2–3 mm. This resolution is expected to be greater when higher transmit frequencies are used, but at the expense of reduced tissue penetration (i.e., the system will be limited to shallower imaging depths). TVI is available on several commercially available ultrasound systems (Doppler tissue imaging [DTI] – Acuson, Mountain View, California; Tissue Doppler imaging [TDI] – Toshiba, Tustin, California); our experience is confined to the Acuson DTI system.

Initial clinical studies examined TVI assessment of myocardial motion in open-chest pigs with coronary occlusion and in the hearts of healthy volunteers.[6] More recent studies have demonstrated the capability of TVI to measure shortening velocity in in-situ skeletal muscle groups in healthy volunteers.[9] In that study, TVI was used to illustrate differences in velocity profile between passive muscle motion and active isometric and isotonic contraction.

Furthermore, it was capable of resolving near-tetanic muscle contraction and could demonstrate the latency, contraction, and relaxation phases of a monosynaptic tendon jerk reflex. This ability to demonstrate the dynamics of skeletal muscle function, coupled with the ability to quantify the velocity of ventricular wall motion, led to the application of TVI in the assessment of skeletal muscle cardiac assist systems.[10]

## TVI of Free Latissimus Dorsi

Tissue velocity imaging studies of cardiomyoplasty subjects are best performed with two operators to minimize variation in transducer angle. One operator is required to maintain a constant angle of insonation and to adjust machine settings, while the other operator adjusts the programmed muscle stimulator parameters. TVI-derived velocity measurements are angle-dependent, and significant error may be introduced by a single operator repositioning the transducer after each reprogramming. Using specific imaging windows, both the free and wrapped portions of the LD muscle can be examined. The most proximal portion of the muscle can be examined using an axillary view. To obtain measurements, conventional two-dimensional imaging is used to locate the contracting part of the muscle through the resected window of the second or third rib. Once the muscle is identified, the transducer is aligned to minimize the angle between the ultrasound beam and the axis of the muscle fiber shortening. In practice, this is difficult to achieve, and it is often not possible to obtain true fiber shortening velocities with TVI. After transducer position is obtained, TVI is activated and a high-speed (50 mm/second) M-mode trace is obtained. Since TVI precision is affected in the lower 10% of a given velocity scale, the imaging scale is set to the most sensitive value that encompasses the observed velocities (this avoids artifact known as *aliasing,* where measured velocities exceed the selected velocity scale). Measurements can also be obtained from the intrathoracic portion of the free LD muscle, using a fourth intercostal space imaging window.

Color M-mode images taken from these windows provide detailed information about the temporal relationship between the burst stimulus and muscle contraction. In our experience, TVI assessment can identify contraction in situations where conventional echocardiography and clinical examination are not sensitive enough to detect contraction. These measurements may be particularly useful for examining graft function early during the stimulation protocol (Fig. 2), where short burst lengths and low pulse amplitudes are usually used. After completion of training, it is possible to measure the muscle shortening and lengthening times.

## TVI of the Muscle Wrap and Myocardium

As with conventional echocardiography, the ability of TVI to resolve muscle wrap from myocardium is variable and is probably dependent on the composition and thickness of the wrap. The parasternal short axis view can usually demarcate the two structures (Fig. 3). TVI can be used using the four

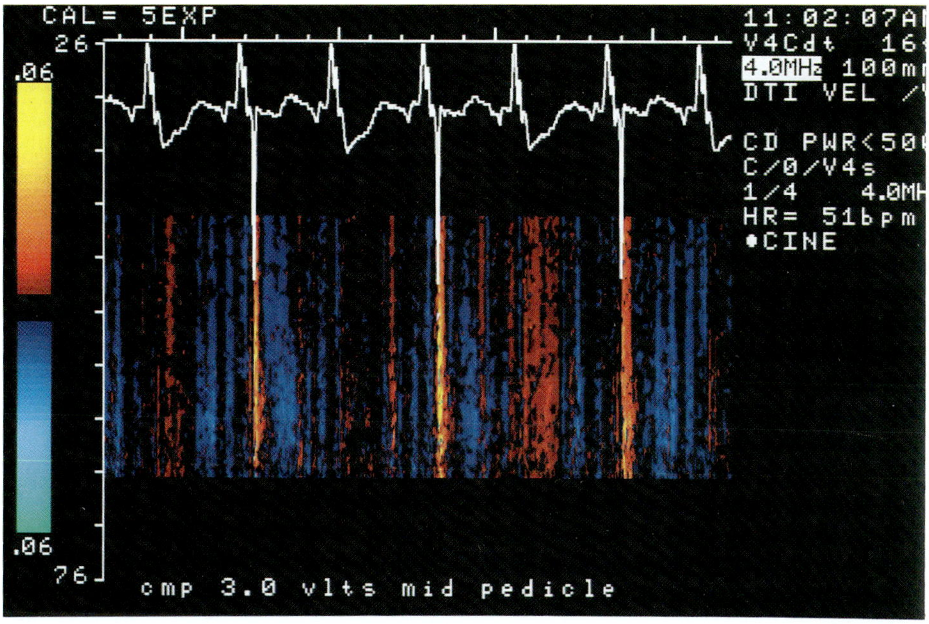


**Figure 2:** *TVI M-mode image of proximal latissimus dorsi at the time of initiation of training. Muscle contraction is clearly seen to coincide with the single stimulus applied on alternate cardiac cycles. The horizontal axis represents time (one tick = 200 ms), the vertical axis tissue depth (one tick = 5 mm).*

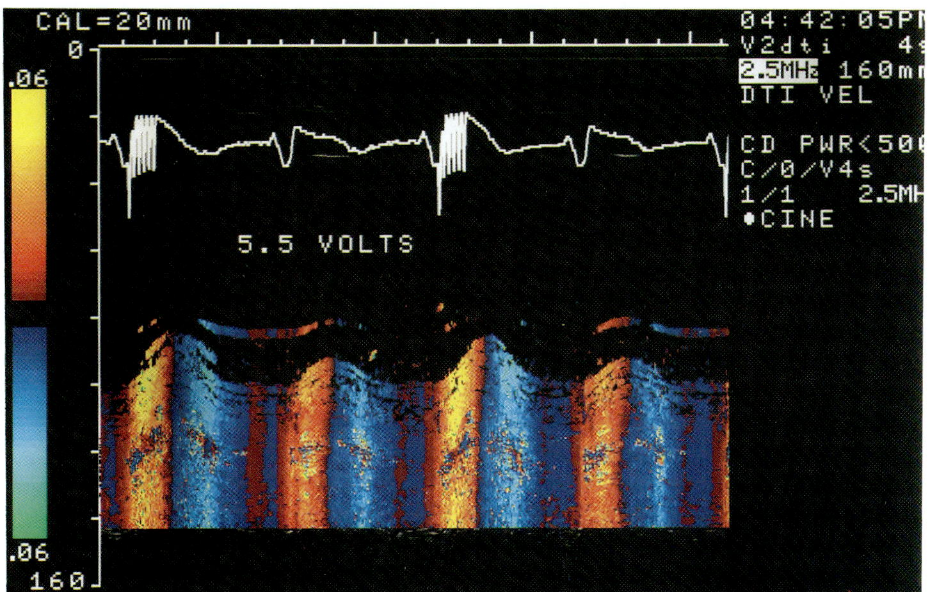


**Figure 3:** *TVI M-mode image of the posterior myocardium and latissimus dorsi wrap. A line of demarcation is just visible between the two structures. Note the beat-to-beat variation in the degree of excursion of the myocardium during systole, and the correspondingly higher coded wall velocities during assisted cycles. The horizontal axis represents time (one tick = 200 ms), the vertical axis tissue depth (one tick = 20 mm).*

standard echocardiographic views to determine the effects of LD contraction on ventricular wall motion. Anterior, inferoposterior, lateral septal, and apical motion are readily assessed. The lateral wall and medial septum cannot be fully assessed since their axis of motion is across rather than along the ultrasound axis in the parasternal short axis and apical four chamber views. As a result of these limitations, TVI is not used as a method of assessing global left ventricular function. The principal application of TVI is in assessing ventricular wall motion during assisted and nonassisted contractions as a measure of energy transmission to the heart from the myograft. TVI assessment of beat-to-beat variation in ventricular wall motion should be principally regarded as a method of assessing muscle function rather than ventricular function. Assessment of the effects of alteration of muscle stimulator programmed parameters is achieved by monitoring inferoposterior wall motion. Off-line analysis provides a plot of mean velocity across the thickness of the posterior wall *versus* time (Fig. 4). From this plot, it is possible to calculate the difference in peak systolic velocity between assisted and nonassisted beats. This value is termed the *assist velocity difference* (AVD).

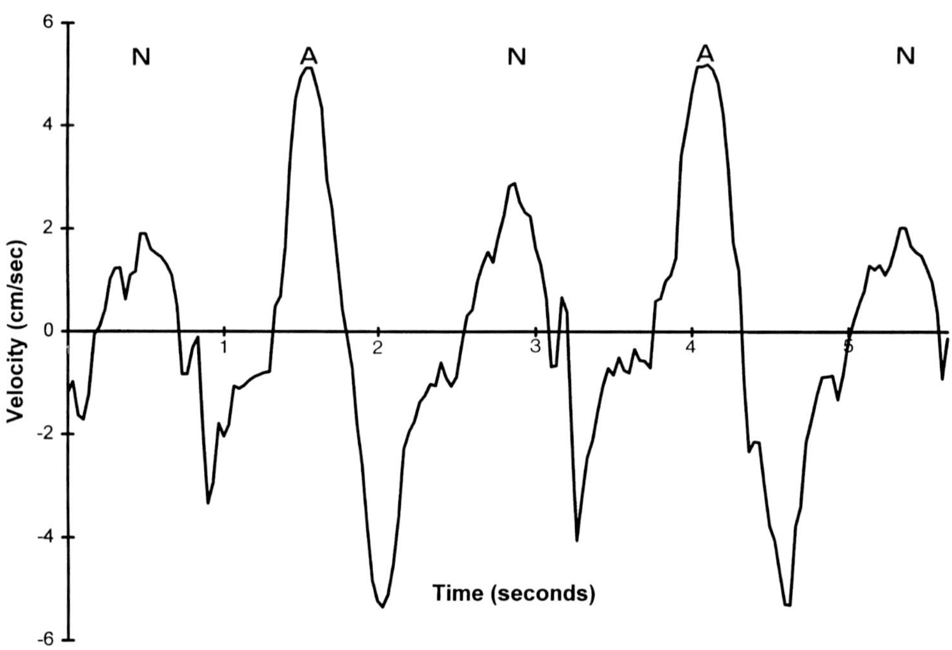


**Figure 4:** *Velocity-time plot obtained by off-line analysis of a TVI M-mode image of posterior wall motion. Wall velocity is approximately 5 cm/sec during systole in the assisted cycles (A), and 2.5 cm/sec during systole in the nonassisted cycles (N).*

## Clinical Application of TVI in Patient Monitoring

Early experience with TVI suggests that it is possible to identify LD dysfunction early after cardiomyoplasty. In one early case, no contraction of proximal latissimus dorsi could be identified using the palpation method on initiation of myostimulation. TVI confirmed that there was no muscle contraction even after maximization of the pulse amplitude (Fig. 5). Weekly monitoring with TVI demonstrated that there was no recovery of function. This patient subsequently failed to improve clinically, did not exhibit any subsequent beat-to-beat variation in ventricular wall motion, and died from progression of underlying disease.

Insight is provided by TVI M-mode images of proximal latissimus dorsi into the relationship between the burst stimulus and muscle contraction. Highest velocity fiber shortening is seen within the first 60 ms of stimulation. It is possible to calculate the muscle shortening and lengthening times from these tracings. In most cases, the shortening/lengthening cycle exceeds 800 ms, which coincides with the diastolic filling period of the next nonassisted cycle at higher heart rates. Further study is necessary to determine whether adaptation (shortening) of the burst stimulus during tachycardia will ameliorate this problem.

TVI can be used to determine the effect of increasing pulse amplitude on ventricular wall motion. This is achieved by measuring the AVD through a range of pulse amplitudes. The relationship between AVD and pulse amplitude is usually sigmoid; at low voltages the AVD is zero, meaning that peak myocardial velocity does not vary between assisted and nonassisted cycles. A threshold is reached at which point the AVD rises above zero, and with increasing voltage continues to rise until a plateau is reached where graft contraction is maximal (Fig. 6). The points of inflexion on this sigmoid curve represent the threshold voltages at which interbeat variation in wall motion is first seen, and at which interbeat variation reaches its maximum. Although the curve is sigmoid in all patients whom we have studied, the points of inflexion vary among patients, suggesting that pulse amplitude should be adjusted according to individual patients' thresholds. This will potentially allow optimization of pulse amplitude, conservation of the stimulator power cell, and may prevent muscle damage from high voltage stimulation. It has yet to be determined whether maximal or submaximal myograft contraction is desirable for long-term stimulation.

Similarly, graphs can be plotted for the ventricle-muscle synchronization delay *versus* AVD (Fig. 7). AVD "optima" using this method does not necessarily occur with synchronization delays optimized to mitral valve closure. It is likely, however, that settings that maximize ventricular wall motion will also optimize augmentation and dynamic assistance. Corroborative hemodynamic studies and examination of pressure-volume relationships will be needed to establish whether TVI optimized myostimulation results in improved cardiac performance.

Although TVI cannot provide an overall index of ventricular function, it can give an assessment of the effects of graft contraction on cardiac displacement and ventricular geometry. Figure 8 is a wall velocity-time graph derived

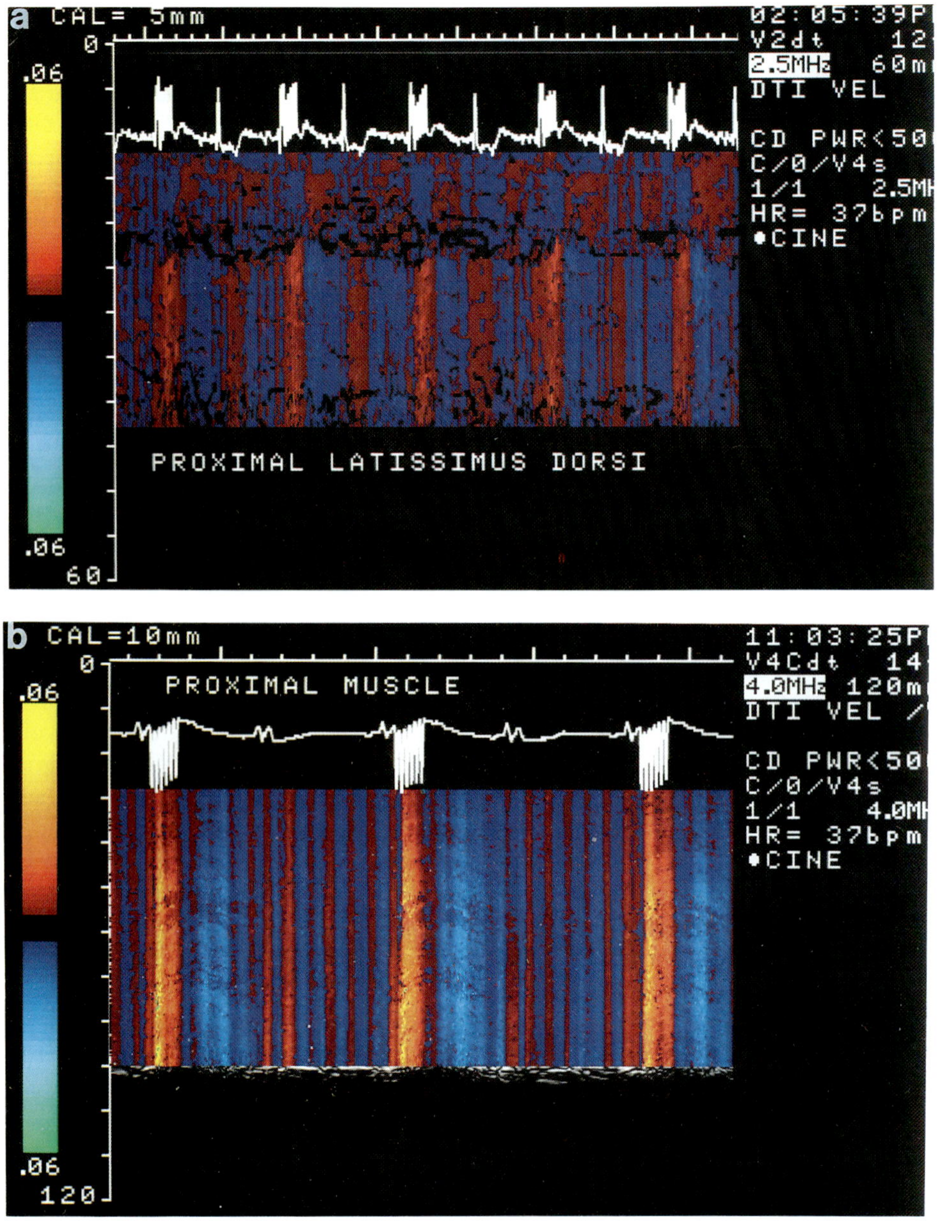


**Figure 5a:** *Muscle failure. This TVI M-mode image shows low-amplitude cyclic movement of proximal latissimus dorsi in time with the cardiac cycle. This is passive, low-velocity motion propagated along the muscle from the heart. There is only a minimal increase in muscle velocity during burst stimulation. One tick = 5 mm.* **Figure 5b:** *In a patient with adequate latissimus dorsi function, beat-to-beat variation in muscle velocity is clearly demonstrated, with higher velocities coded during assisted cycles. The horizontal axis represents time (one tick = 200 ms), the vertical axis tissue depth. One tick = 10 mm.*

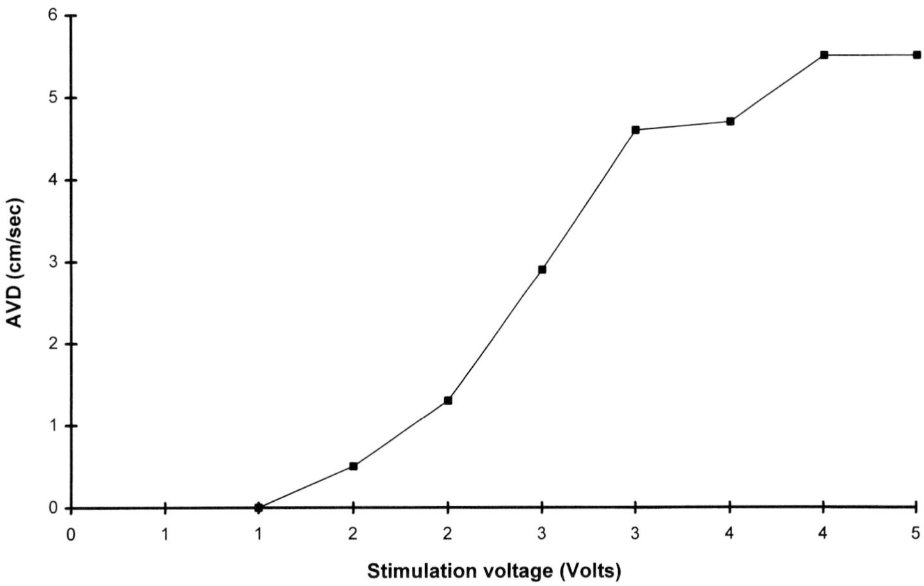


**Figure 6:** *Graph of the assist velocity difference (AVD, see text)* versus *muscle pulse amplitude.*

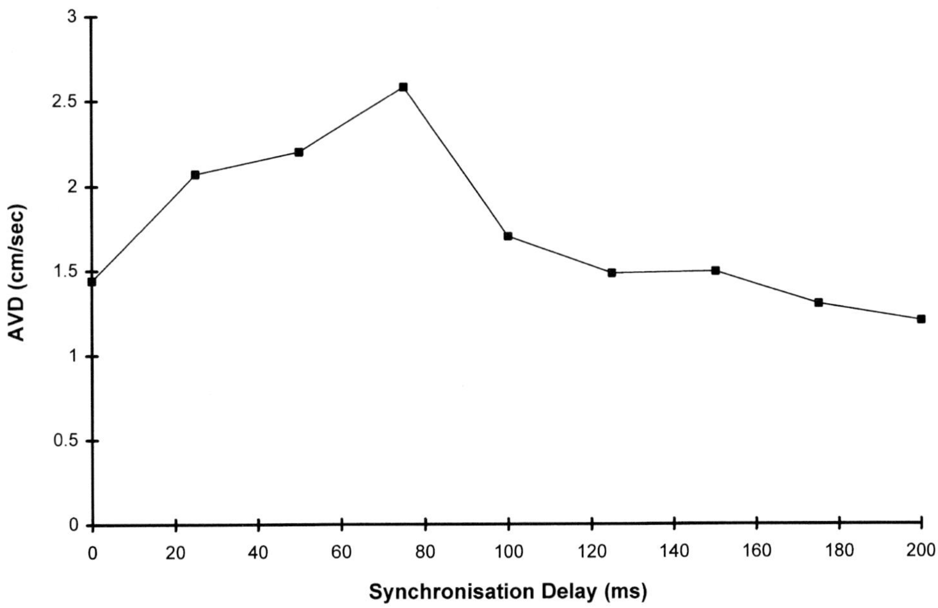


**Figure 7:** *Graph of the assist velocity difference (AVD, see text)* versus *ventricle-muscle synchronization delay.*

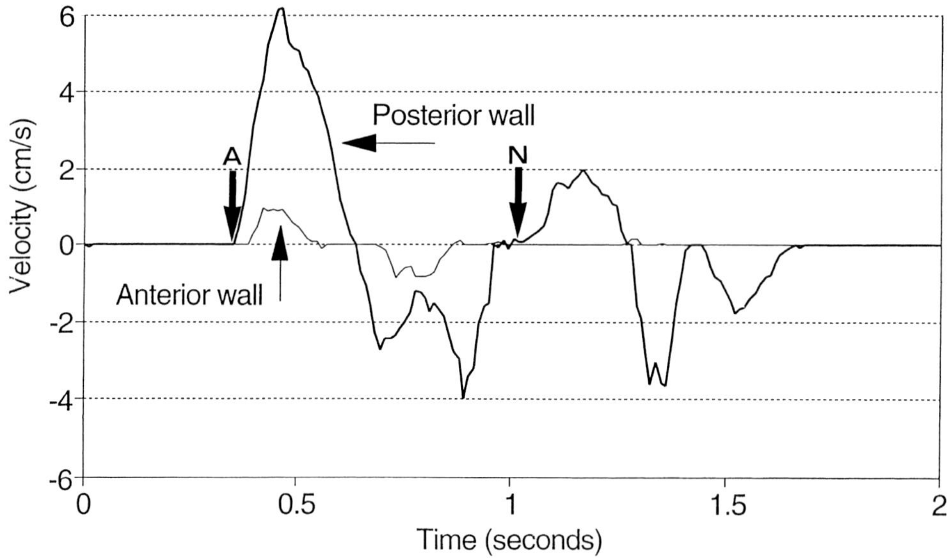


**Figure 8:** *Ventricular wall velocity–time graph derived from TVI M-mode image of anterior and posterior wall motion in a cardiomyoplasty patient with previous anterior myocardial infarction. (A = assisted cycle; N = nonassisted cycle). See main text for explanation of this graph.*

from a patient with previous anterior myocardial infarction after cardiomyoplasty. The graph shows one assisted cycle (left) and one nonassisted cycle (right). The dark line denotes posterior wall motion, the light line anterior wall motion. The posterior wall moves inwards at 2 cm/sec$^{-1}$ during the nonassisted cycle (N), increasing to 6 cm/sec$^{-1}$ during assist (A). This gives an assist velocity difference of $6 - 2 = 4$ cm/sec$^{-1}$. The anterior wall is completely akinetic during the nonassisted cycle, and can therefore be used as a reference point for displacement. It moves at 1 cm/sec$^{-1}$ during assist *in the same direction* as the posterior wall, suggesting overall heart displacement at 1 cm/sec$^{-1}$ anteriorly. In this case, TVI illustrates that displacement accounts for approximately one-quarter of the AVD seen in the posterior wall. In the same patient, two-dimensional TVI images show paradoxical apical motion at peak systole during a nonassisted cycle, which normalizes with graft contraction (Fig. 9). Using the mitral anulus as a reference point for displacement, no displacement was noted in this ultrasound plane.

## Conclusions

Tissue velocity imaging is a new ultrasound technique that provides unique information about LD function and its effects on ventricular wall motion. It overcomes several of the limitations of conventional echocardiographic assessment. First, Doppler techniques are not critically dependent on the echogenicity of the subject. Proximal and midportion LD function can be as-

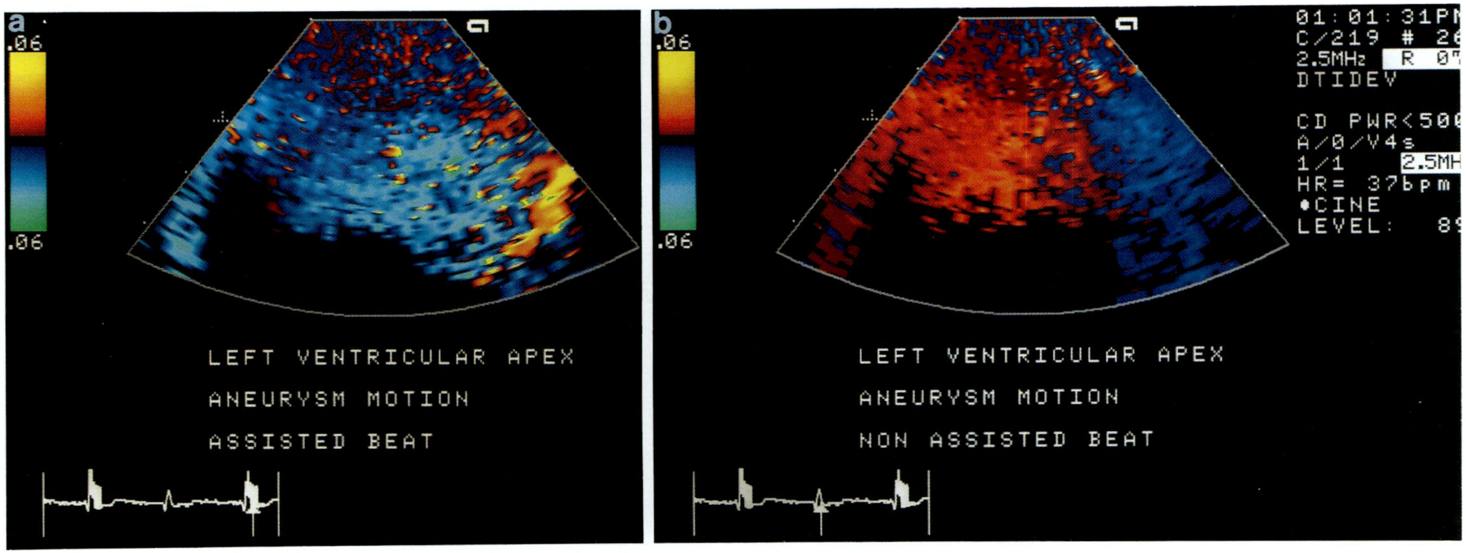


**Figure 9:** *Magnified two-dimensional TVI images of the left ventricular apex taken from an apical four chamber view.* **a.** *During a nonassisted cycle (left), apical motion encodes red, denoting paradoxical motion towards the transducer; the patient has a dyskinetic apex.* **b.** *At the same moment during the assisted cycle (right) apical motion codes blue, denoting a reversal in phase of motion during systole; apical motion has normalized and the apex now moves towards the base of the heart.*

sessed without exposure to ionizing radiation, and detailed temporal assessments of graft contraction and relaxation times can be made. These may in the future form the basis for optimizing the synchronization ratio and burst length adjustment. Ventricular wall velocity can also be measured during assisted and nonassisted cycles, giving an index of transmission of muscle energy to the heart. These variables can be measured under different stimulation settings to optimize muscle stimulator programmed parameters. Assessments can also be made of regional ventricular wall motion and cardiac displacement. TVI monitoring may also have future application in the development and evaluation of muscle training and long-term stimulation protocols, and in the assessment of latissimus dorsi function prior to cardiomyoplasty surgery.

## References


1. Chachques JC, Grandjean PA, Carpentier A: Patient management and clinical follow-up after cardiomyoplasty. *J Cardiac Surg* 6:89–99, 1991.
2. Bocchi EA, Moreira LF, de Moraes AV: Effects of dynamic cardiomyoplasty on regional wall motion, ejection fraction and geometry of the left ventricle. *Circulation* 86(Suppl II):231–235, 1992.
3. Levin HR, Tsitlik J, Halperin H: Optimization of the timing of skeletal to cardiac muscle contraction during dynamic cardiomyoplasty: Analysis using a mathematical model. *J Cardiac Surg* 6:235–244, 1991.
4. Grubb NR, Fleming AD, Sutherland GR, Fox KAA: Optimising muscle synchronization after dynamic cardiomyoplasty: Two educational cases. *Eur J Cardiothorac Surg* 9:45–49, 1995.
5. Moreira LF, Stolf NA, Bocchi EA, et al: Latissimus dorsi cardiomyoplasty in the treatment of patients with dilated cardiomyopathy. *Circulation* 82(Suppl IV): 257–263, 1990.
6. McDicken WN, Sutherland GR, Moran CM, Gordon LN: Colour Doppler imaging of the myocardium. *Ultrasound Med Biol* 18:651–654, 1992.
7. Sutherland GR, Stewart MJ, Groundstroem KWE, et al: Colour Doppler myocardial imaging: A new technique for the assessment of myocardial function. *J Am Soc Echo* 7:441–458, 1994.
8. Fleming AD, McDicken WN, Sutherland GR, et al: Assessment of colour Doppler tissue imaging using test phantoms. *Ultrasound Med Biol* 20:937–951, 1994.
9. Grubb NR, Fleming A, Fox KAA, Sutherland GR: Evaluation of Doppler tissue imaging for the assessment of skeletal muscle function in healthy volunteers. *Radiology* 194:837–842, 1995.
10. Grubb NR, Sutherland GR, Campanella C, Fleming A, et al: Latissimus dorsi muscle: Assessment of stimulation after cardiomyoplasty using Doppler tissue imaging. *Radiology* 199:59–64, 1996.

Chapter 22

# Relationship Between Working Capacity and Activation Frequency of Chronically Stimulated Skeletal Muscle

J.C. Jarvis, H. Sutherland, M.M.N. Kwende, C.N. Mayne, S. Salmons

In the 1980s, conditioning of skeletal muscle reopened the door to providing cardiac assistance from skeletal muscle. While the fatigue resistance of chronically stimulated muscle was correctly presented as being virtually limitless, tests based on the percentage of initial isometric force maintained over time may have given a false impression of the power available from such muscle. Fully transformed muscles are indeed extremely resistant to fatigue, but also very slow to contract and relax. This presents two problems in cardiac assistance. First, the reduction in contractile speed and muscle mass produces a corresponding reduction in power to a level that is adequate but provides little scope for engineering compromises and variations in surgical technique. Second, the slowness of contraction and relaxation seriously limits the volume changes that can be achieved within the space of a cardiac cycle.[1] One of our current objectives, therefore, is to identify patterns of chronic stimulation that can produce muscles that are faster and more powerful, but equally resistant to fatigue. Such advances would benefit the whole field of skeletal muscle assist.

The full extent of the reduction in power output was not recognized until experiments were made to measure the absolute power output during shortening contractions of stimulated skeletal muscles.[1–3] These results showed that under optimum conditions for the extraction of work from fully transformed skeletal muscle, the power available for cardiac assistance was just adequate. On the other hand, the extreme slowness of fully transformed muscle would be a real limitation to synchronous assist, and was the reason for low ejection fractions in skeletal muscle ventricles formed from slow muscle. For example, Acker et al.[4] demonstrated substantial power and flow from chronically stimulated

From Carpentier A, Chachques JC, Grandjean P: Cardiac Bioassist. © Futura Publishing Co, Inc, Armonk, NY, 1997.

skeletal muscle ventricles formed in dogs, but with ejection fractions between a maximum of 40% and (after a few weeks of pumping) only 20%. Such low ejection fractions are likely to be associated with thrombus formation.

It is likewise possible that the benefit afforded by cardiomyoplasty is limited by the slowness of the grafted muscle, both in terms of a limited assistance during systole and in restriction of diastolic filling because of slow relaxation.

There is therefore a pressing need to find out whether it is possible to provide cardiac assistance from skeletal muscle without inducing the extremely slow contractile characteristic of type 1 fibers. Single motor unit studies show that populations of fast fatigue-resistant (type 2A) fibers exist stably in mammalian skeletal muscles. We know that it is possible to produce a stable population of slow (type 1) fibers by electrical stimulation. In fact, because the blood supply and mitochondrial density increase during this process *before* the replacement of fast with slow isoforms of myosin, a fast fatigue-resistant state exists transiently during fast-to-slow transformation. Mabuchi et al.[5] showed that a similar state was reached after 7 weeks of intermittent stimulation, but since the transformation to type 1 fibers normally takes place over 8–10 weeks with continuous stimulation, it was not possible to say that a new equilibrium state had been reached.

The obvious first step towards the maintenance of a fast fatigue-resistant muscle was the use of continuous stimulation at a frequency lower than that which causes complete fast-to-slow transformation. We made stimulators according to our published design[6,7] and completed a time course of the effects of stimulation at 10 Hz or 2.5 Hz for up to 12 weeks. Transformation was both less rapid and less complete when the muscles were stimulated at 2.5 Hz rather than at 10 Hz. Mechanical and histochemical data indicated that the predominantly 2B fiber type population of these muscles was transformed to an intermediate state similar to the 2A type. Muscles stimulated at 2.5 Hz were significantly faster and more powerful than those stimulated at 10 Hz, yet they were just as resistant to fatigue when tested in a series of shortening contractions in which each muscle worked initially at 10 W/kg. In contrast to stimulation at 10 Hz, stimulation at 2.5 Hz failed to induce significant synthesis of type 1 myosin isoforms.[8] We can draw the important conclusion that changes in the bioenergetics of contraction associated with myosin transitions are not a major factor in the development of fatigue resistance. Since induction of type 1 myosin is the major factor responsible for the slowing of contractile speed, it is as undesirable as it is unnecessary.

While the changes brought about by 10 Hz stimulation are complete within 12 weeks, we could not be sure that the same was true for changes induced by 2.5 Hz stimulation. We therefore studied the mechanical characteristics of muscles that had been stimulated continuously at 2.5 Hz ($n = 6$), 5 Hz ($n = 6$), or 10 Hz ($n = 6$) for 10 months, after which it was assumed that the muscles had reached a new stable state under the imposed activity. The results confirm that the intermediate state of transformation observed in the 12-week study is indeed stable over this much longer period for muscles stimulated chronically at 2.5 Hz. An illustrative figure is presented here of the mean maximum power output in single contractions of tibialis anterior muscles within the three groups (Fig. 1). The maximum power is presented as a percentage of that produced by the contralateral unstimulated muscles.

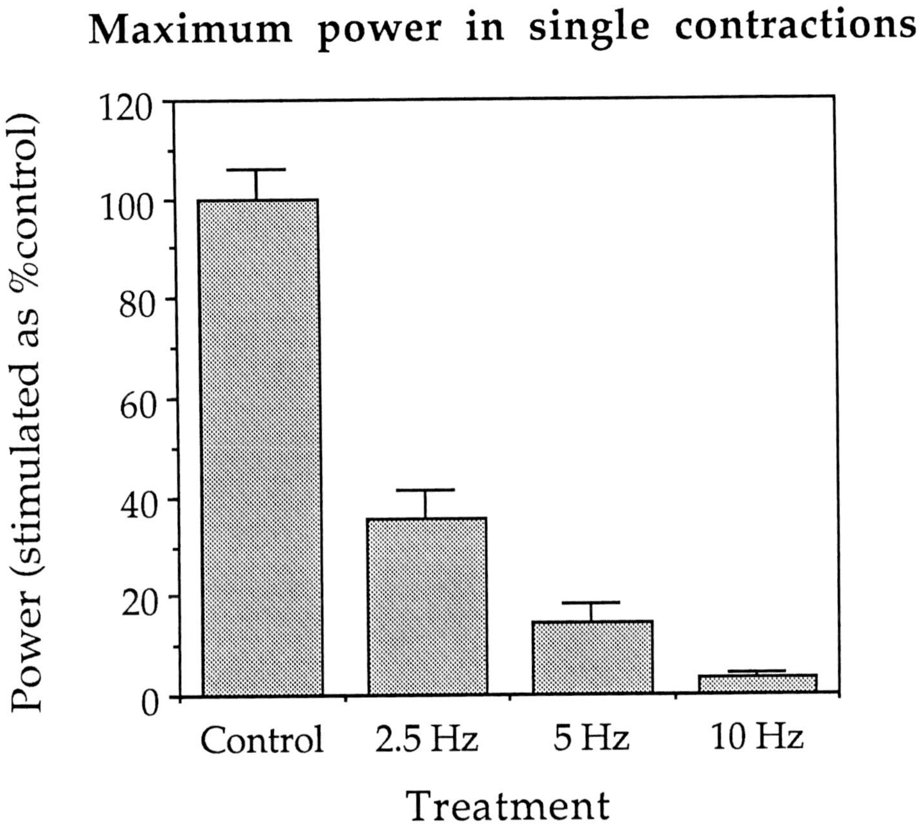


**Figure 1:** *The maximum power in a single shortening contraction of tibialis anterior muscles of adult rabbits stimulated at 2.5 Hz, 5 Hz, or 10 Hz. The columns are plotted as the mean ± SE of the power of the left (stimulated) muscle as a percentage of the right (unstimulated) muscle in the same animal. There were six animals in each experimental group. In the control group (n = 4), neither muscle was stimulated.*

Maximum power output appears to decline exponentially with increasing frequency of continuous activation. The maximum power output of the 10 Hz stimulated muscles is only about 5% of control. This figure is lower than that previously reported for stimulation over 2 or 3 months and suggests that there is some gradual loss of power even after complete fiber type transformation has taken place.

A further striking conclusion is that the aggregate frequency window between normal activity (control) and the frequency that causes complete transformation is very narrow, less than one order of magnitude. Indeed, it seems that if we are to preserve more than 40% of the maximum power of unstimulated muscle, we must not allow our clinical stimulation protocols to exceed an average impulse frequency of 2.5 Hz. In fact, because the force-frequency curve is shifted to lower frequencies in larger mammals, the window may be even narrower in humans.

Since even minor reductions in aggregate frequency may have a significant effect in preserving the power of a stimulated graft, it is important to consider ways of providing adequate cardiac assistance with fewer nerve impulses. An obvious strategy, which may be appropriate in cardiomyoplasty, is to withdraw stimulation of the graft during bed rest. Similar strategies will not be appropriate for skeletal muscle ventricles unless they can be designed to be safe passive conduits. It may be possible to regulate the output of future stimulation devices according to the required degree of assistance.

In conclusion, there are conditions of activation that can establish and maintain fast fatigue-resistant characteristics without driving the muscle in the direction of further adaptive change. With this knowledge, we can work towards clinically useful patterns of stimulation that produce a similar response.

*Acknowledgments:* This work has been supported by grants from the British Heart Foundation, the Science and Engineering Research Council, and the Wellcome Trust. Jonathan Jarvis holds a Beit Memorial Research Fellowship.

## References

1. Salmons S, Jarvis JC: The working capacity of skeletal muscle transformed for use in a cardiac assist role. In Chiu RC-J, Bourgeois IM (eds): *Transformed Muscle for Cardiac Assist and Repair.* Mount Kisco, NY, Futura Publishing Company, Inc, 1990, pp 89–104.
2. Salmons S, Jarvis JC: Cardiomyoplasty: A look at the fundamentals. In Carpentier A, Chachques JC, Grandjean P: *Cardiomyoplasty.* Mount Kisco, NY, Futura Publishing Company, Inc, 1991, pp 3–17.
3. Jarvis JC: Power production and working capacity of rabbit tibialis anterior muscles after chronic electrical stimulation at 10 Hz. *J Physiol* 470:157–169, 1993.
4. Acker MA, Hammond RL, Mannion JD, Salmons S, et al: An autologous biologic pump motor. *J Thoracic Cardiovasc Surg* 92:733–746, 1986.
5. Mabuchi K, Szvetko D, Pinter K, Sreter FA: Type IIB to IIA fiber transformation in intermittently stimulated rabbit muscles. *Am J Physiol* 242:C373–C381, 1982.
6. Salmons S, Jarvis JC: A simple optical switch for implantable devices. *Med Biol Eng Comput* 29:554–556, 1990.
7. Jarvis JC, Salmons S: A family of neuromuscular stimulators with optical transcutaneous control. *J Med Eng Technol* 15(2):53, 1990.
8. Jarvis JC, Brownson C, Sutherland H, Salmons S: Comparison between the effects of continuous long-term stimulation of rabbit muscle at 2.5 Hz and 10 Hz. In Carraro U (ed). *Muscle Driven Devices for Cardiac Assistance:* Commission of the European Communities, 1991.

# Chapter 22

# *Discussion*

**Sir Magdi Yacoub (London):** I have several questions. What is the relationship between these changes in function and changes in muscle, and can you monitor that? Why did you use continuous stimulation at these frequencies? Do you think, for example, that intermittent stimulation at 10 Hz would be equivalent to the lower frequencies? And finally, are these changes permanent? What do you think is the influence of the stimulation program, which will have to be used for generating pressure, on the transformation of the muscle?

**Dr. Jarvis:** We have not quantified the histochemistry yet, but basically the 10 Hz stimulated muscle is fully transformed to type 1. The 5 Hz muscles appear to be 80% and the most variability in fiber type is in the 5 Hz group.

**Sir Magdi Yacoub:** Have you used an intermittent program rather than a continuous?

**Dr. Jarvis:** No, not in a comparable way, not for long-term 10 months.

**Sir Magdi Yacoub:** What do you think is the influence of the stimulation program?

**Dr. Jarvis:** This is clearly an experimental study to see how much we can influence things but I think it might be fair to take from these data that the average frequency is important in the final transformation of the muscle. I think after 10 months, it is final.

**Sir Magdi Yacoub:** What we get, we have forever?

**Dr. Jarvis:** Yes, I think so. One point is that some of the 10 Hz stimulated muscles were showing some damage and the values for mass with the 10 Hz at 10 months were lower than the 10 Hz group of 3 months. So there is some progression.

**Dr. Carpentier:** I think there is a big difference between continuous and intermittent stimulation. However, I congratulate you; this is a very important study because it teaches us that perhaps we should not try to achieve full transformation, in contradistinction to what we thought in the past. But there is a real need for you, if you want to help us, to investigate a train of pulses, because in the past when we did some experiments in continuous stimulation, we developed fatigue, so we are looking for such a study.

**Dr. Jarvis:** My prediction is that if we use the same hertz frequency but in bursts, we will see the same final state but we will maintain mass of the muscle. If we use burst stimulation, we maintain mass of the muscle and that is a good thing because mass is directly related to power.

**Dr. Carpentier:** Yes, but when you are talking about burst stimulation, such as a 1:2 mode or 1:3 mode or 1:4 mode plus the number of impulses per burst, this can make a tremendous difference. So, a lot of variables must be explored.

**Dr. Salmons:** I would like to say that that is precisely why we used continuous frequency to start with. Because you have so many variables when you go into the burst mode. Having established that you can get a sort of dose-related response from the stimulation, now I agree with you it is our job to see what difference it makes when we group these pulses into bursts.

**Dr. Carpentier:** As far as the heart is concerned, it is an intermittent contraction, so we really need something intermittent.

**Dr. Jarvis:** We have a stimulator that we can use in rabbits to do that.

**Sir Magdi Yacoub:** In other clinical applications such as diaphragmatic stimulation, what conditioning program did you use?

**Dr. Letsou:** The pacemaker is placed, no stimulating for 2 weeks and then the conditioning begins at a low frequency of 9–10 Hz for 1 hour per day, and then slowly over 3–6 months, it is increased to full-time pacing.

**Sir Magdi Yacoub:** So when do you start stimulation of the muscle?

**Dr. Letsou:** At 2 weeks.

**Sir Magdi Yacoub:** You said for 1 hour?

**Dr. Letsou:** One hour per day.

**Sir Magdi Yacoub:** That is intermittent?

**Dr. Letsou:** One hour per 24 hours for the first week, then 2 hours per 24 hours the next week, etc.

**Sir Magdi Yacoub:** Do you think it has any role to play in acute phrenic nerve paralysis post surgery?

**Dr. Letsou:** No.

**Dr. Carpentier:** We are all confronted in surgery with phrenic nerve paralysis. So let's concentrate on chronic because you appropriately said it is not for acute situations. However, we have been somewhat disappointed in the past. Each time we asked the question of whether we could use diaphragmatic stimulation, the answer repeatedly was that it does not work. This has been tried in the past 10 years. So could you explain what is the difference between your own experience and the experience of other authors. Is it only the fact that you are conditioning and they are not?

**Dr. Letsou:** We are not the only group doing it. There is a group in Chicago that has been quite successful as well using this protocol. One of the limitations of the technique is the currently available pacing equipment that can be somewhat difficult to work with and unreliable. But our results have been confirmed by several other groups and we are not the only group working in this area, although perhaps we are the most active.

**Dr. Carpentier:** So you think the main contribution you brought was the conditioning?

**Dr. Letsou:** I think the main contribution of this work to skeletal muscle conditioning is that we feel that complete transformation of the muscle is important. That a conditioned state can be induced and maintained over many years and that fatigue is a frequent problem. We see fatigue very frequently. I think one of the important lessons that can be learned is that it was very important to us to have a reproducible measure of muscle function, which I believe may be somewhat less than optimal in LD stimulation and cardiomyoplasty. But there is no real way to tell how effectively you are stimulating a muscle.

**Dr. Moreira:** I think that one important point was the use of LDM electrodes for long-term stimulation. I think that we can obtain good stimulation with low amplitudes with this type of electrode. Therefore, it is a type of stimulation used for cardiomyoplasty as well. I would like to ask you if you had any problem regarding exit blocks over the long term or if you observed problems regarding muscle degeneration or nerve problems with this type of stimulus.

**Dr. Letsou:** In Dr. Glenn's experience in the 1960s, there was one incidence of nerve injury secondary to an electrode being wrapped entirely around the nerve, but other than that, we have not seen any problems with nerve damage or muscle damage.

**Dr. Salmons:** One point should be clarified: you don't learn anything about damage to the muscle by looking at a patient 10 years later. That is far too late. If you want to look for damage induced by stimulation, you have to look at a much earlier stage. There is some stimulation-induced damage and it depends on the regimen that you use.

**Sir Magdi Yacoub:** What is the earliest it can be used clinically? You told us 2 weeks or 1 hour, and in the meantime, are you conditioning?

**Dr. Letsou:** No. Those patients were candidates, the patients with chronic phrenic nerve problems and chronic ventilatory problems but an intact phrenic nerve.

**Dr. Pette:** You showed permanent signs of regeneration and small muscle fiber deterioration. This is also our experience. You see damage because the muscle fibers are not preprogrammed to twitch at such high frequencies, so some of them deteriorate and will be replaced by other muscle fibers. This is an ongoing process, even with very long stimulation periods.

**Sir Magdi Yacoub:** And what a useful thing to have. What is your recommendation? How can we induce the maximum amount of regeneration, for example?

**Dr. Pette:** As long as the muscle has the capacity to regenerate, there is no limit to how long it can go on.

**Dr. Salmons:** The disadvantage of that is that the regenerating cells have rather fast and fatigable characteristics, so I don't think we want to induce regeneration if we can help it. I think there are probably two forms of damage. There is early damage and there is ongoing damage. I think they are different mechanisms.

**Sir Magdi Yacoub:** The regeneration could be programmable again.

**Dr. Salmons:** I would not like to see regeneration, because regeneration means degeneration. It is the sequel of degeneration and I don't think we want to damage the muscle.

**Sir Magdi Yacoub:** You don't want to see degeneration without regeneration.

**Dr. Chachques:** You talk about transformation, but what is important about muscle transformation is to have at least fast twitch fibers at the beginning. So when you show a slide with almost 100% of type 1 fibers, it may be that patients have 80% or 90% of type 1 fibers to begin with. I don't know, but this is perhaps the case as it is for several other muscles where we found a lot of variation between patients.

**Dr. Letsou:** We have many diaphragmatic specimens of humans, and the normal distribution is 50% type 1 and 50% type 2.

**Dr. Chachques:** What kind of variation do you have between patients? It varies between 1 and what?

**Dr. Letsou:** No, there is no real variation; it is pretty standard: 50% type 1 and 50% type 2 in normal human diaphragms.

Chapter 23

# A New Stimulation System for Cardiomyoplasty

Pierre A. Grandjean, Robert Leinders

Dynamic cardiomyoplasty requires that the muscle grafted around the heart chambers contracts during the heart systolic phase. This can be achieved by a system that detects heart contractions and electrically stimulates the grafted muscle to evoke its contraction during the ventricular periods. The "progressive sequential stimulation protocol" necessary to train the muscle to its new task requires a programmable system.[1]

An implantable pulse generator, termed a "Cardio-Myostimulator" (Medtronic® Model SP1005/A), was developed to investigate the cardiomyoplasty procedure[2] and has been described earlier.[3] To date, it has been used in more than 350 cases worldwide. Based on the experience (cumulative experience: >500 years) carefully collected by many investigators in our clinical and experimental investigations with this first-generation system, we developed a new system, aiming at improving the clinical outcome, increasing time between replacements, and easing the implantation and handling during follow-up. The components of this improved system are described below.

## The New Transform™ Cardiomyostimulation System

Similarly to the first-generation system, the new Transform™ cardiomyostimulator (Medtronic Model 4710) is a programmable two-channel system that combines features found in cardiac pacing devices and in neuromuscular stimulators, i.e., output synchronized to sensed or paced cardiac activity and burst of impulses for skeletal muscle stimulation. It consists of a cardiac monitoring and pacing channel and a myostimulation channel, coordinated by a synchronization circuit (Fig. 1).

The heart monitor functions like a demand VVI pacemaker. It is composed of a sense amplifier that monitors the intrinsic heart rate and an output stage that paces the heart as soon as its rate drops below a programmed value (30–120 ppm). The sensing circuit reacts to the intrinsic deflection and slew

From Carpentier A, Chachques JC, Grandjean P: Cardiac Bioassist. © Futura Publishing Co, Inc, Armonk, NY, 1997.

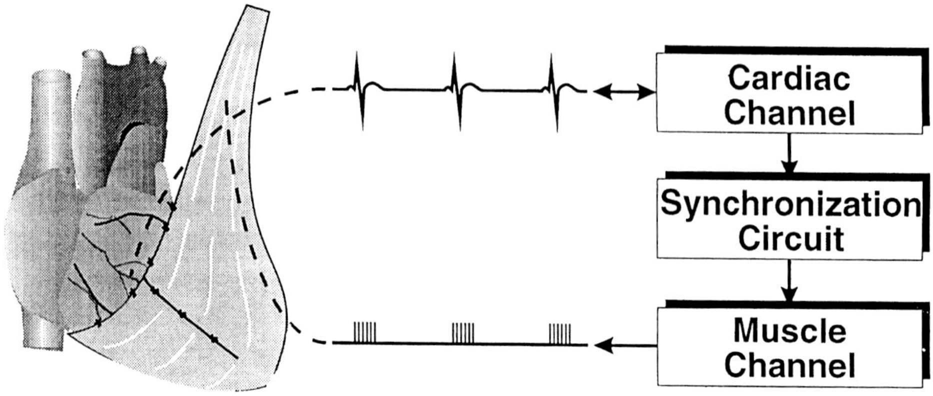


**Figure 1:** *Schematic function of the cardiomyostimulator. Muscle stimulation is activated during the heart systolic phase.*

rate of the ventricular signal collected by unipolar or bipolar myocardial or endocardial electrode(s). The sensitivity of detection is programmable (0.6–5 mV) to ensure reliable QRS detection even in depressed and dilated hearts. As in a demand pacemaker, a cardiac event can be sensed or initiated by the device in case of bradycardia. Basic rate hysteresis can also be selected (40–60 ppm). Polarity is programmable.

The cardiac signal also triggers a synchronization circuit. A delay is then initiated after which the myostimulator outputs a burst of impulses to the muscle via a pair of leads. This synchronization delay is programmable (8–352 ms) to allow for optimal timing of the muscle contractions, which depends on heart conduction velocity, cardiac electrode placement, and heart/muscle complex reaction time (Fig. 2).

To allow for muscle adaptation to its new task, prevent its overuse (e.g., minimize muscle fatigue), and optimize cardiac benefits, the synchronization circuit has some unique safety features (Fig. 3):

- it allows for eight different heart/muscle contraction ratios (from 1/1 to 1/8);
- it prevents muscle overstimulation by limiting the number of muscle contractions per minute (muscle upper rate [MUR] = 65–175 cpm);
- it inhibits muscle output when the R-R interval decreases below a programmable value (synchronization upper rate [SUR] = 105–245 ppm); and
- it also enables muscle synchronization on sensed cardiac events only or on sensed and paced cardiac events.

All of these features are programmable.

The myostimulator outputs balanced charge biphasic pulses. This type of pulse, while ensuring nerve fiber depolarization, prevents or minimizes the risk of neuromuscular tissue and electrode degradation by electrochemical processes. Programmable pulse amplitude (0.1–9 V), pulse width (15–504 μsec), pulse interval (8–242 ms), and number of pulses in a burst (1–14) are available. This high degree of flexibility in programming the myostimulator is necessary because of the way in which neuromuscular tissues react to electrical stimulation. Altering

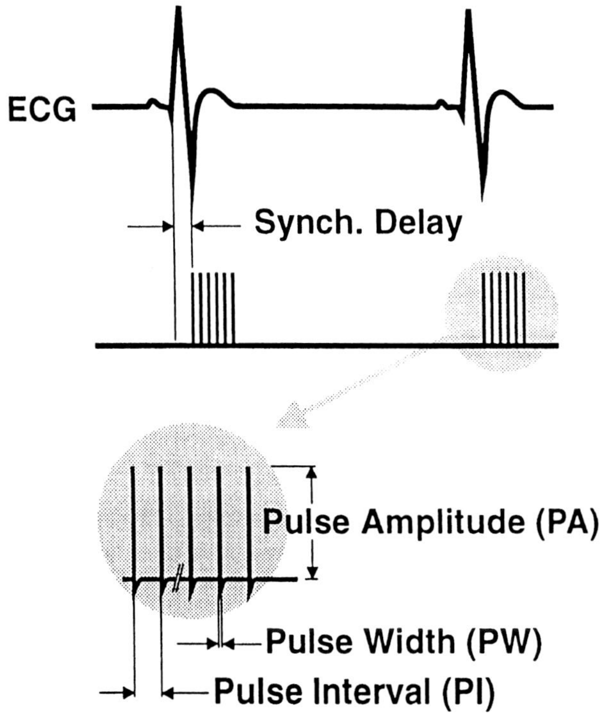


**Figure 2:** *Muscle burst synchronized on ventricular electromyogram. The different muscle stimulation parameters are independently programmable.*

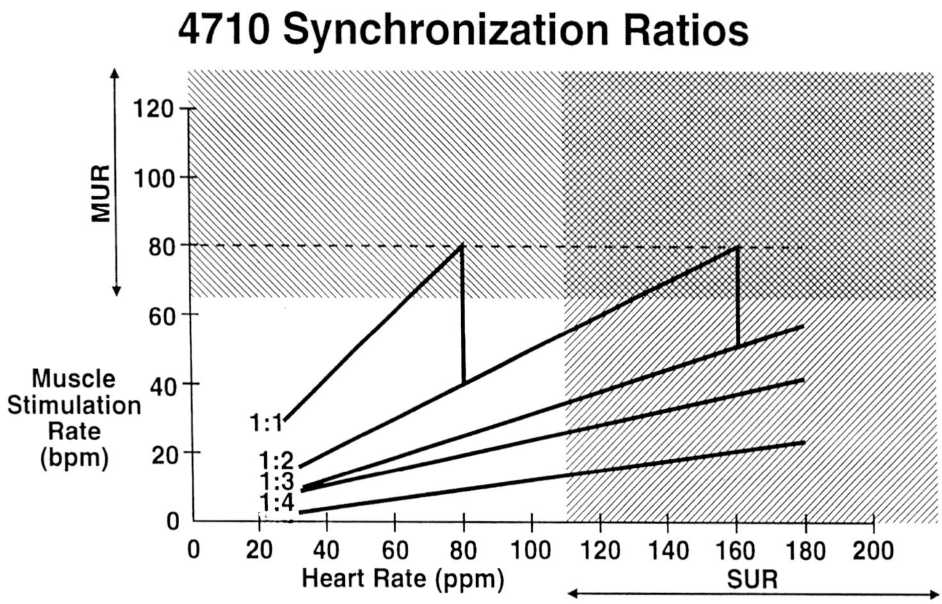


**Figure 3:** *Synchronization function of the cardiomyostimulator. The synchronization (SR) can be programmed from 1/1 to 1/8. SR also automatically increases when reaching the muscle upper rate (MUR) to prevent muscle overstimulation.*

the pulse amplitude or pulse width enables the gradation of the muscle force by varying the number of activated motor units (spatial recruitment). The pulse interval and the number of pulses grade the force by varying the rate of excitation of motor units (temporal summation). As the pulse interval decreases, the force increases to reach a plateau at which the muscle contraction is smooth (fused contraction). Adjusting burst duration by increasing the number of pulses in the burst enables the evoked muscle force to be sustained over a longer period of time. For safety (i.e., to avoid muscle contraction extending during the diastolic phase which could result in ventricular filling impairment), the burst duration can be programmed by adjusting the number of pulses and the pulse interval. Although this tuning may be adequate at a given heart rate (e.g., at rest), diastolic impairment could potentially happen when patients exercise: as the heart rate increases, the systolic contraction time decreases; the muscle contraction rate also increases, leaving less time for rest. This may result in decreased muscle relaxation velocity, which in turn may impede diastolic function. In an attempt to deal with these potential limitations, this new device allows for "fixed" or "adaptive" burst durations (Fig. 4). In the latter case, the burst duration decreases as the heart rate increases as a function of the previous R-R interval, while in the former case, the burst duration remains constant. This programmable feature (14–35% R-R interval) could potentially allow for improved patient exercise performance since the muscle could be allowed to contract at a higher rate without preventing adequate muscle blood perfusion.

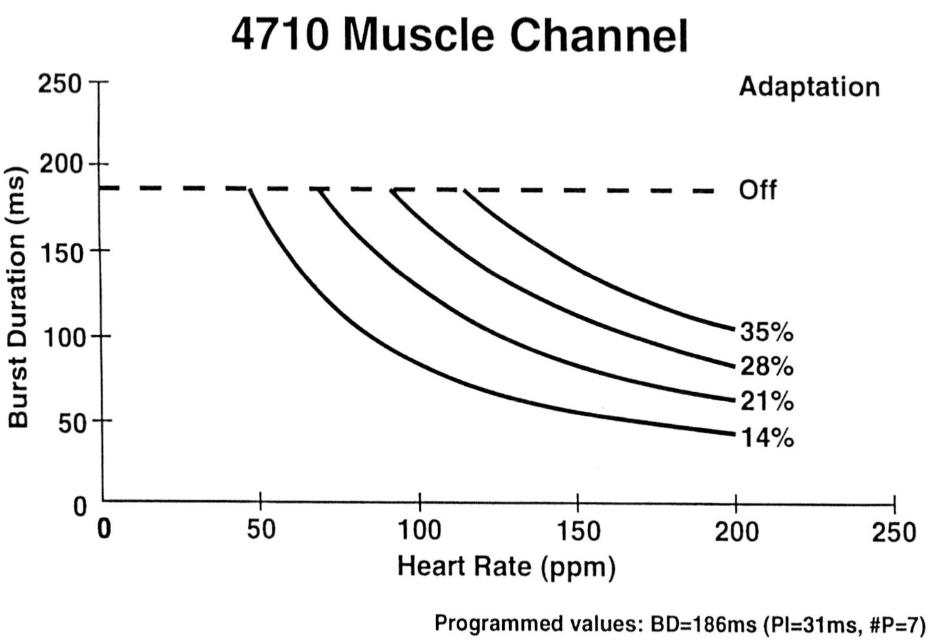


**Figure 4:** *Burst adaptation with heart rate. The muscle burst length can be programmed as being independent of heart rate (adaptation off) or to depend on heart rate (previous R-R interval). In the latter case, burst duration decreases as heart rate increases (four adaptation levels: 14–35% of previous R-R interval).*

The main characteristics of this new Transform™ system (Model 4710) are listed in Table 1 and are compared to the former device (Model SP1005/A).

Parameters are programmable using a standard Medtronic programmer, Model 9710, loaded with the appropriate software cartridge (Model 9756). This system also enables interrogation and monitoring of the pulse generator after implantation (e.g., parameter review, battery check-up, etc.).

A Marker Channel™ feature facilitates determination of times of events in the cardiac and muscle channel. Marker signals transmitted by the pulse generator and electromyogram signals (collected by implanted electrode) can also be printed by the programming system. Both channels of the pulse generator can be independently programmed. To allow for easy patient follow-up, the muscle channel of the pulse generator can also be inhibited by application of a magnet.

Powered by one lithium manganese dioxide battery, this new generation implantable system is enclosed in a small titanium case (Fig. 5). A lateral connector fitted with four ports allows for the connection of four independent unipolar or two bipolar leads without the use of adaptors. An additional safety feature prevents the possibility of misconnecting leads (i.e., connecting a cardiac lead to the muscle channel). This original pulse generator shape, proposed

**Table 1**
Pulse Generators for Cardiomyoplasty

| *Cardiac Channel* | *Model SP1005/A* | *Model 4710* |
|---|---|---|
| modes | VVI, VOO | VVI, VOO |
| P. Amplitude | 3.5 V | 0.9–7.8 V |
| polarity | unipolar | unipolar/bipolar |
| hysteresis | none | programmable |
| *Synchronization* | | |
| ratio | 1:1, 1:2 | 1:1–1:8 |
| upper rate | none | 105–245 ppm |
| delay | 4–250 ms | 8–352 ms |
| event | sense+pace | sense+pace, sense only |
| *Muscle Channel* | | |
| polarity | bipolar | unipolar/bipolar |
| burst length | 185 or 240 ms | programmable (# pulses) |
| adaptation | none | OFF, 14, 21, 28, 35% |
| upper rate | 105 or 55 bpm | 65–175 bpm |
| *Physical* | | |
| size | 62 × 73 × 19 mm | 40 × 67 × 10 mm |
| weight | 95 g | 60 g |
| volume | 75 cc | 32 cc |
| connector | standard | lateral |
| *General* | | |
| battery type | 2 $Li/SOCl_2$ | 1 $LiMnO_2$ |
| longevity | 2 yr (nominal) | 6 yr (nominal) |
| magnet mode | C+M inhibit | M inhibit only |

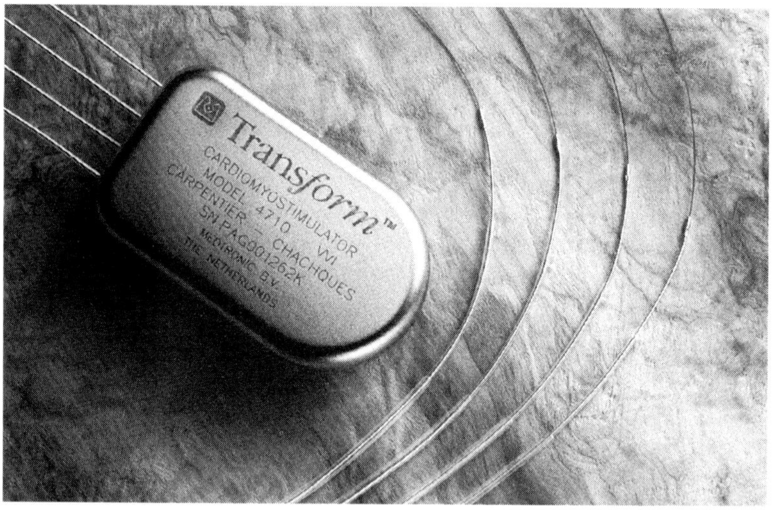


**Figure 5:** *The Transform™ cardiomyostimulator (Medtronic® Model 4710). The lateral connector is under the device.*

by Dr. Carpentier, is aimed at allowing easy implantation under the rectus abdominis muscle. Its small size also allows for placement in the pectoral region.

The lifetime of the device will depend on programmed parameters (pulse amplitude, width, number of pulses, synchronization ratio, electrode impedance) and heart rate., Despite its small size, at standard values, it is estimated that this pulse generator lifetime will exceed 6 years.

## The Muscle Stimulation Leads

The pulse train generator requires leads for cardiac sensing and pacing and leads for muscle stimulation. For cardiac sensing/pacing, epicardial leads or endocardial leads with IS-I connector can be used. At present, long-term muscle stimulation can be achieved only in muscle with preserved neurovascular supply and by depolarization of motor nerve fibers rather than by direct muscle fiber depolarization. Stimulation electrodes must fulfill the following criteria: safety with respect to neural tissues, electrochemical stability, mechanical integrity, reliability, ease of placement, and energy levels compatible with implantable energy sources.

Neuromuscular electrodes can be classified into three main categories, depending on their location: (1) intramuscular (placed in muscle tissues), (2) nerve (perineural, intraneural), and (3) epimysial (placed on muscle epimysium). Since the beginning of our clinical study, we elected to use the intramuscular approach because of its inherent safety towards neural tissues (the nerve main bundle is left undisturbed) while offering ease of placement, stability, reliability, and acceptable energy level.

Our clinical experience to date amounts to more than 700 intramuscular leads (Model SP5528) implanted, accumulating a total of 1,030 device years, the longest implant being 110 months. The performance of this lead has been excellent and no lead failures or breaks have been observed.

Based on these encouraging results, we only made slight modifications to the new leads proposed here. As for the SP5528, the new intramuscular lead (Model 4750, Fig. 6) has a flexible coil made of platinum-iridium alloy contained in a movable polyurethane sheath. The distal part of the electrode ends in the form of a tip that holds a nonabsorbable suture wire with a curved needle for lead insertion and stable positioning. Once the electrode is properly positioned, the insulation sheath is moved forward until its distal end reaches the muscle epimysium. It is then secured with suture and surgical clips.

The lead has been improved with respect to its predecessor to make electrode passage through the muscle tissues less traumatic and to ease insulation sheath sliding. It is also available in different lengths (35–70 cm).

The low profile lead connector is similar in design to the IS-I standard of cardiac leads, with the sealing rings on its body. However, the pin size differs in order to fit the muscle channel of the Model 4710 pulse generator. This feature prevents inadvertent connection of the cardiac lead to the muscle channel.

## Discussion

The new Transform™ cardiomyostimulation system has been successfully used in clinical trials, our experience consists of 300 devices implanted as of September 1996. The device's small size, convenient handling, and ease of pro-

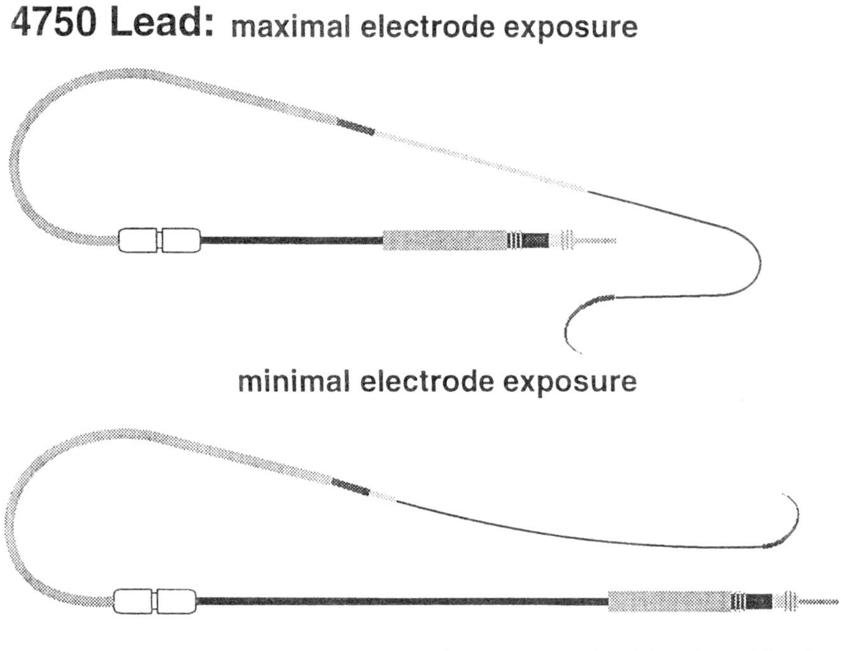


**Figure 6:** *Intramuscular leads (Medtronic® Model 4750) with adaptable electrode exposure.*

gramming have been appreciated by investigators. Its wide range of programming values is the focus of special studies. Of utmost interest will be the testing of new features such as the adaptive burst duration. New modes of muscle stimulation and muscle conditioning are also part of investigations at selected centers.

## References

1. Carpentier A, Chachques JC, Grandjean P: Transformation d'un muscle squelettique par stimulation séquentielle progressive en vue de son utilisation comme substitut myocardique. *CR Acad Sci Paris* 301:581, 1985.
2. Chachques JC, Carpentier A: Postoperative management. In Carpentier A, Chachques JC, Grandjean P (eds): *Cardiomyoplasty.* Mount Kisco, NY, Futura Publishing Co, 1991, pp 131–138.
3. Grandjean P, Chachques JC, Carpentier A: Implantable electronics and leads for muscular cardiac assistance. In RCJ Chiu (ed): *Biomechanical Cardiac Assist: Cardiomyoplasty and Muscle Powered Devices.* Mount Kisco, NY, Futura Publishing Co, 1986, p 103.
4. Grandjean PA: Electrical stimulation of skeletal muscles. In Carpentier A, Chachques JC, Grandjean P (eds): *Cardiomyoplasty.* Mount Kisco, NY, Futura Publishing, 1991, pp 39–62.

Chapter 23

# *Discussion*

**Dr. Curias (Caracas):** I have two questions. First, have you had any breaks of the leads and, if so, how can you diagnose it? Second, what are the parameters that you measure with your equipment?

**P. Grandjean:** A lead break is quite easily noticed by loss of muscle contraction and looking for a change on the ECG. We have performed impedance measurements and we have found that the impedance changed very little. It is a range of less than 3% if we compare the impedance after 2 years, for instance, when we replace the device.

**Unindentified:** What happens if you have a break of the lead in the middle of the muscle? Do you have half of the muscle contracting and the other half not contracting? How can you diagnose the difference?

**P. Grandjean:** We have not experienced such a type of failure.

From Carpentier A, Chachques JC, Grandjean P: Cardiac Bioassist. © Futura Publishing Co, Inc, Armonk, NY, 1997.

Chapter 24

# Electrophysiological Study after Dynamic Cardiomyoplasty

M. A. Radermecker, A. Waleffe, P. Grandjean, R. Limet*

## Introduction

Cardiomyoplasty is a new approach to compensate for cardiac failure and is derived from the concept of skeletal muscle powered cardiac assistance. The technique was introduced in 1985 by Carpentier and Chachques.[1] Since then, more than 300 procedures have been performed worldwide, with encouraging initial results and few reported side effects.[2] Although many fundamental problems remain to be worked out, this initial success and enthusiasm will probably be responsible for an increased role of cardiomyoplasty in the surgical treatment of terminal cardiac pump failure. Currently, few data are available regarding the effects of this procedure on the cardiac electrical activity since the question has never been specifically addressed in an experimental setting. The study was designed to provide preliminary data concerning the electrophysiological characteristics of the heart involved in cardiomyoplasty and the function of the cardiomyoplasty tested under stressful electrophysiological conditions.

## Methods and Material

Six healthy female adults goats (weight 39 ± 6 kg) were studied. The animals were managed following the regulations in the *Guide for the Care and Use of Laboratory Animals,* published by the U.S. Academy of Sciences. One week before surgery, the animals were anesthetized (xylazin, ketamine, halothane, and a mixture of air-$O_2$) for the preoperative electrophysiological study.

Surgery was performed under general anesthesia using a technique previously described.[3] Briefly, anesthesia was induced with xylazin and ketamine.

*With the cooperation of E. Gobin, J. Fourny, and H. Kulbertus.

From Carpentier A, Chachques JC, Grandjean P: Cardiac Bioassist. © Futura Publishing Co, Inc, Armonk, NY, 1997.

Animals were intubated with a cuffed endotracheal tube; anesthesia was maintained with air-$O_2$ and halothane using controlled mechanical ventilation (Servo). After shaving and skin preparation, the surgical field was draped. The left latissimus dorsi muscle was carefully dissected via an oblique left lateral thoracic incision, with particular attention to the neurovascular pedicle. After complete mobilization, stimulating electrodes (Medtronic® SP5528) were implanted and tested for adequate threshold. The proximal electrode (cathode) was inserted just distal (1 to 2 cm) to the division of the neurovascular pedicle. The anode was sewn transversally into the muscle thickness 3 to 5 cm away. The integrity of the neurovascular structure was preserved and incomplete recruitment of the muscular mass on stimulation was avoided. The flap was then transposed into the chest through a second intercostal space window. Thoracotomy in the fourth intercostal space was performed to allow access, after pericardiotomy, to the left side of the heart. An epicardial sensing lead was implanted. Clockwise posterior-anterior cardiomyoplasty was performed. Moderate stretch was applied to the muscle. The chest was closed in standard fashion.

The muscle was stimulated after a 15-day rest period following the Broussais protocol. Voltage was chosen (3 to 5 V) to elicit a palpable contraction in the axillary region. The stimulation protocol began with one pulse, with the addition of supplementary pulses every 15 days up to a maximum of six pulses.

At that point, burst stimulation (30 Hz/185 ms) was delivered at a basic 2:1 mode. All of the animals were alive for the final evaluation, 8 to 9 months later. Electrophysiological studies were performed under general anesthesia. A 9F quadripolar catheter electrode was introduced via the right internal jugular vein and was positioned within the heart under fluoroscopic guidance.

The protocol included the following measurements: basic cycle length (BCL), maximal sinus node recovery time (MSRT) (Fig. 1), effective refractory period of the AV node (AVERP) and the right atrium (RAERP) (Fig. 2), anterograde AV Wenckebach point (AAVWP) determination, and effective refractory period of the right ventricle (RVERP). In addition, one to three extrastimuli were applied to both the atrium and the ventricle during intrinsic

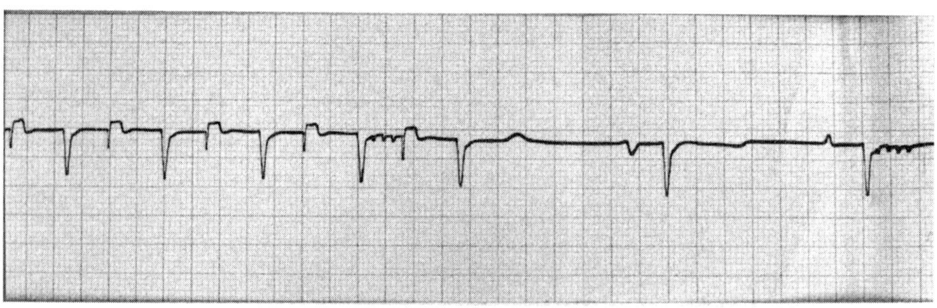

**Figure 1:** *Determination of the right atrial effective refractory period (RAERP) with the CMS ON. The right atrium is paced at 110 BPM, and an extrastimulus is introduced with progressive decrease of the coupling interval. In this case, the extrastimulus is not followed by a P wave indicating that RAERP is reached.*

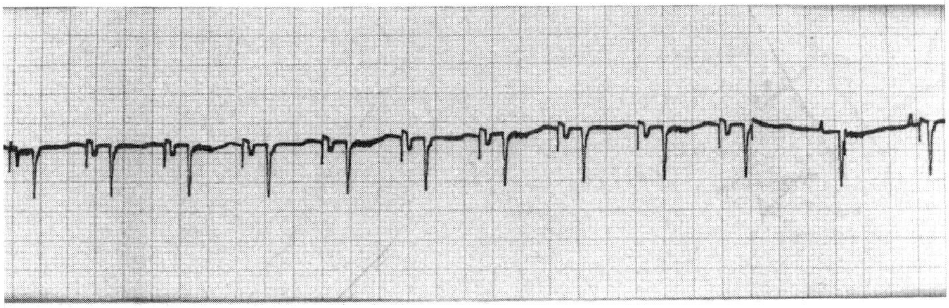

**Figure 2:** *Determination of the maximal sinus node recovery time. Drive at 165 BPM.*

and paced rhythms at increasing rates (Figs. 3a–d). Burst stimulation was applied in the ventricle at a decreasing cycle length until 2:1 capture phenomenon appeared (Figs. 4a,b). During the postoperative electrophysiological testing, the extrastimulation and the burst stimulation were obtained with the cardiomyostimulator off, then again after switching it on. The paired Student *t*-test was used for statistical analysis of the pre- and postoperative data. All data are expressed as mean ± standard deviation.

## Results

The comparison of preoperative and postoperative electrophysiological values (Table 1) did not show significant modifications. Postoperative electrophysiological values were similar when the cardiomyostimulator was on or off.

Pre- and postoperative electrophysiological study in goat 1 was normal. Electrophysiology testing demonstrated considerable electrical stability, even under stressful conditions.

In goat 2, the preoperative protocol was stopped during ventricular pacing. A nonsustained ventricular tachycardia (VT) episode following ventricular extrastimuli was induced. In the postoperative period, however, the study was almost normal: the goat was stable even with high-rate ventricular pacing leading to 2:1 ventricular capture and during electrophysiology testing done with the SP1005 on.

In goat 3, preoperative assessment induced atrial fibrillation requiring external shock on positioning of the electrode in the atrium. When entering the right ventricle, ventricular fibrillation (VF) requiring external shock was induced; VF was also provoked at the onset of ventricular stimulation. The protocol was discontinued. In the postoperative period, atrial fibrillation (AF) was provoked, but resolved spontaneously shortly thereafter. This arrhythmia was concomitant to atrial pacing at 230. Ventricular pacing up to 2:1 ventricular block and high-frequency ventricular pacing did not initiate arrhythmias.

In goat 4, during the preoperative study, a short run of an atrial arrhythmia was induced. In the postoperative period, one spontaneously reverting strip of atrial fibrillation was recorded at the end of an episode of junctional rhythm.

In goat 5, during the preoperative period, although the electrophysiology was almost normal, a spontaneously reverting AF was initiated at the end of the atrial program. In the postoperative period, we noticed a nonsustained VT

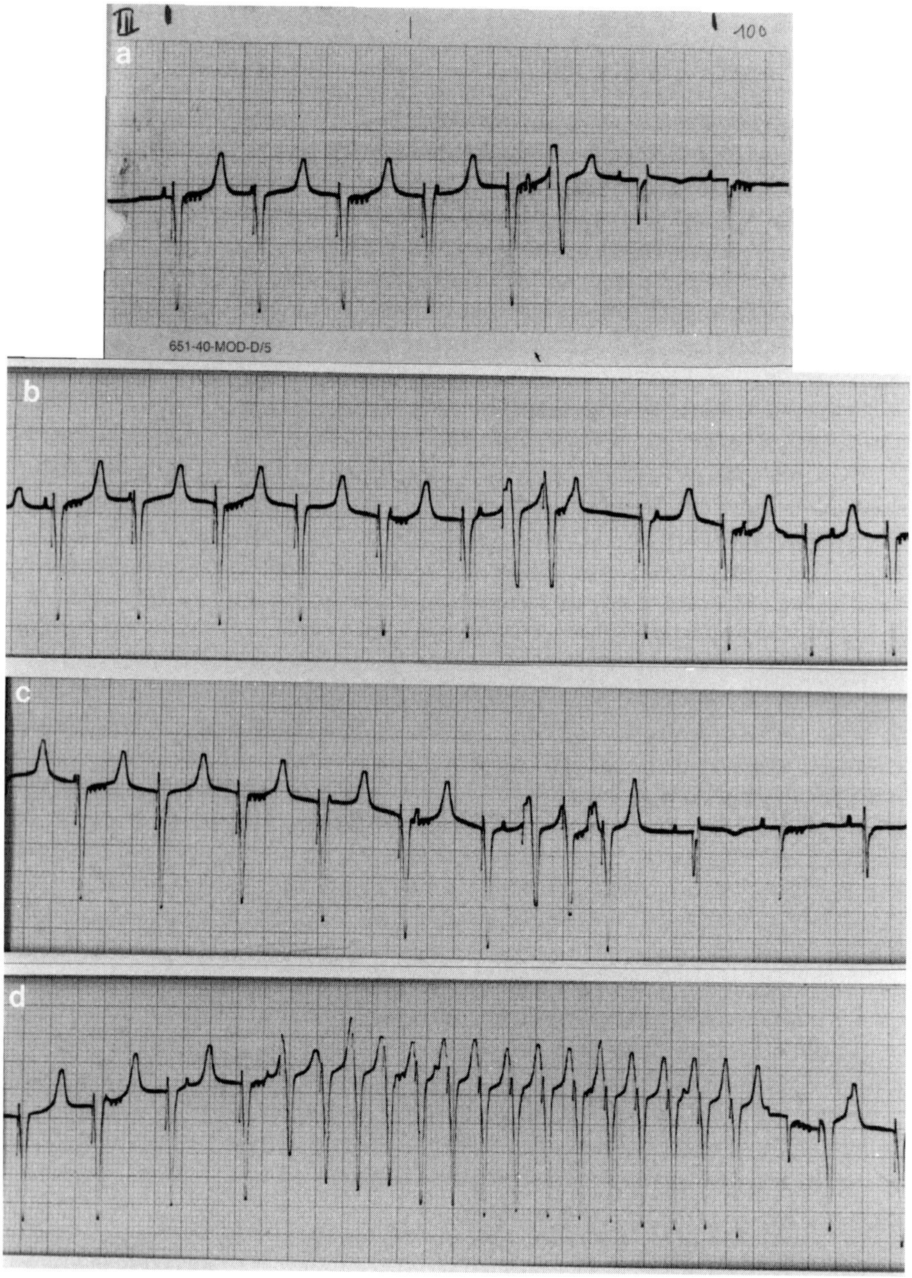


**Figure 3:** ***a–d.*** *Aggressive EP program: introduction of 1 to 3 extrastimuli at the ventricular level with changing drive and extrastimuli coupling. Figure d shows an example of burst pacing at 250 bpm.*

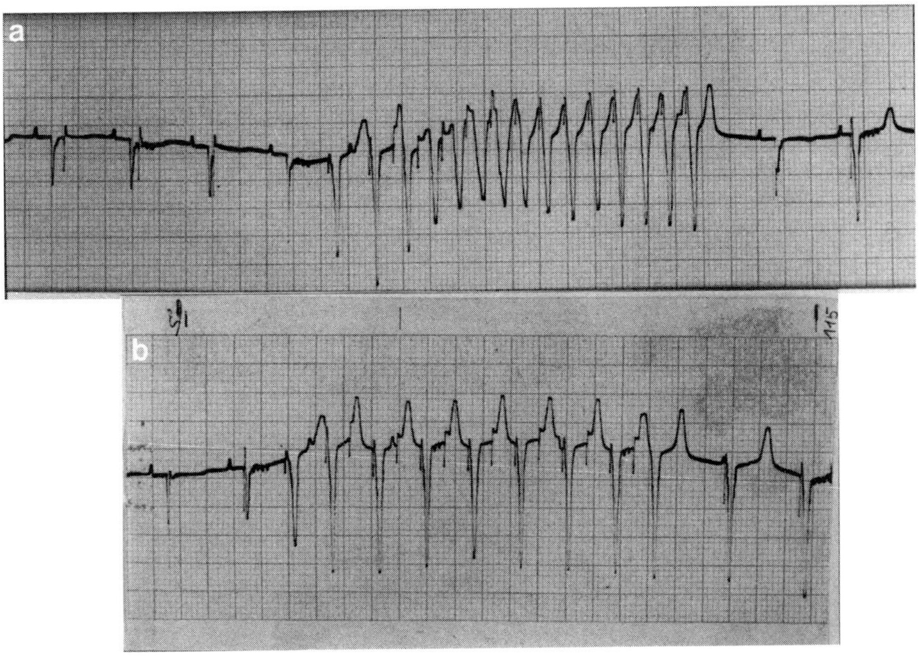


**Figure 4:** ***a,b.*** *In another experiment, burst pacing in the right ventricle at 330 bpm (**a**), increasing the burst frequency (375 bpm) leads to a 2 to 1 capture phenomenon (**b**). The CMS works on 4/1 algorithm.*

**Table 1**
Electrophysiological Data

| | | *G1* | *G2* | *G3* | *G4* | *G5* | *G6* | *M ± SD* | *Stat.* |
|---|---|---|---|---|---|---|---|---|---|
| BCL | before | 857 | 1000 | 857 | 800 | 832 | 769 | 852 ± 80 | p = 0.17 |
| | after | 800 | 909 | 811 | 750 | 682 | 857 | 802 ± 80 | |
| MSRT | before | 1240 | 960 | 1020 | 880 | 1040 | 1100 | 1040 ± 123 | p = 0.48 |
| | after | 1200 | 1000 | 780 | 940 | 940 | 1160 | 1003 ± 156 | |
| AAVWP | before | 170 | 170 | 200 | 190 | 180 | 170 | 180 ± 13 | p = 0.30 |
| | after | 170 | 130 | 230 | 180 | 150 | 150 | 168 ± 35 | |
| AVERP | before | 300 | 440 | 200 | 200 | 360 | 320 | 303 ± 93 | p = 0.18 |
| | after | 320 | 440 | 220 | 300 | 240 | 360 | 313 ± 81 | |
| RAERP | before | — | 240 | 260 | 200 | — | 220 | 230 ± 26 | p = 0.59 |
| | after | — | 240 | 260 | 300 | — | 260 | 250 ± 42 | |
| RVERP | before | 310 | 380 | 240 | 240 | 210 | 320 | 283 ± 62 | p = 0.26 |
| | after | 280 | 400 | 200 | 240 | 200 | 320 | 273 ± 77 | |

See text for abbreviations.

(three complexes) on ventricular positioning of the electrode. During anterograde programmed stimulation, an episode of AF was started and spontaneously resolved by external electric shock. The ventricular stimulation was done with the pace off until burst pacing at a high rate with good stability. During the ventricular refractory period measurement with the pace on, an episode of VF occurred that was resistant to external electrical shock.

In goat 6, preoperative electrophysiology was normal. Postoperative screening did not provoke arrhythmias even under stressful ventricular pacing.

## Summary and Discussion

The occurrence of arrhythmias after cardiomyoplasty remains poorly documented. Although Carpentier and Chachques, who first provided evidence of the feasibility of the technique both in animals and in humans,[1,4] reported no adverse arrhythmic events, the issue has never been systematically addressed in an experimental setting. Available information can only be derived from clinical experience. In a recent retrospective study involving 33 patients surviving the postoperative period (1 month) after cardiomyoplasty and followed from 3 months to 6 1/2 years (mean, 21 months), Chachques et al. showed only one patient dying as a result of a fatal arrhythmia.[5] Due to the mean preoperative NYHA functional class (III–IV) and the known risk of arrhythmic cardiac sudden death, a procedure-related improvement was suspected. Incidentally, this single death out of 33 patients occurred in a young man with advanced valvular heart disease who (objectively) benefited from the procedure with a MUGA scan and echographic evidence of improved cardiac function.[6] Moreira also reported a series of 11 patients receiving cardiomyoplasty in which six showed nonsustained ventricular tachycardia on preoperative Holter recording. The tachycardia subsided in four out of six patients within 6 months after surgery and without antiarrhythmic therapy.[7] In a nonrandomized study, these authors noted an incidence of 0 and 4 fatal arrhythmias, respectively, in 14 operated patients and 17 control patients who were maintained on medical treatment.[8]

Clinical reports from different countries[9,10] have reported several sudden deaths, probably resulting from arrhythmias. These different data collected from the recent literature must be interpreted cautiously and understood in the context of the subgroup of patients concerned, the efficacy of the method, and the current technical approach of this new modality of cardiac assistance. Undoubtedly, a high prevalence of arrhythmia and cardiac sudden death is expected in functional Class III or IV prior to surgery in patients who suffered from ischemic heart disease sometimes associated with aneurysmal dyskinesia or who had a dilated cardiomyopathy.[11] Furthermore, the technique may promote several mechanisms of arrhythmias, in the early postoperative period when only partial assistance is available (conditioning period). On the other hand, an improvement of cardiac performance due to efficient assistance with better matching of myocardial oxygen demand and supply at the fiber level could be associated with regression of frequency of arrhythmia, as reported by Chachques and Moreira.

Cardiomyoplasty itself, besides the immediate consequences of surgery, creates an unusual condition characterized mainly by a close apposition of a paced muscle flap and the diseased heart. It is recognized that a fibrous tissue layer develops at the muscle-epicardium interface, and that the implantation of the sensing electrode and the suture of the latissimus dorsi muscle to the heart may produce a fibrous myocardial scar. All of these sites may promote arrhythmias by creating a substrate for reentry. The effects of mechanical stress in the genesis of arrhythmias is well-recognized by surgeons and should not be underestimated. Once the latissimus dorsi flap has healed around the heart, the force heterogeneity of latissimus dorsi segments and their different situation on the length-tension curve may possibly create nonhomogeneous squeezing of the heart and mechanical stress along the myocardial wall, possibly responsible for arrhythmias. Finally, the use of a cardiomyostimulator and the stimulating electrodes may create an environment enhancing electrical instability. Although the intramuscular stimulating electrodes must be sewed into the muscle body and are situated above the ventricular surface (in the proximal third of the flap that is located in the left thoracic cavity), they may provoke adverse current leak into the underlying myocardium. It was noticed using the SP1005 in bench testing that some cross-talk between the muscle channel and the cardiac pacemaker may occur when the muscle is paced at unusual high amplitude. This cross-talk was due to an electric current flowing during muscle stimulation from the muscle electrode through the body tissues and picked up by the cardiac electrode. This cross-talk current was found to be less than 2.5 mA (0.2 ms pulse width) in routine conditions. With a synchronous burst of 240 ms duration, this current was found to be far below the threshold required for cardiac capture.[12]

Our prospective approach to these questions using a goat model investigated before and after realization of cardiomyoplasty included the use of techniques, materials, and stimulation parameters routinely used in humans. The end-point of the study was to reproduce, before and after surgery, an electrophysiological study of the heart involved in cardiomyoplasty. The potential arrhythmias facilitated by the use of the SP1005 cardiomyostimulator and SP5528 electrodes were specifically addressed. Our data indicate that in this model, the electrophysiological values were not modified by cardiomyoplasty. Endocardial pacing after surgery did not result in increasing the inducibility of arrhythmias and the only fatal VF started with the pacemaker on does not appear to have been specifically initiated by the preceding burst. The aggressivity of our stimulating program was illustrated by the ventricular burst pacing and the frequent achievement of a 2:1 capture at the ventricular level (Figs. 4a,b). The outstanding electrical stability speaks against an arrhythmogenic effect of this procedure via a triggered automaticity mechanism.

In conclusion, the data derived from this experimental model provide evidence that cardiomyoplasty, per se, despite the extensive modifications it induces in the cardiac environment, has little influence on the normal heart electrical stability investigated under stressful electrophysiological conditions. The safety of the SP1005 and associated stimulation devices is also suggested.

## References


1. Carpentier A, Chachques JC: Myocardial substitution with stimulated skeletal muscle: First successful clinical case. *Lancet* 1:1267, 1985.
2. Grandjean PA, Austin L, Chan S, Terpstra B, et al: Dynamic cardiomyoplasty: Clinical follow-up results. *J Cardiac Surg* 6:80–88, 1991.
3. Radermecker MA, Fourny J, Bonnet P, Philippart C, et al: Surgical technique for dynamic cardiomyoplasty and iterative transthoracic biopsies in an experimental goat model. *Eur Surg Res* 25:110–122, 1993.

4. Chachques JC, Grandjean P, Schwartz K, Milhaileanu S, et al: Effect of latissimus dorsi dynamic cardiomyoplasty on ventricular function. *Circulation* 78(Suppl 3):203–216, 1988.
5. Chachques JC, Acar C, Portoghese M, Bensasson D, et al: Dynamic cardiomyoplasty for long-term cardiac assist. *Eur J Cardiothorac Surg* 6:642–648, 1992.
6. Hagege AA, Desnos M, Guerot C, Chachques JC, et al: Dynamic cardiomyoplasty: Long-term clinical results and pathologic study. *Circulation* 80(Suppl 2):670, 1989.
7. Moreira LP, Stolf NAG, Bocchi EA, Barretto AP, et al: Latissimus dorsi cardiomyoplasty in the treatment of patients with dilated cardiomyopathy. *Circulation* 84:257–263, 1991.
8. Moreira LFP, Seferian P, Bocchi EA, Pego Fernandes PM, et al: Surgical improvement with dynamic cardiomyoplasty in patients with dilated cardiomyopathy. *Circulation* 84(Suppl 3):296–302, 1991.
9. Magovern GJ, Christlieb IY, Kao RL: The Alleghany Hospital Experience. In Carpentier A, Chachques JC, Grandjean PA (eds): *Cardiomyoplasty*. Mount Kisco, NY, Futura Publishing Company, 1991, pp 159–170.
10. Odim JNK, Burgess JH, Williams BH, Blundell PE, et al: Pathophysiology of dynamic cardiomyoplasty: A clinico-pathological study. *J Cardiac Surg* 4(5):336–346, 1990.
11. Defibrillation Study Group: Actuarial risk of sudden death while awaiting cardiac transplantation in patients with atherosclerotic heart disease. *Am J Cardiol* 68:545–546, 1991.
12. Grandjean PA, Herpers L, Smits K, Bourgeois IM: Performance of the Cardio-Myostimulator™ and intramuscular leads in the cardiomyoplasty procedure. In Chiu RCJ, Bourgeois IM (eds): *Transformed Muscle for Cardiac Assist and Repair*. Mount Kisco, NY, Futura Publishing Co, 1990, pp 231–240.

Chapter 24

# Discussion

**Dr. Lorusso:** Is your model comparable to the dilated heart in humans? We have been trying to investigate this aspect with our electrophysiological cardiologists, but they tell us that there is no means to predict, prior to surgery, the advent of ventricular fibrillation or ventricular tachycardia in dilated hearts. I don't know whether a goat would be the right model to study this because it has a normal heart instead of a dilated heart.

**Dr. Radermecker:** This model has a normal heart and the correlation with clinical practice must be cautious. We just wanted to see in a normal goat having a cardiomyoplasty procedure the electrophysiological properties of the heart.

**Dr. Lorusso:** Why didn't you try to induce heart failure in goats? We tried inducing heart failure by pacing asynchronously. We had major fibrillation induction. So I do think that heart failure, even in animals, should tell us something more.

**Dr. Radermecker:** We will try to investigate a chronic model of heart failure in animals although it will not be easy to attain that model.

Chapter 25

# Effect of Stimulation Rate on the Blood Flow and Bioenergetics of the Conditioned Latissimus Dorsi Muscle

Kendra K. Gealow, Jianyi Zhang, Eric E. Solien, Richard W. Bianco, Sara J. Shumway

## Introduction

The biochemical adaptation of skeletal muscle in response to electrical stimulation enabling it to perform continuous work is now well documented.[1,2] The sustainable work rate that transformed skeletal muscle is capable of maintaining is not well defined, however. Decreases in muscle performance after several months of stimulation[3] and degenerative changes in muscle morphology have been reported.[4] Stimulation protocols must be optimized so that maximum muscle power is available for cardiac assist but muscle function and long-term viability are not compromised. The sustainable work rate of muscle is determined by its oxidative capacity and the rate of oxygen delivery to the muscle. Our objective was to determine the metabolic response of the transformed muscle to increases in stimulation rate and the effect of stimulation rate on the blood supply to the muscle. In a skeletal muscle ventricle (SMV) model, we measured blood flow to the muscle and used phosphorous nuclear magnetic resonance spectroscopy ($^{31}$P-NMR) to measure the response of high-energy phosphate metabolism to increasing stimulation demands.

From Carpentier A, Chachques JC, Grandjean P: Cardiac Bioassist. © Futura Publishing Co, Inc, Armonk, NY, 1997.

# Methods

## Surgical Model and Training Protocol

SMVs were constructed from the left latissimus dorsi (LD) muscle in dogs ($n = 3$) in accordance with the *Guide for the Care and Use of Laboratory Animals* (NIH Publication No. 85-23, revised 1985). The SMV was configured to work against an implantable mock circulation system (IMC) as described previously.[5] Briefly, the LD is wrapped two times around a 50-cc silicone bladder to form the SMV. The bladder is connected to a compliance chamber by silicone tubing. The system is filled with saline through an access port that also facilitates monitoring of SMV pressure generation. A 4-cm section of the second rib was removed so that the SMV could be positioned subcutaneously but would not protrude from the rib cage. This placement prevents the severe atrophy of the subcutaneous SMV wall due to skin pressure that occurs when the SMV is positioned outside the thorax. The IMC compliance chamber was placed within the chest to prevent additional loading of the SMV due to external pressure on the chamber.

A nerve cuff electrode (Medtronic,® Inc., Minneapolis, MN) was placed on the thoracodorsal nerve for LD stimulation. An implantable 2-mm ultrasonic flow probe (Transonic Systems, Inc., Ithaca, NY) was placed around the thoracodorsal artery to measure LD blood flow. Epicardial electrodes (Medtronic, Inc.) were placed on the left ventricle and connected to the cardiac sensing channel of an implantable, synchronizing pulse train generator (Prometheus™, Medtronic, Inc.). All lines were externalized and the pulse train generator was placed in the pocket of a protective jacket worn by the dogs. The device was externalized because the incompatibility of the pulse train generator with the electromagnetic fields during NMR studies required removal of the device prior to placing the animal within the magnet.

The LD muscle was trained according to the clinical training protocol. A 2-week healing delay was followed by 2 weeks of single pulse stimulation at a rate of 1:1 with the heart. From weeks 4 to 6, two pulses were applied at a rate of 2:1. The number of pulses was increased to three during weeks 6 through 8. For the remaining weeks of the study, the SMV was stimulated at a rate of 2:1 with a 35% contraction duration. Stimulation voltage was set by increasing the voltage just until maximum pressure generation was observed, typically 1–2 volts. Pulse width was 210 μsec and pulse train frequency was 33 Hz. The preload pressure within the IMC was maintained at 20 mm Hg. This low preload does not significantly impair blood flow to the SMV[5] but induces a resting tension that is needed to prevent severe muscle atrophy.[6]

## Study Protocol

$^{31}$P-NMR was performed at 2 weeks following surgery, prior to any training, and again at 6, 10, 14, and 20 weeks. Anesthesia was induced with sodium thiopental and maintained during the study by continuous infusion of sodium methohexital (0.2%). The skin over the area of the SMV was shaved, and a 28-mm diameter surface coil used for radiofrequency transmission and signal detection was sewn directly over the SMV. The animal was then centered in a 40-cm bore, 4.7-tesla magnet interfaced with a CSI console (General Electric). Measurements were conducted at 81 MHz.

An external pulse train generator (SP3080, Medtronic, Inc.) placed away from the magnetic field was connected to the externalized nerve cuff lead using long lead extensions. Stimulation was not synchronized with the heart. Synchronization delay was found to have no significant effect on SMV blood flow or pressure generation in previous studies.[7] To eliminate signal noise due to motion, data acquisition and respiration were gated to the muscle stimulation signal so that spectra were obtained during the muscle relaxation phase. Spectra were obtained during stimulation rates of 40/minute and 80/minute during the 2, 6, 10, and 14-week studies and during rates of 20, 40, 80, 100, and 140 during the 20-week study. The stimulation duration was kept constant at 250 ms. For each stimulation rate, resting spectra were obtained for 5 minutes, and then stimulation was turned on. Acquisition continued through 15 minutes of stimulator. The stimulation was then turned off and additional spectra were acquired during the first 5 minutes of the recovery phase.

At the time of sacrifice, two biopsy specimens were taken from the SMV in the area that would be directly under the surface coil. Control biopsies were taken from the right LD muscle. Biopsies were quickly snap-frozen in methyl butane, cooled in liquid nitrogen, and kept frozen at −70°C. Samples were assayed for total adenosine nucleotide content.

## Data Analysis

The area under the spectral peaks corresponding to inorganic phosphate (Pi), creatine phosphate (CP), and adenosine triphosphate (ATP) were determined by integration. The Pi/CP ratio is used as an indicator of the overall bioenergetic state of the muscle. Pi/CP can be shown to be proportional to adenosine diphosphate (ADP), which is thought to be a regulator of mitochondrial respiration.[8] As ATP is broken down for the transduction of chemical energy into mechanical energy, ADP and Pi are produced. The ATP pool is quickly replenished under nonfatiguing working conditions by the reaction of CP and ADP producing ATP and creatine (Cr). Therefore, the intensities of the ATP peaks remain essentially constant under normal working conditions while the Pi peak increases and CP decreases. Using the ratio of Pi/CP eliminates effects of changes in the signal-to-noise ratio and allows week-to-week comparisons of the muscle's bioenergetic state to be made.

The chemical shift between the Pi and CP peaks was used to calculate pH according to the following equation[9]:

$$\text{pH} = 6.75 + \log\{(\Delta - 3.35)/(5.60 - \Delta)\} \quad [1]$$

where Δ equals the chemical shift between the Pi and CP peaks in parts per million (ppm).

Stroke work, power, and the tension-time index are all useful measures of the performance of the SMV. Stroke work (SW) for the SMV can be calculated from the measurement of the IMC pressure during SMV contraction. Knowing the compliance characteristic of the IMC system, the measured peak pressure is used to estimate stroke volume (SV). SW can then be calculated from:

$$SW = \Delta P \times SV \qquad [2]$$

where $\Delta P$ is the peak pressure minus the resting preload pressure. SMV power output is the product of the SW and the stimulation rate. The tension-time index (TTI) is commonly used as an indicator of myocardial oxygen consumption.[10] For the SMV, TTI is the product of the contraction duration and the mean pressure during contraction.

## Statistical Analysis

Statistical significance of mean differences were analyzed by ANOVA for changes over weeks and for changes with rate during the 20-week study. Paired *t*-tests were performed on weekly data to measure differences between resting and stimulated values.

## Results

The changes in peak intensities occurred within 2 minutes of the onset of stimulation. Each spectra is acquired in approximately 2 minutes, therefore, changes in peak intensities had already occurred by the time the first spectra was acquired after the onset of stimulation. Recovery of resting levels also occurred within one spectral acquisition after stimulation was turned off. The level of Pi/CP varied slightly during the stimulation period but not significantly. The average Pi/CP ratio at rest and during 40/minute and 80/minute stimulation for weeks 2, 6, and 10 are shown in Table 1. At 10 weeks, Pi/CP during stimulation was significantly less than during the 2-week study ($p = 0.03$). Pi/CP did not change significantly during the remaining weeks of the study.

During sustainable, nonfatiguing work, a graded increase in work is expected to cause a graded increase in the Pi/CP ratio.[11] When Pi/CP is plotted as a function of work, a linear relationship exists over the sustainable work range. A change in the slope of this relationship would indicate a change in the oxidative capacity. The variation in the slope of the line defined by the work rates of

**Table 1**
Changes in Pi/CP with Training*

| *Stimulation Rate* | *Pi/CP* 2-Week | *Pi/CP* 6-Week | *Pi/CP* 10-Week |
|---|---|---|---|
| Resting | 0.23 ± 0.08 | 0.20 ± 0.03 | 0.18 ± 0.01 |
| 40/Minute | 0.50 ± 0.26 | 0.36 ± 0.05 | 0.24 ± 0.05 |
| 80/Minute | 0.81 ± 0.42 | 0.52 ± 0.03 | 0.29 ± 0.02 |

*Pi/CP increases during stimulation, however, this increase becomes smaller with training (6-week and 10-week results).

40/minute and 80/minute over the time course of the study is shown in Figure 1. A decrease in the slope of the line indicates a smaller change in Pi/CP when the stimulation rate was increased from 40 to 80/minute. A change in this direction suggests an improvement in the aerobic capacity of the muscle. The slope of Pi/CP versus work rate decreases during the first 4 weeks of training and decreases significantly after 8 weeks of training ($p = 0.03$). No further improvement is seen.

The average resting pH was $7.2 \pm 0.04$ during the 2-week study. It decreased to $7.1 \pm 0.07$ during stimulation, but this decrease was not significant. There was no difference in the pH change during 40/minute stimulation and during 80/minute stimulation. The pH during rest and during stimulation did not change significantly over the course of the study. During the 20-week study, the pH change during all stimulation rates was similar, even at 140/minute, and was not significant.

Pi/CP is shown versus stimulation rate during the 20-week study in Figure 2. For stimulation rates up to 80/minute, the increase in Pi/CP is linear with increasing work rate. Above 80/minute, Pi/CP no longer increases with work rate. The thoracodorsal blood flow (TDBF) at each of the same stimulation rates is shown in Figure 3. TDBF also increases with stimulation rate up to a rate of 80/minute. At rates above 80/minute, TDBF decreases with increasing stimulation rate.

The peak pressure generated by the SMV was highest during 20/minute and 40/minute stimulation. Above the rate of 40/minute, the peak pressure generated by the muscle decreased with increasing stimulation rate. Stroke work performed at 80/minute decreased to 80% ± 20% of the stroke work at 20

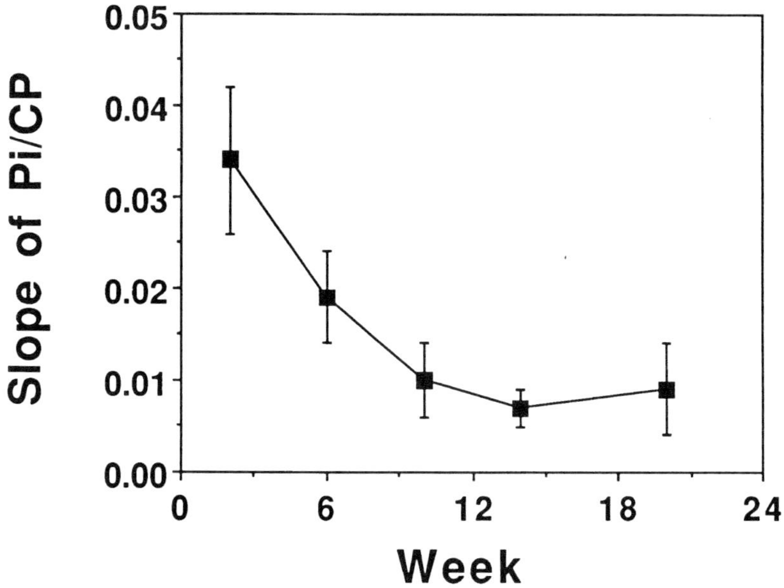


**Figure 1:** *Slope of the Pi/CP and stimulation rate relationship over the course of the study in weeks. Slope values were obtained by plotting Pi/CP versus stimulation rate for the rates of 40 and 80/minute during each study. The decrease in slope indicates an improvement in aerobic capacity.*

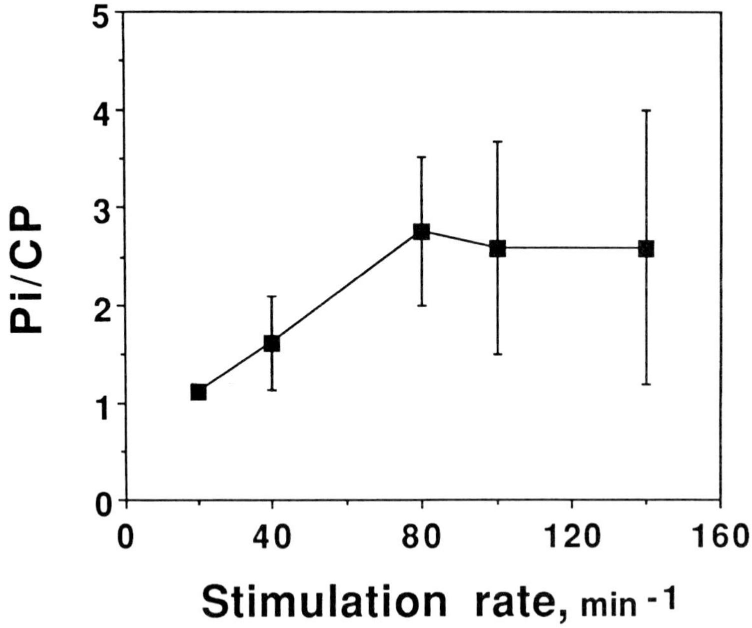


**Figure 2:** *Pi/CP versus stimulation rate during the 20-week study. Up to 80/minute, Pi/CP increases in proportion with stimulation rate. Above this rate, a sudden change in slope occurs. Pi/CP was normalized by the value at 20/minute for each study.*

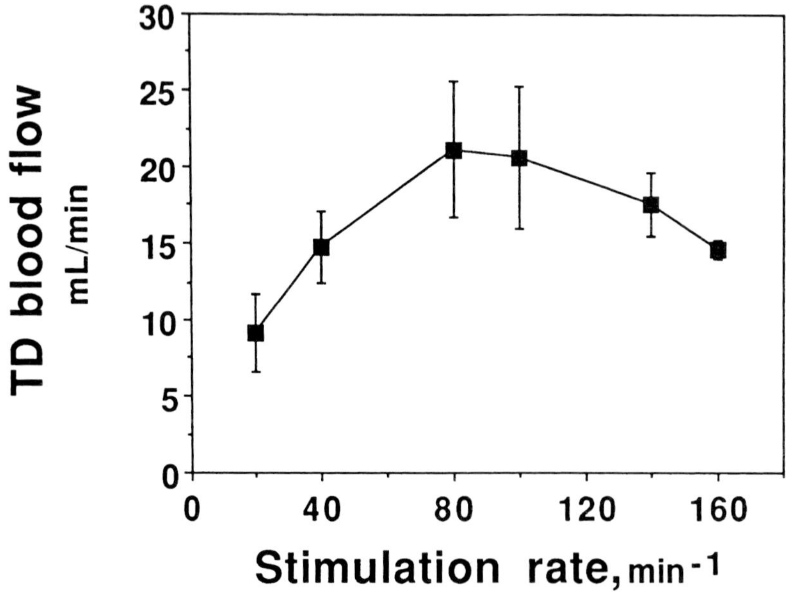


**Figure 3:** *TDBF versus stimulation rate measured at 20 weeks. TDBF is impaired at rates above 80/minute.*

or 40/minute. At 100/minute, the stroke work decreased to 54% ± 19% and at 140/minute to 29% ± 19%.

The ratio of TDBF to TTI represents the ratio of oxygen supply to demand. This ratio is plotted as a function of stimulation rate in Figure 4a. TDBF/TTI increased linearly with stimulation rate. TTI alone does not take into account the

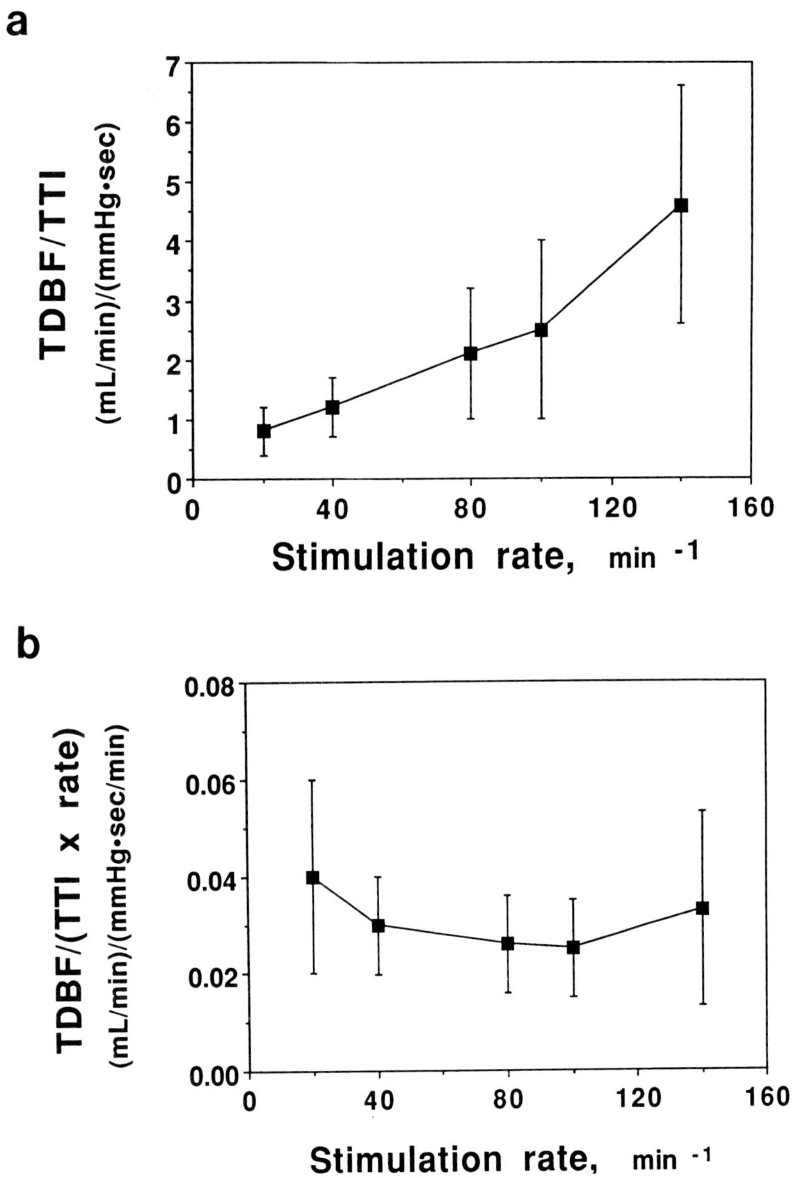


**Figure 4:** ***a:*** *The ratio of TDBF/TTI increases with increasing stimulation rate, indicating that the SW is negatively adjusted to compensate for the lower TDBF at higher rates.* ***b:*** *TDBF/(TTI/rate) decreases with increasing stimulation rate. The supply/demand ratio is maintained.*

rate of contraction, however. The calculated SMV power increased with rates up to 80/minute and decreased above rates of 80/minute. The ratio of TDBF to the product of TTI and rate versus stimulation rate is shown in Figure 4b. The supply-demand ratio is maintained at all rates. The product of TTI and rate versus Pi/CP is shown in Figure 5. TTI/min increases linearly with Pi/CP but undergoes a sudden change in slope when Pi/CP reaches approximately 0.5.

## Histochemical Results

Adenosine nucleotide assay results of biopsies revealed a significantly reduced level of ATP and total adenosine nucleotide (TAN) content in the SMV

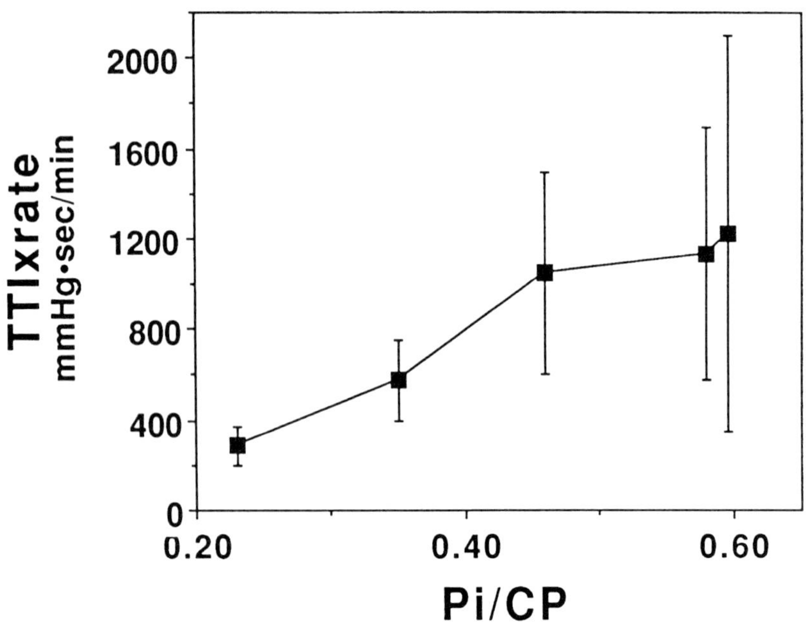


**Figure 5:** *TTI/minute increases linearly with Pi/CP at low work rates. However, a certain maximum is reached at which no further increase in work rate occurs even though Pi/CP continues to increase.*

**Table 2**
ATP, CP, and Total Adenosine Nucleotide (TAN) Content from Biopsy Results Taken from the SMV after 20 Weeks of Stimulation and the Right, Nonstimulated LD*

| | *ATP* | *CP* | *TAN* |
|---|---|---|---|
| Right LD | 4.3 ± 0.2 | 13.9 ± 1.0 | 6.0 ± 0.4 |
| SMV (p<0.001) | 1.9 ± 0.3 | 7.2 ± 1.0 | 3.2 ± 0.4 |

*Values are in nmol/mg wet weight ± standard error.

compared to the right, nonstimulated LD (Table 2). Additional biopsies were taken near the original ATP biopsy site for morphological analysis. These samples were fixed in formalin, embedded in paraffin, and hematoxylin-eosin stained. Increased interfascicular connective tissue was noted, but the change in morphology was not great enough to account for the significant differences in the TAN content in the stimulated and control muscles.

## Discussion

An improvement in the capacity for energy production is apparent after 4 weeks of training but was not significant until after 8 weeks of training. This change corresponds to the reported transformation of myosin type.[12,13] The improvement in the slope of the line defined by Pi/CP versus stimulation rate is in agreement with the positive effect of exercise training on the relationship of work rate and Pi/CP reported by Chance and colleagues.[8] No further improvement occurred with continued chronic stimulation. However, during the first 8 weeks of stimulation, the stimulation to the muscle is progressively increased. From 8 weeks on, the stimulation was held at the same level. Perhaps further progression in the stimulation demand would force further improvements in the oxidative capacity.

Increased acidity is expected at high work loads as anerobic, glycolytic metabolism is activated. However, in slow-twitch muscle, slight increases in pH occur, which are assumed to be the result of hydrogen uptake during the net hydrolysis of CP to Cr and Pi and the absence of lactate production.[14] In our studies, no significant differences in pH were found. This agrees with the finding by Clark et al. of no difference in pH during stimulation of trained and untrained muscle.[15] They suggest this result reflects a lack of pure fast-twitch fibers in dogs.

To determine the limits of the metabolic performance of the muscle trained under this protocol, stimulation rates up to 140/minute were tested. In increasing the rate, the simulation duration was kept constant shortening the relaxation time between contractions. This is the manner in which the SP1005 cardiomyostimulator (Medtronic, Inc.) functions. Because the stimulation duration is fixed and not adaptive, increases in heart rate result in shorter relaxation durations. Up to rates of 80/minute, the TDBF, power output, and Pi/CP all increase linearly with stimulation rate. Above 80/minute, TDBF and power decrease. During a muscle contraction, SMV blood flow is greatly reduced, sometimes to zero.[3] The cyclically contracting muscle is perfused during its resting phase. As stimulation rate increases, the relaxation time and therefore the perfusion time of the muscle becomes shorter. Our results indicated that above the rate of 80/minute, autoregulation mechanisms are unable to further increase muscle blood flow because of the inadequate perfusion time. Compromised oxygen delivery will cause a decrease in the slope of the work rate and Pi/CP relationship.[10] At the rate that blood flow becomes compromised, a sudden change in slope is observed.

The stroke work and TTI of the SMV are the same at 20/minute and 40/minute but decrease when the stimulation rate is increased to 80/minute or greater. This reduction in stroke work is probably a compensatory mechanism acting to maintain adequate ATP levels at higher stimulation rates by reducing stroke work. At the rate of 80/minute, stroke work is reduced, but at this rate power output still increases. Above the rate of 80/minute, stroke work decreases further in trying to compensate for the increased demand, and power output is actually reduced in spite of the higher rate. Both blood flow and power increase with rate up to 80/minute and decrease above 80/minute. The supply/demand ratio, therefore, is maintained at all rates. TTI/minute as an indicator of metabolic demand takes into account both stroke work and the rate at which the work is performed. As work rate increases, Pi/CP increases. A maximum work rate is reached, however, and no further increases in work rate occur even though Pi/CP increases further. This result indicates that above this maximum, the metabolic coupling to work becomes inefficient. This inefficiency, however, is likely to be due primarily to the decrease in blood flow and incomplete relaxation at high stimulation rates rather than a limit of the oxidative capacity of the muscle.

In the study by Clark et al., $^{31}$P-NMR spectra of conditioned and nonconditioned LD was performed during isometric contractions of the in situ muscle. The contractions were at a fixed rate of 54/minute but the on time during the duty cycle was incrementally increased from 200 ms to 800 ms. This range of contraction durations corresponds to a range of relaxation durations of 900 ms to 300 ms. They show that the slope of TTI/minute versus Pi/CP in the control muscle is much lower than the slope of this curve for the conditioned muscle. Their training protocol was 25 Hz pulse trains applied at a rate of 54/minute for 8 weeks. The slope of TTI/minute versus Pi/CP in the conditioned muscle was very steep and showed no sudden change in slope as found in our study. Their results suggest that even at the most demanding duty cycle, the muscle was still functioning within its aerobic range and muscle conditioning had resulted in greatly enhanced aerobic capacity.

An important difference in stimulation protocols may explain this difference in findings. In our studies, the stimulation demand was increased by increasing the stimulation rate but the contraction duration was kept constant. This situation is more similar to how the muscle is currently stimulated for cardiac assist. As heart rate increases, muscle stimulation rate increases, and with a fixed duration, relaxation time is reduced.

Following a contraction, mitochondrial activity will be repaying the developed ATP debt. If the oxidative phosphorylation rate of the mitochondria is such that the metabolic state is returned to its resting level prior to the next contraction, the work rate will be sustainable.[10] The mitochondrial rate is dependent on oxygen delivery. When the stimulation rate is increased, both the time until the next contraction and the oxygen delivery become compromised. Under these working conditions, an upper limit of the sustainable work rate was found. The upper rate is dictated in this case by the oxygen delivery to the muscle. In the practical application of skeletal muscle for cardiac assist, therefore, the effect of the stimulation protocol on muscle perfusion will determine what the maximum stimulation demand can be, not its oxidative capacity. The oxidative capacity of the muscle as shown by Clark et al. does not appear to be the limiting factor.

Another difference in the work performed by the muscle in these two studies is that the contractions were isotonic in the present study and isometric in the study by Clark et al.[15] Bridges et al. also studied the LD in an SMV configuration using $^{31}$P-NMR.[16] This study was performed acutely on untrained muscle. Their results show that the total energy consumption required during isotonic contractions is greater than during isometric contractions because there is a greater energy cost of doing external work. Therefore, the energy costs of performing stroke work in our study would be more demanding than the energy costs of the isometric contractions in the Clark study. Because the energy cost of shortening is greater than the energy cost of maintaining force, skeletal muscle functions more economically during low contraction rates of long duration than high rates of short duration.[17] Because the stimulation rate was kept constant in the Clark study and only the duration of the contraction was increased, the increase in energy cost was really only that of sustaining a tetanic contraction. Increasing the rate of stimulation would have a greater effect on the increase in energy costs. If blood flow were enhanced such that it does not become the limiting factor, a maximum work rate may still exist when the muscle is performing external work.

The reduced levels of high-energy phosphates by biopsy analysis after several weeks of training has also been reported by others.[18,19] Because ATP and CP decreased in the same proportions, the initiation and time course of this decrease was not apparent from the $^{31}$P-NMR spectra. It is unclear whether this decrease is a steady decline of high-energy phosphates that will eventually lead to cell death or if the decrease has reached a plateau at which the muscle is still capable of sustaining normal function. Henriksson et al. found ATP decreased 30% during the first week of stimulation but it remained at this level after 8 additional weeks of stimulation.[17] This study was performed with the muscle in situ, and training consisted of continuous 2 Hz stimulation. Since the stimulation protocol is progressively increased and external work is performed by tetanic contraction in our study, it is not safe to assume that the ATP levels have reached a constant but reduced level. Further work is needed to document the time course of this change and determine whether it poses a threat to chronic muscle viability.

The important finding of this study is that perfusion becomes the limiting factor in determining the sustainable work rate of the LD muscle when stimulated for cardiac assist. However, as a cautionary note, even if perfusion were enhanced, an upper work rate limit may exist when the muscle is performing external work. This upper rate would also depend on whether high rates of short duration contractions or low rates of long duration contractions are used. In terms of power output, there is no advantage in stimulating the muscle above rates of 80/minute because the reduced SW at high rates results in lower power. Furthermore, compromised blood flow may threaten muscle viability.

## References

1. Pette D: Effects of chronic electrostimulation on muscle gene expression. *Sem Thorac Cardiovasc Surg* 3:101, 1991.
2. Salmons S, Henriksson J: The adaptive response of skeletal muscle to increased use. *Muscle Nerve* 4:94, 1981.
3. Anderson DR, Pochettino A, Hammond RL, et al: Autogenously lined skeletal muscle ventricles in circulation: Up to nine months experience. *J Thorac Cardiovasc Surg* 101:661, 1991.

4. Lucas C, Kloosterman E, van der Veen F, et al: Long-term follow-up after dynamic cardiomyoplasty in goats. In Lucas CMHB: The use of the latissimus dorsi muscle for cardiac assist (thesis). Maastricht, Netherlands, Datawyse, University of Maastricht, p 99.
5. Gealow KK, Solien EE, Lang GR, et al: Blood flow to the latissimus dorsi muscle pouch during chronic counterpulsation stimulation. *J Heart Lung Transplant* 11:S306, 1992.
6. Goldspink DF, Easton J, Winterburn SK, et al: The role of passive stretch and repetitive electrical stimulation in preventing skeletal muscle atrophy while reprogramming gene expression to improve fatigue resistance. *J Cardiac Surg* 6:218, 1991.
7. Gealow K: Blood flow, bioenergetics, and mechanical function of the latissimus dorsi muscle when chronically stimulated for cardiac assist (Ph.D. thesis). University of Minnesota, Minneapolis, 1993.
8. Chance B, Leigh JS, Kent G, et al: Metabolic control principles and $^{31}$P-NMR. *FASEB* 45:2915, 1986.
9. Sapega A, Sokolow D, Graham TJ, et al: Phosphorus nuclear magnetic resonance: a non-invasive technique for the study of muscle bioenergetics during exercise. *Med Sci Sports Exerc* 19:410, 1987.
10. Buckberg GD, Fixler DE, Archie JP, et al: Experimental subendocardial ischemia in dogs with normal coronary arteries. *Circ Res* 30:67, 1972.
11. Chance B, Eleff S, Leigh JS, et al: Mitochondrial regulation of phosphocreatine/inorganic phosphate ratios in exercising human muscle. *Proc Nat Acad Sci USA* 78:6714, 1981.
12. Acker MA, Anderson WA, Hammond RL, et al: Oxygen consumption of chronically stimulated skeletal muscle. *J Cardiovasc Surg* 94:702, 1987.
13. Pette D, Mueller W, Leisher E, et al: Time-dependent effects on contractile properties, fiber population, myosin light chains and enzymes of energy metabolism in intermittently and continuously stimulated fast-twitch muscles of the rabbit. *Pflügers Arch* 364:103, 1976.
14. Kushmerick MJ: Energetic studies of muscle of different types. *Basic Res Cardiol* 82(Suppl 2):17, 1987.
15. Clark BJ, Acker MA, McCully K, et al: In vivo P-NMR spectroscopy of chronically stimulated canine skeletal muscle. *Am J Physiol* 254(*Cell Physiol* 23):C258, 1988.
16. Bridges CR, Clark BJ, Hammond RL, et al: Skeletal muscle bioenergetics during frequency-dependent fatigue. *Am J Physiol* 260(*Cell Physiol* 29):C643, 1991.
17. Faulkner JA, Brooks SV: Skeletal muscle fatigue: Implication for circulatory assist pumps. *Sem Thorac Cardiovasc Surg* 3:149, 1991.
18. Henriksson F, Salmons S, Chi MM-Y, et al: Chronic stimulation of mammalian muscle: Changes in metabolite concentrations in individual fibers. *Am J Physiol* 255(*Cell Physiol* 24):C543, 1988.
19. Glatz JFC, Havenith MG, van der Veen FH, et al: Disparity of metabolic and histochemical adaptation following chronic electrical stimulation of canine latissimus dorsi muscle. In: Chiu RC-J (ed): *Transformed Muscle for Cardiac Assist and Repair.* Armonk, NY, Futura Publishing Co, 1990, p 139.

## Chapter 25

# *Discussion*

**Dr. Pette:** Do you think that this 8-week time period fits with the transformation of the myosin level, the fast to slow transition?

**Dr. Gealow:** This time period is basically pretty close to the time period that is reported for the time course of the accepted process. It is interesting to note that for this stimulation protocol, up to the 8 weeks of training, the stimulation was progressively increased and we saw an improvement in the aerobic capacity over that time point.

**Dr. Chachques:** I would like some clarification. When you went to the higher heart rates, did you have any tetany?

**Dr. Gealow:** At the very highest stimulation rate of 140 per minute, the relaxation was incomplete.

**Dr. Chiu:** Is it just the rate, rather than the ratio between the duration of contraction and relaxation? What I mean is, that even if you have the same rate, if your burst duration is short, you probably affect the rate, do you think that was the case? The relaxation period is the issue. You change your burst duration. It might affect the acceptable rate you are talking about.

**Dr. Gealow:** Definitely, it will. In some preliminary studies, I showed that reducing the duration of contraction by 50% has the same effect on high energy phosphate metabolism as reducing the stimulation rate by 50%. So, some balancing of the parameters can be done to try to optimize the stimulation protocols.

Addendum to Chapter 25

# Blood Flow and Bioenergetics of the Electrostimulated Latissimus Dorsi:

## An Update

Kendra K. Gealow, Eric E. Solien,
Richard W. Bianco, Pierre A. Grandjean,
Sara J. Shumway

### Introduction

Since the completion of the previously reported study in Chapter 25, we have continued our investigations in examining the effect of stimulation rate on the blood flow and contractile performance of the trained latissimus dorsi (LD) muscle. In the previous chapter, we reported that an upper rate limit of approximately 80 contractions per minute exists when the pulse train consists of six pulses delivered at 33 Hz. This upper rate limit is expected to be dependent on the duration of the pulse train. Here we summarize more recent studies in which the LD muscle blood flow and contractile response to shorter pulse trains were examined.

### Experimental Methods

Following a 12-week training period, thoracodorsal blood flow (TDBF), contractile force (F), and shortening ($\Delta L$) of the in situ LD of five mongrel dogs were recorded continuously during 60 seconds of stimulation. Stimulation was delivered in 33 Hz trains of two to six pulses at rates randomly varied between 20 to 160 pulse trains per minute. A resting period of 5 minutes was allowed between each stimulation episode to prevent prolonged fatigue.

From Carpentier A, Chachques JC, Grandjean P: Cardiac Bioassist. © Futura Publishing Co, Inc, Armonk, NY, 1997.

## Results

TDBF increased with rate over the entire range tested for pulse trains of two and three pulses ($p$ = 0.03, Fig. 1). TDBF increased with rates up to 120 pulse trains per minute (ptpm) during four and five pulse bursts ($p$ = 0.01 and $p$<0.001, respectively), and decreased at rates above 100 ptpm when six pulses were used.

The stroke work (SW) performed during each contraction was calculated from the measured shortening and force. For rates less than 100 ptpm, SW increased with pulse number ($p$=0.01) ranging from 0.016 ± 0.004 joules during two pulse bursts to 0.122 ± 0.036 joules for six pulse bursts (Fig. 2). When the pulse train rate exceeded 100 per minute, the highest SW on the average occurred when five pulses were used. This SW, however, was reduced compared to the SW performed during five pulse bursts at rates less than 100. The maximum rate at which SW was maintained without evidence of fatigue was 80 ptpm for six pulses, 100 ptpm for five pulses, 120 for four pulses, and greater than 160 ptpm for two and three pulses.

## Discussion

For a given pulse train duration, an upper rate limit exists above which the LD muscle is incapable of sustaining a constant work rate and TDBF declines.

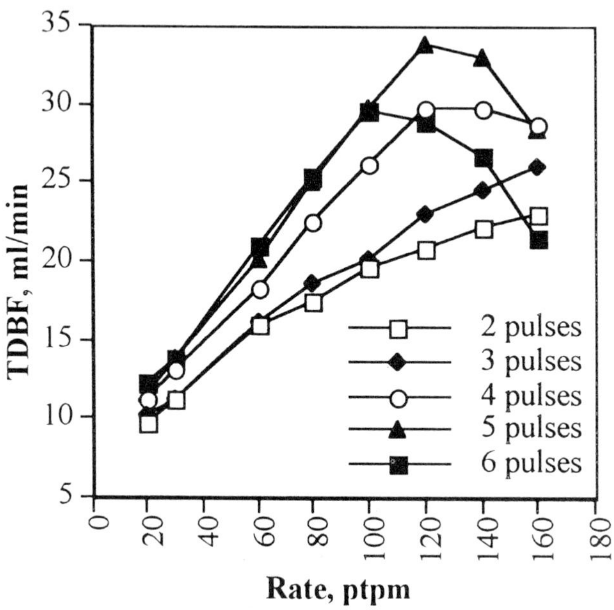


**Figure 1:** *TDBF is shown at each stimulation rate for pulse trains of two, three, four, five, and six pulses. TDBF increases significantly with increasing rate for two and three pulses (p = 0.03). An upper rate limit exists for four, five, and six pulses, above which TDBF decreases.*

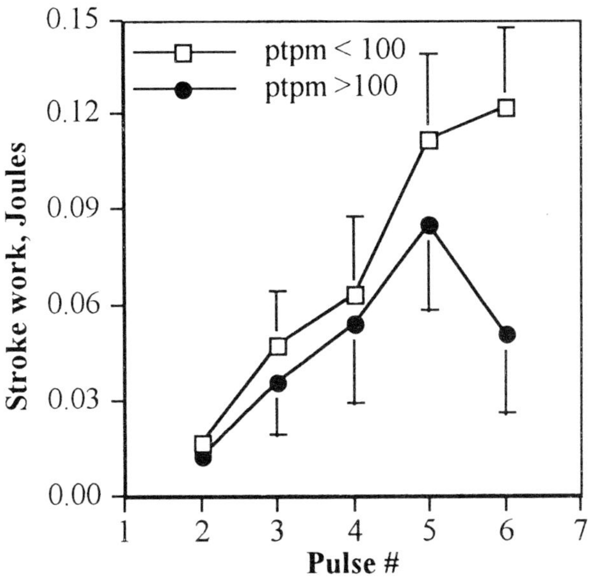


**Figure 2:** *Stroke work (SW) increases with pulse number at rates of less than 100 ptpm* (p = *0.01). At these lower rates, no fatigue occurs and the greatest SW is accomplished with the longest train of six pulses. When the rate exceeds 100 ptpm, the SW decreases during six pulse bursts due to fatigue.*

For very short pulse trains, two or three pulses delivered at a frequency of 33 Hz, the upper rate limit is greater than the maximum rate of 160 ptpm tested in this configuration. As the pulse number increases, the upper rate limit decreases.

In terms of blood flow, an upper rate limit of 80 ptpm was reported in Chapter 25 when the LD muscle was configured into a skeletal muscle ventricle and stimulated with six pulse bursts. This limit is lower than the limit found in the present study, suggesting that the upper rate limit will also depend on loading conditions. In the current study, the LD muscle worked only against an afterload starting from its normal resting length. When the muscle is preloaded, as in our previous study, increased resting tension will cause a higher resistance to blood flow. The increase in TDBF in response to stimulation has been found to be less at high preloads than at low preloads.[1] Therefore, the maximum sustainable work rate of the LD muscle may be further limited by an increase in resting tension.

Our previous results support the recommendation of a 1:2 synchronization ratio when a six-pulse, 33-Hz burst is used. Stimulation at 1:1 when a patient's resting heart rate is approximately 80 bpm can result in prolonged stimulation of the LD muscle above its sustainable working capacity. This may be the cause of muscle compromise observed experimentally[2] and more recently in patients stimulated at 1:1.[3] Stimulation that exceeds the sustainable working rate is likely to lead to chronic injury of muscle cells due to inadequate blood flow or metabolic insufficiency. Knowing the working limitations of the trained LD muscle is important in maximizing the cardiac benefit provided by cardiomyoplasty. Long-term benefit can only be maximized if chronic muscle injury is avoided.

Using a shorter pulse train duration or adaptive duration[4] makes 1:1 stimulation feasible. The LD muscle is able to sustain a higher contraction rate when the contraction duration is shorter. LD stimulation with every cardiac cycle may increase the benefit of cardiomyoplasty, particularly during increased physical activity. A clear understanding of the effects of stimulation mode on LD contractile function and blood flow will allow stimulation parameters to be selected that maximize the dynamic contribution of cardiomyoplasty without compromising muscle function.

## References

1. Gealow K, Solien E, Lang G, et al: Blood flow to the latissimus dorsi muscle pouch during chronic counterpulsation stimulation. *J Heart Lung Transplant* 11: S306–S314, 1992.
2. Lucas C, Kloosterman E, van der Veen F, et al: Long-term follow-up after dynamic cardiomyoplasty. *JACC* 22:758–767, 1993.
3. Kalil-Filho R, et al: Magnetic resonance imaging evaluation of chronic changes in latissimus dorsi cardiomyoplasty. *Circulation* 90(II):102–106, 1994.
4. Gealow K, Solien E, Bianco, R: Importance of adaptive stimulation of the latissimus dorsi muscle in cardiomyoplasty. *ASAIO J* 40:M253–259, 1994.

Chapter 26

# Latissimus Dorsi Structure and Function Following Cardiomyoplasty

John M. Kratz, Wendy S. Johnson, Rupak Mukherjee, Francis G. Spinale*

## Introduction

Dynamic cardiomyoplasty has recently been suggested to be an effective method for the surgical treatment of patients suffering from end-stage heart failure.[1–4] Dynamic cardiomyoplasty is a surgical procedure in which the latissimus dorsi (LD) muscle is wrapped around the heart, providing an endogenous source of force production.[1–7] Using special electrical pacing techniques, the LD muscle is trained with the conversion of fast-twitch fibers to fatigue-resistant slow-twitch fibers.[5–9] Dynamic cardiac assistance is then provided by pacing the LD muscle in synchrony with the intrinsic contractions of the ventricle.[1–6] Dynamic cardiomyoplasty is a potentially attractive treatment for end-stage heart failure in that it overcomes the problems inherent with cardiac transplantation such as the dwindling donor pool and immunosuppression requirements. A large number of patients have been surgically treated using dynamic cardiomyoplasty worldwide and have demonstrated improvements in clinical symptoms of heart failure.[1–4] However, the long-term consequences of chronic electrical stimulation of the LD muscle during dynamic cardiomyoplasty remain unclear. In order for cardiomyoplasty to be considered as a viable therapy for treatment of patients with end-stage heart failure, changes in structure and function of the LD muscle following cardiomyoplasty must be clearly understood. Thus, the overall goal of this project was to determine the specific changes in structure and function that occur within the LD muscle following dynamic cardiomyoplasty.

*With the cooperation of Jie Hu, and Fred A. Crawford.

From Carpentier A, Chachques JC, Grandjean P: Cardiac Bioassist. © Futura Publishing Co, Inc, Armonk, NY, 1997.

## Methods

### Cardiomyoplasty Procedure

Six Yorkshire swine (20–30 kg) were anesthetized using isoflurane (3%/1.5 L/min) and nitrous oxide (0.5 L/minute), and ventilated at a flow rate of 22 mL/kg/min. The animals were placed in left lateral recumbency and the left LD muscle was exposed through an incision performed along the short axis of the muscle. The muscle was dissected free from all insertions and the humeral tendon was cut. Great care was taken to preserve the thoracodorsal neurovascular pedicle. A platinum nerve cuff stimulating electrode (Medtronic Inc., Minneapolis, MN) was positioned around the origin of the thoracodorsal nerve and sutured in place. Next, a thoracotomy was performed at the fourth intercostal space and a window was created by resection of the lateral part of the third rib. The mobilized LD muscle was introduced through this window and positioned within the chest. Careful inspection was performed at this time to ensure that there was no compression and no deformities of the thoracodorsal neurovascular pedicle or nerve stimulating electrode. The pericardium was excised widely and the muscle was wrapped around the circumference of the heart. The LD muscle was carefully positioned to be parallel with the short axis of the left ventricle and sutured to the epicardial surface of the myocardium. A shielded electrode was sutured on the epicardial surface of the left ventricle for sensing ventricular depolarization.[10] The nerve stimulating electrode and the sensing electrode were connected to a myostimulator unit (SP1005, Medtronic Inc.). The thoracotomy was then closed, and the pleural space evacuated of air. The animal was then allowed to recover for 14 days before beginning the stimulation protocol.

Following recovery from the surgical procedure, the muscle was stimulated with incremental increases in pulse duration and frequency which have been well described previously.[1–7,11] The final stimulation settings for this project were a pulse amplitude of 1.5 volts, a pulse duration of 210 ms, and a frequency burst of 185 ms. The muscle underwent chronic electrical stimulation for 6 weeks. Previous studies have clearly demonstrated that this burst frequency and pulse training characteristics successfully prepared the muscle for dynamic assist.[1–6,11] An ECG was obtained on a weekly basis throughout the muscle stimulation protocol to ensure continuous operation of the muscle stimulator. All animals were treated and cared for in accordance with the National Institutes of Health *Guide for the Care and Use of Laboratory Animals.*[12]

### Terminal Study

Following 6 weeks of chronic electrical stimulation of the LD muscle, the animals were returned to the laboratory and anesthetized as described in the previous section. The animal was placed in dorsal recumbency, and the right LD muscle was exposed and removed. This contralateral, unstimulated muscle served as a control for each experiment. Following removal, the LD muscle was immediately placed in chilled, oxygenated Krebs solution and prepared for structural analysis and function studies as described in the following sections. A sternotomy was then performed, and the entire left LD muscle was carefully dissected free from the heart and placed in oxygenated Krebs solution.

Prior to preparation of the control and chronically stimulated muscle for structural studies, a minimum of six muscle strips were harvested from the mid-portion of each muscle and prepared for function studies as described in the following section. In order to examine regional differences in skeletal muscle structure, both the control and the cardiomyoplasty muscle were divided into three regions: **proximal:** 0–4 cm from the origin of thoracodorsal artery; **mid-region:** 4–7 cm from the thoracodorsal artery; **distal:** 7 cm and beyond from the origin of the thoracodorsal artery. Once both muscles had been divided into these regions, 3 × 3 cm cubes of muscle were taken from each of these three regions and prepared for light microscopy, 2 × 2 cm cubes prepared for electron microscopy, and 3 × 3 cm cubes were flash frozen in liquid nitrogen for subsequent hydroxyproline analysis.

## Muscle Fiber Function

Muscle sections (2 mm OD) were taken from the chronically stimulated and control LD muscle and placed in an oxygenated Krebs solution. The muscle strips were mounted in a jacketed muscle chamber (25 mL, 37°C) with one end tied to a fixed post and the other to an isometric force transducer (Grass FT-03, Quincy, MA). After attachment, the muscle strips were stretched in 1-mm increments and the resultant passive tension monitored. Maximal length was defined as the length of the muscle strip at which the passive tension did not decay.[13] For baseline measurements, isometric muscle twitches were elicited by electrical field stimulation at a stimulation frequency of 0.2 Hz. The analog tension signal was digitized at a sampling frequency of 200 Hz (DT2801, Data Translation, Marlboro, MA) and the digitized data stored to disk.

Individual isometric twitches were analyzed off-line for peak tension development (PT), the velocity of tension development (+dT/dt), the velocity of tension relaxation (-dT/dt), the time to peak tension development, the time to 50% relaxation, and the total duration of the twitch. Following the collection of tension data at baseline, the fatigue-resistant properties of the muscle strips were examined by increasing the stimulation frequency to 0.4 Hz, 0.8 Hz, and 1.2 Hz. Peak isometric tension was recorded at each frequency and averaged over a minimum of 20 consecutive twitches. The relative change in the amplitude of the twitches from baseline values was used as an index of muscle fatigue. Following the stimulation protocol, the muscle fiber was cut in cross-section and the cross-sectional area measured. Contraction profile parameters were then normalized to this measured cross-sectional area.[13]

## Light Microscopy

Tissue blocks taken from each region of the control and chronically stimulated LD muscle were immersed in 10% buffered formalin overnight and then embedded in paraplast. Slices of 4-μm thickness were cut from the blocks and mounted on glass slides and stained with hematoxylin and eosin for morphometric analysis. The cross-sectional area of muscle cells within the LD muscle were computed using methods previously described for cardiac muscle.[14]

In order to more carefully examine the distribution and content of extracellular fibrous tissue within the control and chronically stimulated LD muscle, tissue sections were analyzed for the percent area occupied by collagen as described previously by this laboratory.[15] Briefly, 5-μm thick muscle sections were stained using a silver impregnation method and the stained sections imaged on an inverted microscope at a final magnification of 250×.[15] The percent area of collagen was computed from 15 random fields excluding large vascular areas from each section. Mean collagen volume fraction was calculated by averaging the sum of all collagen areas and dividing it by the sum of all extracellular and muscle area and expressed as a percent.

## Electron Microscopy

The muscle samples for electron microscopy were minced finely, immersed in a buffered sodium cacodylate solution containing 2% paraformaldehyde, 2% glutaraldehyde solution, and embedded in Epon resin. Six tissue blocks in the circumferential orientation from each of the three muscle regions were then used to obtain thin sections for electron microscopy. Thin sections were stained with uranyl acetate and lead citrate and examined with a JEOL 100S electron microscope. The central portion of each section was photographed at a calibrated magnification of ×10,000. These electron micrographs were then coded, and this code was not broken until the completion of the study. From the circumferentially oriented micrographs, the percent volume of myofibrils and mitochondria within the skeletal muscle cells was analyzed morphometrically by using a stereology sampling grid consisting of 140 sampling points.[14]

## Collagen Biochemistry

A biochemical assay for hydroxyproline, an amino acid found exclusively in collagen, was performed on the previously frozen muscle sections using methods well described previously.[15,16] The muscle tissue was lyophilized to a constant weight, pulverized in the presence of dry ice, and relyophilized. The ground tissue was then hydrolyzed using 6N hydrochloric acid at 107°C for 16 hours, resuspended in water, and decolorized using activated charcoal. The filtrate was diluted to a convenient volume, and measured spectrophotometrically (550 nm) following reaction with Ehrlich's reagent.[16] Results were expressed as mg hydroxyproline/gram dry weight tissue (mg/gdwt).

## Data Analysis

Comparisons of skeletal muscle function, muscle cell morphology, and collagen content between the control and cardiomyoplasty muscles were performed using multiway analysis of variance. In order to determine regional differences in skeletal muscle structure with chronic electrical stimulation, skeletal fiber location was used as a fixed effect in an analysis of variance model. If the analysis of variance revealed significant differences, pairwise tests of individual group means were compared using Tukey's procedure.[17] Results are presented as mean ± standard error of the mean (SEM). Values of $p<0.05$ were considered to be statistically significant.

## Results

All of the pigs used in this study completed the protocol and the contralateral control and chronically stimulated LD muscle successfully harvested for study. At terminal study, successful stimulation of the chronically stimulated muscle was visually confirmed in all of the surgical preparations prior to harvest.

### Skeletal Muscle Function

A minimum of six muscle fiber samples each were taken from the control and chronically stimulated LD muscle of each pig. A summary of the contraction data obtained from muscle fibers taken from the unstimulated control and chronically stimulated LD muscle is presented in Table 1. At 0.2 Hz, peak tension development was significantly lower in the chronically stimulated muscle fibers. However, there was no difference in this parameter between control and chronically stimulated muscle fibers at higher stimulation frequencies. In the chronically stimulated muscle, the velocity of tension relaxation was lower at all stimulation frequencies compared to control muscle fibers. At increased stimulation frequencies, the time to peak tension was significantly increased in the chronically stimulated muscle fibers compared to controls. The total twitch duration and time to 50% relaxation was significantly prolonged in the chronically stimulated muscle fibers compared to control muscle fibers at all stimulation frequencies.

In order to more carefully examine the fatigue resistance of the skeletal muscle fibers taken from control and chronically stimulated LD muscle, the percent change in peak tension development from 0.2 Hz stimulation frequency was examined. The degradation in peak tension development was significantly greater in the control LD muscle in contrast to the chronically stimulated muscle (Fig. 1). Thus, chronic electrical stimulation of the LD muscle resulted in fatigue resistance and improved muscle fiber contractile function at increased stimulation frequencies. These results demonstrated that 6 weeks of chronic electrical stimulation in this model of dynamic cardiomyoplasty caused functional changes in skeletal muscle performance consistent with conversion of fast-twitch fibers to fatigue-resistant slow-twitch fibers.

In order to address the possibility that regional differences in skeletal muscle fiber contractile function may exist, a subproject was performed in which muscle fibers were harvested from both the mid-region and the distal region of the contralateral control and chronically stimulated LD muscle of two pigs. Contractile performance of control muscle fibers was identical in both regions. In contrast, a 50% reduction in the normalized peak tension development and velocity shortening was observed in muscle fibers taken from the distal region of the chronically stimulated LD muscle. The results from this portion of the

**Table 1**
Latissimus Dorsi Muscle Contractile Function Following Chronic Stimulation

| | *Stimulation Frequency* | | | |
|---|---|---|---|---|
| | *0.2 Hz* | *0.4 Hz* | *0.8 Hz* | *1.2 Hz* |
| Normalized Peak Tension (g/cm$^2$) | | | | |
| Control LDM | 70.34 ± 7.84 | 57.12 ± 6.34 | 44.75 ± 5.20$^+$ | 32.28 ± 3.54$^+$ |
| Chronically stimulated LDM | 51.13 ± 7.51* | 44.73 ± 6.05 | 40.15 ± 5.19 | 35.78 ± 4.39 |
| Normalized Velocity of Tension Development (g/s/cm$^2$) | | | | |
| Control LDM | 309.94 ± 53.47 | 250.54 ± 45.56 | 135.43 ± 18.96$^+$ | 94.73 ± 13.23$^+$ |
| Chronically stimulated LDM | 237.62 ± 51.73 | 196.76 ± 48.99 | 145.12 ± 36.66$^+$ | 103.12 ± 43.60$^+$ |
| Normalized Velocity of Tension Relaxation (g/s/cm$^2$) | | | | |
| Control LDM | 133.19 ± 30.67 | 113.54 ± 27.21 | 82.19 ± 22.62 | 46.28 ± 11.38$^+$ |
| Chronically stimulated LDM | 75.33 ± 15.00 | 62.88 ± 14.06* | 46.62 ± 11.15*$^+$ | 33.23 ± 6.82*$^+$ |
| Time to Peak Tension (ms) | | | | |
| Control LDM | 81.23 ± 3.00 | 78.85 ± 2.47 | 73.95 ± 3.51$^+$ | 73.74 ± 2.92$^+$ |
| Chronically stimulated LDM | 88.41 ± 3.31 | 86.82 ± 3.04* | 84.32 ± 2.43* | 84.07 ± 1.73* |
| Total Twitch Duration (ms) | | | | |
| Control LDM | 348.25 ± 15.17 | 318.41 ± 18.45 | 282.92 ± 21.72$^+$ | 263.71 ± 20.67$^+$ |
| Chronically stimulated LDM | 381.43 ± 9.24* | 366.87 ± 11.04* | 349.87 ± 12.00*$^+$ | 339.23 ± 11.48*$^+$ |
| Time to 50% Relaxation (ms) | | | | |
| Control LDM | 83.67 ± 3.82 | 80.03 ± 3.39 | 75.06 ± 3.22$^+$ | 71.81 ± 3.47$^+$ |
| Chronically stimulated LDM | 96.55 ± 3.59* | 90.23 ± 3.44* | 86.74 ± 1.49*$^+$ | 89.93 ± 3.84*$^+$ |

All values presented as mean ±SEM.

LDM = latissimus dorsi muscle.

*$p<0.05$ vs. control LDM.

$^+p<0.05$ vs. 0.2 Hz.

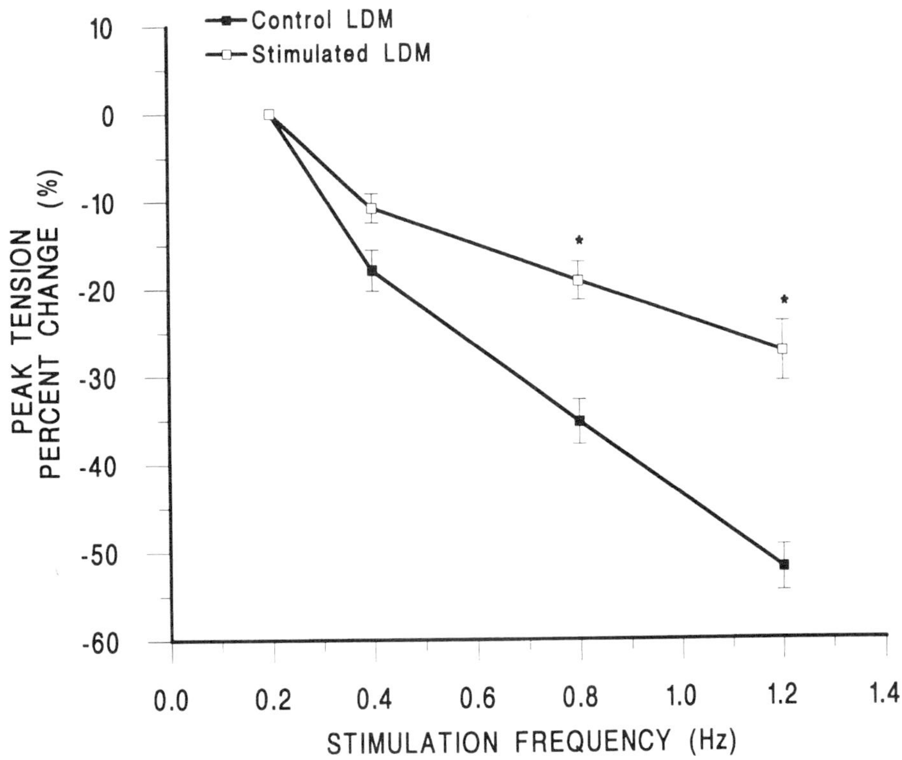


**Figure 1:** *Change in peak tension development as a function of stimulation frequency. The degradation in peak tension development was significantly higher in the control latissimus dorsi muscle (Control LDM) in contrast to the chronically stimulated muscle (Stimulated LDM). Thus, chronic electrical stimulation of the latissimus dorsi muscle resulted in fatigue resistance and improved muscle fiber contractile function at increased stimulation frequencies (*$p < 0.05$ vs. control LDM).*

study are summarized in Table 2. Thus, in contrast to control LD muscle, these results suggest that regional differences in muscle contractile performance occur following dynamic cardiomyoplasty and chronic electrical stimulation. The structural basis for these regional changes in muscle contractile function following 6 weeks of chronic electrical stimulation were examined next.

## Skeletal Muscle Structure

In order to quantify changes in muscle size, muscle fiber cross-sectional area was determined from the proximal, mid-, and distal regions of the contralateral control and chronically stimulated LD muscle. A summary of these results is shown in Table 3. The average cross-sectional area of muscle fibers taken at progressive distances from the LD muscle pedicle remained unchanged in control muscle. However, cross-sectional area of muscle fibers taken from the mid-region of the chronically stimulated skeletal muscle significantly decreased from proximal region values. A further reduction in muscle fiber cross-sectional area was observed in sections taken from the distal portion of the chronically stimu-

**Table 2**
Regional Changes in Muscle Fiber Contractile Function Following Chronic Electrical Stimulation of Latissimus Dorsi Muscle with Cardiomyoplasty

| | *Proximal* | *Distal* |
|---|---|---|
| Normalized Peak Tension (g/cm²) | 51.13 ± 7.51 | 39.00 ± 11.56* |
| Normalized Velocity of Tension Development (g/s/cm²) | 237.62 ± 51.73 | 103.12 ± 43.60* |
| Normalized Velocity of Tension Relaxation (g/s/cm²) | 75.33 ± 15.00 | 36.27 ± 22.09* |
| Time to Peak Tension (ms) | 88.41 ± 3.31 | 95.69 ± 2.98* |
| Total Twitch Duration (ms) | 381.43 ± 9.24 | 440.43 ± 20.61* |
| Time to 50% Relaxation (ms) | 96.55 ± 3.59 | 114.08 ± 5.93* |

All values presented as mean ±SEM.
Stimulation frequency: 0.2 Hz.
n = 2 pigs.
*$p$<0.05 vs. proximal–Wilcoxon test.

**Table 3**
Regional Changes in Latissimus Dorsi Muscle Structure and Biochemical Composition Following Chronic Stimulation

| | *Control* | *Chronically Stimulated* |
|---|---|---|
| Muscle Cell Cross-Sectional Area (μm²) | | |
| Proximal region | 1528 ± 56 | 1110 ± 38* |
| Mid-region | 1813 ± 48 | 1378 ± 42* |
| Distal region | 1883 ± 52 | 836 ± 47*§ |
| Myofibril Percent Volume (%) | | |
| Proximal region | 30 ± 3 | 48 ± 5* |
| Mid-region | 32 ± 4 | 44 ± 3* |
| Distal region | 33 ± 4 | 20 ± 3*§ |
| Mitochondrial Percent Volume (%) | | |
| Proximal region | 12 ± 3 | 20 ± 5* |
| Mid-region | 15 ± 4 | 23 ± 4* |
| Distal region | 16 ± 5 | 30 ± 4*§ |
| Collagen Percent Area (%) | | |
| Proximal region | 5 ± 2 | 9 ± 2* |
| Mid-region | 6 ± 2 | 14 ± 2* |
| Distal region | 5 ± 2 | 18 ± 3* |
| Hydroxyproline Content (mg/gdwt) | | |
| Proximal region | 3.2 ± 0.5 | 7.1 ± 0.5* |
| Mid-region | 4.2 ± 0.6 | 8.6 ± 1.1* |
| Distal region | 5.0 ± 0.9 | 8.0 ± 0.6* |

*$p$< 0.05 vs. control muscle, § $p$<0.05 vs. proximal region.

lated LD muscle. Thus, in contrast to control LD muscle, chronic electrical stimulation for 6 weeks resulted in a reduction in muscle cell cross-sectional area. This cross-sectional area decreased with increased distances from the thoracodorsal neurovascular pedicle.

Representative electron micrographs taken from control and chronically stimulated LD muscle are shown in Figure 2. In control muscle, myofibril units are loosely organized within the muscle cell, and large areas of cytoplasmic space are easily visible (Fig. 2A). In the proximal and mid-regions of chronically stimulated muscle, a dense distribution of myofibrils and mitochondria were clearly visible (Fig. 2B, C). The myofibril content appeared significantly reduced in sections examined from the distal region of chronically stimulated LD muscle

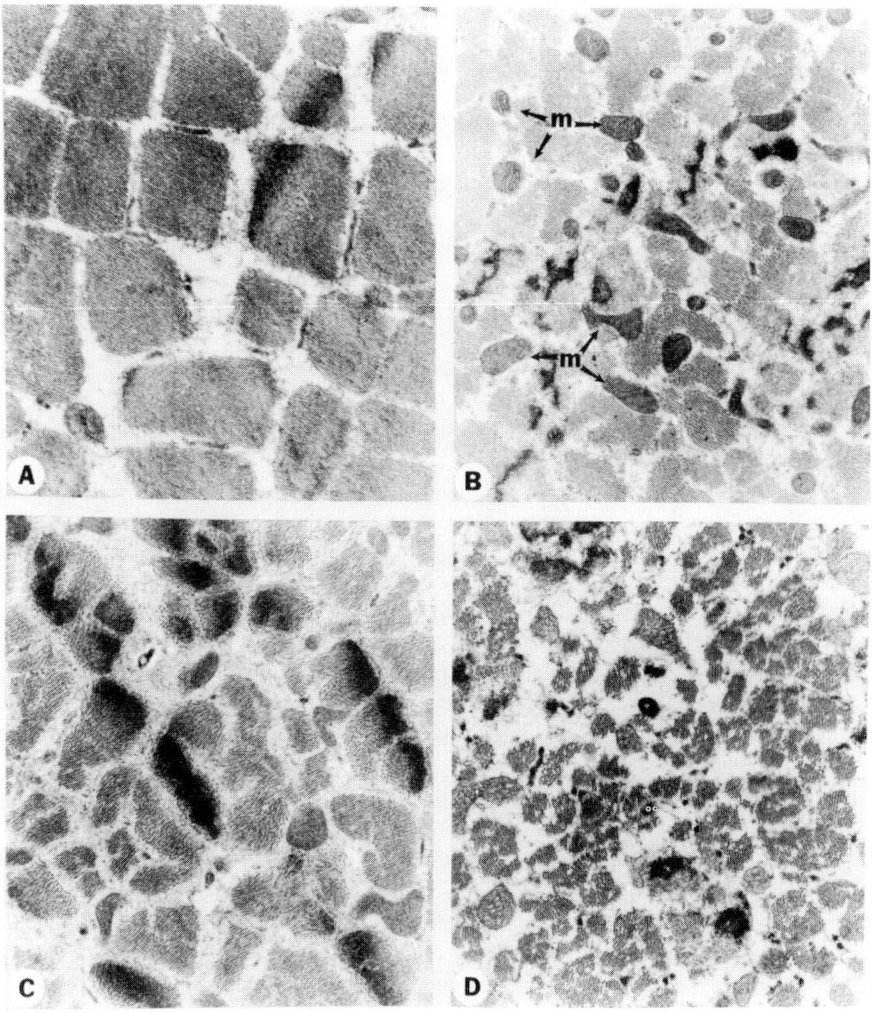


**Figure 2:** *Representative electron micrographs taken in cross-section from unstimulated contralateral control latissimus dorsi muscle (**A**). In this control unstimulated muscle, a loose organization of myofibrils can be observed with a large amount of cytoplasmic space separating the contractile units. (**B**) In cross-sections taken from the proximal region of the chronically stimulated muscle, densely packed myofibrils were observed with a significantly increased number of mitochondria (M-arrows). (**C**) In the mid-region of the chronically stimulated LD muscle, cytoplasmic areas between myofibrils were observed. Mitochondria were readily visible within the cytoplasm surrounding these myofibrils. (**D**) In the distal region of the stimulated muscle, degeneration and myofibrilysis were readily observed within skeletal muscle cells. These ultrastructural changes are consistent with degenerative changes. Quantitative morphometry was performed on electron micrographs obtained from each region of the control and chronically stimulated skeletal muscle and is summarized in Table 3. Original magnification: ×10,000.*

(Fig. 2D). In these distal regions, the myofibril units appeared in disarray and were separated by wide cytoplasmic spaces. In addition, mitochondria exhibited high-amplitude swelling and vacuolization. A total of 970 electron micrographs taken from control and 984 micrographs taken from chronically stimulated LD muscle were subjected to quantitative morphology. The results from this portion of the study are summarized in Table 3. In the control muscle, there were no regional variations in myofibril content or mitochondrial density. In the chronically stimulated LD muscle, regional differences in both myofibril volumes and mitochondrial density were observed. In the proximal and mid-regions of the chronically stimulated muscle, both myofibril and mitochondrial percent volume increased from control values. In the distal region of the chronically stimulated muscle, myofibril volume decreased from proximal and mid-region values as well as from contralateral control values. In contrast, mitochondrial volume percent was increased in the distal region of the chronically stimulated muscle, consistent with mitochondrial swelling and vacuolization. Thus, this ultrastructural study demonstrated that 6 weeks of chronic electrical stimulation with dynamic cardiomyoplasty caused increased myofibril and mitochondrial volumes in the proximal and mid-region of the muscle. However, the distal region of the chronically stimulated LD muscle revealed reduced myofibril volumes and abnormalities in mitochondrial structure.

## Extracellular Structure and Composition

Circumferentially oriented, silver-stained sections of the LD muscle were examined at specific intervals progressing from the pedicle to the distal section of the LD muscle. Representative photomicrographs of sections taken at progressive distances from the muscle pedicle are shown in Figure 3. Examination of sections taken proximal (0–4 cm) to the pedicle revealed a homogenous distribution of muscle cells surrounded by a fine band of collagenous matrix tissue (Fig. 3C). These bands of extracellular material divided the muscle cells into well defined fascicles (Fig. 3D). Sections taken from the mid-region of the latissimus muscle (4–7 cm) revealed focal areas of muscle cell loss with a thickening of the extracellular weave surrounding muscle fascicles (Fig. 3E,F). These zones of fibrosis became more frequent in sections taken from the distal region ( >7 cm from the skeletal muscle pedicle). In these regions, widespread fibrosis with atrophy and dissolution of muscle cells was observed (Fig. 3G,H).

Quantitative morphometry of the silver-stained sections was performed and is summarized in Table 3. A progressive increase in extracellular staining was observed in sections taken from the mid- and distal region of the chronically stimulated LD muscle. The percent area of extracellular staining was significantly increased in the distal region of the chronically stimulated muscle. Examination of the hematoxylin and eosin stained sections of LD muscle taken at progressive distances from the pedicle revealed the absence of a lymphocytic infiltrate. Thus, sections taken from chronic cardiomyoplasty preparations revealed changes in muscle cell size and increased extracellular space in direct proportion to the distance from the LD pedicle. Furthermore, this muscle cell loss and fibrosis did not appear to be associated with a chronic inflammatory response.

In order to more carefully determine the extracellular composition of the chronically stimulated LD muscle, hydroxyproline concentrations were determined and are summarized in Table 3. Hydroxyproline content did not significantly change in any region of the control LD muscle. In the chronically stimulated muscle, hydroxyproline was significantly increased from control values. While hydroxyproline concentrations were higher in the mid- and distal regions of the chronically stimulated muscle compared to the proximal region, these values did not reach statistical significance ($p = 0.35$). Thus, in this model of dynamic cardiomyoplasty, chronic stimulation of the LD muscle for 6 weeks resulted in significantly increased fibrosis based on both histochemical and biochemical measurements.

## Discussion

There are several components of the skeletal muscle that are essential in providing a well-coordinated and forceful contraction on electrical stimulation: the muscle cell itself and the extracellular matrix. The muscle cell is the component responsible for active force production within the skeletal muscle. The extracellular matrix provides the means by which skeletal muscle cell shortening is translated into overall skeletal muscle function. Thus, changes in the composition of the muscle cell and/or the extracellular matrix may significantly influence LD muscle performance with dynamic cardiomyoplasty. Accordingly, the present study examined skeletal muscle structure and function following chronic electrical stimulation with dynamic cardiomyoplasty. To our knowledge, this is the first study that examined the regional changes in LD muscle composition and structure in any model of dynamic cardiomyoplasty. Following 6 weeks of dynamic cardiomyoplasty in pigs, the contractile function of isolated LD muscle fibers revealed slow-twitch characteristics and fatigue resistance. The structure of the chronically stimulated muscle fibers revealed reduced cross-sectional area, and increased myofibril content. However, contractile function of muscle fibers taken from the distal region of the chronically stimulated LD muscle was reduced. In the distal region of the chronically stimulated LD muscle, myofibril volume was decreased and collagen content increased. Thus, in this swine model of cardiomyoplasty, significant regional changes in skeletal muscle structure occur that may significantly influence the overall function of the chronically stimulated muscle and long-term performance with dynamic cardiomyoplasty.

Salmons and Streter demonstrated that skeletal muscle fibers could be converted from fast-twitch fibers to fatigue-resistant slow-twitch fibers using electrical stimulation.[8,9] Using an electrical stimulation training protocol, this past study as well as others have demonstrated that skeletal muscle fibers undergo changes in myosin ATPase isoforms and force development characteristics.[8,9,11,18] In the present study, chronic electrical stimulation of the LD muscle in pigs resulted in skeletal muscle contractile function characteristics consistent with fatigue resistance. Furthermore, the proximal and mid-regions of the chronically stimulated skeletal muscle revealed structural changes (increased myofibril and mitochondrial content) that are consistent with skeletal muscle transformation with electrical stimulation.[8,9] However, in the present

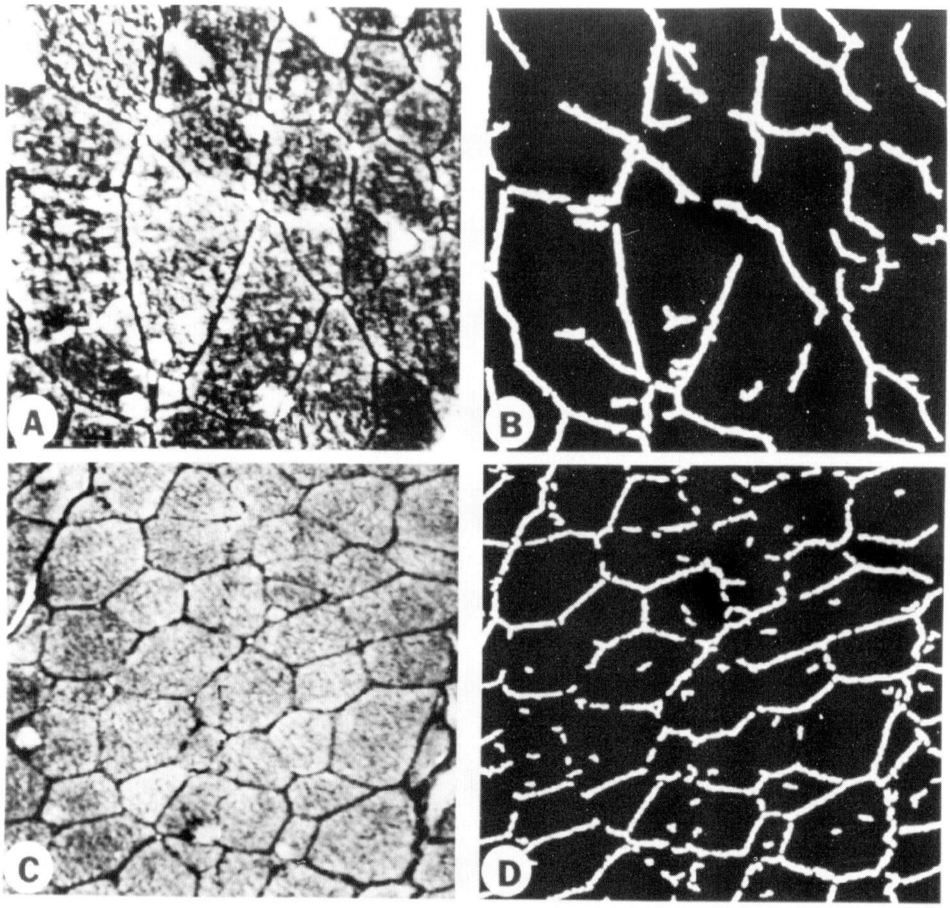


**Figure 3:** *Representative muscle sections taken from control and chronically stimulated LD muscle following silver impregnation staining. Photomicrographs on the left (A, C, E, G) are phase contrast photomicrographs. On the right of each photomicrograph (B, D, F, H) is displayed the same image following input to the image analysis system and digital subtraction. Using this method, the percent area occupied by positive staining extracellular material can be directly quantitated.* ***(A)*** *Section taken from proximal region of contralateral control (unstimulated) LD muscle. The muscle fibers are in cross-sectional orientation and are separated by a fine extracellular latticework.* ***(B)*** *The digital image of the photomicrograph shown in* ***(A)*** *revealed a fine collagenous network surrounding individual muscle fibers.* ***(C)*** *Section taken from proximal region of chronically stimulated LD muscle. Muscle fibers are in cross-sectional orientation and appear to have a reduced cross-sectional diameter compared to unstimulated LD muscle.* ***(D)*** *Digital image of this proximal section revealed an increased abundance of extracellular material surrounding muscle cells. Continued.*

study, skeletal muscle structure and function in the distal region of the chronically stimulated muscle revealed dissimilar characteristics from what was observed in the proximal and mid-regions of the LD muscle. These results for the first time demonstrate that mobilization and chronic electrical stimulation of the LD muscle with dynamic cardiomyoplasty cause region-specific changes in both skeletal muscle structure and function.

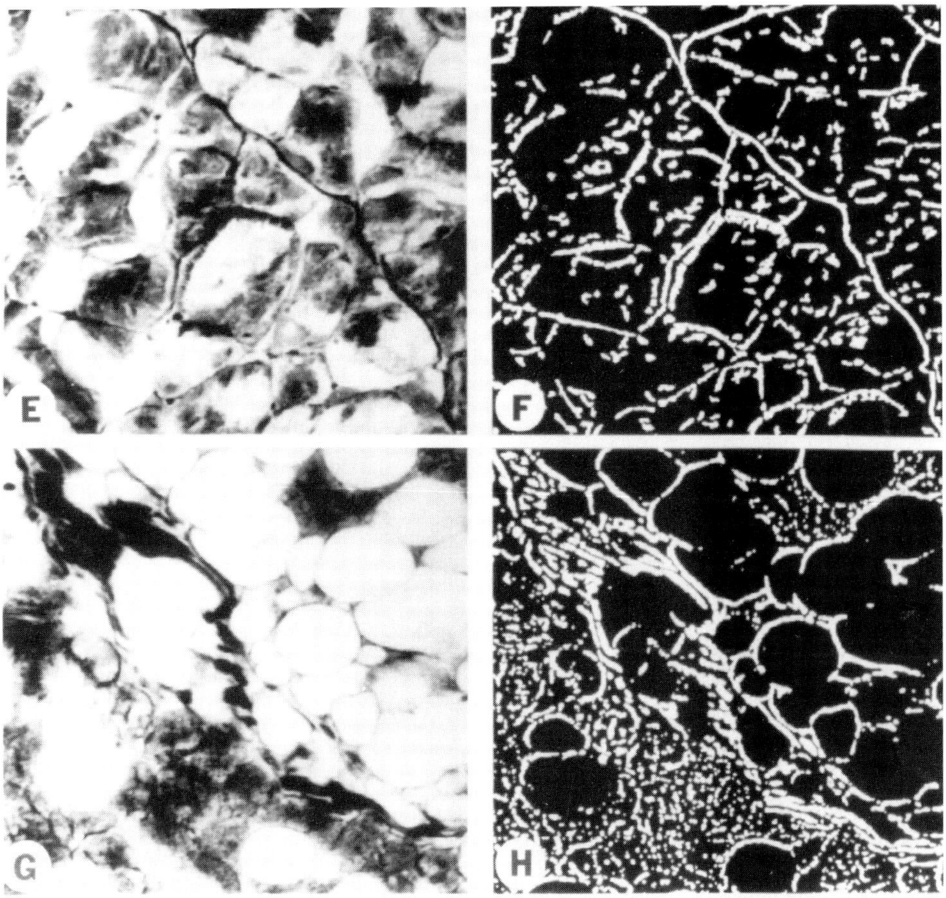


**Figure 3:** *(**E**) Representative photomicrograph of silver stained section from the mid-region of the chronically stimulated LD muscle. Increased vacuole formation was apparent within individual muscle cells. (**F**) Digital subtraction of this image revealed increased extracellular material surrounding individual muscle cells. (**G**) Representative photomicrograph of muscle section taken from distal region of chronically stimulated LD muscle. Large areas of the muscle tissue appear to be replaced by fatty degeneration. Vacuole formation within existing muscle cells was clearly visible. (**H**) The digital image revealed large chords of extracellular staining consistent with collagen fiber formation. Original magnification of all photomicrographs: ×250.*

In the present study, chronic electrical stimulation of the LD muscle with dynamic cardiomyoplasty caused a reduction in skeletal muscle cell cross-sectional area. In a past report by Mannion and colleagues, a similar directional reduction in muscle cell size was observed following 6 weeks of chronic LD muscle in dogs.[11] In this past report, muscle cell cross-sectional area decreased by approximately 30% compared to unstimulated control fibers. In the present study, cross-sectional muscle cell area not only declined following chronic electrical stimulation, but was also reduced in a region-specific manner. In the distal region of the chronically stimulated LD muscle, muscle cell cross-sectional area was reduced by over 25% compared to the proximal and mid-regions. The reduction in peak tension development in the chronically stimulated LD muscle may be due in part to this reduction in muscle cell cross-sectional area.

While results from the present study and past reports demonstrated a reduction in muscle cell cross-sectional area with chronic electrical stimulation, these findings do not necessarily reflect muscle cell atrophy. First, in the present study, myofibril and mitochondrial content in the proximal and mid-region of the chronically stimulated muscle were significantly increased from control, unstimulated muscle. Second, past reports have suggested that the reduction in muscle cell diameter may be an adaptive response to continuous use.[11,18] For example, a smaller fiber diameter will reduce the oxygen diffusion distance across the muscle cell. This may be of particular importance in the chronically stimulated muscle cell, which is more dependent on aerobic metabolism.[8,9,11,19] While the reduction in muscle cell cross-sectional area may be an adaptive response in the proximal and mid-region of the chronically stimulated LD muscle, results from the present study suggest that the reduced muscle cell size in the distal segment of this skeletal muscle may actually be degenerative changes. The structural changes that are discussed in the following section clearly suggest that region-specific changes in skeletal muscle structure occur with dynamic cardiomyoplasty. Thus, while adaptive changes occur within the proximal regions of the skeletal muscle with cardiomyoplasty, degenerative changes may be occurring simultaneously in the more distal region of the chronically stimulated muscle.

Results from the present study clearly suggest that mobilization of the LD muscle and chronic electrical stimulation with dynamic cardiomyoplasty cause a significant reduction in myofibril content and muscle cell diameter in the distal region of this skeletal muscle. In order to determine whether these regional changes in muscle cell structure affected muscle function, the contractile performance of a subset of muscle fibers taken from the distal region of chronically stimulated LD muscle were examined. In muscle fibers taken from this distal region, peak developed tension and velocity of tension development were significantly reduced from proximal region values. Thus, the deterioration in myofibril content and structure of skeletal muscle cells located within the distal region of the chronically stimulated LD muscle was associated with significantly reduced contractile performance.

The extracellular matrix, a three-dimensional collagen latticework, is essential for coordinated force transmission and maintenance of skeletal muscle geometry and alignment. With dynamic cardiomyoplasty, the LD muscle must maintain its conformation around the ventricular chambers in order for appropriate force transmission to occur. Alterations in the extracellular matrix may result in changes in the skeletal muscle geometry that will significantly affect the degree of force delivery to the ventricular chamber. In the present study, significant changes within the extracellular matrix occurred within the LD muscle following 6 weeks of chronic electrical stimulation. Furthermore, these changes within the extracellular space occurred in a progressive fashion: from the proximal to the distal region of the skeletal muscle. With mobilization of the LD muscle and chronic electrical stimulation, a significant increase in collagen content was observed. In the proximal regions, an increased collagenous weave was observed to surround individual muscle cells. This collagenous weave increased in the muscle sections taken from the mid-region of the chronically stimulated LD muscle. In a past report using a similar stimulation protocol, Mannion and colleagues reported a similar qualitative increase in connective tissue.[11] In the present study, the changes within the extracellular space in the distal region of the chronically stimulated LD muscle were in marked contrast to the proximal and mid-regions. In the distal region, increased fibrosis and thick chords of collagenous material coursing through fascicles of muscle cells were observed. Thus, the geometric distribution and structure of the extracellular matrix were significantly different in the distal region compared to more proximal regions of the chronically stimulated LD muscle. One potential mechanism for the increased density and distribution of the extracellular matrix within the distal region of this muscle is replacement fibrosis due to atrophy and loss of skeletal muscle cells. While the mechanism or mechanisms responsible for these changes in extracellular structure with chronic electrical stimulation remain unclear, the present study clearly demonstrated that region-specific changes occur with respect to collagen content and distribution. These regional changes in extracellular structure may significantly influence the performance characteristics of the chronically stimulated LD muscle with dynamic cardiomyoplasty.

The mechanisms responsible for the region-specific changes in skeletal muscle structure with chronic electrical stimulation of the LD muscle are probably due to alterations in blood flow, abnormalities in metabolism, or both. Mobilization of the LD muscle for creation of the cardiomyoplasty results in disruption of blood flow to the regions most distal to the thoracodorsal neurovascular pedicle.[1–10] Thus, the reduced myofibril content and muscle cell size, and increased fibrous weave observed in the distal regions of the chronically stimulated LD muscle may have been due to reduced blood flow. In these distal regions, increased vacuole formation was observed within the cell and within the mitochondria. These vacuoles may represent lipid formation due to a disruption in normal metabolic processes. It is well established that chronically stimulated skeletal muscle has increased oxidative phosphorylation capacity and is dependent on aerobic metabolism.[8,9,18,19] Thus, the appearance of these vacuoles, particularly associated with mitochondria, may be due to a disruption in aerobic metabolism. The specific mechanisms responsible for these changes in skeletal muscle structure within the distal region of the chronically stimulated LD muscle remain speculative. Based on the findings from the present study, future studies aimed at more careful examination of regional changes in blood flow and metabolism would seem appropriate.

## Summary

Dynamic cardiomyoplasty has been demonstrated to provide symptomatic relief in patients suffering from severe congestive heart failure.[1–7] In clinical studies performed worldwide, chronic stimulation of the LD muscle in synchrony with the intrinsic ventricular contraction has been shown to improve left ventricular pump function.[1–7] However, for this surgical treatment of congestive heart failure to gain wider application and acceptance, the structural and functional events that occur within the chronically stimulated skeletal muscle must be understood. In the present study, regional changes in cellular and extracellular structure were observed following chronic electrical stimulation of the LD muscle with dynamic cardiomyoplasty. These regional changes in skeletal muscle structure were associated with regional changes in skeletal muscle contractile function. These region-specific changes in LD muscle structure and function may significantly influence the long-term performance of this skeletal muscle with dynamic cardiomyoplasty. Future studies directed at improving the regional alterations in muscle structure with chronic electrical stimulation and dynamic cardiomyoplasty may be appropriate.

*Acknowledgments:* Supported in part by National Institutes of Health Grant HL45024(FGS), and the Medtronic Corporation, Minneapolis, MN.

## References

1. Magovern GJ, Christlieb IY, Kao RL: The Allegheny Hospital experience. In: Carpentier A, Chachques JC, Grandjean P (eds). *Cardiomyoplasty.* Armonk, NY, Futura Publishing Company, 1991, pp 159–170.
2. Magovern JA, Furnary AP, Christlieb IY, Kao RL, Magovern GJ: Right latissimus dorsi cardiomyoplasty for left ventricular failure. *Ann Thorac Surg* 53:1120–1122, 1992.
3. Moreira LFP, Seferian P, Jr, Bocchi EA, et al: Survival improvement with dynamic cardiomyoplasty in patients with dilated cardiomyopathy. *Circulation* 84(Suppl III):296–302, 1991.
4. Carpentier A, Abry B, Mihaileanu S, Chachques JC: Hôpital Broussais clinical experience. In: Carpentier A, Chachques JC, Grandjean P (eds). *Cardiomyoplasty.* Armonk, NY, Futura Publishing Company, 1991, pp 147–157.
5. Chachques JC, Grandjean P, Schwartz K, et al: Effect of latissimus dorsi dynamic cardiomyoplasty on ventricular function. *Circulation* 78(Suppl III):203–216, 1988.
6. Magovern GJ, Heckler FR, Park SB, et al: Paced skeletal muscle for dynamic cardiomyoplasty. *Ann Thorac Surg* 45:614–619, 1988.
7. Salmons S, Jarvis JC: Skeletal muscle as an adaptive contractile biomaterial for cardiac assistance: Fundamental considerations. *Proceedings of the 14th Annual Conference of the IEEE Engineering in Medicine and Biology Society,* Paris, France, 1992, pp 2798–2799.
8. Salmons S, Streter FA: Significance of impulse activity in the transformation of skeletal muscle type. *Nature* 263:30, 1967.
9. Salmons S, Vrbova G: The influence of activity on some contractile characteristics of mammalian fast and slow muscle. *J Physiol* 201:535, 1969.
10. Carpentier A, Chachques JC: Cardiomyoplasty: Surgical technique. In: Carpentier A, Chachques JC, Grandjean P (eds). *Cardiomyoplasty.* Armonk, NY, Futura Publishing Company, 1991, pp 105–122.
11. Mannion JD, Bitto T, Hammond RL, Rubinstein NA, et al: Histochemical and fatigue characteristics of conditioned canine latissimus dorsi muscle. *Circ Res* 58:298–304, 1986.
12. Institute of Laboratory Animal Resources. Committee on Care and Use of Laboratory Animals: *Guide for the Care and Use of Laboratory Animals.* National Research Council. NIH publication 86–23, 1985.
13. Gordon AM, Huxley F, Julian FJ: Tension development in highly stretched vertebrate muscle fibres. *J Physiol* 184:143–169, 1966.
14. Spinale FG, Zellner JL, Tomita M, Crawford FA, et al: Relationship between ventricular and myocyte remodeling with the development and regression of supraventricular tachycardia-induced cardiomyopathy. *Circ Res* 69:1058–1067, 1991.

15. Spinale FG, Tomita M, Zellner JL, Cook JC, et al: Collagen remodeling and changes in LV function during development and recovery from supraventricular tachycardia. *Am J Physiol* 261(*Heart and Circ Physiol* 30:H308–H318), 1991.
16. Stegemann H, Stalder K: Determination of hydroxyproline. *Clin Chimica Acta* 18:267–273, 1967.
17. Steel RGD, Torrie JH, eds: *Principles and Procedures of Statistics: A Biometrical Approach*. New York, McGraw-Hill, 1980, pp 172–194.
18. Ciske PE, Faulkner JA: Chronic electrical stimulation of nongrafted and grafted skeletal muscles in rats. *J Appl Physiol* 59(5):1434–1439, 1985.
19. Clark BJ, III, Acker MA, McCully K, et al: In vivo $^{31}$P-NMR spectroscopy of chronically stimulated canine skeletal muscle. *Am J Physiol* 254(*Cell Physiol* 23):C258–C266, 1988.

Chapter 27

# The Role of Myogenic Proteins during Conditioning of Skeletal Muscle with Chronic Electrical Stimulation

Steven J. Hoff, Donald F. Pierce, Jr., James R. Stewart*

## Introduction

The use of conditioned skeletal muscle for the augmentation of cardiac function in the failing heart with dynamic cardiomyoplasty has attracted considerable interest. Of paramount importance in the development of cardiomyoplasty is the documentation of morphological changes in skeletal muscle after chronic electrical stimulation.[1] These changes, induced by a program of graded electrical stimulation, include alterations in actin and myosin isoforms, troponin, and calcium ATPase, and mitochondrial volume.[2–6] Most importantly, chronic electrical stimulation results in transformation of skeletal muscle fiber type from predominantly fast-twitch, fatigue-prone type II fibers to predominantly slow-twitch, fatigue-resistant type I fibers.[7–11] Little is known about the molecular mechanisms of these morphological changes that are so important to the development of successful skeletal muscle cardiac assist. Theoretically, a change must eventually occur at the level of the genome to lead to the conversion of terminally differentiated skeletal muscle cells into the fatigue-resistant, cardiaclike fibers required for cardiomyoplasty.

MyoD is one of a family of related proteins that have been shown to be important in the differentiation of determined skeletal myoblasts to terminally differentiated skeletal myotubules.[12–14] Other members of this protein family include myogenin,[15,16] my5,[17] and MRF4.[18] These proteins have a characteristic helix-loop-helix DNA binding motif, reflecting their role as a transcription

*With the cooperation of James A. Atkinson, Charles C. Elkins, Walter H. Merrill, and Harvey W. Bender, Jr.

From Carpentier A, Chachques JC, Grandjean P: Cardiac Bioassist.  Armonk, NY, 1997.

factor. While they are not expressed in normal cardiac muscle, they have been shown to result in terminal differentiation to skeletal muscle when added to immortalized muscle cell lines and fibroblasts.[13,16]

We sought to answer the following questions concerning a possible relationship between these myogenic proteins and the changes seen morphologically in chronically stimulated skeletal muscle used for dynamic cardiomyoplasty:

1. to confirm the expression of two myogenic proteins, MyoD and myogenin, in normal canine skeletal muscle and determine the level of expression in normal canine cardiac muscle.
2. to document the effect of chronic electrical stimulation, with its concomitant changes in skeletal muscle morphology, on expression of myogenic proteins.

## Methods and Materials

### Canine Experiments/Muscle Stimulation

All experimental animals received humane care in compliance with *Principles of Laboratory Animal Care* (National Society for Medical Research) and the *Guide for the Care and Use of Laboratory Animals* (National Institutes of Health publication No. 80-23, revised 1985).

Under general anesthesia, adult mongrel dogs (n=5) underwent bilateral axillary dissection through an oblique incision over the ventral border of the latissimus dorsi (LD) muscle. The neurovascular bundle including the thoracodorsal nerve was identified proximal to its termination on the LD muscle and was encircled bilaterally with the cuffed end of a modified Medtronic skeletal muscle pacing lead (Medtronic model 4080, Medtronic, Inc., Minneapolis, MN). The proximal end of the left lead was capped. The pacing lead to the right was connected to a myostimulator pulse generator (Medtronic model SP1005, Medtronic, Inc., Minneapolis, MN). A pocket was created under the rectus abdominus muscle and the pulse generator was placed within.

Multiple biopsies from the most lateral segment of the LD muscle were obtained from both sides. They were rapidly labeled and quick-frozen in liquid nitrogen. Muscle biopsies were stored at −70°C for later analysis. A single biopsy was retained fresh and used for histopathologic and enzyme histochemical analysis.

### Muscle Stimulation Protocol

Animals were allowed to recover from the operative procedure, and on postoperative day 1, the myostimulator pulse generator was activated using a Medtronic programmer (Medtronic model 7531 RF, Medtronic, Inc., Minneapolis, MN) at the following initial settings: rate = 2 Hz, pulse amplitude <3 volts, pulse width 210 microseconds, pulse duration 185 ms. Over the ensuing 8 weeks, the animals underwent graded stimulation of the right LD muscle according to the protocol used most commonly for the conditioning of skeletal muscle for clinical dynamic cardiomyoplasty.[19] Graded stimulation included stepwise increases in rate from 2 to 10 to 20 and finally 30 Hz at 2-week intervals. The left LD muscle was not stimulated and served as a sham-operated control for each animal. At the end of each 2-week interval, multiple muscle biopsies were obtained from the most ventral aspect of both LD muscles under general anesthesia. At the end of the 8-week stimulation period, the myostimulator pulse generator and leads were removed. Biopsies were obtained from both LD muscles at the time of explantation, and again at 2 weeks and 2 months following the cessation of continuous graded electrical stimulation. Dogs were euthanized at the conclusion of the latter procedure.

## Enzyme Histochemical Analysis

Frozen sections of freshly obtained muscle biopsies were cut at 8 microns and stained using the actomysin ATPase histochemical method.[20] Type IIB fibers stain dark, type I fibers stain light, and type IIA fibers are intermediate. Fiber type was quantitated by an observer blinded to the stimulation protocol by counting the number of fibers of each type in three separate areas of the stain and reporting the average of these values. Fiber typing is reported as the mean % of fibers ± standard deviation.

## RNA Extraction

Total RNA extraction from muscle biopsies was performed using a guanidine isothiocyanate/ultracentrifugation technique.[21] Ice-cold guanidine isothiocyanate (0.67 mL/0.1 gram of muscle) was added to skeletal muscle tissue and the samples were homogenized using a Brinkman tissue homogenizer set at medium speed for 15 seconds. Care was taken to wash the homogenizer with large amounts of water and then a guanidine isothiocyanate wash to avoid cross-contamination. Cesium chloride (2 mL) was added to ultracentrifuge tubes and the lysate carefully layered on top. Tubes were then spun in an ultracentrifuge (Sorvall) at 22°C for 20 hours at 35,000 rpm. The supernatant was removed and the RNA pellet was resuspended in 200 microliters of 0.3 M sodium acetate. Samples were purified using 100%, then 80% ethanol, and RNA quantity was determined by optical densitometry at 260 nm.

## Northern Blot Analysis

Standardized amounts of total RNA were run on a formaldehyde/agarose denaturing gel and Northern blot analysis was performed.[22] cDNA probes were prepared from stock samples of myoD (generously provided by Dr. H. Weintraub, Seattle, WA[23]) and myogenin (generously provided by Dr. E. Olson, Houston, TX[16]). The Northern blot was probed with one $^{32}$P-labeled cDNA, stripped, and probed a second time with the other probe. Equivalent loading of lanes was evident in photographs of UV backlit gels containing ethidium bromide.

## Results

Table 1 shows the results obtained by enzyme histochemical analysis of fiber typing. While control and unstimulated skeletal muscle was composed of approximately 19% type I by week 8 of the stimulation protocol, type I fibers constituted nearly 85% of all muscle fibers ($p<.05$). In addition, there was evidence of "detransformation" of fiber types after cessation of stimulation. This process appears to be slower than the changes seen with stimulation and remained incomplete, with 44% type I fibers by 10 weeks after the cessation of chronic stimulation.

Figure 1 summarizes the results of myogenic gene expression in muscle stimulated chronically. MyoD and myogenin RNA are expressed in LD muscle before the institution of the stimulation protocol and in unstimulated control muscle. There is expression of myoD (Fig. 1A) and myogenin (Fig. 1B) RNA at 2 and 4 weeks following the initiation of electrical stimulation. Their expression becomes undetectable by the sixth week of the stimulation protocol. This loss of expression of myogenic proteins remains even after 2 months following the cessation of stimulation.

## Discussion

The morphological changes that occur in skeletal muscle subjected to chronic electrical stimulation have been well characterized. These include changes in fiber type and contraction characteristics,[7–11] actin and myosin,[2,3] troponin,[3,4] mitochondria content,[6] and sarcoplasmic calcium-ATPase.[5] Effects of chronic electrical stimulation on metabolism have also been described.[24–26] The diversity of contractile protein isoforms is essential to the maintenance of plasticity in tissue that must constantly adapt to changing environmental stimuli. Chronic electrical stimulation of LD muscle used for cardiomyoplasty demonstrates that such plasticity is present in differentiated skeletal muscle.[27] Our data confirm the graded change in response to electrical stimulation and result in the conversion of predominantly fatigable type II fibers into fatigue-resistant type I fibers in canine LD muscle. In addition, we observed the incomplete resolution of these

**Table 1.**
Quantitation of Fiber Type after Electrical Stimulation

| *Week* | *Control* | *Stimulated* | *p Value* |
|---|---|---|---|
| 0 | 17.8 ± 2.2 | 19.0 ± 3.1 | 0.497 |
| 2 | 17.0 ± 2.1 | 26.5 ± 8.2 | 0.156 |
| 4 | 19.8 ± 3.3 | 40.5 ± 8.3 | 0.001 |
| 6 | 19.0 ± 1.6 | 50.5 ± 12.0 | 0.001 |
| 8 | 19.4 ± 3.9 | 85.5 ± 18.3 | 0.006 |
| 10 | 20.0 ± 3.7 | 63.7 ± 39.2 | 0.195 |
| 16 | 18.2 ± 2.3 | 42.5 ± 27.6 | 0.431 |

All values are % type I fibers ±SD. *p* values are stimulated vs. control (two-tailed Fisher's exact).

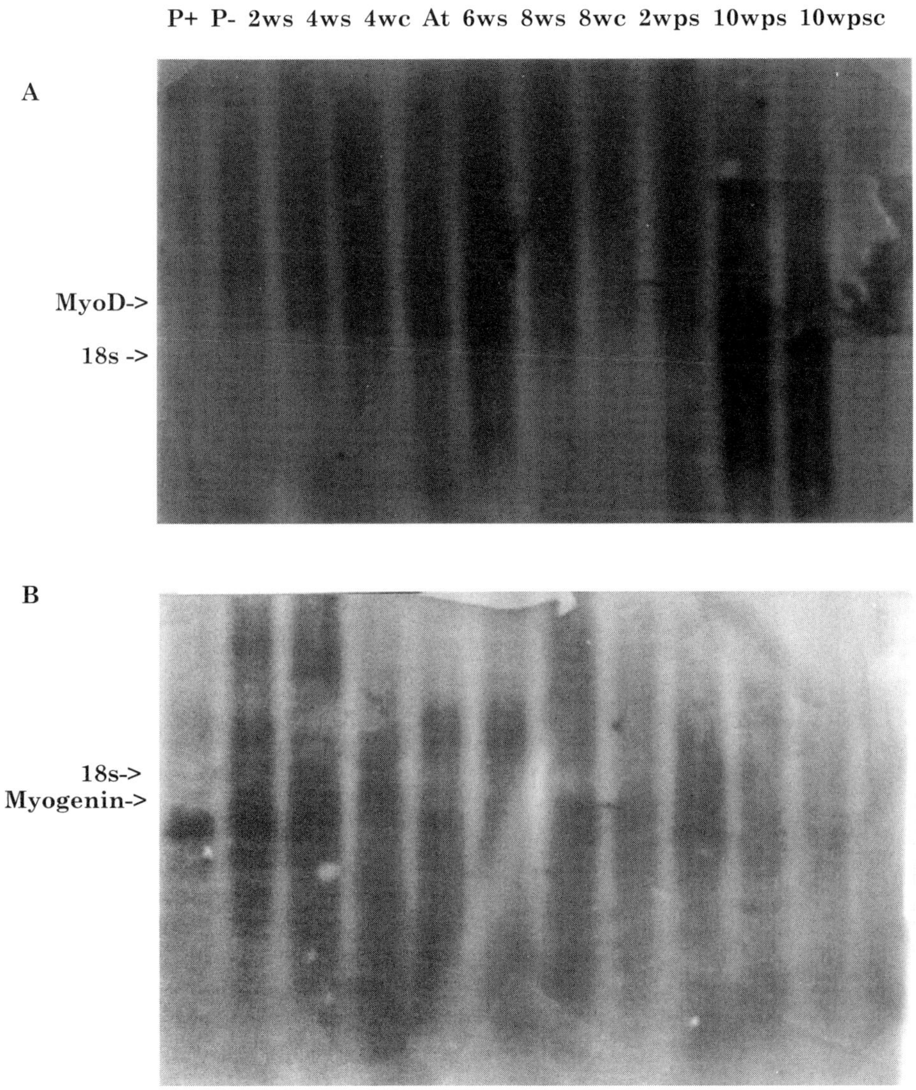


**Figure 1:** *Northern blot analysis of myoD (A) and myogenin (B) mRNA expression in canine skeletal muscle. Samples are of total RNA extracted from skeletal muscle biopsies during graded electrical stimulation and from contralateral, unstimulated skeletal muscle controls.* **Lane 1,** *prestimulation with implanted electrode (P+);* **Lane 2,** *control (P-);* **Lanes 3 and 4,** *2 and 4 weeks of stimulation (2ws, 4ws);* **Lane 5,** *4 week control (4wc);* **Lane 6,** *atrial control (A+);* **Lanes 7 and 8,** *6 and 8 weeks of stimulation (6ws, 8ws);* **Lane 9,** *8 week control (8wc);* **Lane 10,** *2 weeks post stimulation (2wps);* **Lanes 11 and 12,** *10 weeks post stimulation and control (10wps, 10wpsc). All lanes were loaded with 10 μg of total RNA and hybridized with $^{32}$P-labeled myoD (A) or myogenin (B) cDNA probes.*

changes after the cessation of electrical stimulation, previously described by Eisenberg and colleagues in a model of rabbit hindlimb stimulation.[28]

Some important limitations of this model relative to clinical myoplasty deserve note. Canine LD muscle used in this model is stimulated in situ. No dissection of the body of the LD muscle was performed, which occurs during mobilization for clinical cardiomyoplasty. In the clinical situation, a 2-week latent period is generally used to allow the intramuscular collaterals already present in the LD muscle to replace blood supply from perforators along the chest wall when the muscle is in situ.[29] Factors associated with local tissue ischemia and angiogenesis induced by this process may affect myogenic protein expression, either directly or indirectly. This will require investigation before these data may be interpreted for clinical myoplasty. In addition, this model takes advantage of the fact that the muscle remains in a state of passive stretch that may be different than the muscle used in clinical myoplasty.[30] Finally, evidence exists that there are intramuscular differences in fiber type among various segments of the LD muscle.[11,31] We took care in biopsying only the ventral segment of the muscle, thereby controlling for this confounding variable.

Although myogenic proteins are not expressed typically in normal mammalian cardiac muscle, Miner and colleagues developed a line of transgenic mice that expressed myoD in their developing hearts.[32] This forced expression led to lethal morphological changes associated with the activation of skeletal muscle-specific structural and regulatory genes. The presence of regulatory proteins such as myoD exacting similar regulatory control over cardiac muscle-specific development has recently been proposed.[33] However, differences in the embryonic origin of skeletal and cardiac muscle and variations in their responsiveness to growth factor signals suggest these regulatory effects would be expressed much earlier in muscle development than seen in the skeletal muscle system.

The effect of electrical activity on myogenic proteins has been well characterized. Its effect seems to be closely related to changes in acetylcholine receptors.[34–36] In addition, factors such as c-myc have recently been shown to influence myogenic protein-initiated muscle differentiation.[37] MyoD and myogenin have also been shown to be involved in muscle regeneration.[38] Cytosolic growth factors are also involved in the regulation of the effects of myogenic proteins.[33,39]

The exact cellular events that result in the morphological changes seen after electrical stimulation remain to be elucidated. By more clearly understanding these mechanisms, we may be able to alter the cellular messages to the genome required for these morphological changes. Optimization of fiber type transformation to ensure the most efficient muscle for fatigue-resistant work would be possible. Alteration in the electrical stimulation, cytosolic milieu, or genetic signal via transfection techniques could also be evaluated. Any or all of these may help improve the functional results and clinical outcome for patients treated with dynamic cardiomyoplasty.

## References

1. Salmons S, Sreter FA: Significance of impulse activity in the transformation of skeletal muscle type. *Nature* 263:30–34, 1976.

2. Carraro U: Contractile proteins of fatigue-resistant muscle. *Semin Thorac Cardiovasc Surg* 3:111–115, 1991.
3. Pattison CW, Cimming DVE, Jones DGC, et al: Variable adaptation of molecular mechanisms in relation to the use of autologous striated muscle to augment myocardial function. *Cardiovasc Res* 23:593–600, 1989.
4. Hartner KT, Pette D: Fast and slow isoforms of troponin I and troponon C. *J Biochem* 188:261–267, 1990.
5. Leberer E, Hartner KT, Brandl CJ, et al: Slow/cardiac sarcoplasmic reticulum $CA^{++}$-ATPase and phospholamban mRNAs are expressed in chronically stimulated rabbit fast-twitch muscle. *Eur J Biochem* 185:51–54, 1989.
6. Eisenberg BR, Salmons S: The reorganization of subcellular structure in muscle undergoing fast-to-slow type transformation. *Cell Tissue Res* 220:449–471, 1981.
7. Pette D: Effects of chronic electrostimulation on muscle gene expression. *Semin Thorac Cardiovasc Surg* 3:101–105, 1991.
8. Pette D, Simoneau JA: Chronic stimulation-induced alterations in phenotypic expression and functional properties of skeletal muscle. In Chiu RCJ, Bourgeois I: *Transformed Muscle for Cardiac Assist and Repair.* Futura Publishing Co. Inc, Mt Kisco, NY, 1990, pp 129–137.
9. Ianuzzo CD, Hamilton N, O'Brien PJ, Desrosiers C, et al: Biochemical transformation of canine skeletal muscle for use in cardiac-assist devices. *J Appl Physiol* 48:1481–1485, 1990.
10. Havenith MG, van der Veen FH, Glatz JFC, et al: Monitoring of muscle fiber type of canine latissimus dorsi muscle during chronic electrical stimulation by enzyme and immunohistochemistry. In Chiu RCJ, Bourgeois I: *Transformed Muscle for Cardiac Assist and Repair.* Futura Publishing Co. Inc, Mt. Kisco, NY, 1990, pp 53–61.
11. Mannion JD, Bitto T, Hammond RL, et al: Histochemical and fatigue characteristics of conditioned canine latissimus dorsi muscle. *Circ Res* 58:298–304, 1986.
12. Weintraub H, Davis R, Tapscott S, et al: The myoD gene family: Nodal point during specification of the muscle cell lineage. *Science* 251:761–766, 1991.
13. Davis RL, Weintraub H, Lassar AB: Expression of a single cDNA converts fibroblasts to myoblasts. *Cell* 51:987–1000, 1987.
14. Olson EN: MyoD family: A paradigm for development? *Genes Dev* 4:1454–1461, 1990.
15. Wright WE, Sassoon DA, Lin VK: Myogenein, a factor regulating myogenesis, has a domain homologous to myoD. *Cell* 56:607–617, 1989.
16. Edmonson DG, Olson EN: A gene with homology to the myc similarity region of MyoD1 is expressed during myogenesis and is sufficient to activate the muscle differentiation program. *Genes Dev* 3:628–640, 1989.
17. Braun T, Bober E, Buschhausen-Denker G, et al: Differential expression of myogenic determination genes in muscle cells: Possible autoactivation by the Myf gene products. *EMBO J* 8:3617–3625, 1989.
18. Rhodes SJ, Konieczny SF: Identification of MRF4: A new member of the muscle regulatory factor gene family. *Genes Dev* 3:2050–2061, 1989.
19. Chachques JC, Grandjean PA, Carpentier A: Patient management and clinical follow-up after cardiomyoplasty. *J Cardiac Surg* 6:89–99, 1991.
20. Dubowitz V: In: *Muscle Biopsy: A Practical Approach,* 2nd ed. Bailliere Tindall, London, 1985.
21. Chirgwin JM, Przybyla AE, MacDonald RJ, et al: *Biochemistry* 18:5294–5306, 1979.
22. Lehreach H, Diamond D, Wozney J, et al: *Biochemistry* 16:4743–4755, 1979.
23. Weintraub H, Tapscott SJ, Davis RL, et al: Activation of muscle specific genes in pigment, nerve, fat, liver, and fibroblast cell lines by forced expression of MyoD. *PNAS* 86:5434–5438, 1989.
24. Clark BJ, Acker MA, McCully K, et al: In vivo $^{31}P$-NMR spectroscopy of chronically stimulated canine skeletal muscle. *Am J Physiol* 254:C258–C266, 1988.
25. Acker M, Anderson WA, Hammond RL, et al: Oxygen consumption of chronically stimulated skeletal muscle. *J Thorac Cardiovasc Surg* 94:702–709, 1987.
26. Henriksson J, Salmons S, Lowry OH: Chronic stimulation of mammalian muscle: Enzyme and metabolic changes in individual fibers. *Biomed Biochem Acta* 5:S445–S454, 1989.

27. Bandman E: Contractile protein isoforms in muscle development. *Dev Biol* 154:273–283, 1992.
28. Eisenberg BR, Brown JMC, Salmons S: Restoration of fast muscle characteristics following cessation of chronic stimulation. *Cell Tissue Res* 238:221–230, 1984.
29. Hudlicka O: Anatomical changes in chronically stimulated skeletal muscles. *Semin Thorac Cardiovasc Surg* 3:106–110, 1991.
30. Goldspink DF, Easton J, Winterburn SK, et al: The role of passive stretch and repetitive electric stimulation in preventing skeletal muscle atrophy while reprogramming gene expression to improve fatigue resistance. *J Cardiac Surg* 6:218–224, 1991.
31. Sola OM, Herring S, Zhang G, et al: Significance of the biopsy site of the latissimus dorsi muscle for fiber typing. *J Heart Lung Transplant* 11:S315–S319, 1992.
32. Miner JH, Miller JB, Wold BJ: Skeletal muscle phenotypes initiated by ectopic MyoD in transgenic mouse heart. *Development* 114:853–860, 1992.
33. Olson EN: Regulatory mechanisms for skeletal muscle differentiation and their relevance to gene expression in the heart. *Trends Cardiovasc Med* 5:163–170, 1992.
34. Eftimie R, Brenner HR, Buonanno A: Myogenin and MyoD join a family of skeletal muscle genes regulated by electrical stimulation. *PNAS* 88:1349–1353, 1991.
35. Dutton EK, Simon AM, Burden SJ: Electrical activity-dependent regulation of the acetylcholine receptor delta-subunit gene, MyoD, and myogenin in primary myotubules. *PNAS* 90:2040–2044, 1993.
36. Witzmann V, Sakmann B: Differential regulation of MyoD and myogenin mRNA levels by nerve-induced muscle activity. *FEBS Lett* 282:259–264, 1991.
37. Miner JH, Wold BJ: C-myc inhibition of MyoD and myogenin-initiated myogenic differentiation. *Mol Cell Biol* 11:2842–2851, 1991.
38. Fuchtbauer EM, Westphal H: MyoD and myogenin are co-expressed in regenerating skeletal muscle of the mouse. *Dev Dyn* 193:34–39, 1992.
39. Olson EN: Interplay between proliferation and differentiation within the myogenic lineage. *Dev Biol* 154:261–272, 1992.

# Chapter 27

## *Discussion*

**Dr. Schwartz:** Myogenin and myoD are obviously not so abundant in the cell and of course it is very difficult to probe them in a very specific way. This was apparent in your northern blot where obviously you had a very high level of background, which in some parts obscured the specific message. So I wanted you to comment a little more, if possible, on the technical considerations. Why do you have such a big level in the line that was indicated At, meaning atria, which was not supposed to have the expression of any of these proteins? You still had a very significant base that was higher than the supposed message. Could you comment a little more on that?

**Dr. Hoff:** The technical aspects of the northern blot analysis were controlled by staining the gel bromide and looking at the gels under UV light. We were able to show that the loading of the lanes was standardized. I apologize if these blots did not project very well. Because of the relatively small percentage of myoD and myogenin, mRNA, and the total RNA, we had to probe the blot relatively hot to produce a signal and that explains, in part, the relatively high background.

**Dr. Schwartz:** Did you do total RNA or poly RNA?

**Dr. Hoff:** These experiments are with total RNA and I think an interesting corroborating study, which is one that we plan to do, will be a similar study looking at poly RNA.

**Dr. Chachques:** I noticed that at 8 weeks, you had half of the fibers that were still type 1 fibers. This is in contradiction to the accepted findings of Dr. Salmons, which showed a complete reversibility of the muscle after this delay.

**Dr. Hoff:** Dr. Salmons also showed that these changes are completely reversible. Our data are a little different from that. We cut off the experiment rather arbitrarily at 8 weeks after the cessation of stimulation and I suspect that had we continued it somewhat longer than that we would have seen a complete reversal of fiber type back to a more normal expression. One side benefit from this model would be the ability to study different pacing protocols and the

From Carpentier A, Chachques JC, Grandjean P: Cardiac Bioassist. © Futura Publishing Co, Inc, Armonk, NY, 1997.

change in fiber type both with stimulation and after the cessation of stimulation or with certain delays.

**Dr. Pette:** Of course it is normal that myoD and myogenin are not really expressed in other muscle fibers. The only fact is MRF4 which persists. The sensitivity of the method you used is the lowest possible. This should be done on the single fiber level because what you have seen is probably regeneration, satellite cell proliferation, and formation of new myotubes. You cannot be sure, when you have reversion, that this does not take place and see any changes or any expression of these factors.

**Dr. Hoff:** That is a valid point. The myogenic proteins that I have talked about—myogenin, myoD, MRF4, and myo5—may, from a semantic standpoint, be a little different from the isoforms we see with various growth factors or even contractile proteins. And their effects are probably one small part of a very complex skeletal muscle regulatory system. We are currently looking at studies that would, in this particular pacing protocol, correlate what we have seen with levels of muscle injury or regeneration.

**Dr. Gagneau (Quebec):** I would like to know about your cDNA. Is it dog cDNA?

**Dr. Hoff:** The cDNA that we use is human. But the laboratory that we obtained it from has used it in dogs and there is a good homology between the two. The probes that we use are human probes, but they worked very well for canine tissue.

**Dr. Gagneau:** Is it the cDNA sequence of the myoD gene?

**Dr. Hoff:** Yes.

**Dr. Schwartz:** I would expect that there would be a high level of homology between the two.

**Dr. Salmons:** I never lose an opportunity to agree with Dirk Pette and I agree with him about the possibility that regeneration is what is being observed here. This relates to my question, which is: why should a sequence of myogenic determination factors, which we know intervene at the point where myoblasts become committed to making embryonic muscle? Why should that set of helix proteins be involved in the fast-slow transition which, as we know, is a transition between two adult forms of muscle?

**Dr. Hoff:** We have shown an association between these regulatory proteins and changes among skeletal muscle contractile isoforms that we can't understand at this point because it is very complex. We know that the expression of these regulatory proteins is important in the differentiation from myotubules to the differentiated skeletal muscle. It may be that some repression of their regulation is important in the genetic message to the relatively plastic muscle which has isoforms of all these different types to regulate expression of different isoforms that might be better used in cardiomyoplasty.

**Dr. Pette:** Just a short reply. Myogenic factors are not only expressed when the muscle stems get committed. They are expressed also during myogenesis for a rather long time. And we also know that muscle does not only contain satellite cells but in addition stem cells, which may be turning into satellite cells.

**Dr. Schwartz:** And also, I think that as you stated yourself, these are preliminary results that really need to be confirmed by using very specific techniques. PCR is obviously, as suggested by Dirk Pette, one of the possibilities of working on messenger DNA only.

Chapter 28

# Effect of Mobilization and Stimulation on pH and Temperature in Pedicled Latissimus Dorsi Flaps Used for Cardiac Assist

Robert R. Lazzara, Dennis R. Trumble, Changping Duan, James A. Magovern

## Introduction

The latissimus dorsi (LD) muscle is used clinically for the performance of dynamic cardiomyoplasty (CMP), a surgical treatment for congestive heart failure.[1,2] The LD muscle is also used experimentally as a mode of cardiac assist, utilizing a variety of surgical techniques in a number of different experimental models.[3,4] During LD surgical mobilization there is concern that significant muscle ischemia occurs. Some authors have speculated that muscle ischemia, necrosis, and subsequent fibrosis may in part explain the equivocal clinical results obtained with dynamic CMP.[3,5,6] Studies documenting decreased blood flow to the LD following surgical mobilization generally rely on perfusion studies of blood flow.[5,6] Although blood flow may be reduced, the amount of perfusion remaining after surgical mobilization of the LD muscle may be adequate to meet the metabolic demands of the muscle when it is quiescent. This study was undertaken to determine the acute changes in temperature and tissue pH that occur following surgical mobilization of a pedicled LD flap.

## Methods

Five mongrel dogs were used. All animals received humane care in compliance with the *Guide for the Care and Use of Laboratory Animals* published by the NIH (publication No. 8523, revised 1985). Animals were sedated with acepromazine (0.25 mg/kg), and general anesthesia was induced with pentothal (20

From Carpentier A, Chachques JC, Grandjean P: Cardiac Bioassist. © Futura Publishing Co, Inc, Armonk, NY, 1997.

mg/kg). Anesthesia was maintained with 1–2% isoflurane. A longitudinal incision was made over the anterior border of the LD muscle. The muscle was then mobilized by creating subcutaneous flaps, ligation of intercostal perforators, and transection of tendinous insertions. The origin of the muscle and thoracodorsal neurovascular pedicle were left intact. A left thoracotomy was performed with subperiosteal resection of the fifth rib. The pericardium was opened and tacked to the chest wall. A modified bipolar paraneural lead (Model 4545, Medtronic, Inc., Minneapolis, MN) was placed adjacent to the thoracodorsal nerve and secured in place with 4-0 silk. Threshold voltage and current were measured in all animals and found to be <1.5 volts and 1.5 mAMPs, respectively. Two unipolar sensing leads (Model 6917A-53T, Medtronic, Inc.) were placed 1 cm apart on the right ventricle.

Muscle pH was measured utilizing a Khuri tissue pH monitor (Model 740110, Vascular Technology, Inc., Chelmsford, MA). The pH monitor consists of an IBM PC compatible laptop computer that digitally displays pH in pH units and temperature in degrees Celsius. The pH probe is a microneedle, steel-jacketed pH glass electrode that is inserted directly into tissue (Fig. 1). The thermistor probe is placed simultaneously just adjacent to the pH probe (Fig. 1). The pH probes were calibrated with standard buffer solutions and referenced using a 3M KC1 agar gel bridge, which contacted a silver chloride reference needle.

The pH and temperature were obtained in the distal third of the muscle. Baseline pH and temperature were obtained immediately after surgical inci-

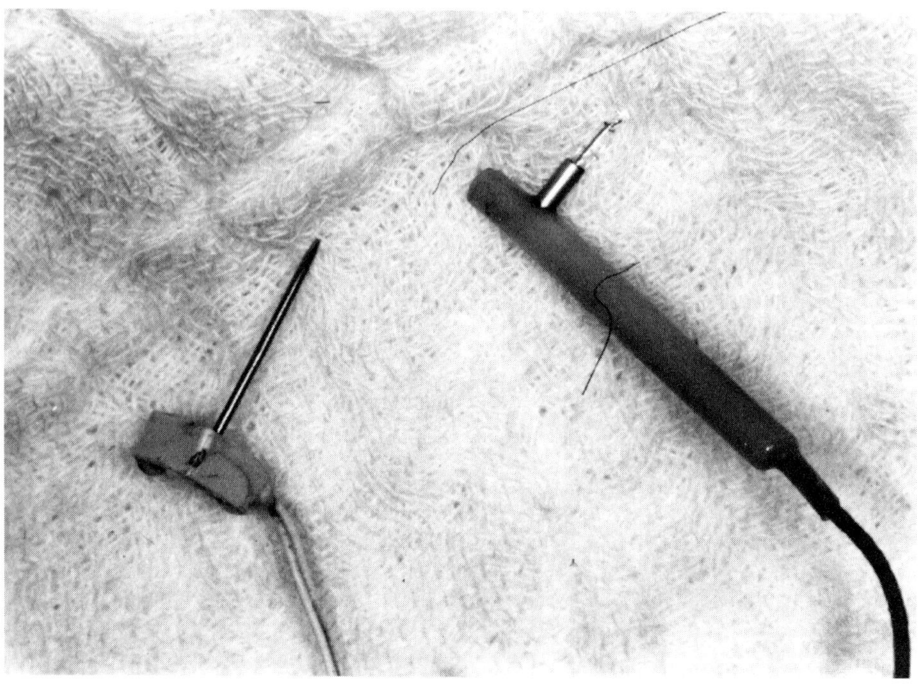

**Figure 1:** *The pH and Thermistor probe in the dog. Probes were placed directly into muscle in the distal third of the latissimus dorsi flap.*

sion, and pHs and temperatures were then obtained following complete surgical mobilization of the LD muscle. This entailed mobilization of subcutaneous flaps, ligation of intercostal perforators, and transection of tendinous insertions using sharp dissection with only the thoracodorsal neurovascular pedicle remaining as the sole vascular supply. The pH was then measured with the LD stimulated at a rate of 60 contractions per minute using single spike stimulation. The pH and temperature were then measured following burst stimulation. Burst stimulation was initiated at a pulse amplitude of 3 volts, a pulse width of 210 μsec, a frequency of 50 hertz, and a burst duration of 30% of the R-R interval. Single pulse and burst stimulation were performed for 1 minute, following which pH and temperature were measured in the distal third of the muscle. The LD muscle was rested for 15 minutes between stimulation protocols to allow for normalization of pH.

Biopsy samples were obtained in two animals before muscle mobilization, after acute stimulation, and after 6 or 12 weeks of chronic burst stimulation. All muscle samples were quickly frozen. Serial transverse frozen sections, 8 μm thick, were cut on a cryostat and stained for myofibrillar adenosine triphosphatase (ATPase) with acid (pH 4.3) preincubation. The slides were reviewed, and two to five representative muscle bundles were evaluated on each stain. The percent slow and fast fibers was calculated by averaging the counts from the representative muscle bundles. In the muscle sections, a fiber was counted as a slow fiber if it stained darkly. Hematoxylin and eosin were used on selected sections and reviewed for degenerative muscle fibers. Statistical analyses were performed utilizing repeated measures of ANOVA for analysis of pH and temperature means ($p<0.05$ was considered significant). Numerical results are expressed as ± standard deviation.

## Results

Baseline pH measured following skin incision was 7.31 ± 0.08. The corresponding temperature at this time was 32.4 ± 0.68°C. Complete surgical mobilization of the pedicled LD flaps resulted in very little change in pH (7.32 ± 0.07). Temperature of the LD muscle decreased to 28 ± 2.1°C; however, this was not statistically significant. Following single pulse stimulation at threshold levels for 1 minute, pH of the pedicled LD flap decreased to 7.25 ± 0.10 and temperature increased slightly to 29 ± 3.0°C. The changes noted after single pulse stimulation from baseline were not significant. Burst stimulation at a pulse amplitude of 3 volts and a synchronization ratio of 1:4 with the native heart rate resulted in a significant decrease in tissue pH in the distal third of the LD muscle (6.98 ± 0.3, $p<0.05$). Temperature at this time did not change significantly from baseline (29.0 ± 3.0°C). Changes in pH and temperature following mobilization, single pulse stimulation, and burst stimulation are shown in Table 1 and illustrated in Figures 2 and 3. Figure 4 compares a biopsy from a left LD muscle obtained prior to complete surgical mobilization with a biopsy specimen taken 6 weeks later from the same muscle site. The 6-week specimen was obtained after a 5-day delay period followed by chronic electrical stimulation at 3 volts, a pulse width of 210 μsec, and a

**Table 1**
Effect of Surgical Mobilization and Electrical Stimulation on Latissimus Dorsi pH and Temperature in Dogs

| | *Baseline* | *Following Mobilization* | *Single Pulse Stimulation* | *Burst Stimulation* |
|---|---|---|---|---|
| pH | 7.31 ± .08 | 7.32 ± .07 | 7.25 ± .10 | 6.98 ± .13* |
| Temperature (°C) | 32.4 ± .68 | 28 ± 2.1 | 29 ± 3.0 | 28.9 ± .50 |

*$p<.05$ from baseline.

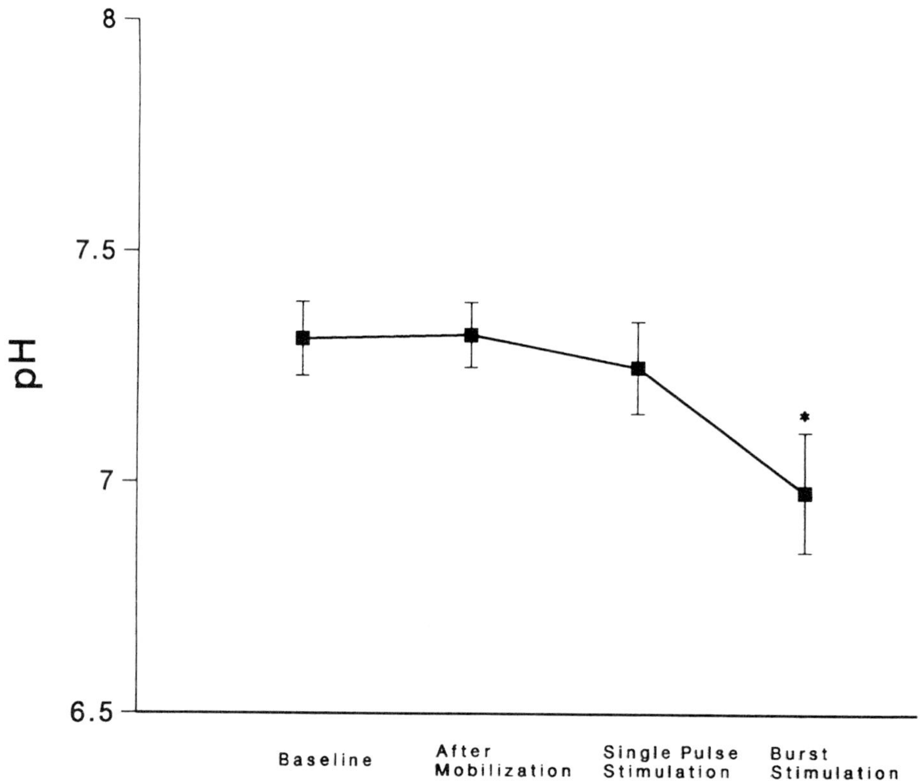


**Figure 2:** *Change in pH in the distal third of the latissimus dorsi flap. The pH attained following burst stimulation is significantly lower than pH at baseline.*

frequency of 30 Hz at a rate of 30 contractions per minute with an Itrel myostimulator (Model 7420, Medtronic, Inc.). Comparison of the specimens reveals an absolute increase in type I fibers from 45% to 59%. No evidence of necrosis or fibrosis on routine hematoxylin and eosin staining are seen despite the temporary muscle acidosis (pH<6.73) caused by burst stimulation 6 weeks previously. Figure 5 illustrates a specimen obtained following surgical mobilization, acute stimulation, a 5-day delay period, and a 3-month

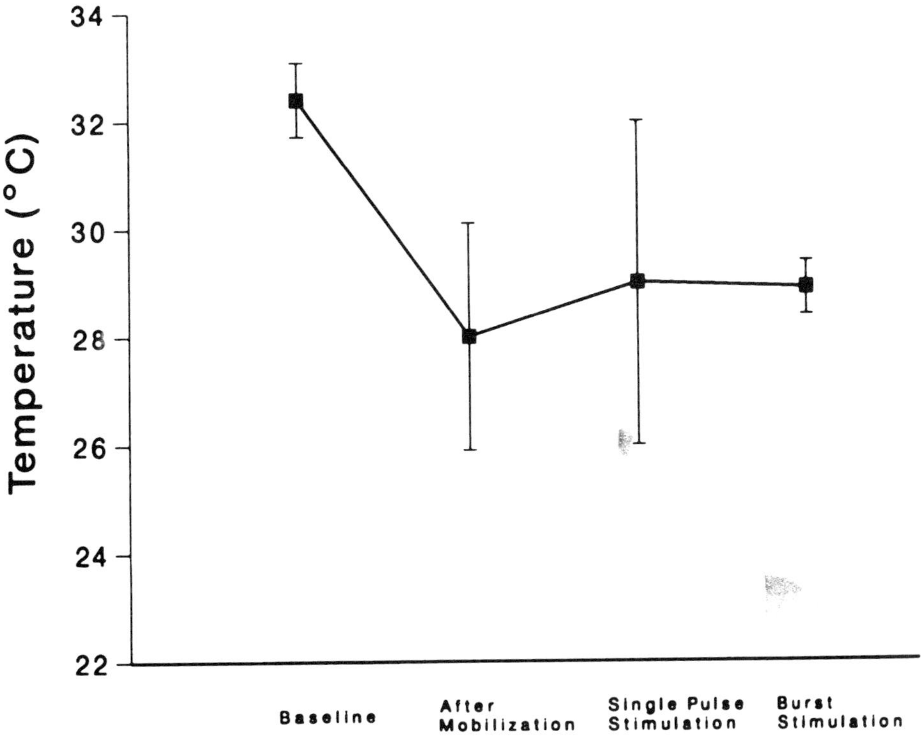


**Figure 3:** *Changes in temperature following surgical mobilization and electrical stimulation of latissimus dorsi flap.*

burst stimulation conditioning protocol. The specimen shows that 81% of the muscle fibers are type I. Hematoxylin and eosin stains show normal muscle bundles with no fibrosis or necrosis.

## Discussion

Latissimus dorsi muscle is currently used clinically for performance of CMP and experimentally utilizing a variety of techniques to perform cardiac assist. Previous work has been done documenting the effect of surgical mobilization on the development of ischemia and necrosis in the LD muscle. There is significant concern that surgical mobilization with division of all blood supply except the thoracodorsal neurovascular pedicle results in significant flap ischemia and subsequent flap necrosis and death, particularly in the distal portion of the LD muscle. If ischemia is produced at the time of surgical mobilization with subsequent flap necrosis and death, this may in part explain the equivocal clinical results that have been obtained thus far utilizing clinical cardiomyoplasty. Tobin and associates used laser Doppler Fluximetry and color change to study perfusion and documented a significant decrease in perfusion to the distal LD flap following intercostal perforator ligation.[6] This flow de-

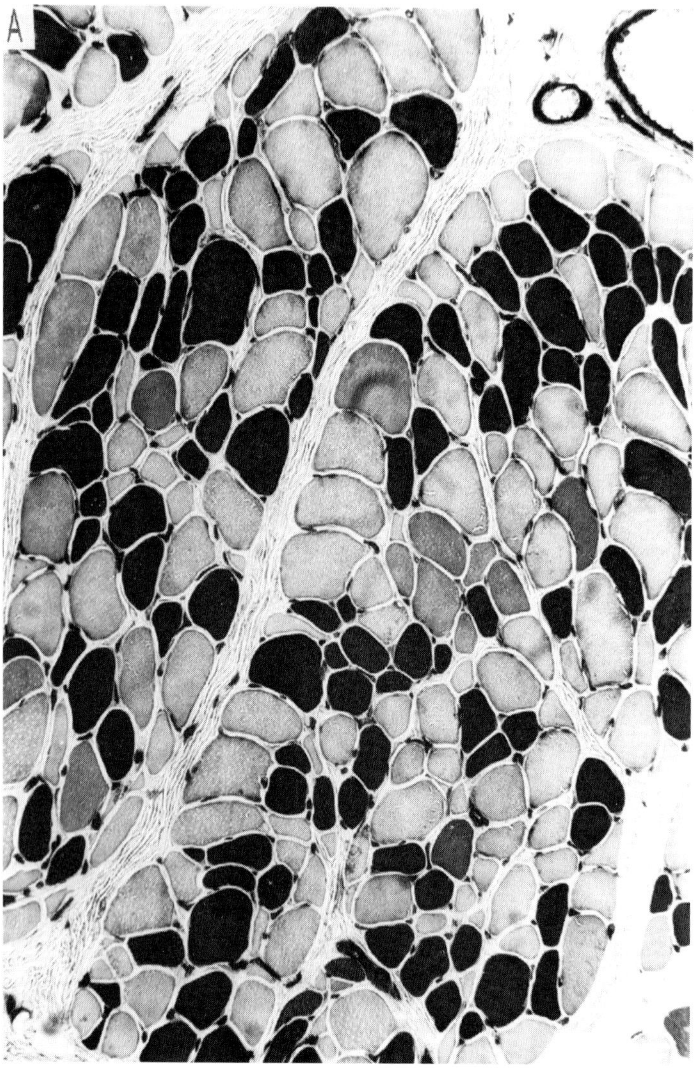


**Figure 4:** *Biopsy specimens (×10) comparing myosin ATPase staining obtained **(A)** prior to surgical mobilization and **(B)** 6 weeks following electrical conditioning. Specimen **(A)** was obtained after inducing a pH of 6.73 following burst stimulation.Continued.*

pression persisted following repeat studies in 1 week. Tuchek documented a 52.8% decrease in blood flow following collateral ligation of the LD muscle in a group of canines.[7]

To our knowledge, the effect on tissue pH and temperature in pedicled LD flaps utilized for cardiac assist has not yet been studied. A decrease in blood flow has been documented following surgical mobilization of the LD muscle, but decreased blood flow and true tissue ischemia may not correlate. Tissue pH directly reflects the balance of metabolic supply and demand, with maintenance of pH representing viable tissue. Baseline pH in this study was mea-

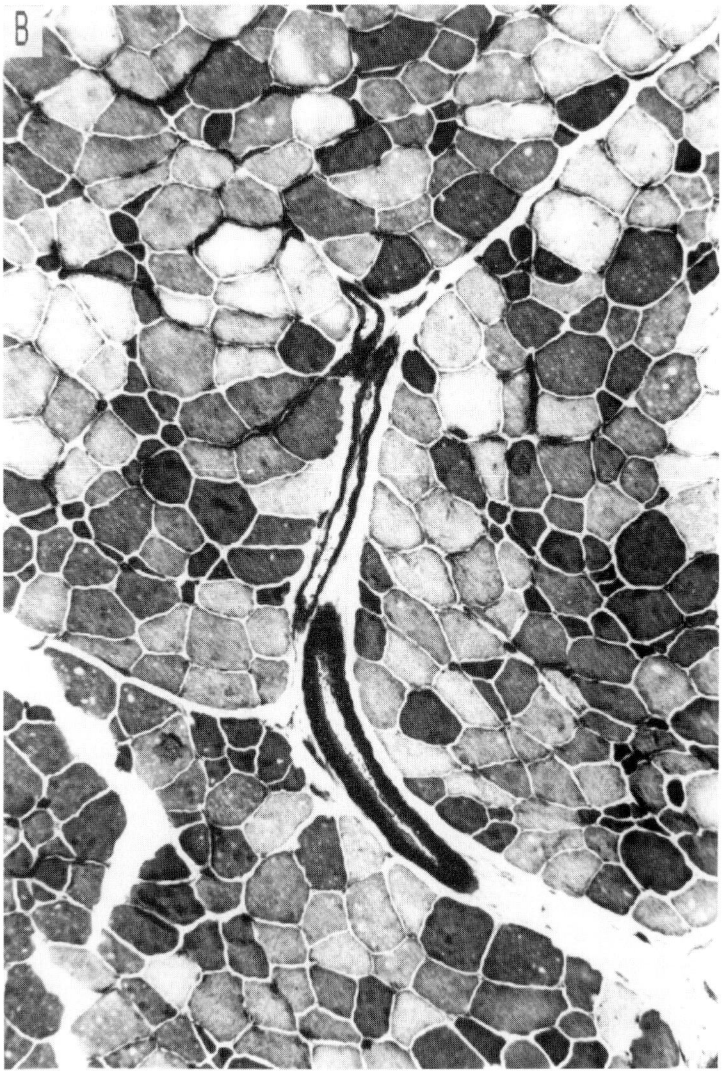


**Figure 4B.**

sured at 7.31 ± 0.08. Following complete surgical mobilization with interruption of all collateral vessels with the exception of the thoracodorsal neurovascular pedicle, pH was 7.32 ± 0.07. Clearly, surgical mobilization in this group of animals did not have a profound effect on initiating muscle ischemia as determined by comparison of pH. Since clinical and experimental use of the LD muscle requires single pulse stimulation to assess threshold voltage and current, our studies also included the effect of single pulse stimulation on pH in the distal LD flap following surgical mobilization. Single pulse stimulation resulted in a decrease in pH to 7.25 ± 0.10. Our protocol called for continuous stimulation for 1 minute with single pulse stimulation. In general, threshold

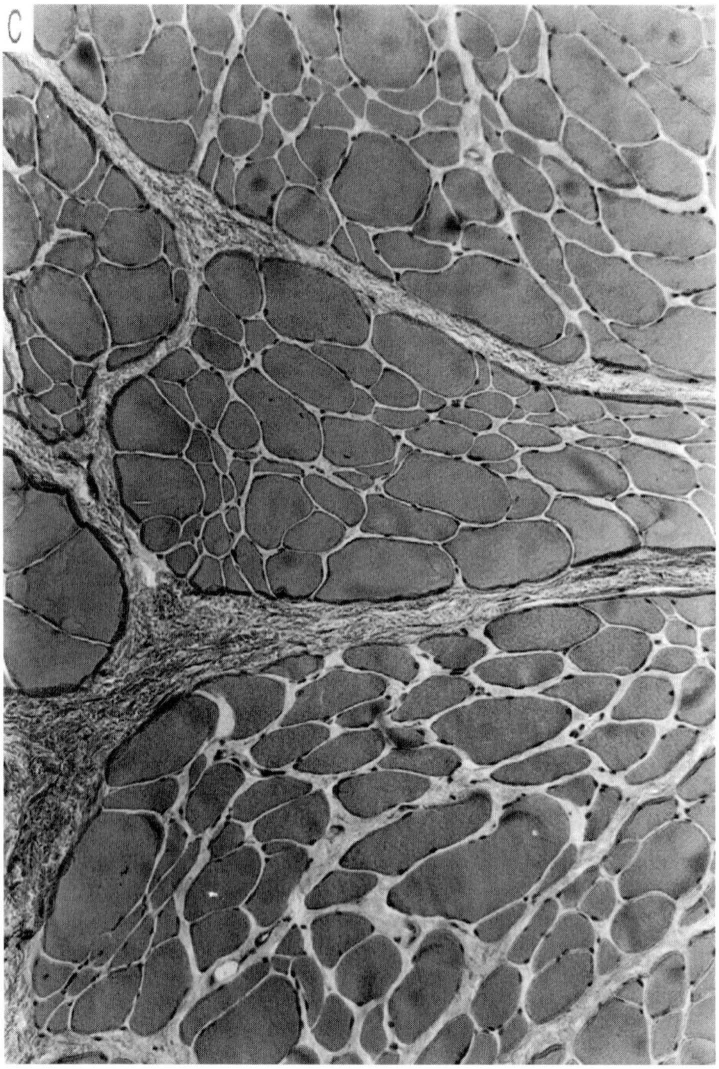


**Figure 4** *(continuation): Biopsy specimens comparing hematoxylin and eosin staining were obtained* **(C)** *prior to surgical mobilization (×10) and* **(D)** *6 weeks following continuous electrical stimulation (×25). Specimen* **(C)** *was obtained after inducing a pH of 6.73.*

testing clinically does not persist for a full minute. Therefore, the pH decrease seen after single pulse stimulation for 1 minute may not be as great if stimulation persisted for only a few seconds. Burst stimulation of the LD muscle performed immediately after surgical mobilization resulted in a significant drop in pH to 6.98 ± 0.13. No significant differences were noted in temperature from baseline.

These results indicate that despite ligation of important collateral vessels during the surgical mobilization of the LD muscle, blood flow is adequate

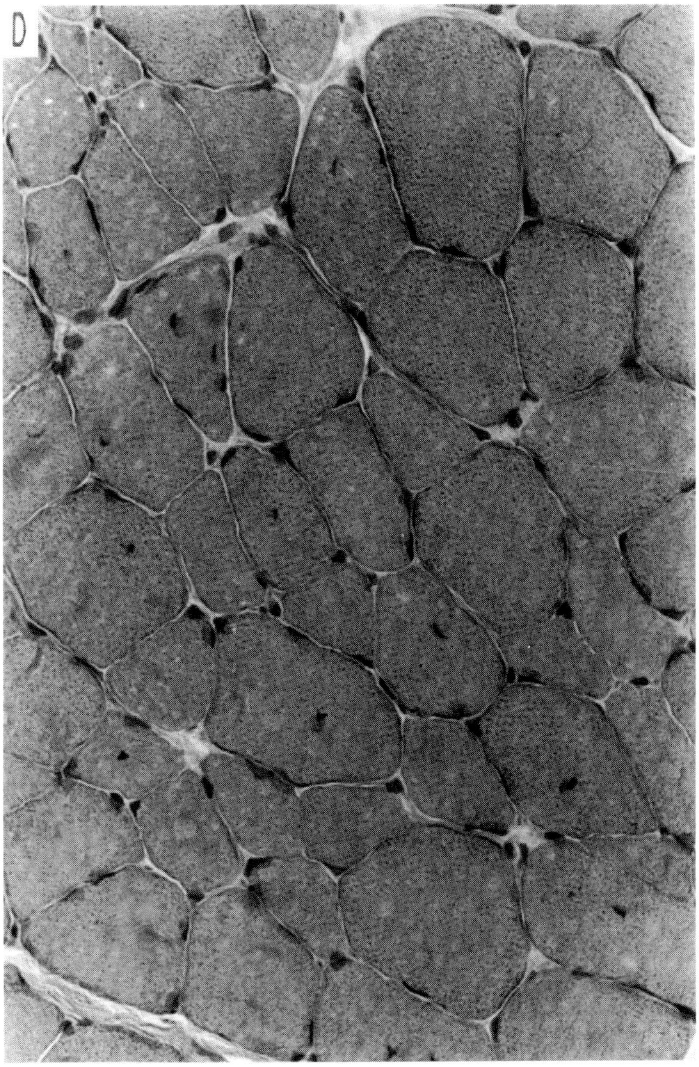

**Figure 4D.**

to maintain the metabolic needs of a quiescent muscle. Electrical stimulation with a single pulse at this time resulted in a small but not significant drop in pH. However, burst stimulation, even at synchronization ratios of 1:4 with the native heart rate, results in a dramatic and profound drop in pH indicative of an imbalance between the needs of the muscle and perfusion. What effect does the acute drop in pH from the single pulse or burst stimulation at the time of surgery have with regard to long-term muscle function and viability? Specimens taken from the distal LD muscle following 6 and 12 weeks of electrical conditioning (Figs. 4 and 5) show an increase in type I fibers and no significant histological damage, which demonstrates that the LD muscle

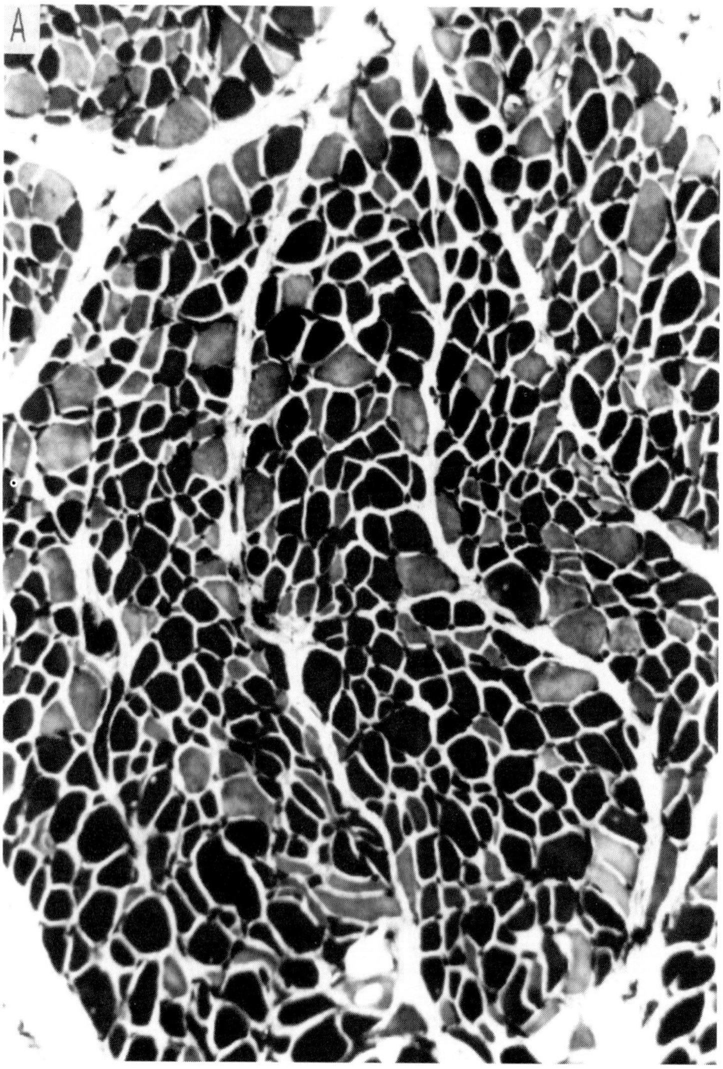


**Figure 5A:** *Biopsy specimen (×10) comparing myosin ATPase staining obtained (**A**) 3 months after initial surgical mobilization and chronic electrical conditioning. Eighty-one percent of the fibers are type I. The pH following burst stimulation at the time of initial surgery was 7.06.*

can tolerate an acute drop in pH for a short period of time with complete recovery. However, persistent burst stimulation of a freshly mobilized LD would likely damage the LD muscle and lead to necrosis and fibrosis. On the basis of these results, we would recommend careful attention to operative technique and gentle handling of the LD muscle during surgical mobilization and threshold testing. Burst stimulation, however, should be avoided pending a vascular delay.

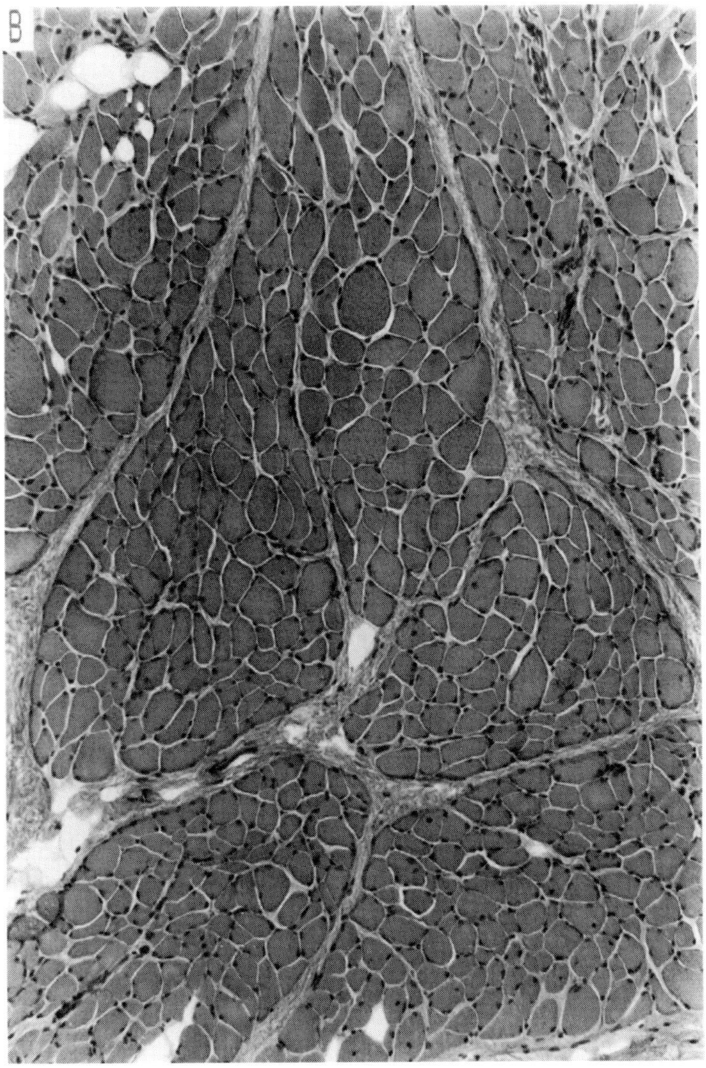

**Figure 5B:** *Biopsy specimen (×10) showing (**B**) hematoxylin and eosin staining obtained 3 months after initial surgical mobilization. The pH following burst stimulation at the time of initial surgery was 7.06.*

## References

1. Magovern GJ, Heckler FR, Park SB, et al: Paced skeletal muscle for cardiac assist. *Ann Thorac Surg* 45:614–619, 1988.
2. Chachques JC, Grandjean PA, Carpentier A: Latissimus dorsi dynamic cardiomyoplasty. *Ann Thorac Surg* 47:600–604, 1989.
3. Pochettino A, Spanta AD, Hammond RL, et al: Skeletal muscle ventricles for total heart replacement. *Ann Thorac Surg* 212:345–352, 1990.

4. Pattison LW, Cumming AVE, Williamson A, et al: Aortic counterpulsation for up to 28 days with autologous latissimus dorsi in sheep. *J Thorac Cardiovasc Surg* 102:766–773, 1991.
5. Mannion JD, Velchik M, Alave A, et al: Blood flow in conditioned and unconditioned latissimus dorsi muscle. *Proceedings of the Second Vienna International Workshop on Functional Electrostimulation,* 1985, p 28.
6. Tobin G, Gu JM, Tobin AE, et al: The anatomic basis for latissimus dorsi cardiomyoplasty flap loss. *Proceedings of the Cardiovascular Science and Technology Conference,* 1991, p 28.
7. Tuchek JM, Lonchyna VA, Pifarre R, et al: Sympathectomy improves blood flow in latissimus dorsi muscle used for dynamic cardiomyoplasty. *Proceedings of the Cardiovascular Science and Technology Conference,* 1992, p 244.

Chapter 28

# *Discussion*

**Dr. John Katz (Charleston):** Did you compare results for more proximal versus distal muscle in your studies?

**Dr. Lazarra:** No, we did not.

**Dr. Lonchyna (Chicago):** We could probably predict that with burst stimulation you would have acidosis in the distal flap. I would like to ask: Did you follow up on what the recovery was like and if the pH returned to normal and how long it took to recover following the burst implantation?

**Dr. Lazarra:** pH returned to normal after approximately 15 minutes.

**Dr. Chachques:** Have you tried, perhaps during the same experiment, with papaverine or a similar technique to improve blood flow to your flap and again test the pH with burst stimulation?

**Dr. Lazarra:** An excellent idea, but one that we have not yet pursued.

**Dr. Chachques:** Am I correct in understanding that the temperature dropped from 32° to 28° when you mobilized the muscle but the pH stayed the same?

**Dr. Lazarra:** That is correct.

**Dr. Chachques:** That would imply that, in fact, the distal muscle was becoming acidotic or ischemic, would it not? Normal tissues, when cooled, if not ischemic, should show a rise in pH. That has been well shown in the heart.

**Dr. Lazarra:** That is true.

**Dr. Chachques:** So, was this muscle ischemic after mobilization?

**Dr. Lazarra:** Well, it depends on how you quantify ischemia and that is what we are attempting to do here by utilizing the pH.

**Dr. Adim (Boston):** Based on your pH technique, I am curious to find out from you what period of vascular delay would prevent this pH change with burst stimulation.

**Dr. Lazarra:** Experimentally, we utilized a 1-week vascular delay, but clinically, we think that a 2-week vascular delay is preferable.

**Dr. Tobin (Louisville):** It is becoming increasingly clear to all of us that the distal muscle is highly vulnerable to ischemia. In your studies, did you simply look at a central zone of the distal third of the muscle or were you able to go through an echelon of zones to more precisely define the area at risk?

**Dr. Lazarra:** These were initial studies and we utilized just the central area of the distal third.

**Dr. Pette:** I just would like to make a comment. The drop in pH, of course, may be deleterious to the muscle with regard to the calcium sequestration because calcium and protons exchange over the sarcoplasmic reticulum membrane. Therefore, a drop in pH and an increase in protons in the cytosome would impair the calcium pump function dramatically.

Chapter 29

# Vasoreactive Responses of the Human Latissimus Dorsi Artery

## Implications in Cardiomyoplasty

Catherine Chardigny, Juan-Carlos Chachques, Tony J. Verbeuren, Jean-Noel Fabiani, Alain Carpentier

### Introduction

Benefits of cardiomyoplasty cannot be sought until 3 to 4 weeks after the procedure. Therefore, candidates for this operation usually require pharmacological support to emerge. Biomechanical support after cardiomyoplasty is directly related to the quality of latissimus dorsi (LD) muscle flap contractility, which depends on the arterial supply. Numerous conditions can alter blood supply to the LD muscle flap: (1) low perioperative cardiac output, (2) technical problems, such as injury, excessive tension, or twist of the vascular pedicle, and (3) vasoconstriction due to inotropic drugs introduced in the postoperative period. The aim of this study is to assess the vasoreactivity of the artery of the LD muscle to different agents used in the clinical setting.

### Materials and Methods

#### Arterial Segments

Human LD muscle artery (n=24) segments were collected from five patients undergoing thoracic vascular surgery. Table 1 summarizes the clinical characteristics of these patients.

One to 2 centimeters of the first collateral branch of the LD artery, near the pedicle, were carefully removed and immediately placed in a container with oxygenated physiological salt solution (Krebs) at 4°C. The time delay from the operating room to the laboratory was 0.5–1 hour.

From Carpentier A, Chachques JC, Grandjean P: Cardiac Bioassist. © Futura Publishing Co, Inc, Armonk, NY, 1997.

**Table 1**
Clinical Characteristics of Patients Undergoing Thoracic Vascular Surgery

| | |
|---|---|
| **Clinical Characteristics of Five Patients** | |
| Age (years) | 49.8 ± 4.6 |
| Sex (male/female) | 4/1 |
| **Preoperative Medication** | |
| Diltiazem | 1 |
| Glyceryl trinitrate | 1 |
| Enalapril | 1 |
| **Anesthetic Protocol** | |
| Flunitrazepam | 5 |
| Phenoperidine | 4 |
| Fentanyl sulfate | 1 |
| Pancuronium bromide | 4 |
| Atracutium dibesylate | 1 |
| Nicardipine | 1 |
| Sodium nitroprusside | 1 |
| Phenylephrine | 1 |

The vessel was then pinned out in a dish coated with silicone rubber, and the surrounding adipose tissue was removed under magnification. The vessel was then cut into 3-mm long segments that were then suspended on wires in organ baths. The number of rings taken from each vessel varied from four to six. The Krebs solution had the following composition (mM): NaCl 118.3, KCl 4.7, $NaHCO_3$ 25, $MgSO_4$ 1.2, $KH_2PO_4$ 1.2, $CaCl_2$ 2.5, glucose 11. The solution was aerated with a gas mixture of 95% $O_2$ – 5% $CO_2$ at 37°C.

## Organ Bath Technique

Artery ring segments were mounted on two stainless steel wires in a 20-mL water-jacketed glass organ bath (Figs. 1 and 2). The upper wire was attached to a force transducer (EMKA Technologies, Paris, France). The lower wire was fixed to a micrometer (Palmer Bioscience, Sheerness, England). A normalization procedure was performed to standardize baseline resting length. The normalization procedure determined the circumference of each vessel at a pressure of 100 mm Hg as previously described.[1] This method allows maximum tension development while standardizing resting tension independent from vessel diameter. Ring segments were allowed to relax for 120 minutes and were rinsed many times in the organ bath in oxygenated, normothermic Krebs solution at this optimal resting length.

## Protocol and Drugs

Agents used for this study are listed in Table 2. Solutions were prepared daily and discarded after each experiment. Initial solubilization and dilutions were realized with distilled water. Arterial segments were contracted using

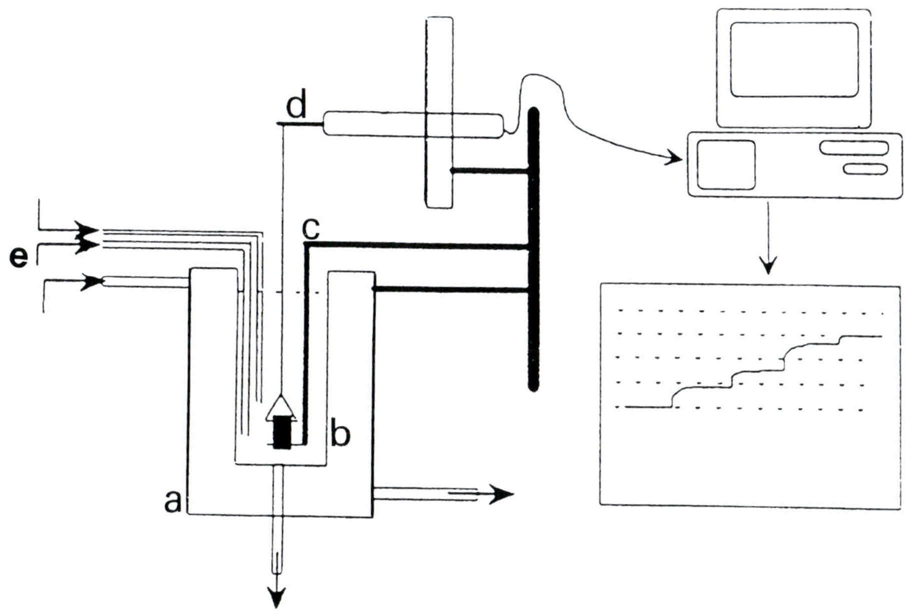


**Figure 1:** *Organ bath apparatus. a = 20-mL water-jacketed glass organ bath; b = artery ring segment mounted on two stainless steel wires; c = lower wire fixed to a micrometer; d = upper wire attached to a force transducer; e = Krebs + 95% $O_2$ - 5% $CO_2$ + 37°C.*

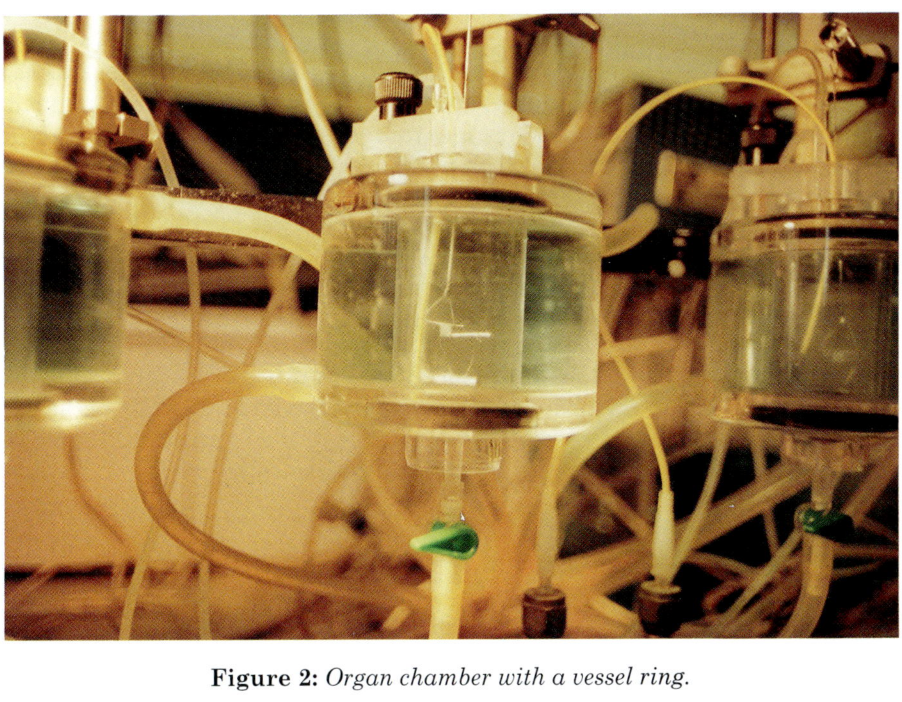

**Figure 2:** *Organ chamber with a vessel ring.*

**Table 2**
Listing of Drugs Used and Their Pharmacological and Cardiovascular Effects

| *Drug* | *Pharmacological Effects* | *Cardiovascular Effects* |
|---|---|---|
| Potassium chloride | membrane depolarization | smooth muscle contraction |
| Epinephrine | $\beta_1$ & $\beta_2 > \alpha$ | vasoconstriction inotropic + |
| | $\alpha > \beta_1$ | vasoconstriction |
| Phenylephrine | $\alpha$ | vasoconstriction |
| Isoprenaline | $\beta_1$ & $\beta_2$ | vasodilation inotropic + |
| Dopamine | DA1 & 2 | renal artery vasodilatation |
| | $\beta$ | inotropic + |
| | $\alpha$ | vasoconstriction |
| Dobutamine | $\beta_1$ | inotropic + |
| Enoximone | phosphodiesterases inhibitor | inotropic + vasodilation |

Potassium chloride (Sigma Chimie, St. Quentin Fallavier, France), epinephrine (epinephrine hydrochloride, Sigma Chimie, St. Quentin Fallavier, France), norepinephrine (arterenol hydrochloride, Sigma Chimie, St. Quentin Fallavier, France), phenylephrine (Neosynephrine*, Merck Sharp and Dohme-Chibret, Paris, France), isoprenaline (Isuprel*, Sterling-Winthrop, Clichy, France), enoximone (Perfane*, Merrell Dow, Levallois, France), dopamine (3-hydroxytyramine, Sigma Chimie, St. Quentin, Fallavier, France), and dobutamine (Dobutrex*, Lilly France, Lyon, France.)

potassium chloride 100 mM (KCl) in order to obtain maximum smooth muscle contraction (100%), rinsed and allowed to equilibrate after contraction. The first step of the study was the screening of the effects of the different drugs on the artery at its optimal resting tension: constriction or dilation or no effect.

*Contraction*

Contraction-response curves were then obtained by adding increasing concentrations of constrictor substance to the organ bath fluid in 0.5 log unit steps. Each step was made when previous maximum contraction was achieved and stabilized. One constrictor agent was studied with each segment. At the end of each test, injection of KCl was applied in order to obtain a reference contraction (the results were expressed as percent of KCl maximal contraction).

*Relaxation*

A submaximal precontraction before relaxation test was induced by norepinephrine $10^{-7}$ M. Relaxation response-curves were obtained by adding increasing concentrations of vasodilator substance to the organ bath fluid in 0.5 log unit steps. One dilator agent was studied with each segment.

## Data Analysis

Forces generated by the vessels were digitalized by a personal computer using the Moise 3 software package (EMKA Technologies, Paris, France). Several parameters were studied in order to characterize arterial segment reactivity: (1) Type of response: contraction or dilation or no effect. (2) Absolute maximum contraction force, expressed as milligram weight, was recorded for each segment and for each constrictor agent. (3) Contraction force was normalized to the maximum contraction with KCl ($10^{-1}$ M) and expressed as percent of KCl contraction. (4) Normalized relaxation force, expressed as a percent of dilation on a vessel precontracted by norepinephrine. (5) Sensitivity, measured by effective drug concentration producing 50% of maximum contraction ($EC_{50}$) or dilation ($IC_{50}$). $EC_{50}$ was calculated from contraction response curves generated by a sigmoidal curve model for every ring segment. $EC_{50}$ parameter was determined by nonlinear curve fitting regression with the simplex algorithm (Caceci and Cacheris, 1984) using the Michaelis and Menten equation (1913): $E = (E_{max} \times C^n)/(EC^n + C^n)$ with E = contraction, $E_{max}$ = maximum contraction, C = concentration, EC = $EC_{50}$, n = Hill's coefficient.

## Results

### *Resting Vessels Parameters*

Twenty-four ring segments were used in this study, obtained from five patients. Resting tension, diameter, and weight are summarized in Table 3. Three segments did not respond to potassium chloride and were eliminated for further tests.

### *Classification of Responses*

The screening of the effects of the different drugs on the artery permitted us to distinguish vasoconstrictors (epinephrine, norepinephrine, phenylephrine), and vasodilators (dobutamine, enoximone). No significant effect was assessed with dopamine or with isoprenaline.

### *Maximum Contraction Force*

The highest maximum contraction force was obtained, respectively, with epinephrine, phenylephrine, norepinephrine, and potassium chloride (Fig. 3).

**Table 3**
Comparison of Diameter and Resting Force

| *D100 (mm)* | *Resting Tension (g)* | *Weight (mg)* |
|---|---|---|
| 0.8 | 6.1 | 6 |
| 0.9 | 6.2 | 6.8 |
| 1.2 | 5.5 | 10.4 |
| 1 | 4.5 | 7 |
| 0.8 | 5.9 | 6.1 |
| = 0.9 ± 0.07 | = 5.6 ± 0.3 | = 7.3 ± 0.8 |

D100 = internal diameter at transmural pressure of 100 mm Hg.

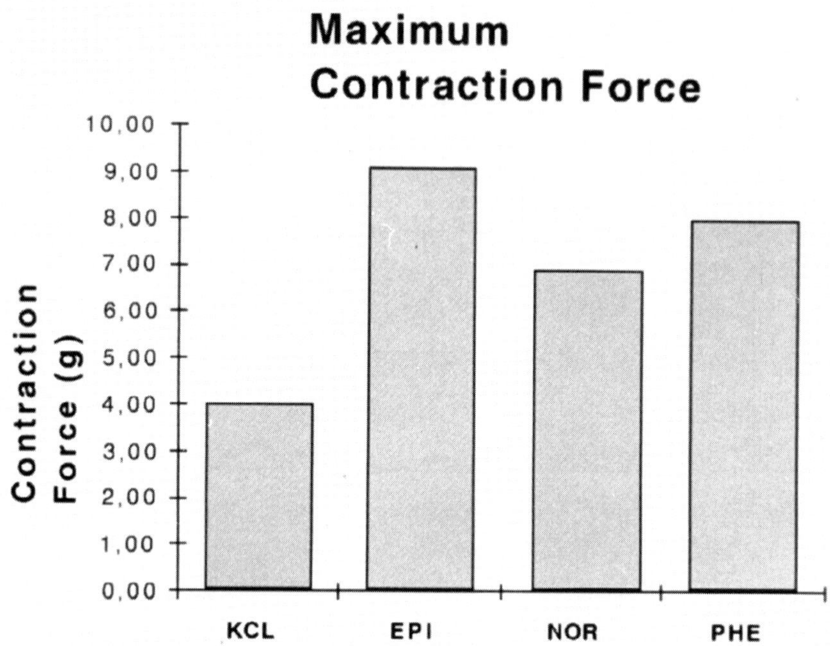


**Figure 3:** *Maximum contraction force of the latissimus dorsi muscle artery in response to potassium chloride, epinephrine, norepinephrine, phenylephrine. KCl = potassium chloride; EPI = epinephrine; NOR = norepinephrine; PHE = phenylephrine.*

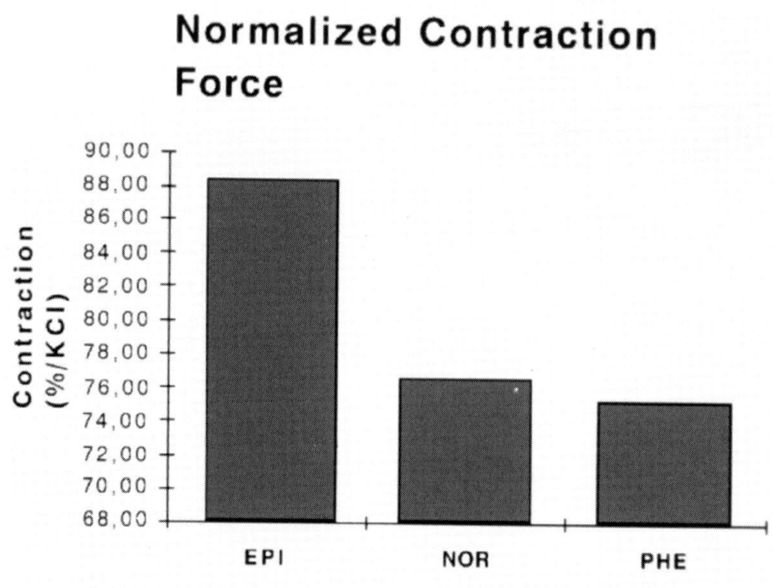


**Figure 4:** *Normalized contraction force of the latissimus dorsi muscle artery in response, respectively, to epinephrine, norepinephrine and phenylephrine. KCl = potassium chloride; EPI = epinephrine; NOR = norepinephrine; PHE = phenylephrine.*

*Normalized Contraction Force*

The highest normalized contraction force, expressed as a percent of KCl, was obtained, respectively, with epinephrine, norepinephrine, and phenylephrine (Figs. 4 and 5).

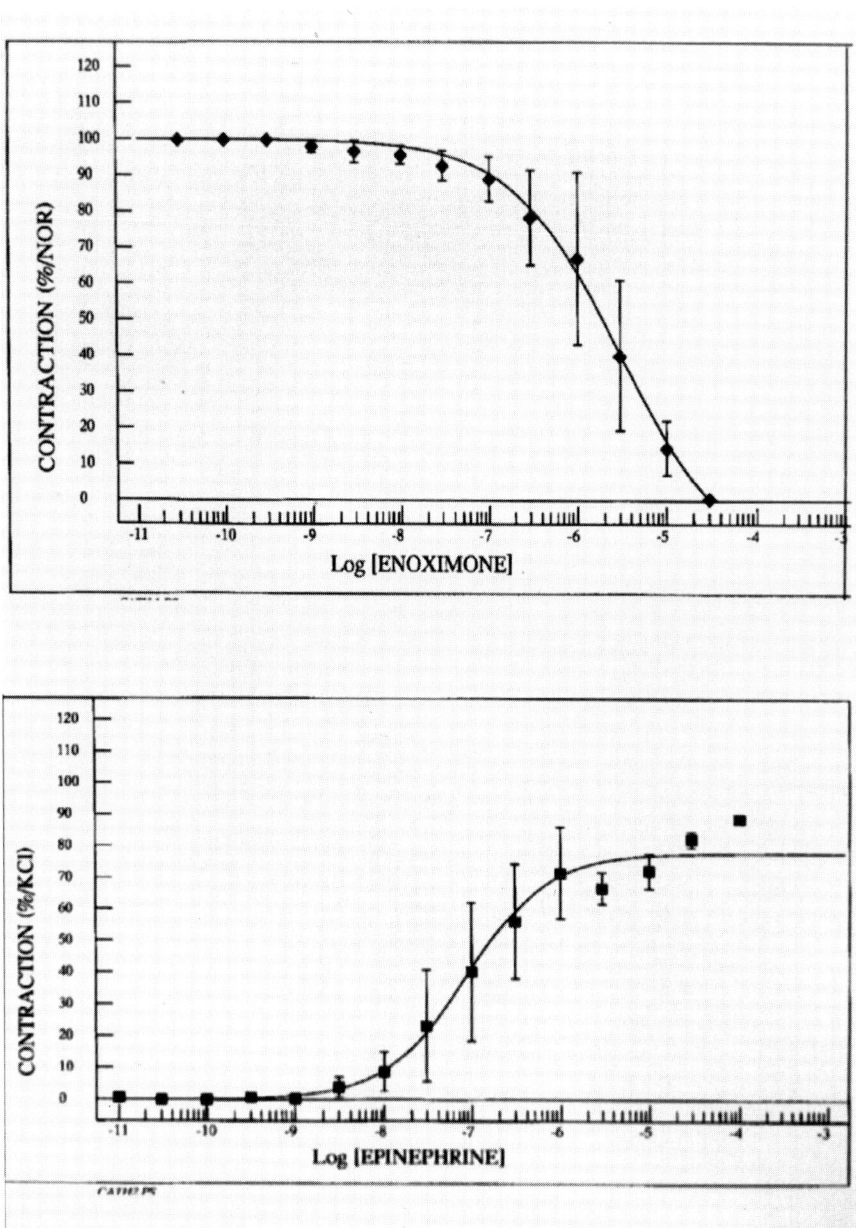


**Figure 5:** *Concentration-response curves to enoximone and to epinephrine. KCL = potassium chloride; NOR = norepinephrine.*

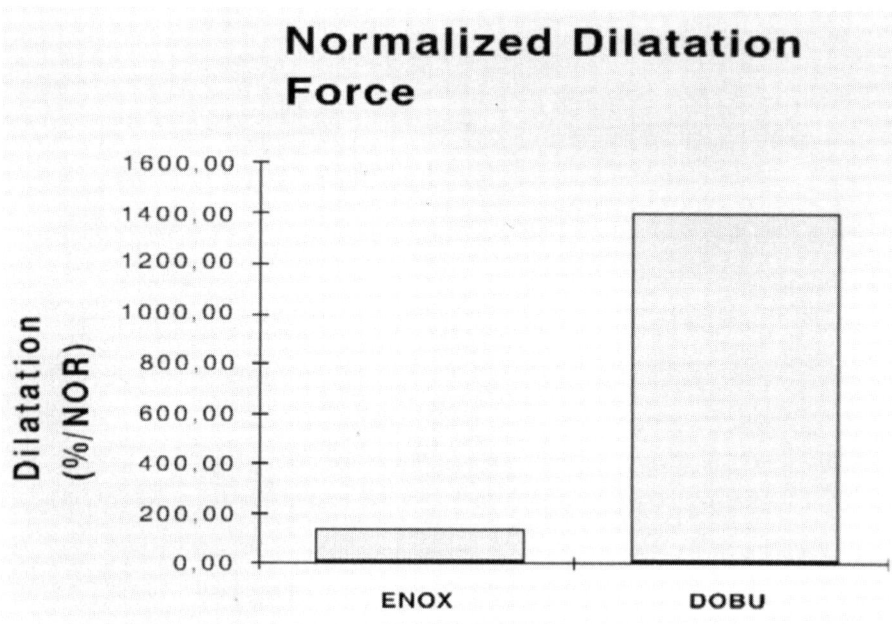


**Figure 6:** *Normalized dilation force of the latissimus dorsi muscle artery in response, respectively, to enoximone and dobutamine. NOR = norepinephrine; DOBU = dobutamine; ENOX = enoximone.*

*Normalized Relaxation Force (Percent of Relaxation on Precontracted Vessel)*

It was higher in response to dobutamine than to enoximone (Figs. 5 and 6).

*Sensitivity*

The most powerful constrictor, corresponding to the lowest $EC_{50}$, was norepinephrine, followed by epinephrine and phenylephrine. The most powerful dilator corresponding to the lowest $IC_{50}$, was enoximone, followed by dobutamine.

## Discussion

*Methodology*

The use of arterial ring segments suspended under isometric tension in the controlled environment of an organ bath provides a precise method to measure changes in circumferential force caused by vasoconstrictor or vasodilator agents.[1] A long incubation period and multiple rinsings of the segments before applying the different pharmacological agents are very important because of the eventual impregnation of the vessels by preoperative and perioperative anesthetics and cardiovascular drugs given to the patients in this study[2] (see Table 1). Some authors demonstrate the limits of this experimental model and prefer to study vessels on cannulated and pressurized segments.[3]

### *Choice of the Latissimus Dorsi Muscle Artery*

The primary vascular supply of the latissimus dorsi is the thoracodorsal artery. This vessel is a branch of the subscapular artery that originates from the axillary artery. The diameter in vivo is usually 0.8 to 1 mm. Histologically, it is a muscular artery (Fig. 7).

Several reports have pointed out differences between the peripheral arteries that may cause differences in contractile properties: the number of receptors on the vascular smooth muscle cell membrane, signal transduction pathway of the receptors, size of the blood vessels, and thickness and histological composition of the media.[4,5]

Cardiomyoplasty benefits are influenced by technical aspects and by skeletal muscle flap response to electrical stimulation.[6,7] Absence of a left ventricular ejection fraction increment occurs in patients with important muscle flap ischemic compromise after the operation. This event demonstrates the importance of the skeletal muscle contractile state for cardiomyoplasty effectiveness and shows the necessity to preserve normal muscle flap perfusion in the immediate postoperative period. Moreover, patients need to be stable enough on medical therapy to maintain normal cardiac output to withstand a

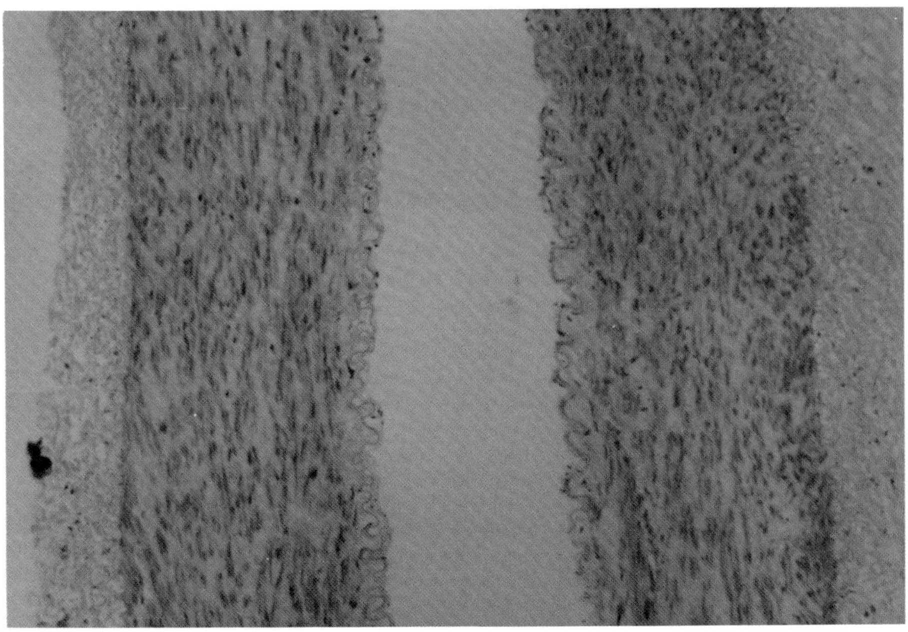

**Figure 7:** *Histological structure of the latissimus dorsi muscle artery showing the muscular media.*

waiting period of 6 to 8 weeks before effective skeletal muscle flap adaptation. Inotropic treatment may compromise the vascularization of the LD muscle flap. Fitzgerald et al.[8] studied cardiac and peripheral arterial responses to isoprenaline in vivo with the Doppler technique. Isoprenaline is a beta adrenoreceptor agonist activating both $beta_1$ and $beta_2$ adrenoceptor sites and is expected to cause dilation and increases in blood flow in certain arteries. The increase in systolic blood pressure together with a fall in diastolic blood pressure represent the classic responses to nonselective beta adrenoreceptor stimulation. They demonstrated different levels in response among different vessels—common femoral artery and posterior tibial artery. The increase in diameter of vessels following the infusion of isoprenaline depends on the density of the $beta_2$ adrenoreceptor population in the different arterial beds and on the extent of reflex sympathetic neurohumoral activation with the resultant alpha adrenoceptor activation, which again depends on the density of alpha receptors in different vascular beds.

## Conclusion

In conclusion, the main interest of this study is to demonstrate variable responses to inotropic drugs commonly used in the clinical setting as inotropic support. Epinephrine seems to be a strong vasoconstrictive agent, but on the contrary, enoximone is drastically vasodilative. These data suggest guidelines for postoperative management of cardiomyoplasty. Obviously, this is a preliminary study and further experiments are necessary to confirm these results and to determine the optimal treatment to be used in the clinical setting.

## References

1. Dignan RJ, Yeh T, Dyke CM, et al: Reactivity of gastroepiploic and internal mammary arteries: Relevance to coronary artery bypass grafting. *J Thorac Cardiovasc Surg* 103:116, 1992.
2. Wyse DG, McMartin G, Mullinger B: Responses of human peripheral arteries to agonists: Similarities and differences. *Fed Proc* 44:331, 1985.
3. Lew MJ, Angus JA: Wall thickness to lumen diameters ratios of arteries from SHR and WKY: Comparison of pressurised and wire-mounted preparations. *J Vasc Res* 29:435, 1992.
4. Van Son JA, Smedts F, Vincent JG, et al: Comparative anatomic studies of various arterial conduits for myocardial revascularization. *J Thorac Cardiovasc Surg* 99:703, 1990.
5. Massa G, Johansson S, Kimblad PO, et al: Might free arterial grafts fail due to spasm? *Ann Thorac Surg* 5:94, 1991.
6. Chachques J-C, Grandjean PA, Carpentier A: Latissimus dorsi dynamic cardiomyoplasty. *Ann Thorac Surg* 47:600, 1989.
7. Moreira LFP, Bocchi EA, Stolf NAG, et al: Current expectations in dynamic cardiomyoplasty. *Ann Thorac Surg* 55:299, 1993.
8. Fitzgerald DE, O'Shaughnessy AM: Cardiac and peripheral arterial responses to isoprenaline challenge. *Cardiovasc Res* 18:414, 1984.

Chapter 30

# Sympathectomy Improves Blood Flow in Latissimus Dorsi Muscle for Dynamic Cardiomyoplasty

J. M. Tuchek, V. A. Lonchyna, R. Pifarre, R. Izquierdo*

## Introduction

It is estimated that nearly 3 million people in the United States and 15 million worldwide suffer from congestive heart failure (CHF).[1,2] Nearly 500,000 new cases are diagnosed in the US each year. This number is likely to increase not only because myocardial infarction patients now survive longer with impaired ventricular function[1] but because the age of the general population is steadily increasing. Even now, CHF is the most common medical discharge diagnosis for patients over 65 years of age.[1] There is a 15–60% annual mortality rate for patients with all functional classes of CHF[3] and nearly 200,000 patients die annually from CHF in the US.[1] It is estimated that in the US 10,000 patients each year develop end-stage CHF with an alarming 50% 1-year mortality.[4] Prognosis is even worse in patients refractory to standard medical management.[5,6]

Congestive heart failure is the inability of the heart to deliver a sufficient quantity of blood to meet the body's metabolic demands. End-stage heart failure carries a dismal prognosis and patients have few options once conventional surgical options have failed and medical therapy has been optimized.[6,7] Cardiac transplantation has revolutionized the surgical treatment of end-stage cardiac failure, but the number of potential recipients far outnumber the available donors. Due to strict selection criteria and the donor shortage, only a small percentage of end-stage CHF patients undergo cardiac transplantation, which may be their only hope for improved quality of life and survival.[7]

Dynamic cardiomyoplasty is an alternative to cardiac transplantation. [8–10]Dynamic cardiomyoplasty is a surgical procedure in which a skeletal muscle, usually the latissimus dorsi (LD) muscle, with an intact neurovascular bundle is wrapped around one or both ventricles of the failing heart. Pulse

*With the cooperation of M. R. Johnson, M. Gerdisch, and J. X. Thomas.

From Carpentier A, Chachques JC, Grandjean P: Cardiac Bioassist. © Futura Publishing Co, Inc, Armonk, NY, 1997.

training (synchronized burst electrical stimulation with a specialized pacemaker) converts the LD muscle from a fast-twitch, glycolytic, fatigable muscle to a slow-twitch, oxidative, fatigue-resistant muscle very similar physiologically and histochemically to myocardium. The trained muscle can then assist the failing heart by synchronously contracting with the myocardium to augment ventricular function. Since the first clinical case performed in France in 1985 by Carpentier and Chachques, more than 250 patients have undergone dynamic cardiomyoplasty worldwide. Much research has been done to perfect the technical aspects of this procedure. Although patients may subjectively improve following dynamic cardiomyoplasty, few studies have shown definitive hemodynamic improvement.

The use of muscle flaps is commonplace in surgery today. They are used to cover exposed vital structures, repair cosmetic defects, or aid in healing wounds needing improved blood supply. The use of a functional muscle flap requires an intact neurovascular bundle.

The LD muscle is a broad, fan-shaped muscle with its origin from the iliac crest and the surface of the external oblique inferiorly to the thoracolumbar fascia and the spines of the lower six vertebrae posteriorly. The muscle inserts into the lesser tubercle of the humerus. It causes abduction and medial rotation of the arm. The LD muscle is divided into three major segments: the transverse, oblique, and lateral segments.

In order for the LD muscle to serve as a potential cardiac assist device, its neurovascular supply must be preserved. The main blood supply to the proximal LD muscle is from the thoracodorsal artery, which usually divides into segmental branches to supply the transverse, oblique, and lateral segments of the LD muscle.[9–11] The blood supply to the distal LD muscle is primarily from the posterior paravertebral perforating vessels with collateral flow from a branch of the artery to the serratus anterior and the paraspinal muscle collateral branches. The LD muscle receives motor innervation from the thoracodorsal nerve,[10–12] which follows the muscle's vascular supply. This neurovascular bundle is surrounded by fatty connective tissue. The nerve typically has a proximal trifurcation that usually enters each of the LD muscle segments separately.

The dissection of the LD muscle involves a lengthy skin incision along the lateral border of the muscle. The LD muscle insertion on the humerus is left intact and the thoracodorsal neurovascular bundle is carefully preserved. The collaterals, however, are ligated as the dissection proceeds. Upon cutting the collateral vessels, it is common to see ischemia of the distal LD muscle so much so that after 1 week, some of the distal LD muscle may remain noncontractile and fibrotic.[13] Paradoxical lengthening of the distal LD muscle due to excessive loading of the portion of the muscle with decreased blood flow may occur.[14] Thus, distal LD muscle ischemia may result in less than optimal function of the wrapped muscle flap.

If blood flow to the distal LD muscle could be improved, flap viability and function should be enhanced. We hypothesized that sympathectomy of the thoracodorsal artery would improve the blood supply of the LD muscle flap before and after ligating the collateral vessels. Sympathectomy may be performed by surgical and/or chemical means. Because the sympathetic fibers lie in the adventitia of the thoracodorsal artery,[15,16] stripping the adventitial layer for 1–2 cm would disrupt this nervous network. It is well known that phenol sympathectomy chemically disrupts the autonomic network and increases regional blood flow.[10] Because so much of the LD blood supply is from the intercostals, the effect of sympathectomy on LD blood flow following transection of the intercostals remains unclear. The purpose of this study was to evaluate the effects of sympathectomy on blood flow to the LD muscle before and after transection of the collateral vessels.

## Methods

Six mongrel dogs 20–30 kg were anesthetized with Rompun and Chloralose with small supplemental doses of Chloralose given as needed to maintain adequate anesthesia (Table 1). The dogs were intubated and ventilated with 21% $FIO_2$ Bird respirator. A femoral arterial line was placed to monitor ABGs and blood pressure. Temperature, blood gases, and blood pressure were kept constant throughout the experiment.

The LD muscle was exposed and the LD neurovascular bundle was identified and isolated. An appropriately sized electromagnetic blood flow probe (Carolina Medical Electronics) was placed around the thoracodorsal artery and baseline blood flow was measured and recorded on a Gould 2800 recorder.

Using a meticulous dissecting technique, the proximal thoracodorsal artery was sympathectomized via circumferential stripping of a 1.5 cm length of the artery's adventitial layer. To ensure complete sympathectomy, five drops of 10% phenol were then placed on a segment of umbilical tape and applied circumferentially to the stripped area. LD muscle blood flow was again measured.

Following sympathectomy, the entire LD muscle was mobilized. The collaterals were transected via suture ligature and the LD insertions were transected, insuring complete collateral flow disruption. The LD muscle was placed in its normal anatomic position to maintain muscle length-tension relationships constant and LD blood flow was again measured.

Similar measurements were made in six sham-sympathectomy dogs that were time-matched controls. All flows were normalized to LD muscle weight and reported in mL/min/100 gm of LD muscle weight. The LD muscle flap was weighed at the completion of the experiment.

**Table 1**
Amounts Needed to Maintain Adequate Anesthesia

| *Canine Model Anesthesia* | *Concentration* | *Dose* |
|---|---|---|
| Rompun (Xylazine) | 20 mg/cc | 0.45 mg/kg, IM |
| Alpha Chloralose | 50 mg/cc | 75–100 mg/kg IV |

## Results

The control dogs' baseline LD blood flow was 7.01 ± 0.71 mL/min/100 gm LD muscle weight, which was similar to the sympathectomized dogs' baseline LD blood flow of 7.30 ± 0.78 mL/min/100 gm.

Following sympathectomy, LD muscle blood flow increased to 9.59 ± 1.20 mL/min/100 gm (an increase of 31.4%). In the sham control group, LD muscle blood flow decreased to 5.83 ± 0.66 mL/min/100 gm after the same 30-minute period (a decrease of 16.8%).

After the LD muscle origins were cut and the muscle's collateral blood flow transected, blood flow in the sham control LD muscle decreased even further to 3.31 ± 0.36 mL/min/100 gm, a total decrease of 52.8% from the baseline flow. On the other hand, the sympathectomized LD muscle blood flow decreased only to 6.91 ± 0.90 mL/min/100 gm, a total decrease of 5.3% from the baseline flow (Table 2).

## Discussion

Over the years, plastic surgeons have become skilled in using the LD muscle for reconstruction of the breast, chest wall, head and neck regions, arm, back, and abdomen. Due to its long neurovascular pedicle with the ability to mobilize the LD muscle with its neurovascular supply intact, LD muscle myocutaneous flaps in humans experience partial necrosis less than 5% of the time. In addition, in cadaver dissections, no significant atherosclerotic changes have been found in the thoracodorsal artery supplying the LD muscle.[17] Because of the blood flow from the thoracodorsal artery, the LD muscle can recover from the initial ischemia seen after collateral vessels are ligated if given a sufficient time for vascular delay.[18] Unfortunately, more than 60% of the LD muscle receives its blood supply from distal perforators.[13] Thus, after cutting the collaterals, blood flow decreases by up to 70% in the distal portion of the LD muscle flap.[19]

The LD muscle anatomy in dogs is similar to that in humans and thus is a good model for use in LD studies.[20] The muscle is large and relatively thin, allowing it to be easily wrapped around the heart. Anatomic variations are uncommon and the muscle is easily dissected. There are few functional defects to the patient after the muscle has been removed from its anatomic position.[21]

**Table 2**
Sympathectomized Latissimus Dorsi Muscle Blood Flow

| | *Mean Blood Flows ± SEM (mL/min/100 gm)* | | |
|---|---|---|---|
| *Group* | *Baseline* | *Sham/Sympathectomy* | *Collaterals Tied* |
| Control | 7.01 ± 0.71 | 5.83 ± 0.66 | 3.31 ± 0.36 |
| Sympathectomy | 7.30 ± 0.78 | 9.59 ± 1.20$^{+}$ | 6.91 ± 0.90$^{+}$ |

$^{+}p<0.025$ when compared to control group.

Dynamic cardiomyoplasty has been purported to improve patient symptoms for a variety of reasons. Dynamic cardiomyoplasty may alter the progression of CHF by decreasing systolic and diastolic wall tension and thus limiting cardiac dilation. It may truly augment cardiac output and decrease pulmonary capillary wedge pressure, thus decreasing patient symptoms. However, although dynamic cardiomyoplasty decreases patient symptoms, evidence to date does not show clear-cut hemodynamic improvement in dynamic cardiomyoplasty patients.[7–10] Certainly, if the distal LD muscle becomes ischemic following the procedure, the hemodynamic benefit of cardiomyoplasty, whatever its mechanism, may be lost.

Patients with moderately severe CHF have elevated resting efferent sympathetic nerve activity to skeletal muscle[12] and elevated sympathetic nervous activity during exercise.[22] Exercise produces excessive skeletal muscle vasoconstriction in CHF patients secondary to neurohumoral reflexes[11] and sympathetic nervous system activation.[23] Such increased sympathetic activity might exacerbate the ischemia seen in the distal LD muscle of CHF patients during (and possibly following) dynamic cardiomyoplasty. We hypothesized that blocking the excess sympathetic tone to the LD muscle could favorably affect LD blood flow and decrease LD muscle ischemia. This effect may also be important in other potential uses of the LD muscle, including skeletal muscle ventricles, aortic counterpulsation, dynamic patches for ventricular aneurysms, and the treatment of some congenital heart diseases.

Early in this century, sympathectomy was found to produce vasodilation in the arterioles of the rabbit ear.[24] In 1949, phenol was first used to perform a chemical sympathectomy.[25,26] Sympathectomy has increased blood flow in human subjects in some studies.[26–29] More recent studies have shown that sympathectomy increases blood flow and decreases total peripheral resistance in nonischemic limb studies.[30] Studies using radioactive microspheres have shown that sympathectomy results in relaxation of smooth muscle fibers in blood vessels.[31,32] Sympathectomy may increase limb blood flow secondary to the opening of AV fistulae.[31,32] Sympathectomy in ischemic canine hindlimbs increased AV shunting in one study but there was no improvement in total capillary blood flow.[33] Doing a sympathectomy may open multiple arteriovenous fistulae in the LD muscle, resulting in a decrease in peripheral resistance and an increase in LD muscle blood flow.[34,35] However, whether sympathectomy actually increases nutritive muscle blood flow remains controversial.

The benefit of sympathectomy may lie in the stimulation of increased collateral blood flow due to the increased pressure gradient created by vasodilation in the 6 to 8 weeks following sympathectomy.[35] Following dynamic cardiomyoplasty, this same 6 to 8 week hyperemic period with increased collateral flow may be enough to decrease or reverse the ischemia seen after taking down the LD muscle. This is the period used clinically in dynamic cardiomyoplasty patients to allow the LD muscle to adhere to the heart, to pulse train the muscle with the implanted pacemaker, and in some cases develop neovascularization. Pulse training during this time changes the LD skeletal muscle to a slow-twitch, oxidative, fatigue-resistant muscle with increased capillary density and increased mitochondrial volume fraction.[36–40] The increase in capillary density may be enhanced by the increase in blood flow after sympathectomy. In our study, sympathectomy clearly improved blood flow to the LD muscle by 31% prior to cutting the collaterals and it preserved the muscle's baseline blood flow following collateral ligation.

Intraoperative arterial vasospasm is due not only to autonomic nervous system stimulation but also to a myogenic reaction[41] that would not be blocked by sympathectomy. Thus, papaverine (which causes vasodilation via smooth muscle relaxation) may be synergistic with sympathectomy's vasodilatory effects.[42] Consequently, the combined use of topical papaverine for short-term and sympathectomy for longer term effects on blood flow to the distal LD muscle during and following dynamic cardiomyoplasty should be explored.

## Conclusion

If one could develop an effective skeletal muscle ventricle using the LD muscle to assist the pumping function of a failing heart, one could eliminate the need for transplant. The ability of the LD muscle to convert chemical power to mechanical power is greater than any man-made device presently being used. Dynamic cardiomyoplasty does not carry with it the infectious complications, possibility of mechanical failure, or rejection potential that an implantable man-made pump does. It also does not carry with it the need for immunosuppression and thus the immunosuppressive side effects that cardiac transplant patients suffer. In addition, the ischemic myocardium may derive collateral blood flow directly from the LD muscle wrap.[40,43,44] Thus, the need to maximize LD muscle blood flow may be important for reasons other than LD muscle contractile function.

We have shown that sympathectomy increases blood flow to the LD muscle. However, several studies will be required before clinical testing is feasible. We are currently using microsphere technology to better quantify the effects of sympathectomy on LD muscle blood flow. It will also be important to determine the effect of sympathectomy on LD muscle blood flow in dogs with end-stage CHF in contrast to the normal dogs that were studied here. Perhaps the effects will be even more pronounced due to the increased baseline sympathetic outflow in subjects with CHF. Further studies will also need to explore the long-term effects of sympathectomy on LD muscle blood flow in contrast to the immediate effects that were studied here.

Sympathectomized LD muscle preps also need to be evaluated with pulse training and after the muscle is wrapped both acutely and chronically. If in fact the ischemic LD muscle is part of the reason equivocal hemodynamic results are being seen in dynamic cardiomyoplasty, any effort to increase blood flow to the LD muscle through sympathectomy or other means could favorably alter the results of dynamic cardiomyoplasty in canine experiments and in human studies.

## References

1. Packer M: Prolonging life in patients with congestive heart failure: the next frontier. *Circulation* 75(Suppl IV)1–3, 1987.
2. Orie JE: Dynamic cardiomyoplasty: A possible alternative treatment of congestive heart failure. *Semin Thoracic Cardiovasc Surg* 3(2):98–100, 1991.

3. Kannel WB, Plehn JF, Cuppler LA: Cardiac failure and sudden death in the Framingham Study. *Am Heart J* 115:869–875, 1988.
4. Franciosa JA, Wilen M, Zuseke S, Cohn JN: Survival in men with severe chronic left ventricular failure due to either coronary heart disease or idiopathic dilated cardiomyopathy. *Am J Cardiol* 51:831–836, 1983.
5. McKee PA, Castelli WP, McNamara PM, et al: The natural history of congestive heart failure: The Framingham Study. *N Engl Heart J* 285:1441–1446, 1971.
6. Wilson JR, Schwartz JS, St. John Sutton M, et al: Prognosis in severe heart failure: Relation to hemodynamic measurements and ventricular ectopic activity. *J Am Coll Cardiol* 2:403–410, 1983.
7. Bontemps L, Itti R, Delahaye F, Jegaden O, et al: Evaluation of stress ejection fraction in patients with severely reduced left ventricular function before and after cardiomyoplasty. *Eur J Nucl Med* 18(8):648, 1991.
8. Magovern G: Introduction to the history and development of skeletal muscle plasticity and its clinical application to cardiomyoplasty and skeletal muscle ventricle. *Semin Thoracic Cardiovasc Surg* 3(2):95–97, 1991.
9. Sola OM, Haines LC, Kakulas BA, et al: Comparative anatomy and histochemistry of human and canine latissimus dorsi muscle. *J Heart Transplant* 9:151–159, 1990.
10. Walsh JA, Glynn CJ, Cousins MJ: Blood flow, sympathetic activity and pain relief following lumbar sympathetic blockade or surgical sympathectomy. *Anaesth Intens Care* 13:18–24, 1984.
11. Wilson JR, Mancini DM, Rein AJ, Georgopoulos L: Exercise produces excessive skeletal muscle vasoconstriction in patients with heart failure (abstract) *Circulation* 82(4):733, 1990.
12. Oren RM, Zavala DC, Schobel HP, Berg WJ, et al: Resting muscle sympathetic nerve activity predicts exercise capacity in human heart failure (abstract). *Circulation* 82(4):692, 1990.
13. Tobin G, Gu J, Tobin A, Barker J, et al: The anatomic basis for latissimus dorsi cardiomyoplasty flap loss (abstract). *Proceedings:* Cardiovascular Science and Technology Conference, 1991, p 69.
14. Levin HR, Curtis W, Tsitlik JE, Sullivan WD, et al: Alterations in regional mechanics and blood flow can explain lack of benefit during cardiomyoplasty (abstract). *Circulation* 84:1412, 1991.
15. Miller ME: *Guide to Dissection of the Dog,* 3rd ed, Ithaca, New York, 1952, pp 149–156.
16. Evans HE, Christensen GC: *Miller's Anatomy of the Dog,* 2nd ed, 1979, pp 1042–1053.
17. Bartlett SP, May JW Jr, Yaremchuk MJ: The latissimus dorsi muscle: A fresh cadaver study of the primary neurovascular pedicle. *Plastic Reconstructive Surg* 67(5):631–636, 1981.
18. Mannion JD, Velchik M, Hammond R, Alavi A, et al: Blood flow characteristics of conditioned and unconditioned canine latissimus dorsi muscle (abstract). Second Vienna Muscle Symposium, p 28, 1985.
19. Durham L, Michael LH, Laurie GM: Regional perfusion of latissimus dorsi pedicle flaps in dynamic cardiomyoplasty (abstract). *Proceedings of Cardiovascular Science and Technology Conference,* Dec 91, p 77.
20. Tobin GR, Schusterman M, Peterson GH, Nichols G, et al: The intramuscular neurovascular anatomy of the latissimus dorsi muscle: The basis for splitting the flap. *Plastic Reconstructive Surg* 67(5):637–641, 1981.
21. Laitung JK, Peck F: Shoulder function following the loss of latissimus dorsi muscle. *Br J Plastic Surg* 32:275, 1979.
22. Sullivan MJ, Kuhn CM, Charles HC, Negro-Villar R, et al: Skeletal muscle adrenergic activation is increased at rest and during exercise in chronic heart failure (abstract). *Circulation* 84(4):296, 1991.
23. Leuenberger U, Sinoway L, Davis D, Baily R, et al: Norepinephrine spillover is elevated even with low intensity dynamic exercise (abstract). *Circulation* 82(4):693, 1990.
24. Bernard C: Influence du grand sympathetique sur la sensibilité et sur la calorification. *C R Soc Biol (Paris)* 3:163–164, 1851.

25. Brunn J, Mandl F: Die Paravertebrale Injektion Zur Bekämpfung Visceraler Schmerzen. *Wiener Klin Wochensch* 37:511–514, 1924.
26. Haxton HA: Chemical sympathectomy. *Br Med J* 1026–1028, 1949.
27. Silverman NA: Left ventricular function changes after cardiomyoplasty in patients with dilated cardiomyopathy (letter to the editor). *J Thoracic Cardiovasc Surg* 101(7):156–157, 1991.
28. Lantsberg L, Goldman M: Lower limb sympathectomy assessed by laser Doppler blood flow and transcutaneous oxygen measurements. *J Med Engineering Technol* 14(5):182–183, 1990.
29. Stewart DJ, Münzel T, Jürgen H, Bassenge E: Discrepancy between initial and steady-stage resistance vessel responsiveness to short-term nitroglycerine exposure in the hindlimb of conscious dogs. *J Cardiovasc Pharmacol* 12:144–151, 1988.
30. Vulpio C, Borzone A, Iannance C, Agnes S, et al: Lumbar chemical sympathectomy in end-stage of arterial disease: Early and late results, Angiology. *J Vasc Dis* 89:948–952, 1989.
31. Cronenwett JL, Lindenauer SM: Direct measurements of arteriovenous anastomotic blood flow after sympathectomy. *Surgery* 82:82–89, 1977.
32. Scarpino JH, Delaney JP: Lumbar sympathectomy and arteriovenous shunting. *Surg Forum* 22:176–178, 1971.
33. Strandness DE, Sumner JR: Therapy of occlusive arterial disease. In ed(s): *Hemodynamics for Surgeons.* New York, Grune & Stratton, 1975, pp 317–341.
34. Cronenwett JL, Lindenauer SM: Hemodynamic effects of sympathectomy in ischemic canine hindlimbs. *Surgery* 87(4):417–424, 1980.
35. Cronenwett JL, Shellito JL, Luce JL, et al: Interaction of hindlimb blood flow, AV shunting and AV oxygen difference. *J Surg Res* 36(3):223–229, 1984.
36. Salmons S, Vrbova G: The influence of activity of some contractile characteristics of mammalian fast and slow muscle. *J Physiol* 201:535–549, 1969.
37. Cotter MA, Hudlicka O, Pette D, et al: Changes of capillary density and enzyme pattern in fast rabbit muscles during long-term stimulation. *J Physiol* 230:34–35, 1973.
38. Cousins MJ, Wright CJ: Graft muscle, skin blood flow after epidural block in vascular surgical procedures. *Surg Gynecol Obstet* 133:59–64, 1971.
39. Hudlicka O, Brown M, Cotter M, et al: The effect of long-term stimulation of fast muscles on their blood flow, metabolism, and ability to withstand fatigue. *Pflügers Arch* 369:141–149, 1977.
40. Mannion JD, Magno MG, Buckman PD, et al: Acute muscle stimulation after latissimus dorsi cardiomyoplasty increases collateral blood flow from skeletal muscle to chronic ischemic myocardium (abstract). *Proceedings: Cardiovascular Science and Technology Conference,* Dec 1991, p 81.
41. Samson RH, Gupta SK, Scher LA, et al: Arterial spasm complicating distal vascular bypass procedures. *Arch Surg* 117:973–975, 1982.
42. Galt SW, Cronenwett JL: The interaction of vasodilating drugs and sympathetic blockade in normal and ischemic canine hindlimbs. *J Vasc Surg* 13(6):861–866, 1991.
43. Mannion JD, Buckman PD, Magno M, et al: Collateral blood flow to the myocardium from skeletal muscle in goats. Abstracts, Coronary Physiology, *FASEB* 5(4):A695, 1991.
44. Mannion JD, Magno MG, Buckman PD, et al. Acute muscle stimulation after latissimus dorsi cardiomyoplasty increases collateral blood flow from skeletal muscle to chronic ischemic myocardium (abstract). 18th ESAO Congress, *Intern J Artificial Org* 14(9), 1991.

Chapter 31

# Improved Viability of Latissimus Dorsi Muscle for Heart Wrap

Patricia C. Keelen, John H. Barker, Johannes M. Frank, Gary L. Anderson, Gordon R. Tobin

## Introduction

Since cardiomyoplasty procedures were first proposed, the latissimus dorsi (LD) muscle has become the muscle of choice for wrapping a failing heart.[1] Most research done in cardiomyoplasty has centered on such things as hemodynamic improvements[2–4] and skeletal muscle transformations.[5,6] Throughout all of this research, little attention has been paid to the surviving length of the LD muscle when it is used in cardiomyoplasty procedures.

Reconstructive surgeons have long used the LD muscle as a workhorse for coverage of large tissue defects. It is regularly used for reconstructions of the breast,[7] chest wall,[8] head and neck,[9] and in free tissue transfers.[10] Their experiences have shown them that if the entire LD muscle is raised in a single surgical procedure—as is done in cardiomyoplasty—the distal portion of the muscle will almost always become ischemic and go on to necrose. To avoid this problem, reconstructive surgeons often use only the proximal LD muscle.

In cardiomyoplasty, the entire length of the LD muscle is needed to wrap the often dilated heart. Depending on the muscle length and degree of heart dilation, a pericardial patch must sometimes be used in order to complete the wrap.[11] Regardless of whether a patch is needed, a healthy, well-perfused distal portion of the LD muscle is essential for optimal function of the wrap. Therefore, any distal LD muscle necrosis would not only effectively reduce the length of an already insufficient amount of tissue, but would also interfere with the mechanical function of an important part of the wrap.

Perhaps the most important advance in flap surgery was when surgeons recognized the importance of planning their flaps within the parameters of the naturally occurring vasculature of the donor tissue. Surgeons began designing

From Carpentier A, Chachques JC, Grandjean P: Cardiac Bioassist. © Futura Publishing Co, Inc, Armonk, NY, 1997.

flaps in which blood supply through the pedicle directly nourished all of the tissue within the flap.[12] For this, an in-depth knowledge of vascular anatomy is essential.[13] This improvement of knowledge and technique decreases the probability that ischemia-induced necrosis will occur. However, there are times when even these methods do not enable surgeons to design flaps that will meet the structural parameters of a given defect. For example, there may be no donor site that will provide a flap or combination of flaps to fill a certain defect, or the surgeon may need a very large flap for which there can be no reliable blood supply throughout. In situations such as these, a staged procedure known as delay can be used to help prevent necrosis.[12,14–29]

Delay consists of rendering a tissue partially ischemic by ligating some of its blood supply. It is left for 7–20 days (hence the term *delay*), and then lifted as a flap in a second intervention. Clinically, delay is used mainly in skin, and consequently, the majority of research on delay has been in skin flap models.[12,14–29] There is active controversy as to whether delay should be used in skeletal muscle because no one has conclusively proven its effectiveness in preventing muscle flap necrosis.[30,31]

Though delay has proven to be reliable in consistently preventing skin flap necrosis, the mechanisms by which it acts are not fully understood. Experimental studies indicate that microcirculatory changes—either in the form of vascular reorganization[12,14,25] or as the result of metabolic[22,26] or other changes[15–20,22–25,27,28] within the tissue—play an important role in the mechanisms by which delay prevents necrosis.

In the present study, we had two goals. The first was to determine whether delay prevents necrosis in skeletal muscle. The second was to develop a model in which we could directly observe and quantitatively analyze delay-induced microvascular changes with the hope of discovering the mechanisms by which delay benefits tissue.

## Materials and Methods

### Model

The male homozygous (hr/hr) hairless mouse was chosen due to the thin structure of its LD muscle, which allows direct microscopic observation and measurement of skeletal muscle microcirculation using high magnification video microscopy. The muscle measures 200 μm thick, 2.0 cm long, and 1.2 cm at its widest point.

The vascular anatomy of the hairless mouse LD muscle is similar to that of humans. It presents a single neurovascular pedicle (thoracodorsal artery, vein, and nerve) and has a segmental blood supply arising from perforating vessels and nerves.

### Flap Construction

Twelve male homozygous hairless mice (30–35 g; 24–28 wk) were divided into two groups: delayed (n=5) and nondelayed (n=7). For all manipulations of the animals, pentobarbital (60 mg/kg; ip) anesthesia was used.

In both groups, the left LD muscle was exposed through a paraspinal incision. In the delayed group, 10 days prior to flap creation, 2–4 vessel perforators feeding the muscle were ligated. The principal vascular pedicle (arising from the thoracodorsal artery, vein, and nerve) and a single distal perforator were left intact, creating a bipedicle blood supply similar to that of a bipedicle skin flap. In nondelayed animals, all perforators, including the distal perforator, were ligated in a single procedure, leaving the muscle solely dependent for its blood supply on the vascular pedicle (Fig. 1). Thus, the two groups were different only in that the distal perforator in the delayed group was divided in a second operation, whereas in the nondelayed animals it was ligated simultaneously with the other perforators.

To prevent vascular ingrowth into the LD muscle from nearby tissues, the muscle was wrapped in an inert plastic film.[33] After each procedure, the LD muscle was sewn back into its original bed (9-0 nylon) and the skin incision closed with (6-0 nylon) interrupted sutures.

## Observation and Measurement

Observation of flap necrosis was performed using high magnification (×60) video microscopy. The LD muscle was gently extended and held in place over a small platform by eight suture (9-0 nylon) loops placed equidistantly

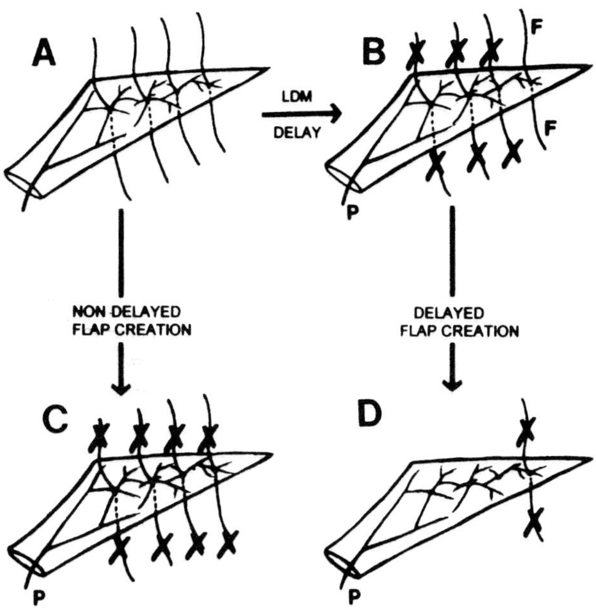


**Figure 1:** *(A) Latissimus dorsi muscle (LDM) with all of its blood supply—pedicle (P) and perforators (F)—intact. (B) LDM made partially ischemic (delayed) by ligating all but two vessel groups (P & F) 10 days prior to flap creation. (C & D) All vessels except pedicle ligated, creating a nondelayed (C) and a delayed (D) LDM flap.*

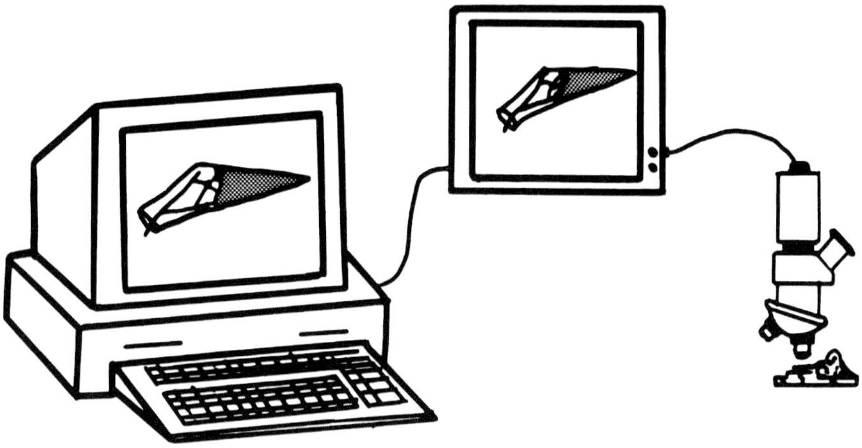

**Figure 2:** *To observe and quantify latissimus dorsi muscle flap necrosis, the anesthetized animal is placed on the stage of a vital microscope. The muscle is epi-illuminated and observed at high (×60) magnification. This image is displayed and filmed using a monitor and video camera. Computer-assisted digitized planimetry is used to quantify necrosis.*

around the perimeter of the muscle. The mouse was placed on the stage of a stereomicroscope (Zeiss Stemi SV 6), and the LD muscle was observed and recorded using a video camera (Microimage Video Systems, RGB/YC/NTSC, Boyentown, PA) and monitor (Trinitron Color Video Monitor, Sony Model No. PVM-1943MD).

The video images were transferred to a personal computer where quantification of necrosis was performed 5 days after flap creation using digitized planimetry (Fig. 2). Percent necrosis was calculated from total flap surface area and necrotic area ($mm^2$).

## Protocol

Figure 3 shows the experimental protocol. At day 0, LD muscle flaps were created in both delayed and nondelayed animals. Ten days prior to this, the LD muscles of the delayed animals were partially elevated. Five days after flap creation, necrosis measurements were taken in both groups.

### *Animal Maintenance*

The mice were housed in individual cages in a room with controlled temperature (24°C). All animals were maintained on commercially available, balanced rodent food and tap water ad libitum. Upon completion of the experiments, the animals were sacrificed with an overdose of pentobarbital (100 mg/kg; ip). All handling of animals was performed in accordance with the In-

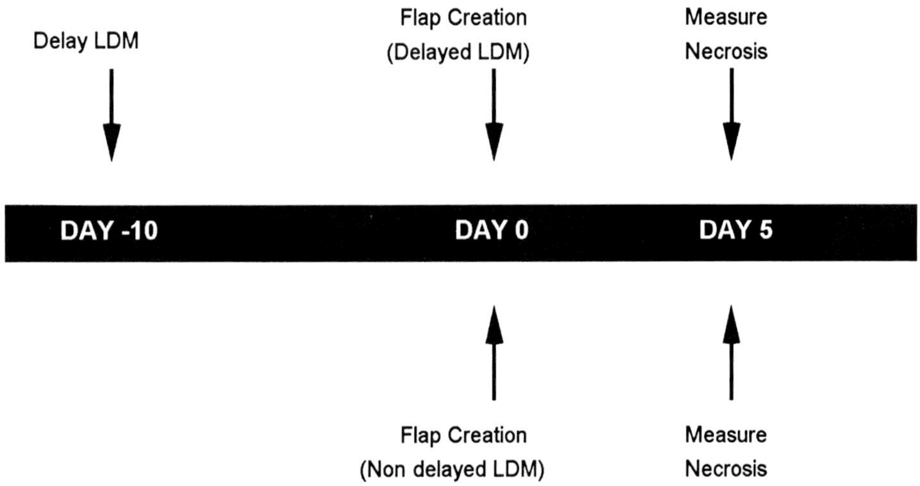


**Figure 3:** *The time course of the experiment consists of creating the latissimus dorsi (LDM) flap (day 0) and subsequently measuring the amount of necrosis (day 5) in both delayed and nondelayed groups. In the delayed group, the LDM is partially elevated 10 days prior to flap creation.*

stitutional Animal Care and Use Committee (IACUC) guidelines at our AAALAC-approved institution.

## Statistics

The results from this experiment were statistically analyzed using Student's *t*-test and are presented as mean ±SEM.

# Results

## Quantitative Results

The results from our experiment show that delay significantly decreased the amount of LD muscle necrosis from 57 ± 9% in nondelayed flaps to 22 ± 3% in delayed flaps (Fig. 4).

## Qualitative Results

The homozygous (hr/hr) hairless mouse LD muscle is an excellent model in which to study microcirculatory changes occurring throughout delay. It is sufficiently thin to permit high magnification epi-illumination for observation and measurement of vascular parameters with the perforators left intact.

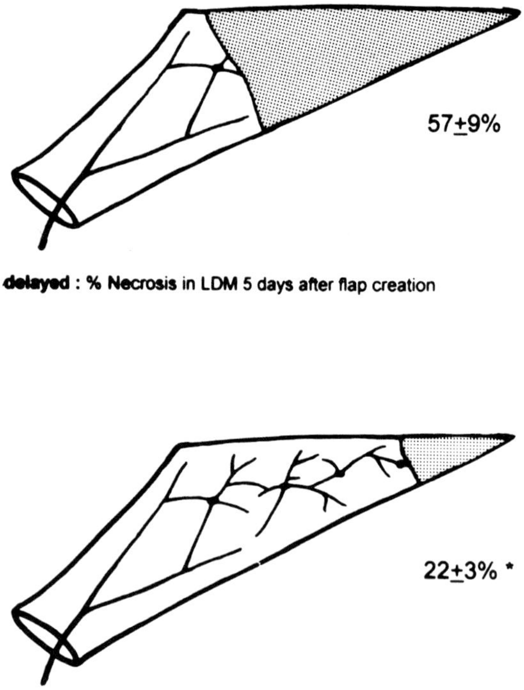


**Figure 4:** *Delay significantly (p<0.01) reduces LDM flap necrosis compared to nondelayed flaps.*

## Discussion

In reconstructive surgery, distal flap necrosis due to ischemia continues to be a problem. In recent years, importance has been placed on knowledge and recognition of vascular anatomy in flap design. This attention to vascular structures has drastically improved the success rate of flap surgeries. However, there are circumstances in which such knowledge is insufficient for providing a desired surgical result. In these cases, a surgeon can use delay to prevent flap necrosis.

Although the methods used to produce delay vary slightly from flap to flap, basically delay consists of dividing part of the blood supply to a tissue prior to flap creation. The time period of delay between the first and second operations remains primarily a matter of surgeon's preference. In our study, we decided on a delay of 10 days based on literature describing delay in skin flaps and on our own clinical experiences.

The first part of our experiment was designed to answer questions about the effectiveness of delay in skeletal muscle. The method we used in delaying the flap was based on the bipedicle method of delaying skin.[12,14–18,20–23,25–28] In this technique, parallel skin incisions are made, and the area designed to be the flap is undermined. The skin flap is left on two pedicles for up to 3 weeks and then isolated on a single pedicle for transfer. In the hairless mouse LD muscle model, we ligated all vessels feeding the muscle except for its anatomic vascular pedicle and the most distal intercostal perforator. The muscle was left with this bipedicle blood supply for 10 days, at which time the distal perforator was ligated to create a single pedicle flap. This "flow-through" method of delaying the LD muscle was effective in increasing survival length of the flap. We found that delay significantly reduced necrosis from 57 ± 9% in nondelayed flaps to 22 ± 3% in delayed flaps.

Over the years, numerous experimental flap models have been designed and many measuring techniques used to quantify tissue perfusion. Dye injections have been used to determine flap survival length,[28] functional flow changes during delay have been measured using microspheres,[18,27,29] xenon washout,[19] and oxygen levels.[22] The fact that all of these are indirect methods of analyzing the microcirculation has led to contradictory results.

Based on the varying results from these indirect measuring techniques, several hypotheses concerning the mechanisms by which delay prevents necrosis have developed. Gillies described delay in tubed pedicle skin flaps, and he claimed that delay causes a reorientation of vessels along the long axis of the flap.[17] German,[12] Milton,[24] and Braithwaite[14] agree that vascular anatomic changes are the key to the delay effect. Others think that delay enhances circulation by causing vasodilation,[15,16] ischemia,[23–25] inflammation,[22,26] denervation,[23] or decreased shunting away from nutritional circulatory pathways.[27]

Probably all of these, either directly or indirectly, contribute to the beneficial effects of delay. The one element common to all of these hypotheses is the importance placed on the microcirculation, where nutritional exchanges within the tissue occur. The second goal of our experiment was to develop an animal model in which we could study the mechanisms of delay at the microcirculatory level. The two principal factors that came into play in selecting a model were (1) that the animal's muscle presents a vascular anatomy similar to that of humans, and (2) that the muscle must be one in which it is possible to make direct observations and measurements of microcirculatory changes throughout delay. After pilot studies in which we also considered the LD muscles of rats, hamsters, and gerbils, we decided that the hairless mouse LD muscle best meets these two criteria. It is ideal for making direct observations and measurements of microvascular parameters such as vessel lengths, diameters, directionality, and tortuosity. To make these measurements, the same system described above (Fig. 2) for quantifying necrosis can be employed.

The results of this experiment suggest that delay could be useful for enhancing LD muscle surviving length in cardiomyoplasty procedures. The portion of the LD muscle that is at risk for necrosis is the distal muscle—also an important area in terms of wrap function. Delaying the muscle prior to elevating it on its neurovascular pedicle could help ensure optimal contractile function of the wrap. In experiments currently under way in our lab, we are using the hairless mouse LD muscle microcirculation model to gain a better understanding of the mechanisms by which delay acts to prevent skeletal muscle necrosis. This knowledge will be used to develop alternative treatment modalities for reproducing the beneficial effects of delay, both for cardiomyoplasty and reconstructive surgeries.

## References

1. Hume WI: Construction of a functioning accessory myocardium. *Transactions of the Southern Surgical Assoc* 79:200, 1968.
2. Lee KF, Dignan RJ, Parmar JM, et al: Effects of dynamic cardiomyoplasty on left ventricular performance and myocardial mechanics in dilated cardiomyopathy. *J Thorac Cardiovasc Surg* 102:124, 1991.
3. Carpentier A, Chachques JC, Acar C, et al: Dynamic cardiomyoplasty at seven years. *J Thorac Cardiovasc Surg* 106:42–52, 1993.
4. Magovern GJ, Heckler FR, Park SB, et al: Paced skeletal muscle for dynamic cardiomyoplasty. *Ann Thorac Surg* 45:614, 1988.
5. Macoviak JA, Stephenson LW, Armenti F, et al: Electrical conditioning of in situ skeletal muscle for replacement of myocardium. *J Surg Res* 32:429, 1982.
6. Mannion JD, Velchik M, Hammond R, et al: Effects of collateral blood vessel ligation and electrical conditioning on blood flow in dog latissimus dorsi muscle. *J Surg Res* 47(4):332, 1989.
7. Bostwick J, Vasconez LO, Jurkiewicz MJ: Breast reconstruction after radical mastectomy. *Plast Reconstr Surg* 61:682, 1978.
8. Tobin GR: Segmentally split pectoral girdle muscle flaps for chest-wall and intrathoracic reconstruction. *Clin Plast Surg* 17(4):683, 1990.
9. Tobin GR, Mavroudis CA, Howe WR, et al: Reconstruction of complex thoracic defects with myocutaneous and muscle flaps: Application of new refinements. *J Thorac Cardiovasc Surg* 85:219, 1983.
10. Maxwell GP, Stueber K, Hoopes JE: A free latissimus dorsi myocutaneous flap. *Plast Reconstr Surg* 62:462, 1978.
11. Chachques JC, Grandjean P, Carpentier A: Latissimus dorsi dynamic cardiomyoplasty. *Ann Thorac Surg* 47:600, 1989.
12. German W, Finesilver EM, Davis JS: Establishment of circulation in tubed skin flaps: An experimental study. *Arch Surg* 26:27, 1933.
13. Callegari PR, Taylor GI, Caddy CM, et al: An anatomic review of the delay phenomenon: I. Experimental studies. *Plast Reconstr Surg* 89(3):397, 1992.
14. Braithwaite F: Some observations on the vascular channels in tubed pecicles II. *Br J Plast Surg* 4:28, 1952.
15. Cutting CB, Robson MC, Koss N: Denervation supersensitivity and the delay phenomenon. *Plast Reconstr Surg* 61(6):881, 1978.
16. Finseth F, Cutting C: An experimental neurovascular island skin flap for the study of the delay phenomenon. *Plast Reconstr Surg* 61(3):412, 1978.
17. Gillies H: Experience with tubed pedicle flaps. *Surg Gynecol Obst* 60:291, 1935.
18. Guba AM: Study of the delay phenomenon in axial pattern flaps in pigs. *Plast Reconst Surg* 63(4):551, 1979.
19. Hendel PM, Lilien DL, Buncke HJ: A Study of the pharmacologic control of blood flow to delayed skin flaps using xenon washout. Part II. *Plast Reconst Surg* 71(3):399, 1983.
20. Hoffmeister FS: Timing of transfer of flaps in reconstructive surgery. *Surg Gynecol Obst* 108 (1):68, 1959.
21. Hoopes JE, Su CT, Im MJ: Enzymatic responses to skin flap elevation following a delay procedure. *Plast Reconstr Surg* 66(3):369, 1980.
22. Jonsson K, Hunt TK, Brennan SS, et al: Tissue oxygen measurements in delayed skin flaps: A reconsideration of the delay phenomenon. *Plast Reconst Surg* 82(2): 328, 1988.
23. Jurell A: Adrenergic nerves and the delay phenomenon. *Ann Plast Surg* 17:493, 1986.
24. Milton SH: The effects of "delay" on the survival of experimental pedicled skin flaps. *Br J Plast Surg* 22:244, 1969.
25. Myers MB, Cherry G: Mechanism of the delay phenomenon. *Plast Reconst Surg* 44(1):52, 1969.
26. Murphy RC, Lawrence WT, Robson MC, et al: Surgical delay and arachidonic acid

metabolites: Evidence for an inflammatory mechanism: an experimental study in rats. *Br J Plast Surg* 38:272, 1985.
27. Reinisch JF: The pathophysiology of skin flap circulation: The delay phenomenon. *Plast Reconst Surg* 54(5):585, 1974.
28. Suzuki S, Issihiki N, Ogawa Y, et al: The minimal requirement of circulation for survival of undelayed and delayed flaps in rats. *Plast Reconst Surg* 78(2):221, 1986.
29. Kerrigan CL: Skin flap failure: Pathophysiology. *Plast Reconst Surg* 72(6):766, 1983.
30. Heckler F: Isolation of skeletal muscle for biomechanical circulatory assist. *Semin Thorac Cardiovasc Surg* 3(2):128, 1991.
31. Williams NS, Patel J, George BD, et al: Development of an electrically stimulated neoanal sphincter. *Lancet* 338(8776):166, 1991.
32. Pittman RN: Oxygen delivery and transport in the microcirculation. In McDonagh PF (ed): *Microvascular Perfusion and Transport in Health and Disease.* Basel, Karger. p 60, 1987.

Chapter 31

# Discussion

**Dr. Salmons:** This is a very nice scientific study and certainly addresses some of the questions that people should have been addressing a long time ago. The one disadvantage, to me, of your model is that this is such a thin muscle that many of the fibers are going to be able to obtain adequate oxygen by diffusion from surrounding tissues. And so the necrosis you are getting is an underestimation of what actually takes place.

**Dr. Keelen:** Actually, we took that into account in this experiment and all of the muscles were wrapped in inert plastic films.

**Dr. Lorusso (Italy):** We have been performing some other experiments concerning the ischemia of the latissimus dorsi muscle in Maastricht and we started the latissimus dorsi stimulation just 24 hours after cardiomyoplasty using a low pacing frequency. After 2 weeks, we sacrificed eight goats and we did not see any muscle necrosis. Don't you think that very slight contraction could induce hyperemia that in turn could counteract collateral vessel severance?

**Dr. Keelen:** Yes, perhaps some of the mechanisms by which delay protects the muscle are related to ischemia due to reduction in the blood supply of the muscle. I think that a low-level stimulation also produces a certain amount of ischemia, which will then allow the muscle to have some of the same vascular reaction that delay would have, and thus protect it from necrosis.

**Sir Magdi Yacoub (London):** This is a very elegant study in more ways than one. You mentioned something about microvascularization; can you tell us how you studied microvasculature, how you looked at it? You speculated that you have other means of influencing microvasculature; what are they?

**Dr. Keelen:** We studied the microvasculature by taking high magnification pictures of the muscle fields. Those images are transferred to the computer and then we can actually trace the vessels all the way down to the capillary level. We can measure vessel length, vessel diameter, muscle tortuosity, and we can look at changes in directional. Once we understand exactly what the microvascular changes are, then we can look at things such as pacing and various vasoactive or neuroactive drugs to see if we can emulate the effects of delay.

**Dr. Carpentier:** Today, we know that there are two ways to enhance vascularization. One is to delay division of distal vessels as you showed. The other is early stimulation using low-rate stimulation. However, Dr. Salmons told us that it is not good to stimulate and simultaneously distend the muscle. Could you elaborate, Dr. Salmons?

**Dr. Salmons:** It is well known from exercise physiology that if you exercise muscles in such a way that they are activated as they are being stretched, you get damage. For example, you damage a muscle much more by stepping downstairs than by stepping upstairs if you look at the quadriceps because the weight of the body actually stretches the muscle. The same thing has been established in stimulation and stretching. If you are simultaneously stretching a muscle and stimulating it you get a lot of damage.

**Dr. Carpentier:** What would be your recommendation?

**Dr. Salmons:** Probably staging it.

**Dr. Carpentier:** Beginning by distension or beginning by stimulation?

**Dr. Salmons:** I have not thought this through yet, but I think probably beginning with distension and adding stimulation at a later stage. If you look at a very late stage, by that time, regeneration has taken place. You never know how much damage has occurred. You may well say it does not matter by then, but of course there is some fibrosis that is left behind.

**Dr. Carpentier:** But fibrosis is not the same as necrosis!

**Dr. Salmons:** If you stretch the muscle, you do actually stimulate a formation of collagen by existing cells, but if you damage the muscle, you get replacement of muscle tissue by fibroblasts, collagen and fat, so you actually have a loss of muscle. I think I would prefer to have a little connective tissue and not lose the muscle.

**Dr. El Oakley (Manchester, UK):** We have some very interesting findings: 12 weeks following mobilization of latissimus dorsi muscle in sheep, if you mobilize the muscle or tenotomize it by cutting collateral supply without stimulation, the muscle is not damaged at all. The muscle structure is almost completely preserved. The problem arises only if you add stimulation; then, you have a severe degree of muscle damage. I just wonder why we are noticing such a difference with your work. Is it because we looked only 12 weeks after the mobilization, or is it because the experiments were done with sheep?

**Dr. Keelen:** In mice, I always had severe necrosis when I divided the entire collateral supply in a single operation.

**Dr. Frazier:** Is it easy for plastic surgeons to use mice?

**Dr. Keelen:** Actually, they are used in our lab for studying microcirculation in skin, they were the smallest animals that we had around and we needed something very small and very thin to look at the microcirculation in muscle.

**Dr. Subramanian (New York):** Could you tell us, if you increase the delay period, do you get an incremental value of the flap viability?

**Dr. Keelen:** I did not do that in this study. From reading the literature, it suggests that there is actually a window in which delay is effective. If you delay a piece of tissue for too long and then lift it as a flap, you get as much necrosis as you did if you just lift it acutely. This has been done in skin and not in muscle.

**Dr. Tobin (Louisville, KY):** I would like to answer the question about the sheep muscle compared with the microvascular model that has just been presented. There is substantial variability in the anatomic extent of the collateral blood supply from the intercostal perforators. We have looked at virtually all experimental and domestic animal models for this purpose. It turns out that among these animals, dogs and small rodents correspond most closely to human beings in terms of the extent of the collateral blood supply, whereas pigs, sheep, and other animals have substantially less blood supply coming from intercostal perforators. So the answer to your question is that there is a very real anatomical difference among the species studied.

**Dr. Carpentier:** Discrepancies have been noticed in the various experiments reported. They are due to the many variables involved. The size of the muscle and type of vascularization, the technique of dissection, and the degree of stretching and the mode of stimulation are four variables among others, and of course the timing and duration of the experiments also play an important role. In most experiments, only two variables were explored, i.e.: either mobilization + stimulation, or stretching + exercise, or stretching + stimulation, and so on. If we are to make progress in our understanding of muscle function, all of these variables must be taken into consideration and investigated in each experiment.

Chapter 32

# Optimization of Latissimus Dorsi Performance in Cardiomyoplasty by Anabolic Steroids

D. Fritzsche, R. Krakor, S. Lange*

## Introduction

Since its clinical introduction by Carpentier and Chachques in 1985,[1] cardiomyoplasty has become the object of intensive clinical and theoretical research. The procedure has thus far been performed on more than 300 patients worldwide, and initial results are encouraging. It is therefore not inappropriate to consider whether cardiomyoplasty could develop into a viable alternative to heart transplantation, in particular where the latter form of therapy is contraindicated. To date, however, there has been no conclusive proof of the manner in which cardiomyoplasty works. Although clinically impressive improvements in NYHA stage or survival rates have been demonstrated, attempts at providing objectifiable hemodynamic parameters have been disappointing. The effect of cardiomyoplasty could, on one hand, consist of a direct increase in ventricular contractility (the "squeezing" effect).[2,8,9] One factor tending to support this hypothesis is the measurable increase in left ventricular ejection fraction. On the other hand, a rise in contraction amplitude of the left ventricular posterior wall has been observed even in the "off" mode. The muscle wrapped around the heart appears to lead to a decrease in wall tension, which contributes to a reduction in oxygen consumption according to Laplace's law, and thus to an optimization of contraction parameters.[3,9] Probably, it is the combination of both effects that leads to the remarkable improvement in the patients' clinical condition. The hemodynamic benefit of cardiomyoplasty thus depends in a decisive way on two variables: the force capacity and the thickness of the latissimus dorsi (LD) muscle.

The values of both of these variables, however, decline significantly in the course of the conditioning process: force capacity and thickness are sacrificed in favor of increased resistance to fatigue. If it were possible to use pharmacological

*With the cooperation of G. Asmussen, A. Kaufmann, P. Zapf, J. Berkei, and R. Widera.

From Carpentier A, Chachques JC, Grandjean P: Cardiac Bioassist. © Futura Publishing Co, Inc, Armonk, NY, 1997.

means to induce a "thicker" and "stronger" muscle than is obtainable using electrical conditioning alone, then a combined pharmacological/electrical approach could be expected to provide distinct hemodynamic benefits for the patient. This was the line of thinking that prompted us to investigate the effect of anabolic steroids on the contraction parameters of stimulated LDs.

## Methods and Materials

The study was carried out on 12 female adult merino sheep with an average weight of 45.5 kg. The surgery performed on all of these experimental subjects was in strict accordance with the guidelines of the Federal Republic of Germany's legislation for the prevention of cruelty to animals: the law of 18.08 1986 (Bundesgesetzblatt I, p. 1319), as amended by article 5 of the law of 20.06. 1990 (BGB1. I, p. 1080) and article 3 of the law of 20.08.1990 (BGB1. I, p. 1762). Premedication consisted of 0.03 mg/kg atropine + 1.0 mg/kg diazepam. Narcosis was induced with 0.22 mg/kg xylacine (Rompun®) plus 11.0 mg/kg ketamine (Ketanest®) and maintained by appropriate doses. All animals received twice-daily injections of an analgesic (Tramal®) for 8 days postoperatively.

After a postoperative recovery period of 10–14 days, the left LD muscles of the animals were conditioned using a myostimulator (ITREL®, Medtronic). Stimulation parameters were increased gradually over a period of 12 weeks, reaching a burst of 30 Hz and a pulse amplitude of 10.5 V. In the 14th week, the contraction parameters were investigated and all LD muscles were biopsied. During the conditioning phase, six sheep received weekly injections of an anabolic hormone (Metenolon); these sheep constituted group B. The remaining six sheep were subjected to electrical conditioning alone and formed group A. The control group consisted of the right LD muscles of all 12 sheep; these LD muscles, which had not been conditioned, underwent identical investigations to those carried out on the left LD. A large cutaneous incision was made superficial to each left LD and the muscle was prepared as far as the humeral origin, keeping the neurovascular bundle intact and severing the costal insertion completely. Approximately 1 cm of the distal portion was wrapped around a metal rod and secured with a continuous suture. The rod was connected via a thin wire to a force transducer (Hottinger Baldwin Meßtechnik; Z6-4), which was attached to a freely rotatable holder, thus permitting easy determination of optimal pre-tension of muscle fibers. The signals from the force transducer were fed into a computer and sampled at a frequency of 1,000 Hz. The humerus was secured against a rod set into the operating table, permitting clean isometric contraction sequences to be obtained. The skin of the animal was attached to an oval-shaped metal plate placed over the operating field. The basin thus formed was filled with isothermic (39°C) normal saline solution to protect the muscle from fatigue due to undercooling. A biopsy specimen (approximately 1 cm) was taken from a defined region of the LD (constant across all subjects) and was cryogenically preserved for the use in later histochemical and immunohistological tests. Once the operating field had been prepared, the LD muscles were first stimulated with 7.5 V and burst frequencies of 5, 10, 15, 20, and 30 Hz until contraction became tetanic. The contraction parameters were then investigated under impulses of up to 10.5 V, with burst frequencies marginally exceeding those required to induce tetanism. Finally, the conditioned muscles were subjected to a 90-minute fatigue test. Upon completion of the bilateral investigations, the LD muscles were severed at the humeral origin and weighed. Curve analysis was then performed by computer. Of special interest were:

| | |
|---|---|
| • contraction time: | KZ (ms) |
| • half relaxation time: | HRT (ms) |
| • frequency required to induce tetanism: | VFR (Hz) |
| • contraction amplitude at VFR: | $F_{max}$ VFR (kp) |
| • contraction amplitude under supramaximal stimulation patterns: | $F_{max}$ (kp) |
| • steepness of force development | dF/dt (kp/s) |

The values calculated were checked for significance using Student's *t*-test.

## Results

As expected, the chronic electrostimulation resulted in near complete transformation of fast type II fibers to slow type I fibers. The ratio of type I to type II was 65%/35% for group A, 99.9%/0.1% for group B, and 21.3%/78.7% for the control group A. (Figs. 1A–C, 2).

KZ at VFR was 345.3 ± 11.9 ms in group A and 432.3 ± 54.7 ms in group B, in contrast to 186.3 ± 6.66 ms and 247.8 ± 82.0 ms, respectively, for the corresponding control group muscles ($p<0.001$). There was a corresponding increase in HRT at VFR: the values were 170 ± 36.2 ms for group A and 163.1 ± 13.9 ms for group B versus 93 ± 7.94 and 107.6 ± 60.5 ms ($p$=ns) for the control muscles. The maximum contraction amplitude under stimulation at 7.5 V and tetanic frequencies ($F_{max}$ at VFR) was 1.15 ± 0.7 kp in group A and 4.13 ± 1.2 kp in group B ($p<0.05$). The values measured for the corresponding control muscles were 4.27 ± 0.57 kp and 4.95 ± 1.1 kp ($p$ = ns) (Fig. 3).

The conditioned LD muscles of group A reached a force velocity dF/dt at VFR of 0.64 ± 0.23 kp/s; the corresponding value for group B was 4.9 ± 1.97 kp/s ($p<0.05$). The control group muscles displayed dF/dt values of 13.5 ± 0.74 kp/s and 15.5 ± 2.18 kp/s. Renewed determination of the same contraction parameters, this time under supramaximal stimulation patterns (10.5 V, burst frequency >VFR), produced the following results. Contraction time was 383.6 ± 83.7 ms for group A and 494.17 ± 30.5 ms for group B, compared with control group values of 161 ± 19.52 ms and 253.83 ± 98.1 ms, respectively ($p<0.05$). HRT also showed a clear increase, but this result fell short of the threshold of statistical significance. Maximum force capacity was determined at 4.23 ± 0.55 kp in group A and 6.0 ± 3.14 kp in group B ($p$ = ns). Under identical stimulation conditions, the control muscles were stronger in group A (6.1 ± 2.3 kp), but weaker in group B (5.25 ± 1.57 kp; $p$ = ns). (Fig. 4).

The maximal force velocity for group A was calculated at 6.7 ± 1.05 kp/s compared to a control value of 16.4 ± 1.36 kp/s ($p<0.01$). The corresponding

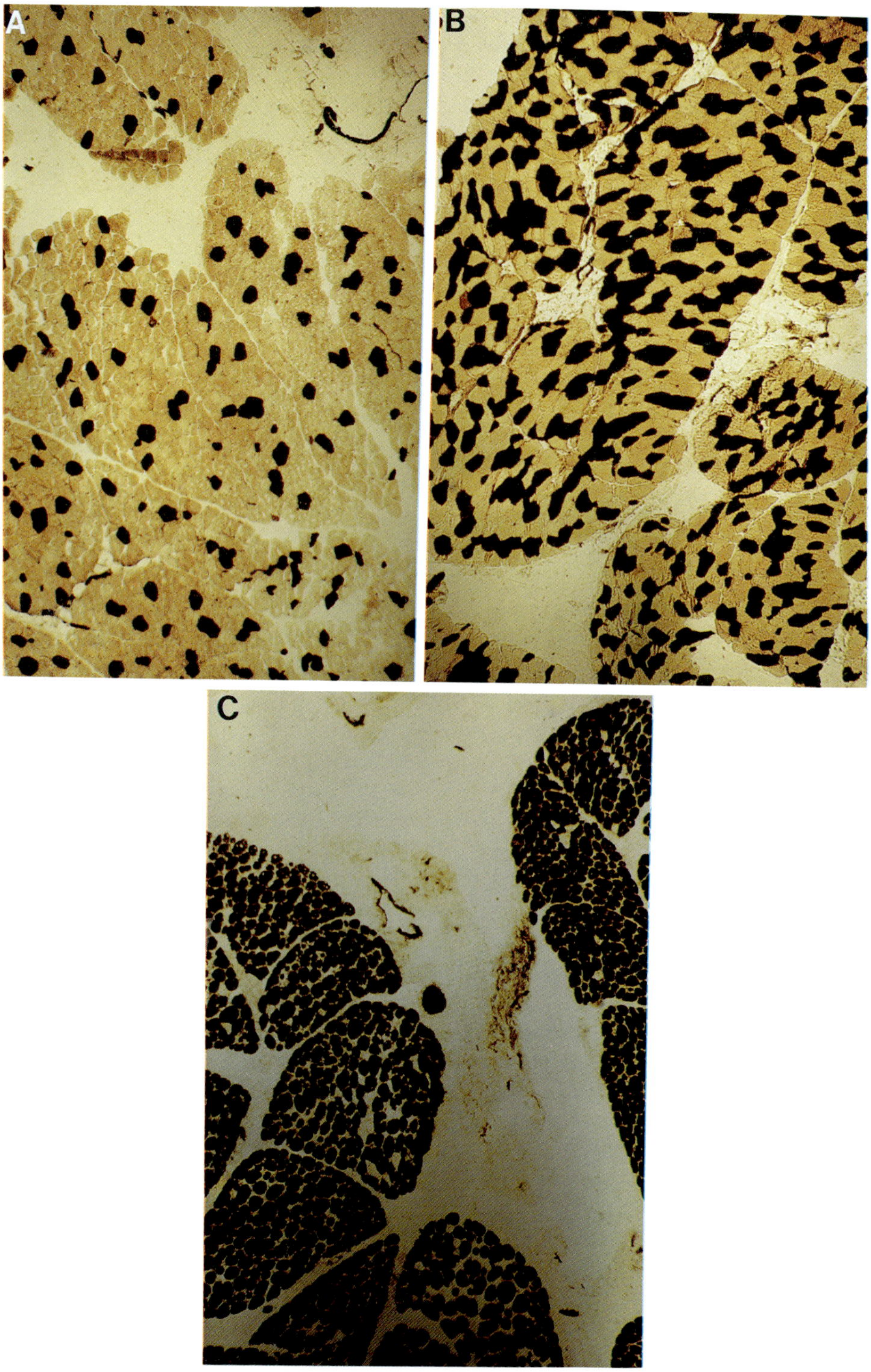


**Figure 1:** ***A***. *Control muscle; in acid ATPase type I fibers are stained dark.* ***B***. *LD preparation of group A.* ***C***. *LD preparation of group B.*

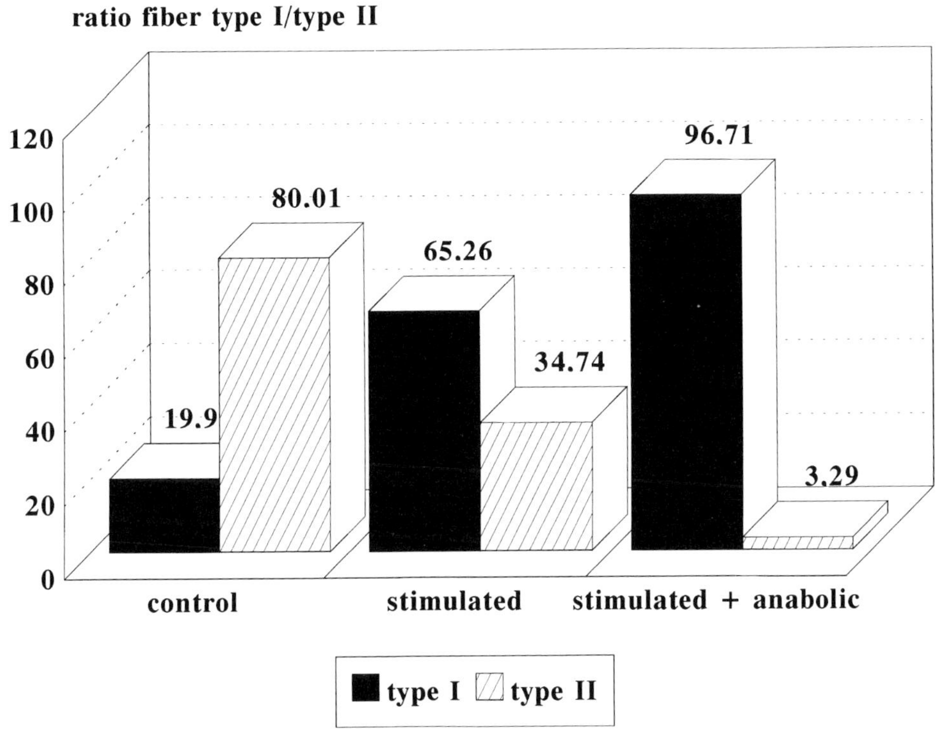


**Figure 2:** *The ratio of type I/II fibers was gradually increased by electrostimulation and anabolic treatment.*

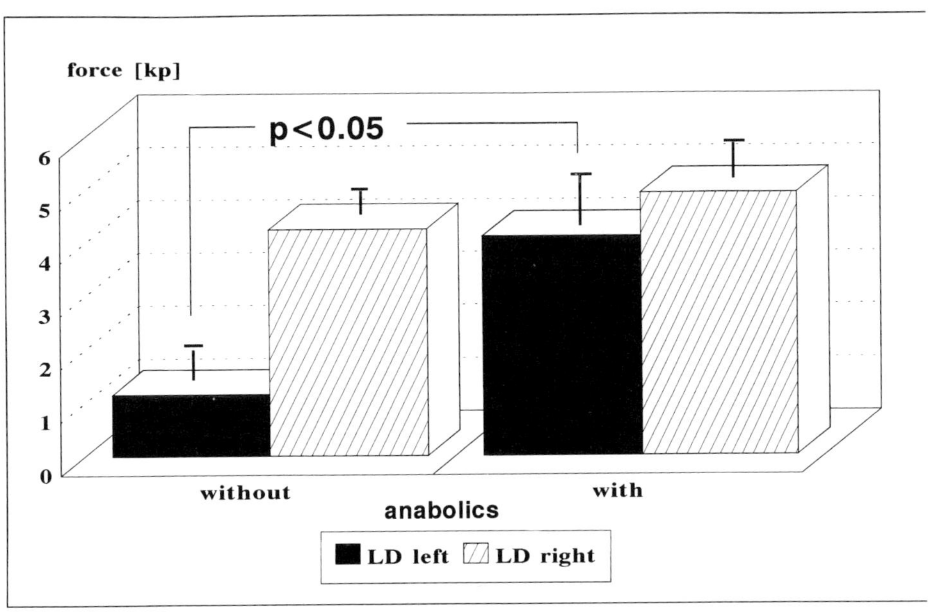


**Figure 3:** *Maximal force capacity under stimulation patterns that were just tetanic.*

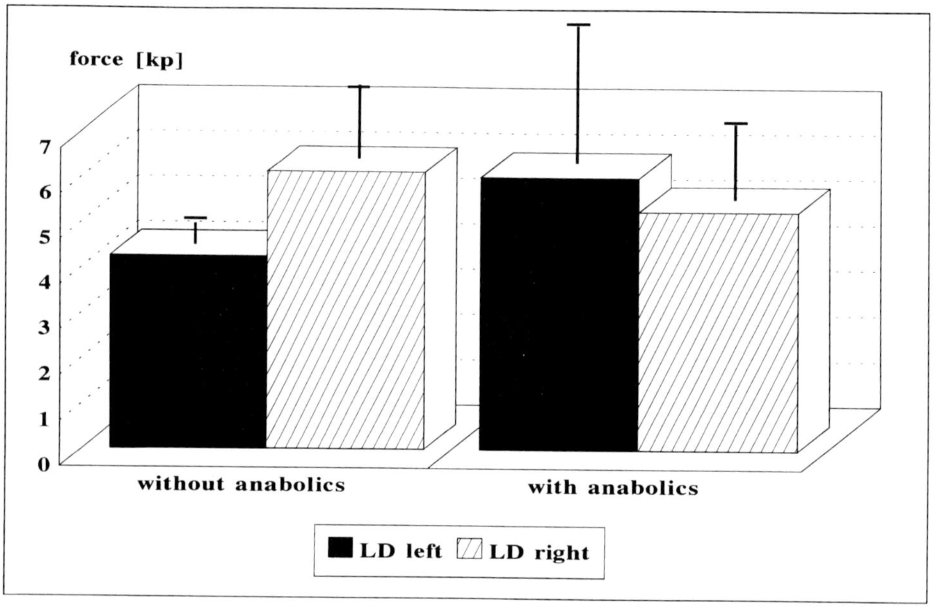


**Figure 4:** *Maximal force capacity at supramaximal stimulation for both group A and group B muscles.*

value for group B was 5.13 ± 2.19 kp/s in contrast to a control value of 15.8 ± 2.16 kp/s ($p<0.05$). In the fatigue test, none of the muscles in groups A and B displayed any falloff in contraction amplitude during the 90 minutes the test lasted. The contraction amplitude of the control group muscles declined after 2.25 min (±28 s) to 80% of the initial values. The muscle weight of the stimulated LD muscles in group A was 172.6 ± 10.0 g versus 155 ± 7.51 g for the control muscles. In group B, there was a remarkable increase in muscle weight: 249.17 ± 91.4 g versus 145.67 ± 57.96 g ($p<0.05$) (Fig. 5).

The relative increase in weight of the conditioned muscles in group A was 11.7 ± 1.06% and in group B, 79.97 ± 40.8% ($p<0.05$). The values for the muscle weight per 50 kg body weight of the animal were as follows: in group A, 172.6 ± 10 g versus 155 ± 7.51 g; in group B, 247 ± 43.8 g versus 155.6 ± 39.2 g ($p<0.05$). The calculated maximal force capacity per 100 g muscle tissue did not differ significantly between the two groups. The value for group A was 2.42 ± 0.17 kp/100 g versus 3.87 ± 1.46 kp/100 g (control muscles); in group B, 2.52 ± 0.48 kp/100 g versus 3.95 ± 1.45 kp/100 g ($p$ = ns) (Fig. 6).

Light microscopic and electron microscopy investigations of the liver parenchyma taken from the animals of both groups showed no irregularities. In particular, no fatty deposits, mitochrondrial swellings, or signs of connective tissue infiltration were observable in the anabolically treated animals.

The average relative weight gain of all animals amounted to 7% over the duration of the experiment, and can be explained by the general conditions (diet, exercise) under which the animals were kept. The weight gain of the anabolically treated animals was not significantly greater or more rapid than that of the untreated animals (Fig. 7).

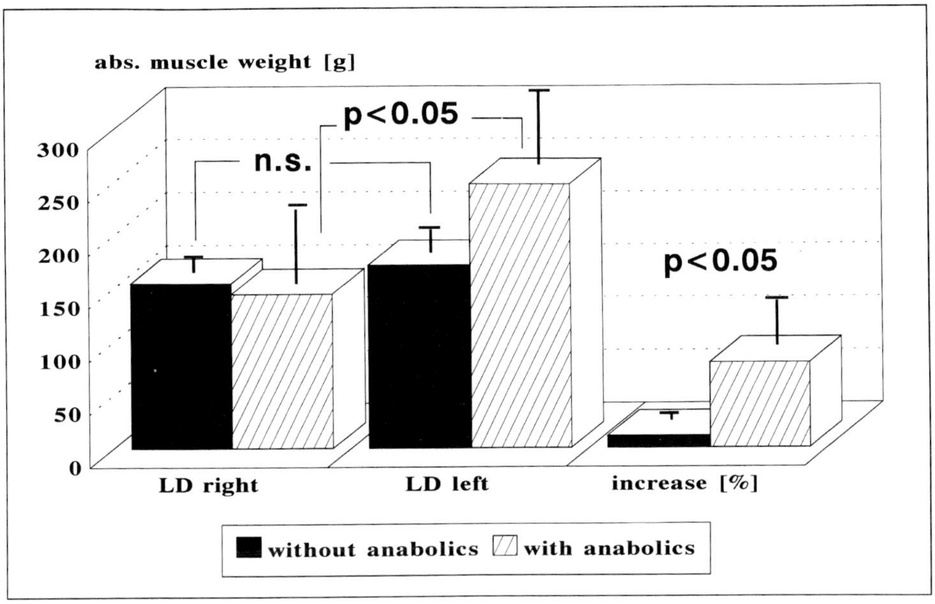


**Figure 5:** *Average muscle weight for both groups and its relative increase during the conditioning process.*

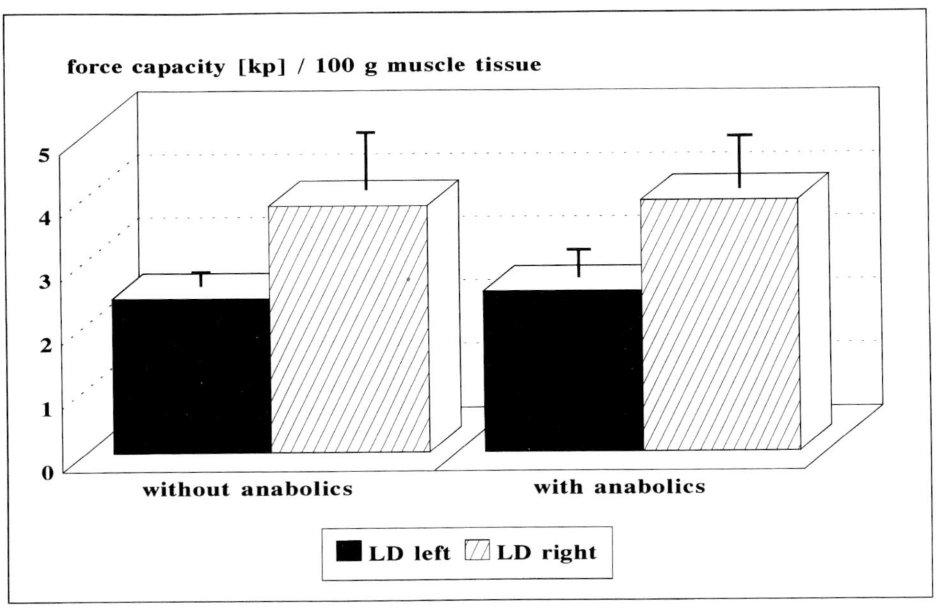


**Figure 6:** *Average force capacity related to 100 g muscle tissue.*

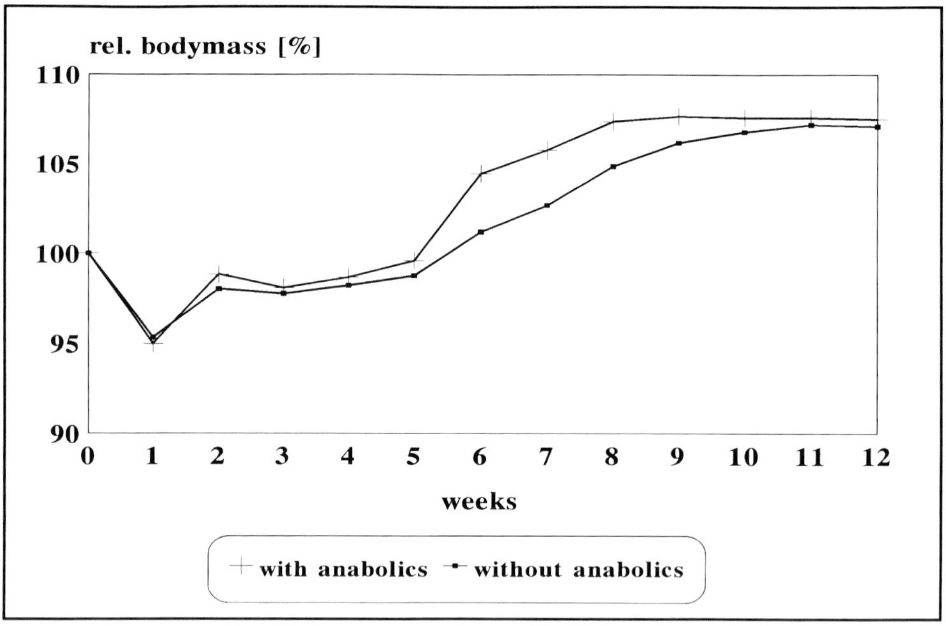


**Figure 7:** *Relative increase in body mass of each group (differences in % of the initial values).*

## Discussion

Since its initial introduction by Carpentier and Chachques in 1985, dynamic cardiomyoplasty has aroused considerable clinical interest and is now in the clinical trial stage as an option in the surgical treatment of terminal cardiac insufficiency. A more rapid implementation of cardiomyoplasty as an alternative to heart transplantation is presently hindered by a number of experimental and clinical observations that have been made; we will discuss a selection of these in connection with the results of our study. The process of fast-to-slow twitch transformation via chronic electrostimulation has been extensively described for skeletal muscle of various species.[4,5,12,13] The induced resistance to fatigue is accompanied on the one hand by a significant reduction in force capacity. On the other hand, a loss of mass has been described in the chronically stimulated muscle, apparently due to a localized degenerative process in which connective tissue replaces previously contractile tissue. Dynamic cardiomyoplasty leads to a measurable increase of left ventricular ejection fraction, although this increase is not correlated with the patient's clinical improvement.[11] Apparently, the wrapped muscle has a synergistically acting and objectifiable "squeezing" effect on ventricular performance.[8]

There can be no doubt that the regional wall mobility of the insufficient heart is measurably greater during the LD contraction cycle.[9] However, it has also been observed that the contraction amplitude of the left ventricular posterior wall is greater in the "off" mode of the cardiomyostimulator than in the preoperative findings (Lange, oral communication). This may mean that a lessening of the wall tension of the insufficient, dilated heart is brought about by the mere passive presence of the wrapped muscle. According to Laplace's law, this should lead to a reduction in myocardial oxygen consumption.

These considerations lead us to believe that, in the ideal case, the loss of force capacity and muscle mass induced in the LD by chronic electrostimulation should be able to be counteracted pharmacologically.

As far as we are aware, no studies have previously been performed on the effects of anabolics on the conditioning process of the LD, with the exception of the work of Dr. Hohenhaus from the research group led by L. W. Stephenson.[7] Apparently, it was the general nonacceptance of anabolic steroids by the medical profession that led to the rejection of such studies. However, in light of investigations into anabolic side effects carried out at the former East German Research Institute for Physical Culture and Sport at Leipzig, we conclude that side effects can be expected to occur primarily in the growing organism as a function of dosage levels and length of treatment. Given the average age and life expectancy of patients for whom cardiomyoplasty is a clinical option, the dangers of anabolic side effects would appear to lose much of their significance. In fact, in our investigations, we found no evidence of either systemic or hepatocellular changes such as might have been feared to result from anabolic steroid administration. In the context of the conceptual framework sketched out above, and in the light of the experimental results thus far obtained, a discussion of the results of the present study appears warranted.

Interestingly enough, it was only in group B that a ratio of type I/type II fibers of 99.9%/0.1% was obtained. Given that electrostimulatory conditioning was identical in both groups, we had been expecting a complete transformation in group A as well. It is possible that anabolic steroids accelerate the process of fiber transformation and thus that the end-state had not been reached in group A by the end of the 12-week conditioning phase. This, however, would contradict observations made by other authors who were able to describe an almost complete transformation within 12 weeks.[13] Muscle tissue deterioration was not observed in either group. The record of the contraction and relaxation times of all muscles displays a clear reduction in the contraction times of both groups of conditioned LD muscles with the left LD muscles of group A reaching the maximum contraction amplitude faster than those of group B. This finding was not statistically significant. One possible explanation might be the lower proportion of type I fibers in group A. From a neurophysiological point of view, it was interesting that KZ and HRT of the unconditioned right LD muscles of group B were prolonged by an average 60–90 ms in comparison to those of group A, although histochemical and immunohistochemical tests detected only slight changes.

Under tetanic stimulation patterns, the left LD muscles of group A were in general weaker than those of group B. This difference was significant when stimulation was performed at a voltage of 7.5 V. Even intra-individually, the conditioned LD muscles were weaker than the unconditioned control muscles. In group A, the loss of maximal force capacity was significant; in group B, it was less marked, and under maximal stimulation (10.5 V), the left LD muscles actually displayed a higher force development than the contralateral muscles. The maximal force capacity of the contralateral control muscle remained unchanged in both group A and group B. This means that anabolic steroids per se do not appear to have any protein-synthesizing or "training" effect on the unstimulated LD in terms of a force increase. However, the use of anabolic steroids antagonized the loss of maximal force capacity in the course of the transformation process.

No differences in maximal force capacity per 100 g muscle tissue occurred in our study. In other words, the increase in contractile potential must be due solely to the mass increase of the conditioned muscles of group B. The protein-anabolic effect was not observable in the absence of chronic stimulation (contralateral muscles). The chief effect of the anabolic steroids consisted of an increased synthesis of structural and functional proteins. Apparently, the steroids also have a synergistic effect on the extent and completeness of the transformation process.

The results achieved—the antagonizing of the loss of force and mass while maintaining full resistance to fatigue—are highly desirable in the context of dynamic cardiomyoplasty, since both a strengthening of the "squeezing" effect and a significant reduction in wall tension can be expected. Further animal studies, with a primarily hemodynamic orientation, will be required to provide evidence for this hypothesis.

## References


1. Carpentier A, Chachques JC: Myocardial substitution with a stimulated skeletal muscle: first successful clinical case. *Lancet* 76:1267, 1985.
2. Chachques JC, Grandjean PA, Bourgeois I, Carpentier A: Dynamic cardiomyoplasty to improve ventricular function. In Unger F (ed): *Assisted Circulation 3,* Springer-Verlag Berlin Heidelberg, 1989.
3. Chagas ACP, Moreira LF, da Luz PL, Camarano GP, et al: Stimulated preconditioned skeletal muscle cardiomyoplasty; an effective means of cardiac assist. *Circulation* 80(Suppl III):202–208, 1989.
4. Cumming DVE, Pattison CW, Yacoub MH: Autologous skeletal muscle and cardiac assistance. *Ann Cardiac Surg* 75:82, 1989.
5. Goldspink DF, Easton J, Winterburn SK, Williams PE, et al: The role of passive stretch and repetitive electrical stimulation in preventing skeletal muscle atrophy while reprogramming gene expression. *J Cardiac Surg* 6:218–225, 1991.
6. Grandjean PA, Austin L, Chan S, Terpstra B, et al: Dynamic cardiomyoplasty: clinical follow-up results. *J Cardiac Surg* 6:80–89, 1991.
7. Hohenhaus E, Pochettino A, Hammond RL, Niinami H, et al: The effect of anabolic steroids on isometric and fatigue characteristics of unconditioned and conditioned canine latissimus dorsi muscle. *4th World Symposium on Transformed Muscle for Cardiac Assist,* Oct. 3–6 Palm Springs, CA, 1990.
8. Hooper TL, Niinami H, Hammond RL, Lu HP, et al: Skeletal muscle ventricles as left atrial-aortic pumps: Short-term studies. *Ann Thorac Surg* 54:316–22, 1992.
9. Lange R, Sack FU, Saggau W, Vahl C, et al: Performance of dynamic cardiomyoplasty related to the functional state of the heart. *J Cardiac Surg* 6:225–235, 1991.
10. Moreira LF, Seferian P, Bocchi A, Pego-Fernandes PM, et al: Survival improvement with dynamic cardiomyoplasty in patients with dilated cardiomyopathy. *Circulation* 84(Suppl):296–302, 1991.
11. Moreira LF, Stolf NA, Jatene AD: Benefits of cardiomyoplasty for dilated cardiomyopathy. *Semin Thorac Cardiovasc Surg* 3:140–44, 1991.
12. Pattison CW, Cumming DVE, Clayton Jones DE, Goldspink G, et al: Review article: Variable adaption of molecular mechanism in relation to the use of autologous striated muscle to augment myocardial function. *Cardiovasc Res* 23:593–600, 1989.
13. Pette D: Activity-induced fast to slow transition in mammalian muscle. *Med Sci Sports Exercise* 16:517–528, 1984.

Chapter 32

# *Discussion*

**Dr. Carpentier:** How do you explain the difference between the left and the right latissimus dorsi? Are there right-handed goats and left-handed goats?

**Dr. Fritzsche:** In force capacity, I would say yes. We explain the differences between the left and the right muscle, because of the transformation process, because of the conditioning.

**Dr. Carpentier:** By using steroids, you probably increase oxygen consumption, which may lead to a higher oxygen demand and therefore may worsen function of the heart. Have you analyzed oxygen consumption?

**Dr. Fritzsche:** Well, we did not investigate that directly, but the average weight gain of the animals amounted to 7%.

**Dr. Carpentier:** Can you elaborate a little bit more on the possible side effects?

**Dr. Fritzsche:** Possible side effects could be fatty deposits, swelling, or any connective tissue infiltration within the layers, but we did not observe anything.

**Dr. Chachques:** Did you use the opposite muscle in each animal as a control?

**Dr. Fritzsche:** The corresponding right latissimus dorsi muscle, yes.

**Dr. Chachques:** Did you try removing the anabolic steroid to see if the effect was still there?

**Dr. Fritzsche:** No, the experiment was finished at the point of the investigation of the contraction parameters and they were still on steroids.

**Dr. Salmons:** We looked at the interaction between stimulation and anabolic steroids during the 1970s. We found that the stimulated muscle was quite unaffected and that it was the unstimulated muscle that showed an anabolic ef-

From Carpentier A, Chachques JC, Grandjean P: Cardiac Bioassist. © Futura Publishing Co, Inc, Armonk, NY, 1997.

fect. In addition, the anabolic effect was restricted to certain muscles. I advise people to be very cautious about such studies because there are many potential pitfalls. For example, there is no significance in looking at mass alone because of potential salt and water retention. You can get edema in the muscle, which can increase the mass. You have to look at protein content, dry weight, or force. And although you seem to get an increase in force, it is not significant. One of the reasons that the anabolic steroids have fallen into disrepute is because the idea that they actually increase muscle mass is a myth. They have so many other side effects; I have mentioned salt water retention, and they also interrupt pituitary secretion. My study was one of the few that demonstrated that the muscle mass increases proportionally to the body mass. Many muscles, particularly limb muscles, have a mass that is proportional to body mass. And what most people have found is that anabolic steroids increase body mass. So, it is very important to normalize your results against the body mass.

**Dr. Fritzsche:** That is what we did.

**Dr. Salmons:** Let me add that it depends not only on the muscle, but also on the species and whether it is male or female; and furthermore, in my experience, it even depended on the time of year. Because aromatic enzymes can be induced into the brain at specific times of the year in animals, you have to be extremely careful about drawing conclusions from this.

**Dr. Fritzsche:** Dr. Salmons, I have read a lot of papers from Liverpool in the last year or so. It is true that you found quite the opposite to our findings, but please keep in mind that both studies are not comparable. You used rabbits; we used sheep. You used other steroids; we used metalone. You used a continuous burst stimulation of 10 hertz; we used a burst stimulation, etc. And you finally concluded that, last but not least, you found a clear response to anabolic steroids in terms of the wet weight, maximum cross-section area, and the maximum isometric tension. Am I correct?

**Dr. Salmons:** Yes.

**Dr. Fritzsche:** And your results became very clear after 12 weeks and not after 4 weeks. Is that correct?

**Dr. Salmons:** Yes.

**Dr. Schwartz:** Dr. Fritzsche, your data concerning the histochemistry were very impressive because all of the fibers appeared to be transformed. However, the size of the fibers did not seem to be increased a great deal in comparison to the controls and yet you have a big increase in mass. How do you reconcile this?

**Dr. Fritzsche:** I don't have the exact data here with me that are going to be published. I believe that the fiber sizes showed a slight decrease, but an enormous increase in the capillarization. That is to say, the number of capillaries per fiber increased, but the fibers themselves showed a very slight decrease.

**Dr. Schwartz:** But you have an increase in muscle mass.

**Dr. Fritzsche:** An enormous increase in muscle mass.

**Dr. Schwartz:** So, if the fiber size is not increased, would that mean that you have more fibers or that you have more water?

**Dr. Fritzsche:** The investigations are not yet finished and we are continuing with our investigations.

# Part IV

## Alternative Techniques

Chapter 33

# Latissimus Dorsi Muscle Expansion Prior To Cardiomyoplasty

Juan Carlos Chachques, Michel Tapia, Marc Radermecker, Michel Pellerin, Alain F. Carpentier

## Introduction

The efficacy of cardiomyoplasty is related to the relationship between the heart and the transposed latissimus dorsi (LD) muscle. A complete myocardial wrapping provides maximal assistance, when the LD muscle flap surface area is sufficient to cover completely both the left and the right ventricles. As demonstrated in experimental and clinical studies, systolic augmentation during synchronous LD muscle flap contraction and an improved diastolic pressure-volume relationship allow the re-establishment of cardiac reserve and prevent further cardiac dilatation.[1–4]

The application of this knowledge to human clinical practice is limited by the impossibility to completely cover the heart due to lack of available LD muscle flap surface area and cardiomegaly. This situation is a constant finding in patients with a cardiothoracic ratio of >0.60, and a left ventricular end-diastolic diameter of >75 mm. Several hypotheses to solve this problem were studied at Broussais Hospital. Among them were double flap cardiomyoplasty, optimal dissection and mobilization of the thoracodorsal neurovascular bundle, progressive denervation by ameroid compression, and LD muscle flap expansion and stimulation prior to surgery. The latter has merited our closest attention and is the subject of the present study.

Use of balloon expanders to increase the surface of subcutaneous and cutaneous layers has been widely used in plastic and reconstructive surgery. This technique has been reliable and effective.[5–7] We have adapted this principle, with technical modifications, to potentiate the LD muscle surface area and contractility in a cardiomyoplasty model.

From Carpentier A, Chachques JC, Grandjean P: Cardiac Bioassist. © Futura Publishing Co, Inc, Armonk, NY, 1997.

The purpose of this experimental study was to analyze the qualitative and quantitative modifications of an LD muscle flap resulting from a previous balloon expansion.

Four specific issues were evaluated: (1) modification of the LD muscle flap surface, (2) the effects of preoperative LD muscle electrostimulation, (3) consequences of the division of the LD muscle flap peripheral blood supply, and (4) preliminary results of human application and surgical experience.

## Methods and Materials

The experimental data were obtained from the study of five adult goats in which LD muscle silicone expanders were implanted. The balloon expanders were triangular and were made of silicone (Sigma Medical, France). Their size and shape were specially designed according to the LD muscle anatomy. The maximal inflation volume was 900 mL. The device was connected to a valved chamber allowing progressive percutaneous inflation of the balloon. The edges of the device allowed for suturing to the intercostal muscles in order to avoid displacement. Two electrodes (Medtronic® model SP5528) were located on the external surface of the expander to electrostimulate the LD muscle flap (Fig. 1).

Five alpine goats (mean weight, 52 kg) were used. General anesthesia was induced by intravenous administration of propofol (5 mg/kg) and maintained by inhalation of isoflurane (2.5 vol/100 mL). Surgery was performed on the animal in the right lateral decubitus position. A 10–15 cm left paravertebral incision was performed to provide direct access to the LD muscle thoracolumbar aponeurosis. This fascia was opened longitudinally and the dissection was carried out beneath the distal half of the LD muscle. Collaterals from the intercostal arteries to the LD were divided. Superiorly, blunt dissection was conducted to the level of the tip of the scapula. In this manner, a space was created beneath the LD muscle to introduce and place the expander that was secured to the chest wall with interrupted polypropylene sutures. The thoracolumbar aponeurosis was carefully closed and a subcutaneus pocket was created to allow the implantation of an Itrel® myostimulator (Medtronic® pacing system), which was connected to the LD muscle pacing leads.

The postoperative filling of the expander began 1 week following surgery by progressive injection of saline solution up to 500 mL at 8 weeks.

Postoperatively, the LD muscle was electrostimulated, using a graded stimulation protocol, increasing the number of impulses in the burst stepwise over 4 weeks in order to achieve transformation without producing fatigue. The final myostimulation state 1 month postoperatively was as follows: burst of six pulses, burst frequency of 30 Hz, pulse amplitude between 8 and 10 volts, and 40 bursts per minute.

The LD muscle surface area was measured by planimetry, at implantation of the balloon expander and 10 weeks later. The electrophysiological data included LD muscle threshold of contraction and muscle impedance. Biopsy samples of the complete section area of the LD were obtained in the proximal and distal parts of the muscles, 10 weeks following balloon implantation. These specimens were submitted for routine analysis including hematoxylin, eosin, and trichrome histological staining. Statistical analysis of the data was expressed as mean ±SD.

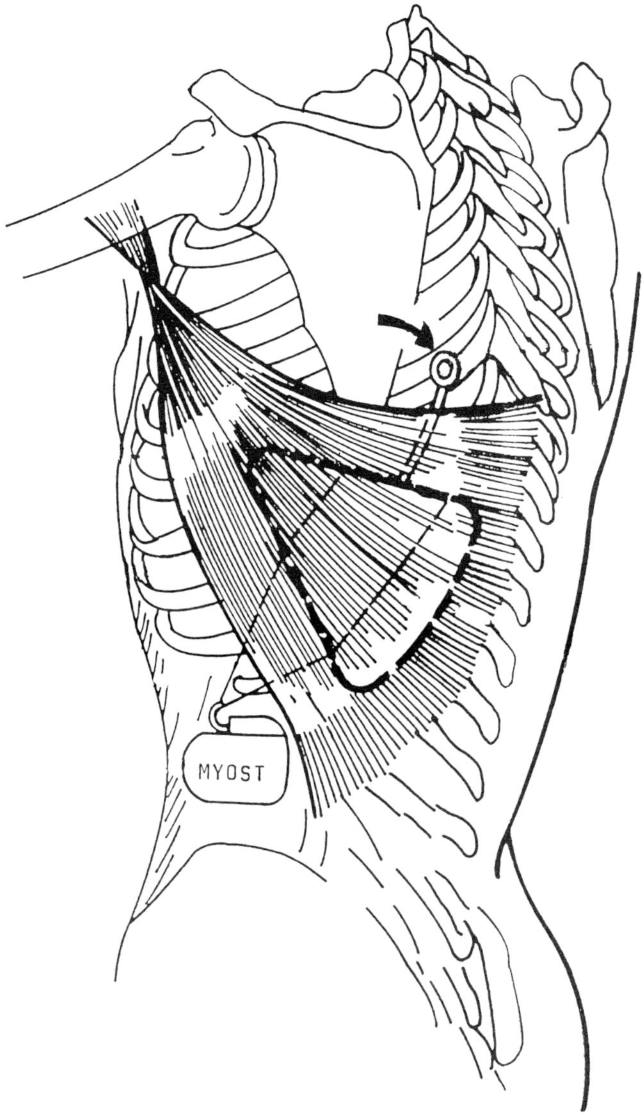


**Figure 1:** *Balloon expander implanted beneath the LD muscle, including a valved chamber (arrow) for progressive percutaneous inflation, and two pacing leads connected to an Itrel® (Medtronic) myostimulator (MYOST).*

## Results

The inflation of the expander was well tolerated and achieved in an 8-week interval. The position of the expander remained stable throughout the study and no surgical wound complications were encountered. The evaluation of the LD muscle surface area after 10 weeks demonstrated a significant increase of the LD muscle surface from $175 \pm 12$ cm$^2$ to $229 \pm 17$ cm$^2$ ($+ 31 \pm 4\%$, $p<0.05$) (Table 1).

**Table 1**
Evaluation of the Latissimus Dorsi Muscle

| | *Intraoperative* | *Postoperative (2 months)* | |
|---|---|---|---|
| Latissimus dorsi muscle area | 175 ± 12 $cm^2$ | 229 ± 17 $cm^2$ | + 31 ± 4% $p < 0.05$ |
| Twitch (threshold) | 2.1 ± 0.2 volts | 1.9 ± 0.2 volts | NS |
| Recruitment | 5.4 ± 0.4 volts | 4.6 ± 0.3 volts | NS |
| Impedance | 1526 ± 78 ohms | 342 ± 62 ohms | $p<0.05$ |

Thresholds and impedance were measured through the electrodes of the expander. NS = not significant.

After complete dissection, the LD muscle flap looked healthy and thicker. At the expander-muscle interface, a thin fibrous tissue layer had developed that did not seem to interfere with muscle contractility. The electrophysiological values remained stable as far as first twitch threshold and full recruitment threshold were concerned (Table 1). Muscle impedance decreased at 10 weeks (from 1,526 ± 78 ohms to 342 ± 62 ohms, $p<0.05$). The reduction of impedance between the leads could be explained by an increased contact area between the pacing electrodes (fixed on the external surface of the balloon) and the LD muscle following inflation of the expander.

The analysis of biopsy samples revealed histological integrity of muscle fibers that had maintained their mean diameter. There was no change in muscular and neurovascular anatomy (Fig. 2). A thin layer of connective fibrous tissue was found on the deep surface of the LD muscle flap.

## Discussion

The clinical experience in reconstructive surgery with balloon expanders has already shown the efficiency of this technique in progressively increasing the surface area of soft tissues and muscles. This process is safe and reversible.[5,7] This phenomenon is quite similar to the abdominal wall overdistension during pregnancy and does not demonstrate late functional damage.

It was therefore felt that the use of this technique could be used to augment LD muscle surface area and would improve cardiac wrapping in cardiomyoplasty procedures. This study has shown that using a silastic expander inflated with 500 mL of saline solution, a 31% increase in LD muscle surface area can be obtained.

Due to the specific design of the expander (for the purpose of cardiomyoplasty), this technique improves the muscle flap not only quantitatively but also qualitatively. Indeed, the positioning of the expander implies that collaterals from intercostal and lumbar arteries are suppressed. This delay certainly modifies results in vascular adaptation of the principal thoracodorsal supply.

It is known that the natural anastomoses that exist between the proximal

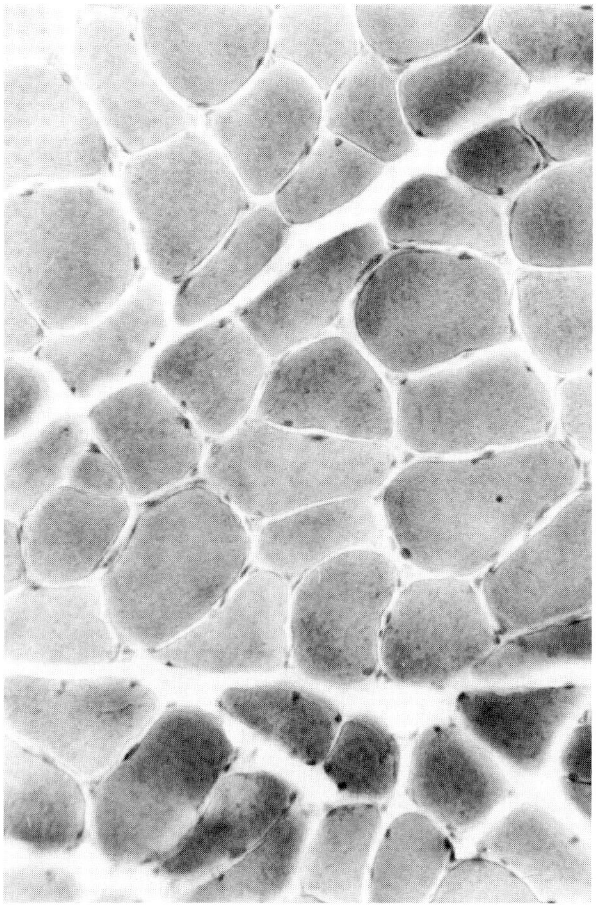

**Figure 2:** *Histological study of the LD muscle following expansion associated with electrostimulation, showing preserved myofibrillar structure, with normal fiber diameter.*

thoracodorsal blood supply and the peripheral blood vessels originate from the intercostal and lumbar arteries. In an acute setting, however, the distal border of the LD muscle flap is usually cyanotic, suggesting reduced blood flow. The positioning of the expander beneath the LD muscle therefore prepares the muscle for exclusive vascularization from the thoracodorsal pedicle and development of collaterals to the distal aspect of the LD muscle flap.

Furthermore, the progressive increase in the balloon expander volume slowly overstretches the LD muscle and consequently increases its tension. It has been shown[8] that overstretching not only promotes the transformation of type 2 glycolitic to type 1 oxydative fatigue-resistant muscle fibers, but also results in physical reinforcement of the muscle due to the better actin myosin length-tension relationship. Furthermore, in our experimental study, the LD muscle was stimulated with a progressive protocol. This was done to avoid overdistension of the muscle and to acquire fatigue resistance from electrical stimulation. Preconditioning of the LD muscle flap in situ prior to surgery not only results in complete muscle transformation but also in an optimal bioenergetic profile and a preserved muscle physiology.

These considerations support the concept of an in situ muscle preparation with a balloon expander and associated myostimulation system. This management may provide the LD muscle flap with an improved biomechanical performance and better cardiac assistance.[9]

## Clinical Experience

Recently, a 900 mL expander was used preoperatively at Broussais Hospital, 10 weeks before cardiomyoplasty, in two patients with refractory congestive heart failure (one ischemic and one idiopathic cardiomyopathy) with dilated hearts (cardiothoracic ratio >0.60). The progressive inflation of the device was well tolerated and resulted in muscle augmentation as well as an increased vascular supply of the distal margin of the LD muscle flap. Vascularization was excellent without any sign of distal ischemia.

Both muscles were used to perform a complete myocardial wrap in both patients, in spite of massive cardiomegaly. The postoperative course was uneventful and there were no complications related to balloon expansion.

## Conclusion

Potential benefits of an LD muscle expansion associated with electrostimulation 2 months prior to cardiomyoplasty are: (1) increase in muscle surface, (2) training of muscular fibers and preservation of muscular tone, and (3) division of the distal vascular supply at the time of implantation may potentiate vascularization from the LD muscle main pedicle. LD muscle expansion should be considered prior to cardiomyoplasty in cases of extreme heart dilatation.[10,11]

## References


1. Chachques JC, Grandjean P, Schwartz K, Mihaileanu S, et al: Effect of latissimus dorsi dynamic cardiomyoplasty on ventricular function. *Circulation* 78 (Suppl 3):203–216, 1988.
2. Carpentier A, Chachques JC, Acar C, Relland J, et al: Dynamic cardiomyoplasty at seven years. *J Thorac Cardiovasc Surg* 106:42–54, 1993.
3. Bellotti G, Moraes A, Bocchi E, Arie S, et al: Late effects of cardiomyoplasty on left ventricular mechanics and diastolic filling. *Circulation* 88 (part 2):304–308, 1993.
4. Cho PW, Levin HR, Curtis WE, Tsitlik JE, et al: Pressure-volume analysis of changes in cardiac function in chronic cardiomyoplasty. *Ann Thorac Surg* 56:38–45, 1993.
5. Slavin SA: Improving the latissimus dorsi myocutaneous flap with tissue expansion. *Plast Reconstr Surg* 93:811–824, 1994.
6. Argenta LC, Marks MW, Grabb WC: Selective use of serial expansion in breast reconstruction. *Ann Plast Surg* 11:188–195, 1983.
7. Morykwas MJ, Marks MW, Argenta LC: Surface area and tissue volume increases with differential expansion. *Ann Plast Surg* 28:311–314, 1992.
8. Goldspink DF, Easton J, Winterburn SK, Williams PE, et al: The role of passive

stretch and repetitive electrical stimulation in preventing skeletal muscle atrophy while reprogramming gene expression to improve fatigue resistance. *J Cardiac Surg* 6 (Suppl):218–224, 1991.
9. Adamopoulos S, Coats AJS, Brunotte F, Arnolda L, et al: Physical training improves skeletal muscle metabolism in patients with chronic heart failure. *J Am Coll Cardiol* 21:1101–1106, 1993.
10. Chachques JC, Acar C, Portoghese M, Bensasson D, et al: Dynamic cardiomyoplasty for long-term cardiac assist. *Eur J Cardiothorac Surg* 6:642–648, 1992.
11. Carpentier A, Chachques JC, Grandjean P (eds): *Cardiomyoplasty.* Futura Publishing Co, Mount Kisco, New York, 1991, pp 1–280.

Chapter 33

# Discussion

**Dr. George Magovern (Pittsburgh):** We did a number of experiments similar to this using a breast implant, but what we found is that if you kept this over a period of time, the muscle that was expanded became fibrotic. That was in the experimental animal. We kept them going for at least a year. This may be a different concept if you are doing it for a shorter period of time. But certainly if you leave it in over a long period of time, you will get fibrosis just over the part that is over the expanded area. How long preoperatively have you done this?

**Dr. Chachques:** We implant this balloon for 2 months, no more. And we know from the plastic surgeons that in 2 months, the fibrosis is minor and reversible. So the solution is not to implant for more than 2 months. We see only a thin layer of fibrosis and not an organized reaction. And also motion of the LD around the balloon prevents fibrosis just as in women with this kind of prosthesis, in order to avoid fibrosis, massage is recommended. So we think that, with electrostimulation and 2 months of implantation, fibrosis should not be a problem.

**Dr. Magovern:** This would be a good opportunity also to perform a biopsy on the skeletal muscle in congestive failure preoperatively.

**Dr. Chachques:** We did this in goats. The LD was of good quality, with a thin layer of fibroblasts.

**Dr. Magovern:** From a physiological aspect, cardiologists say that things happen in the skeletal muscle of congestive heart failure patients and that may make it an opportunity to use such a device.

**Dr. Mikaeloff:** How much expansion do you expect to get from this preparation?

**Dr. Chachques:** In animals, we had 30% so far. So we expect the same kind of increase of surface in patients. This procedure is very safe for the patient.

**Dr. Herman (Israel):** What you are doing is training the muscle in situ. What have you achieved in goats in your training period in situ? It has been proposed

From Carpentier A, Chachques JC, Grandjean P: Cardiac Bioassist. © Futura Publishing Co, Inc, Armonk, NY, 1997.

in the past that the training period is much better when done in situ than when it is done on the free flap.

**Dr. Chachques:** We worked for 5 years, between 1980 and 1985 on in situ stimulation of the LD muscle. We performed this procedure on three patients prior to surgery. The advantage of stimulation prior to surgery is to transform the LD to a fatigue-resistant state. But this transformation is reversible during the waiting period of adhesions between the LD and the heart, so it is not a clear advantage.

**Dr. Herman:** I agree with you because I did 30 sheep with local stimulation as training period and the results were that some of them had a lot of fibrosis and some of them increased the muscle mass.

**Dr. Stanley Salmons (University of Liverpool):** This procedure is based on another adaptive feature of muscle, which is that the fibers, if lengthened, will add sarcomere to the ends. And that is something that there is a lot of literature on. But there are two sources of damage and I would like to offer it as a word of warning. One is that if you expand the muscle too rapidly, it can add sarcomeres to the ends of the fibers and you will get damage. And the other is when you introduce the stimulation in combination with the expansion. I don't think you did this but when others attempted it, it was a surefire recipe for damage. It has been found in both exercise and stimulation alone but the combination of stretch and stimulation is extremely damaging. You won't see it at 8 weeks because there has been a lot of regeneration taking place. And I think what you should do is look at the early stages, for example after 9 days of expansion, to check whether there is any actual histological damage.

Chapter 34

# Cardiomyoplasty and Defibrillator:

## A Combined Treatment for Heart Failure

David Francischelli, David Peterson, Paul M. Stein, Kendra K. Gealow and Pierre A. Grandjean

## Introduction

Sudden (unexpected) cardiac death is responsible for 40% to 50% of the total mortality in most clinical studies of patients with end-stage heart failure.[1] Despite improvements in cardiac pump function, cardiomyoplasty patients may still be prone to sudden death. Therefore, combining cardiomyoplasty and antitachyarrhythmia therapies in some patients may improve both the mechanical and the electrical dysfunctions of the failing heart.[2,3] Concerns when combining these two therapies are that the muscle stimulation burst from the cardiomyostimulator (CMS) would be interpreted by the implantable defibrillator (PCD®, Medtronic) as ventricular tachycardia (VT) or ventricular fibrillation (VF) episodes, and that the muscle stimulation would interfere with VT or VF therapies. The objectives of this study were to: (1) evaluate if an implantable defibrillator and a cardiomyostimulator could be implanted, without complication into the same animal, (2) test for any interaction between the two devices, and (3) test if the DFTs (defibrillation thresholds) change as the skeletal muscle used for cardiomyoplasty is converted to fatigue resistant.

## Methods

### Defibrillator Implantation

The Medtronic Jewel® Model 7219C implantable defibrillator was used in this study (Fig. 1). It is a fourth-generation defibrillator that can sense and distinguish VT and VF, and provide the appropriate pacing or high-voltage therapy

From Carpentier A, Chachques JC, Grandjean P: Cardiac Bioassist. © Futura Publishing Co, Inc, Armonk, NY, 1997.

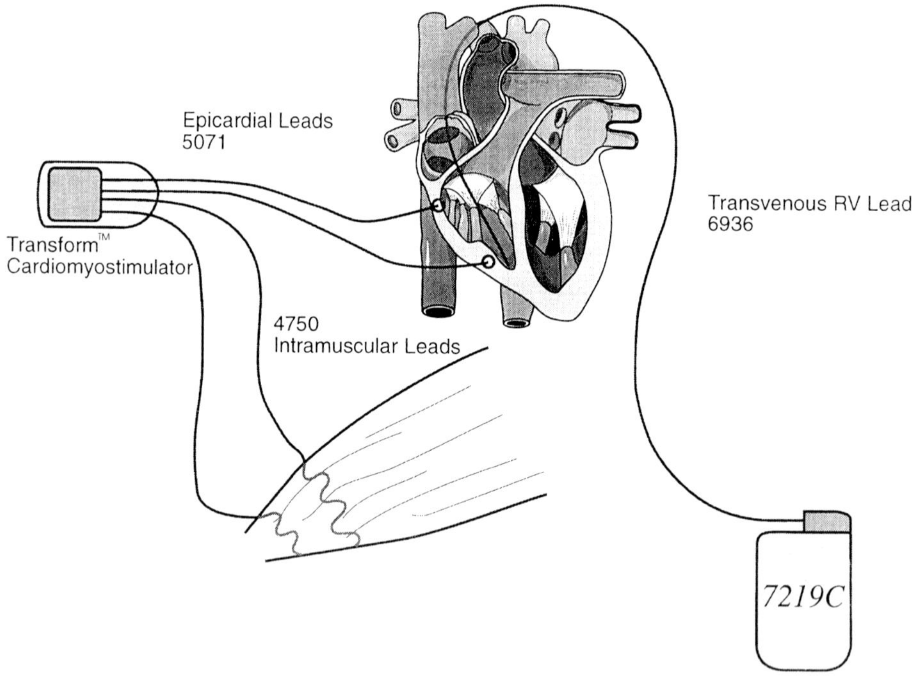


**Figure 1:** *Diagram of implanted devices: Transform® cardiomyostimulator system and anti-tachyarrhythmia (Model 7219C) system.*

to terminate the arrhythmia. The device also incorporates event storage capabilities, which aid the physician in evaluation of arrhythmias and therapies. The Medtronic 6936 transvenous lead incorporates a bipolar sensing/pacing lead at the tip, and a high-voltage coil that is positioned in the right ventricle. Defibrillation shocks are initiated between this coil and the PCD® can.

Five mongrel female dogs (>24 kg) were implanted with the system described above. The PCD® was positioned subcutaneously in the left pectoral area, and the defibrillation threshold (DFT) was evaluated by a binary search method.

## Cardiomyoplasty Procedure

After obtaining an acceptable DFT, cardiomyoplasty was performed using the technique described by Carpentier and Chachques.[4] Two intramuscular leads (Medtronic Model 4750) were woven into the left latissimus dorsi (LD) muscle. The LD muscle was then wrapped around the heart and the leads were connected to the Transform® cardiomyostimulator (Medtronic Model 4710), which was placed in the left abdomen. The Transform® system (see Fig. 1) is a dual channel, implantable pulse train generator that can be programmed via telemetry. Muscle stimulation and synchronization parameters are programmable to optimize cardiac assistance.

## Follow-Up and Measurements

The animals were followed for 14 weeks. During that period, a number of measurements were made at regular intervals to investigate DFTs, lead positions, and proper functioning of the devices. A timeline for these measurements is shown in Figure 2.

## Defibrillation Thresholds

DFTs were measured using a binary search method on weeks 0, 4, and 14. On week 0, this was done before and after the cardiomyoplasty procedure.

## X-Ray of Lead Positions

Lead positions were verified by x-ray. In order to verify that leads did not become dislodged, lateral and dorsoventral radiographs were taken after initial implant and on weeks 2, 4, 6, 8, and 14.

## Defibrillation Under Fluoroscopy

It was hypothesized that a high-voltage defibrillation shock may induce a tetanic contraction of the cardiomyoplasty muscle wrap and impede cardiac output. To investigate this hypothesis, all animals underwent 34-J mono- and biphasic defibrillation shocks during week 7. Before, during, and after each shock, lateral videofluoroscopy was performed and aortic pressure was monitored so that any excessive contraction of the LD muscle could be visualized.

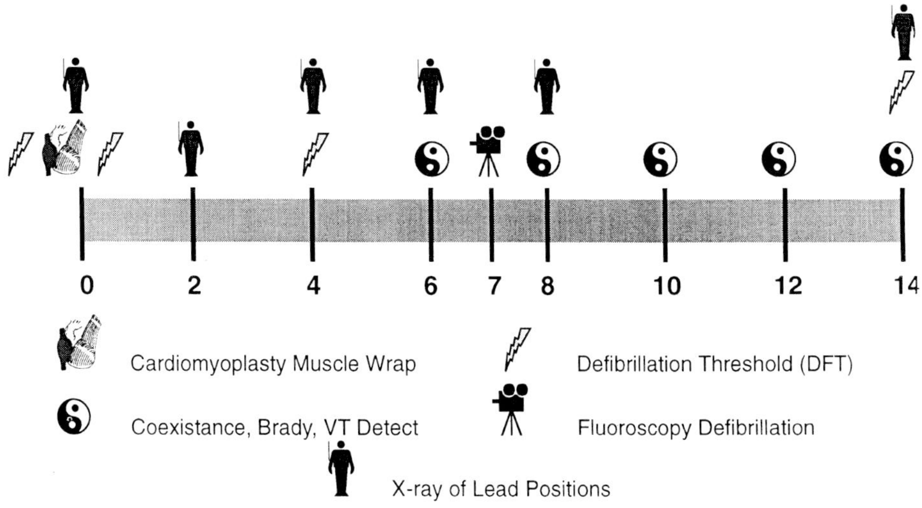


**Figure 2:** *Timeline and measurements performed on each animal.*

## Bradycardia Pacing

Both the CMS and PCD® are capable of pacing the heart in the VVI mode. To demonstrate that bradycardia pacing is possible with this system, each device was, in turn, programmed to maximum pacing amplitude and pulse width, and a lower rate that was greater than the animal's intrinsic heart rate.

## VT Detection/Therapy

The PCD® system is capable of detecting ventricular tachycardia and providing three different pacing therapies as well as cardioversion. In order to simulate VT, the VT detection interval was set to a value greater than the animal's intrinsic RR interval. The PCD® was allowed to detect VT and provide the three different pacing therapies (ramp, ramp+, burst).

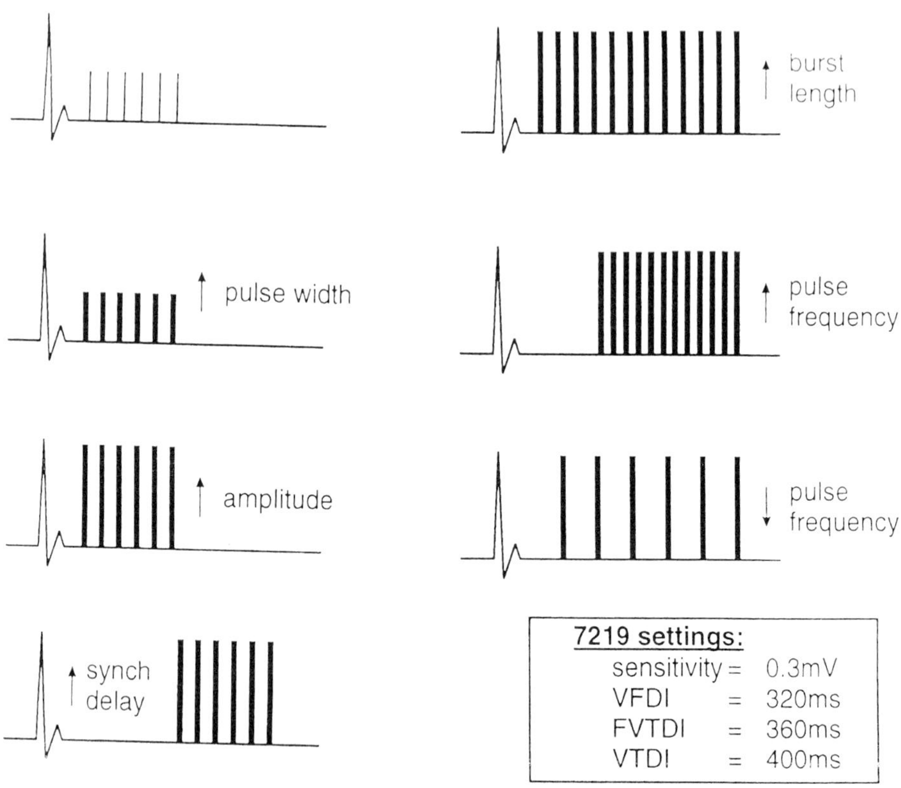


**Figure 3:** *Parameter settings of cardiomyostimulator (Model 4710) and PCD® (Model 7219C) systems during acute coexistence tests: muscle burst amplitude, pulse width, synchronization delay, burst length, and frequency were varied devices possible interactions.*

## Coexistence Tests

The muscle stimulation pulses from the CMS are a relatively high-amplitude signal that may be sensed by the PCD® and result in overdetection. The coexistence tests consisted of two components:

1. **Acute coexistence tests** were designed to test *worst case* situations of muscle burst (high amplitude and pulse width, relatively large distance from the R wave, and very high PCD sensitivity; see Fig. 3). To test for possible frequency dependency, the pulse interval was also varied. The IPGs were programmed to 18 different settings while the animal was awake. Both bipolar and unipolar muscle stimulation modes were tested.
2. **Chronic coexistence tests** monitored cross-talk 24 hours per day, while the IPG parameters were set to more realistic values (normal burst characteristics and 7219C sensitivity set to 0.6 mV). This was accomplished via the event recording capabilities of the PCD. The 7219C was programmed to record the last five VT or VF episodes along with 5 seconds of EGM before arrhythmia confirmation. The number of VT and VF episodes since the previous reset were also recorded. Twice weekly, the PCD was interrogated, and all stored data were evaluated for indication of cross-talk.

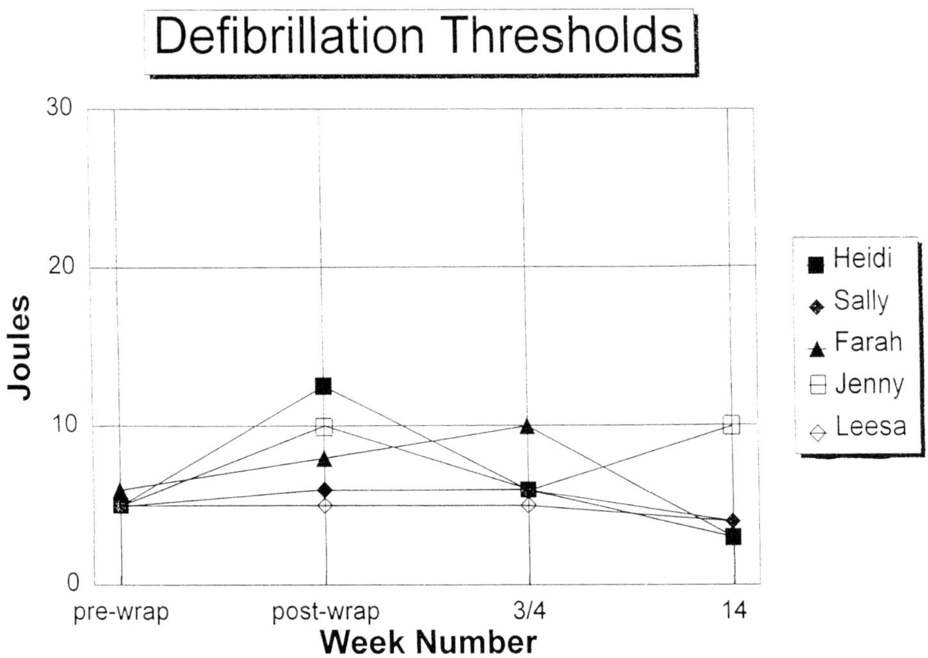


**Figure 4:** *Operative and postoperative defibrillation thresholds (DFT) at 0, 4, and 14 weeks. There was no significant difference in DFT over time.*

## Results

### Defibrillation Thresholds

There was no significant difference in DFT over time ($p$=0.0116). The defibrillation thresholds for each animal are shown in Figure 4. The slight, nonsignificant (Student's $t$-test; $p$=0.078) increase in DFT immediately after the cardiomyoplasty procedure is most likely due to the long anesthesia time (4–5 hours) associated with the surgery. The DFTs return to near baseline at the week 4 monitor, and remain there until termination at 14 weeks.

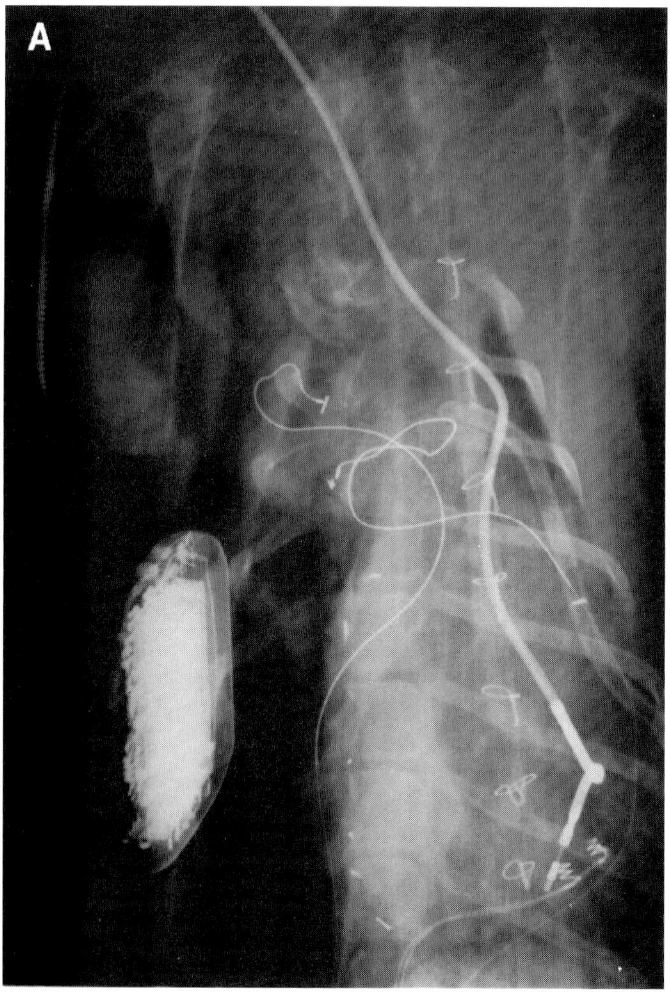


**Figure 5:** *Operative (**A**) and postoperative (**B,** 14 weeks) radiographies show no evidence of lead dislodgement. These findings were confirmed at necropsy. Continued.*

## X-Ray of Lead Positions

There was no evidence of significant lead movement or dislodgement in any animal throughout the course of the study. This was verified by visual inspection during necropsy. Representative x-rays taken after initial implant and at termination are shown in Figure 5.

## Fluoroscopy Defibrillation

Defibrillation under cine fluoroscopy showed no evidence of excessive muscle contraction or impairment of cardiac output due to the muscle wrap. The

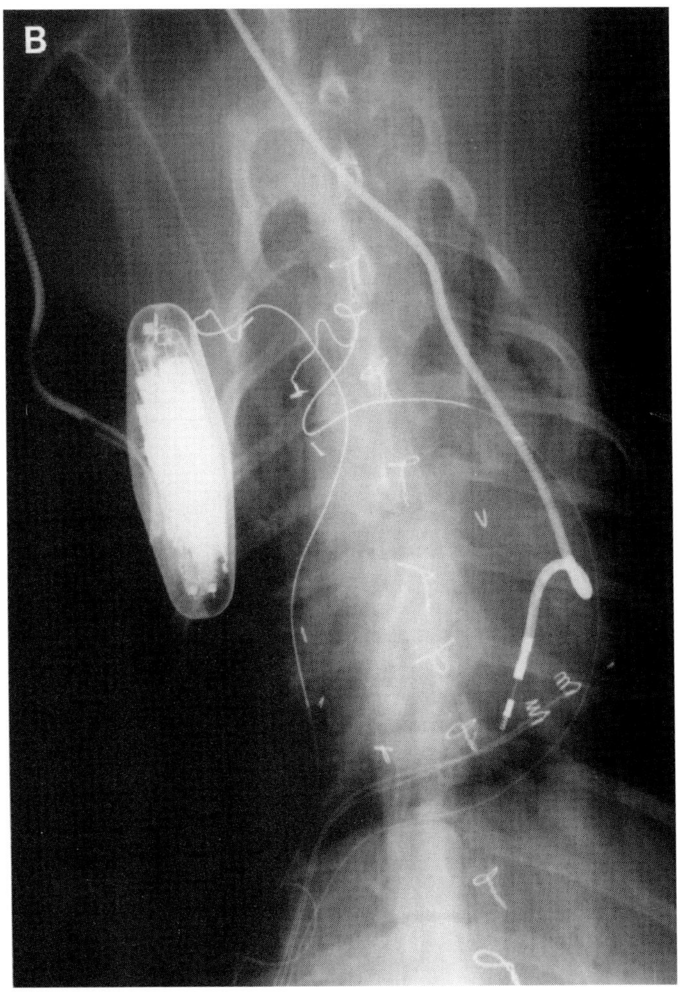


**Figure 5B**

heart returned to its normal position with a few seconds of the shock. Following the shocks, most animals were asystolic and required bradycardia pacing from the PCD® for a few beats. This is common after a defibrillation shock.[5] However, once intrinsic (nonpaced) contractions started, there was no evidence of electromechanical dissociation (EMD) as viewed from the fluoroscopy or blood pressure waveforms.

## Bradycardia Pacing

The muscle burst did not interfere with delivery of therapy. In *all* cases, the CMS and the PCD® were able to independently pace the heart in VVI mode while the other device functioned as programmed.

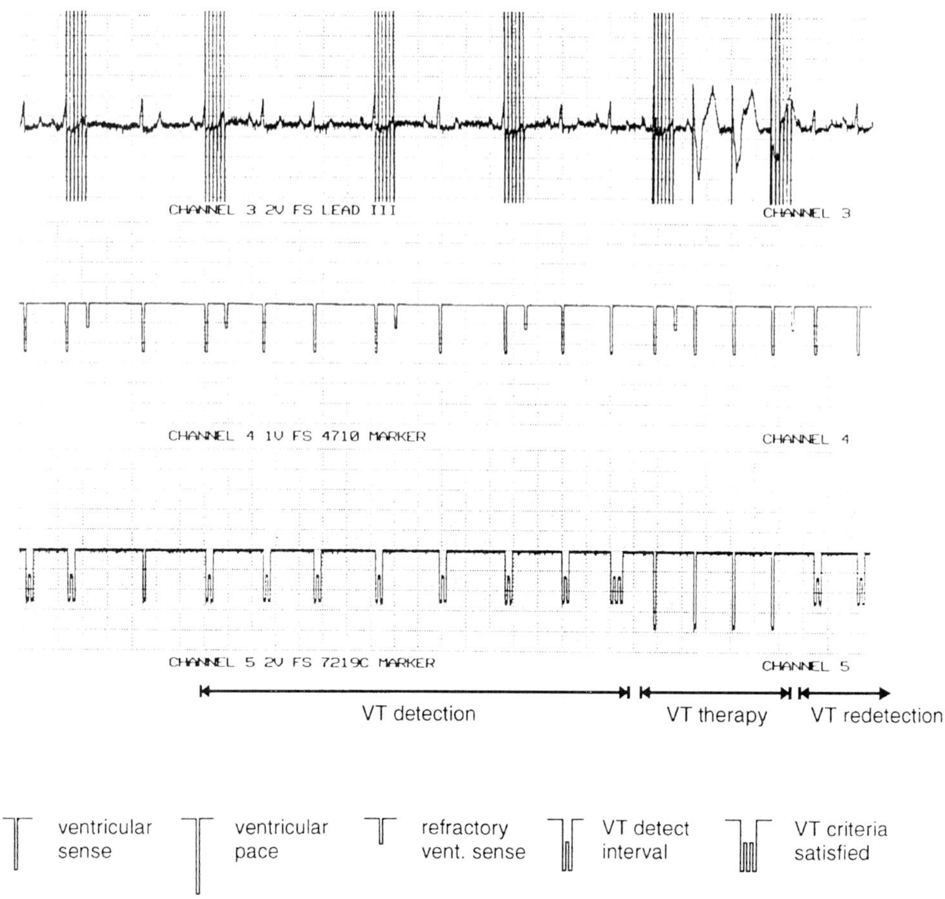


**Figure 6:** *Typical chart recorder tracings of the PCD® detecting VT and delivering antitachy pacing therapy while the CMS continues to stimulate the latissimus dorsi muscle as programmed (PCD® therapy = ramp +, initial # pulses = 1; sequence # = 4).*

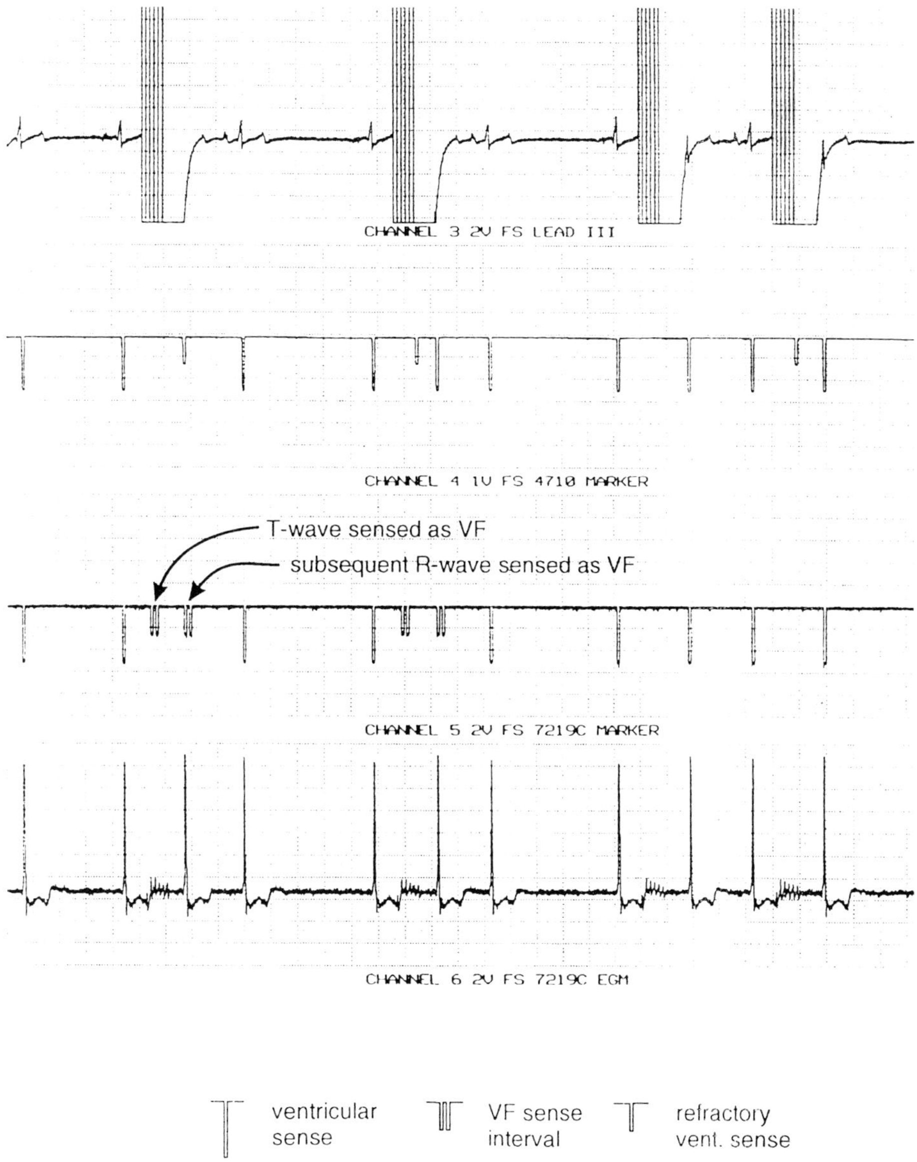


**Figure 7:** *Device coexistence tests showed that incidence of cross-talk was greater when the muscle channel was programmed for unipolar rather than bipolar stimulation. During worst case tests, the cross-talk was manifested by an oversensing of T waves due to superposition of the burst with T wave. Under normal conditions (muscle amplitude: 2–5 V; PCD® sensitivity: 0.6 mV), the cardiomyostimulator never interfered with the PCD® function.*

## VT Detection/Therapy

The muscle stimulation did not interfere with the PCD®'s ability to detect VT, or to deliver appropriate therapy. In *all* cases, the PCD® was able to detect VT based on rate, and deliver three tiers of anti-tachy pacing therapy. A typical tracing is shown in Figure 6.

## Coexistence Tests

### *Acute Coexistence*

There was a significantly greater incidence of cross-talk when the CMS was programmed to unipolar than bipolar muscle stimulation (chi square; $p<0.0001$). The results of the acute coexistence tests showed that during these worst case tests, this cross-talk was always manifested as an oversensing of T-waves due to a superposition of the burst with the localized T wave (see Fig.

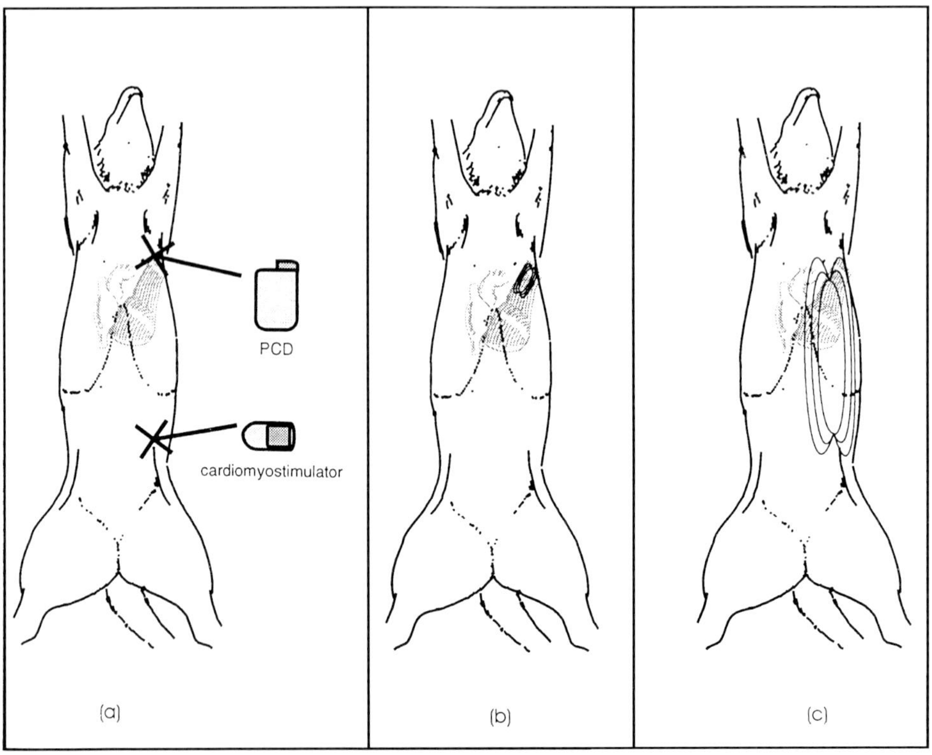


**Figure 8:** *The PCD® system is placed subcutaneously in the left anterolateral side near the midaxillary level, and the cardiomyostimulator (CMS) is located subcutaneously over the rectus abdominus muscle (**a**). When the CMS is programmed to bipolar muscle stimulation (**b**), the electrical field generated is well localized between the two intramuscular electrodes. However, when programmed to unipolar muscle stimulation (**c**), the electrical field extends to the CMS can and this increases the probability of interacting with the PCD® device.*

7). There was no correlation between oversensing and weeks post-implant, burst frequency or synchronization delay.

The reason for this increased oversensing associated with the burst is best shown by Figure 8. Bipolar muscle stimulation results in a tight and localized electric field between the two intramuscular leads. However, a unipolar configuration will generate a field between the intramuscular cathode and the CMS can. This field passes through the right ventricle and the PCD® sensing/pacing lead and could result in PCD® oversensing of T waves associated with a muscle burst.

### *Chronic Coexistence*

The cardiomyostimulator never interfered with the PCD® function. Evaluation of *all* stored episode data showed that with the IPGs programmed to normal values (2–5 V burst amplitude; 210 μs pulse width; 0.6 mV 7219C sensitivity), there was no evidence of oversensing T waves and no correlation with the muscle burst (i.e., the burst was never sensed by the PCD®). Therefore, during the normal operations of the two devices, there were no adverse interactions.

### *Histopathology*

Histopathology showed no evidence of shock-induced myocardial or LD muscle tissue damage. There were normal adhesions between cardiac and LD muscle tissues, and all leads were well fixed.

## Conclusions

The results of this study showed that it is feasible to implant both an implantable defibrillator (Medtronic Model 7219C) and a cardiomyostimulator (Medtronic Model 4710) into the same host. The cardiomyostimulator was able to provide LD muscle stimulation during periods of normal sinus rhythm and bradycardia. The cardiomyoplasty system did not prevent the PCD® from detecting and delivering appropriate therapy for VT and VF arrhythmias, and the DFTs remained fairly stable over the 14-week study. Histological analysis showed no evidence of shock-induced damage to myocardial or LD muscle tissue.

Throughout the course of the study, the PCD® did not sense the muscle burst under normal operating conditions. However, due to the orientation of the electric fields, there was a greater incidence of T-wave sensing associated with the burst in unipolar mode. This was easily remedied by appropriate programming of the PCD® sensitivity and confirmed by the Marker Channel™ available with both systems.

Clinical studies are currently under way to confirm the safety, effectiveness, and compatibility of combined cardiomyoplasty and PCD® therapies. In order to minimize the potential for cross-talk: (1) the cardiomyostimulator should always be set to a bipolar muscle configuration, (2) the sensitivity of the

PCD® should be set to twice (2x) the minimum value which precludes sensing of P and T waves, and (3) the ability of the PCD® to reliably detect VF at this sensitivity setting should be verified in the electrophysiology lab.

## References

1. NHLBI Report of the Task Force on Research in Heart Failure, May 94.
2. Bocchi EA, Moreira LPF, de Moraes AV, Bacal F, et al: Arrhythmias and sudden death after dynamic cardiomyoplasty. *Circulation* 90:5:II-107–II-111, 1994.
3. Gorgels APM, Vos MA, Smeets JLRM, Wellens HJJ: Ventricular arrhythmias in heart failure. *Am J Cardiology* 70:37C-43C, 1992.
4. Carpentier A, Chachques JC: Cardiomyoplasty: Surgical technique. In Carpentier A, Chachques JC, Grandjean P (eds): *Cardiomyoplasty*. Futura Publishing Co, Inc, Mount Kisco, NY, 1991, pp 105–122.
5. Waldecker B, Brachman J, Schmitt C, Killat H, et al: Heart rhythm after conversion of ventricular tachyarrhythmia by internal shock delivery. *Z Kardiol* 83:283–292, 1994.

Chapter 35

# Serratus Anterior Aortic and Ventricular Myoplasties:

## The Anatomic Basis for Human Application

Gordon R. Tobin, Anne-Elise Tobin,
Ardeshir Hakami*

### Introduction

This chapter discusses the anatomic basis in man for use of the serratus anterior muscle as a new motor unit for cardiac assist. It introduces applications of the serratus anterior alone and in combination with the latissimus dorsi (LD) muscle to both aortic counterpulsation and cardiomyoplasty. These applications overcome two of the major obstacles that have prevented human application of muscle wraps for aortic counterpulsation. First, they have the ability to form wraps that preserve all aortic branches, including those supplying the spinal cord, thus avoiding the risk of paraplegia. Second, they also have the ability to wrap the entire thoracic aorta, thus overcoming previous limitations of volume displacement.

### Background

To date, the LD muscle has been the most thoroughly studied and virtually the only clinically applied motor unit for cardiac assist procedures. The diaphragm and rectus abdominis have also been proposed and used experimentally.[1,2] However, wrapping the descending aorta with any of these three muscles requires dividing the aortic origin of the intercostal arteries, thus interrupting the blood supply to the spinal cord in humans and risking cord ischemia and paraplegia. Also, the diaphragm and rectus abdominis wrap the ventricles incompletely and fail to reach and wrap the ascending and proximal

*With the cooperation of John H. Barker, A. David Slater, and Laman A. Gray, Jr.

From Carpentier A, Chachques JC, Grandjean P: Cardiac Bioassist. © Futura Publishing Co, Inc, Armonk, NY, 1997.

descending aorta. Thus, only the latissimus dorsi serves well for cardiomyoplasty and none of these muscles are adequate for aortomyoplasty.

Recently, we proposed using the serratus anterior muscle as a new motor unit for cardiac assist applications.[3] Our studies of human serratus anterior anatomy showed this muscle to be especially well suited for descending aortomyoplasty and counterpulsation because its highly segmental morphology and neurovascular anatomy permits surgical splitting of the muscle segments to wrap the aorta between its intercostal side branches without dividing them.[4] Thus, the intercostal branches that also supply the spinal cord are preserved, and the disastrous neurological complication of paraplegia can be avoided. This eliminates a major barrier to human application of the diastolic counterpulsation principle by aortic muscle wraps.

A second major barrier to human application of the diastolic counterpulsation principle has been the limited volume displaced by the experimental muscle wraps used previously. This barrier is also eliminated by serratus anterior wraps because the entire thoracic aorta can be wrapped by use of extended applications of these motor units. The right serratus muscle will wrap the ascending aorta, the left serratus muscle will wrap the upper descending aorta, and a left LD muscle can wrap the remaining descending aorta to the diaphragm.

This chapter will fully define the anatomic basis of serratus anterior and combined serratus anterior-latissimus dorsi muscle wraps for cardiac assist applications and it will describe the surgical crafting and transfer of these motor units to the aorta and heart for ascending aortomyoplasty, descending aortomyoplasty, and cardiomyoplasty.

## Methods

We studied the morphology and neurovascular anatomy of 22 fresh and 13 preserved human cadaver serratus anterior muscles by dissection and specimen angiography following arterial perfusion with barium sulfate 2:1 in 5–10% gelatin solution using the method described by the senior author.[4,5] We also studied intrathoracic transfer dimensions for cardiac assist applications of serratus anterior and serratus anterior-latissimus dorsi muscle combinations by dissections and transfers of these muscles to the aorta and heart. We measured the ability of neurovascular pedicle and flap length to provide wraps of the descending aorta, arch, ascending aorta, and heart. Functional neuroanatomy was studied in a clinical setting by selective nerve stimulation in five patients during transfer of serratus anterior and combined serratus anterior-latissimus dorsi muscle flaps to repair intrathoracic defects.

## Results

### Muscle Morphology

The serratus anterior muscle was strictly segmental in all specimens, with each segment corresponding to its rib of origin. There were $8.6 \pm 0.8$ ($X \pm SD$) segments with variable presence on ribs 1 and 8–10.

## Nerve Anatomy

In all specimens we found little anatomic variation of the long thoracic nerve, the motor nerve to the muscle. It was always a single trunk on the external surface of the muscle with segmental branches to each muscle segment. The entire muscle was supplied by this nerve and its segmental branches. Thus, the muscle can be paced and transformed either by nerve trunk or by direct muscle stimulation. In patients undergoing thoracotomy, main trunk stimulation contracted the entire muscle, and selective stimulation of each branch contracted only the supplied segment.

## Vascular Anatomy

The origin of the vascular pedicle to the serratus was variable (Fig. 1). In 89% of muscles, the trunk of origin was the thoracodorsal vessels (Figs. 1A and B), either in common with the circumflex scapular vessels from the subscapular trunk or independent of them. Within this group, the trunk of origin was the subscapular-thoracodorsal vessels, in common with circumflex scapular branches and branches to the LD muscle in 73% of total muscles. In the remainder of this group, the trunk of origin was the thoracodorsal vessels, in common with the latissimus dorsi pedicle but independent of the subscapular-circumflex scapular trunk in 16% of total muscles. In 9% of muscles, the vascular pedicle origin was the lateral thoracic, not the thoracodorsal vessels, and there was no common blood supply to the LD muscle (Figs. 1C and D). In 2% of muscles, a double pedicle was found—one each from the thoracodorsal and lateral thoracic vessels that supplied approximately equal portions of the muscle. Regardless of origin, the serratus anterior vascular pedicle followed closely the long thoracic nerve on the muscle external surface and also gave independent branches to each muscle segment. In the 89% of specimens with a common thoracodorsal supply, the serratus anterior and LD muscles could be simultaneously transferred on this single vascular pedicle (Figs. 2B and C). In the 9% of specimens with the serratus supplied by the lateral thoracic vessels, simultaneous use of the serratus and LD would require independent transfer of each flap or their respective pedicles (Fig. 2A).

We also studied the neurovascular anatomy of the LD muscle. The findings confirmed our previous reports of the proximal branching of the thoracodorsal pedicle at the neurovascular hilum and segmental pattern of intramuscular supply to the proximal one-third of the muscle.[5–8] This branching pattern allows surgical splitting into two or three segments at the level of the neurovascular hilum and distal splitting into four to six segments near the origin along the spine and the 12th rib.[7]

## Arc of Rotation

Due to close proximity of origin for subscapular, thoracodorsal, and lateral thoracic vessels, the arcs of rotation of the serratus anterior and combined ser-

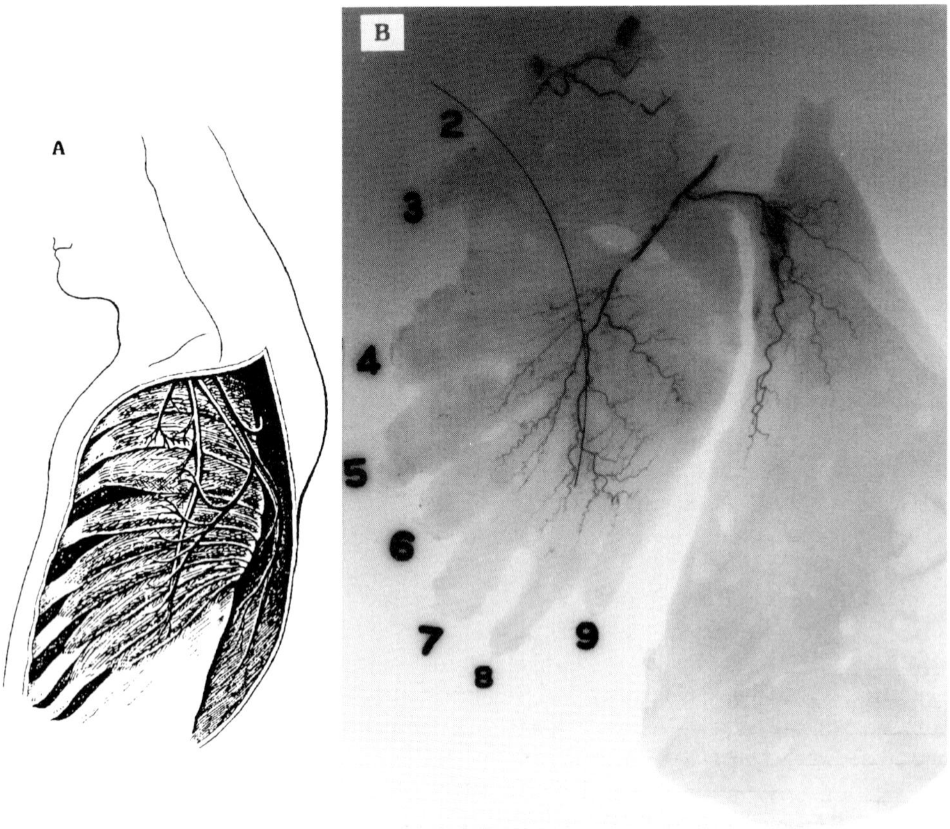


**Figure 1 A, B:** *Figures* **A** *and* **B** *show the most frequent (89%) vascular pedicle pattern, which is a common thoracodorsal vascular pedicle to both serratus anterior and latissimus dorsi muscles, with independent nerve trunks. This allows the muscles to be simultaneously transferred on the common vascular pedicle when both are used. Continued.*

ratus anterior-latissimus dorsi muscle transfers were virtually unaffected by the anatomic variations described above, as all pedicle origins permitted essentially equivalent arcs of rotation when the muscle flaps were transferred. When passed through a second or third rib window, both serratus anterior muscles reach transversely across the midline to the contralateral midclavicular line. When transferred diagonally, both right and left serratus anterior muscles reach the distal borders of the heart, but are not able to circumferentially wrap it. When transferred caudally, both serratus anterior muscles just reach the ipsilateral diaphragm. This arc of rotation allows either serratus anterior to wrap the ascending aorta and to cover either the anterior or the posterior surface of the heart. In transferring the left serratus to the descending aorta, the clinically useful arc of rotation is shortened somewhat compared

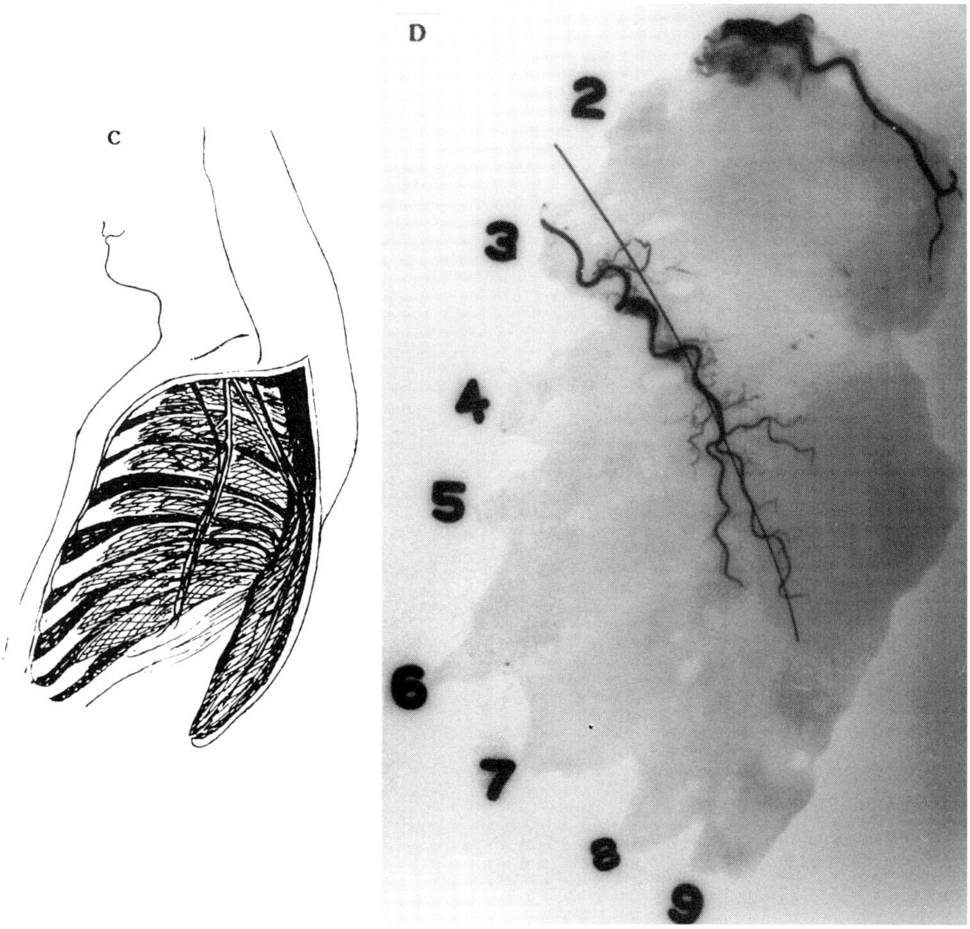


**Figure 1 C, D:** *Figures* **C** *and* **D** *show the second most common vascular pedicle pattern (9%), in which there are independent lateral thoracic and thoracodorsal vascular pedicles to each muscle, as well as independent nerve trunks. The muscle flaps must be separately transferred if both are needed. In the radiographs (Figs.* **B** *and* **D***), the wire marks the course of the long thoracic nerve.*

with its anatomic reach due to the fact that the muscle segments must be oriented transversely to provide a wrap that is perpendicular to the descending aorta. This limits aortic coverage to the level of the eighth or ninth intercostal vessel origin depending on the number of serratus segments present. Therefore, the serratus wrap usually covers the first 15–17 cm of the descending aorta distal to the left subclavian origin. When fully mobilized combined serratus anterior-latissimus dorsi muscles are transferred, the LD extends substantially more distally. When passed through a second or third rib window and the diaphragm at the aortic hiatus, the LD reaches the sacral promontory and could wrap the abdominal aorta to the level of the bifurcation. Thus, it eas-

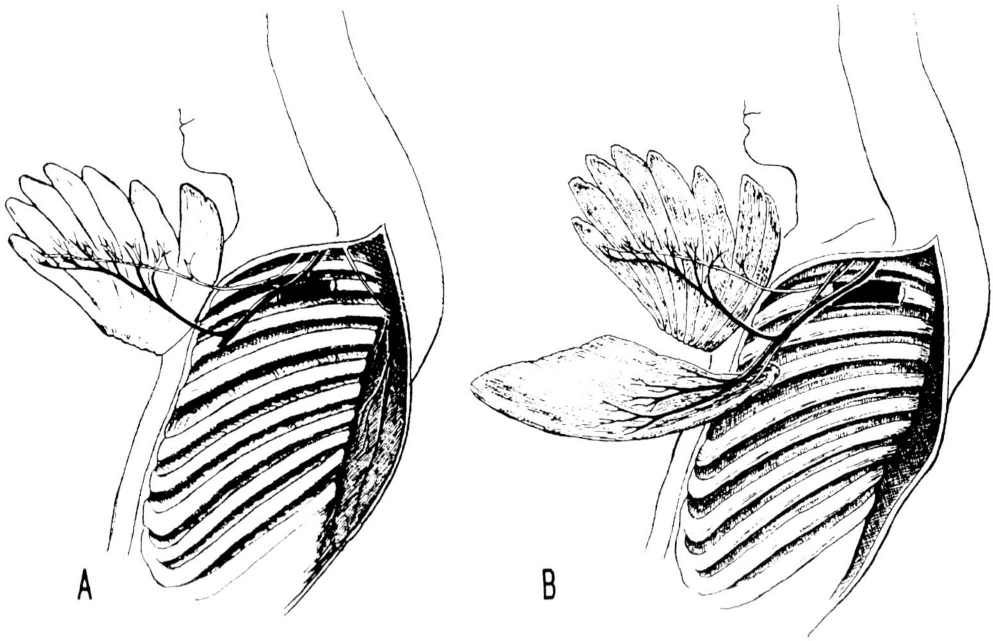


**Figure 2 A, B:** *Transfer of only the serratus anterior motor unit is shown in* **A** *and transfer of the combined serratus anterior-latissimus dorsi motor units is shown in* **B** *and* **C**. *Continued.*

ily can wrap the thoracic aorta between the distal segment of the serratus wrap and the diaphragm.

## Surgical Applications

The anatomic features that we found allowed us to design several new cardiac assist procedures based on the serratus anterior motor unit. In each of these procedures, the muscle origin and insertion are fully detached for island pedicle transfer on their neurovascular pedicles and passed through a second rib resection window to the recipient site on the aorta or heart.

When a common thoracodorsal pedicle to both serratus anterior and LD is present and only the serratus anterior motor unit is to be transferred, the latissimus branch is divided distal to its origin on the thoracodorsal trunk (Fig. 2A) In clinical cases we have shown that latissimus viability is maintained following this maneuver due to collateral circulation to the latissimus from the intercostal perforating vessels, collateral vessels around the scapula, and cutaneous perforators.[7,9] When combined serratus anterior-latissimus dorsi motor units are transferred, they may be carried on the same thoracodorsal vascular pedicle in over 89% of cases (Figs. 2B and C). In clinical cases we have shown that this thoracodorsal supply alone is sufficient to maintain viability of both transferred motor units.[7,9] The motor nerves to both muscles are in immediate

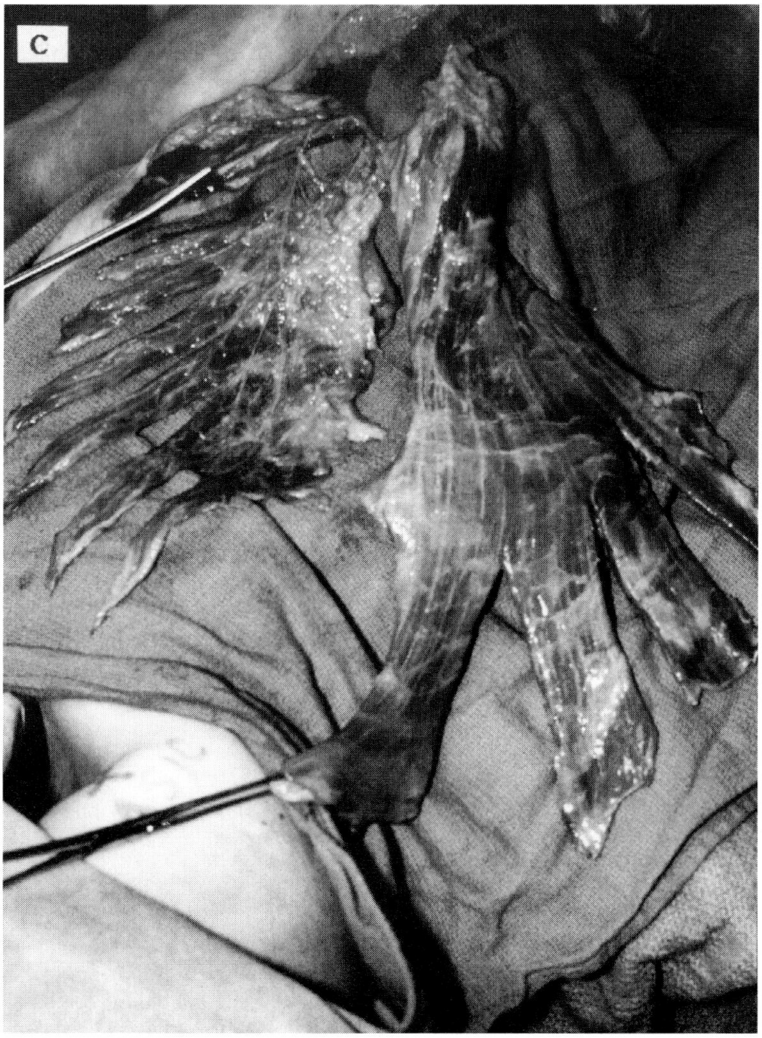


**Figure 2C:** *Both the serratus and the distal latissimus muscles have been surgically split for wrapping between aortic intercostal branches. Detailed knowledge of the neurovascular pedicle anatomy and its variations is essential for technical execution of these transfers.*

proximity in sites in the axilla and remain so in transfer, as the long thoracic nerve is on the superficial surface of the serratus anterior and the thoracodorsal nerve is on the deep surface of the latissimus dorsi muscle. We found that they can both be simultaneously encompassed and stimulated with a single nerve trunk electrode for transformation and cardiac assist as well as stimulated separately and independently.

The cardiac assist procedures that we designed and the optimal motor unit transfer for each of these procedures are summarized below, followed by a more detailed description of each specific procedure.

## Proximal Descending Aortomyoplasty

The region from the left subclavian origin to the eighth or ninth intercostal vessel origin is done with a left serratus anterior wrap, which is split between muscle segments to pass between the preserved aortic intercostal branches.

## Total Descending Aortomyoplasty

The entire thoracic descending aorta from the left subclavian origin to the diaphragm can be wrapped with the left combined serratus anterior-latissimus dorsi motor units, using the serratus anterior in the proximal location as described above and the LD muscle to wrap the lower thoracic aorta between the

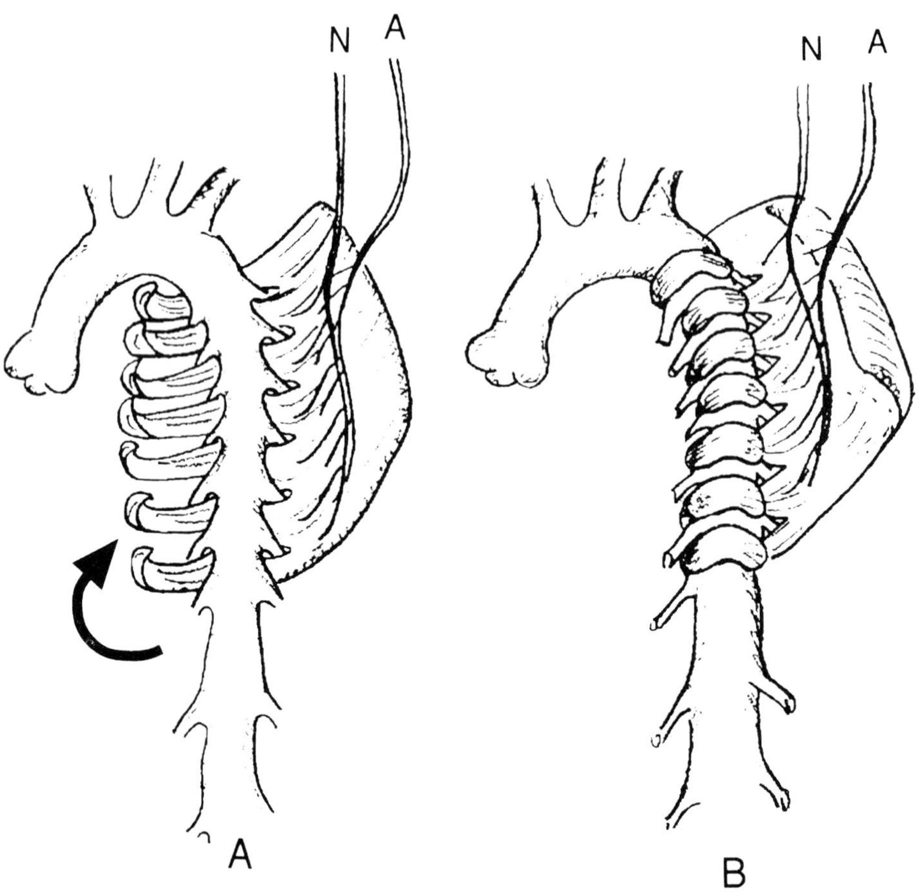


**Figure 3:** *The surgical technique of left serratus anterior descending aortomyoplasty using a counterclockwise wrap is illustrated in* **A** *and* **B**, *and demonstrated in* **C, D,** *and* **E.** *The aorta is mobilized from surrounding structures, preserving the intercostal and other branches* (**C**), *the split serratus anterior muscle segments are passed between these vessels* (**D**), *and the wrap is completed and inset* (**E**). *Continued.*

eighth or ninth intercostal vessels and the diaphragm. The LD muscle is split distally into three to six tails, as needed, to pass between the preserved aortic branches in this region.

## Ascending Aortomyoplasty

The ascending aorta (and optionally the arch between major branches to the head and arms) is wrapped with the right serratus anterior muscle. The left serratus anterior could be used for the ascending aorta equally as well, but it is best reserved for descending aortomyoplasty.

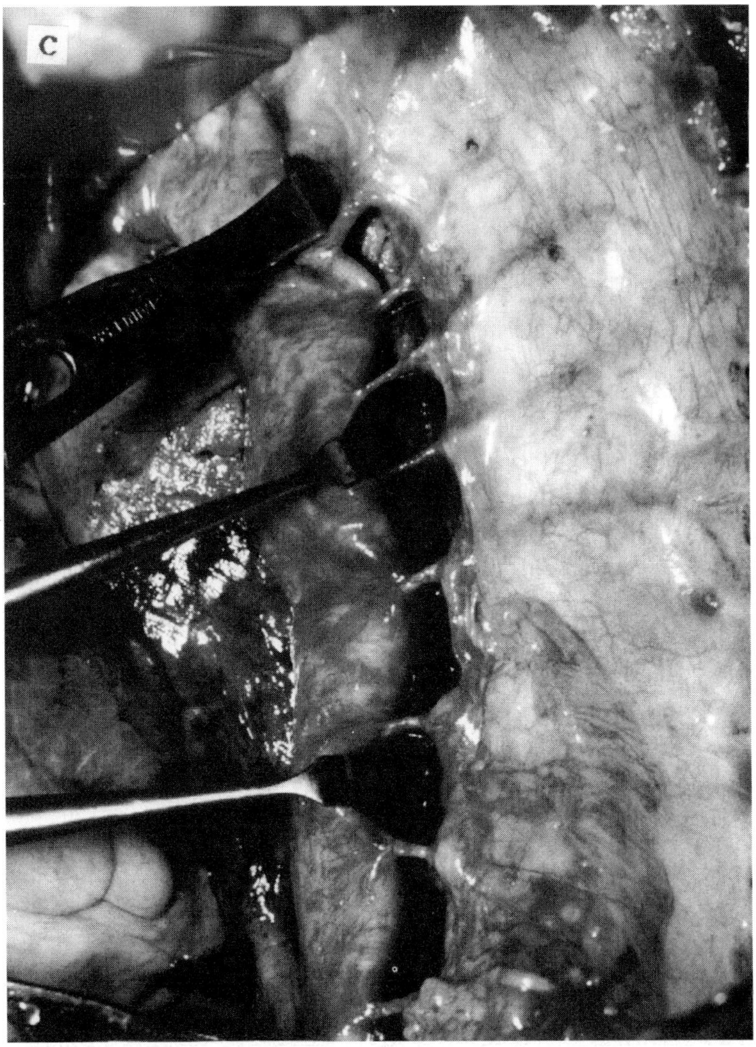

**Figure 3C.** ***Continued.***

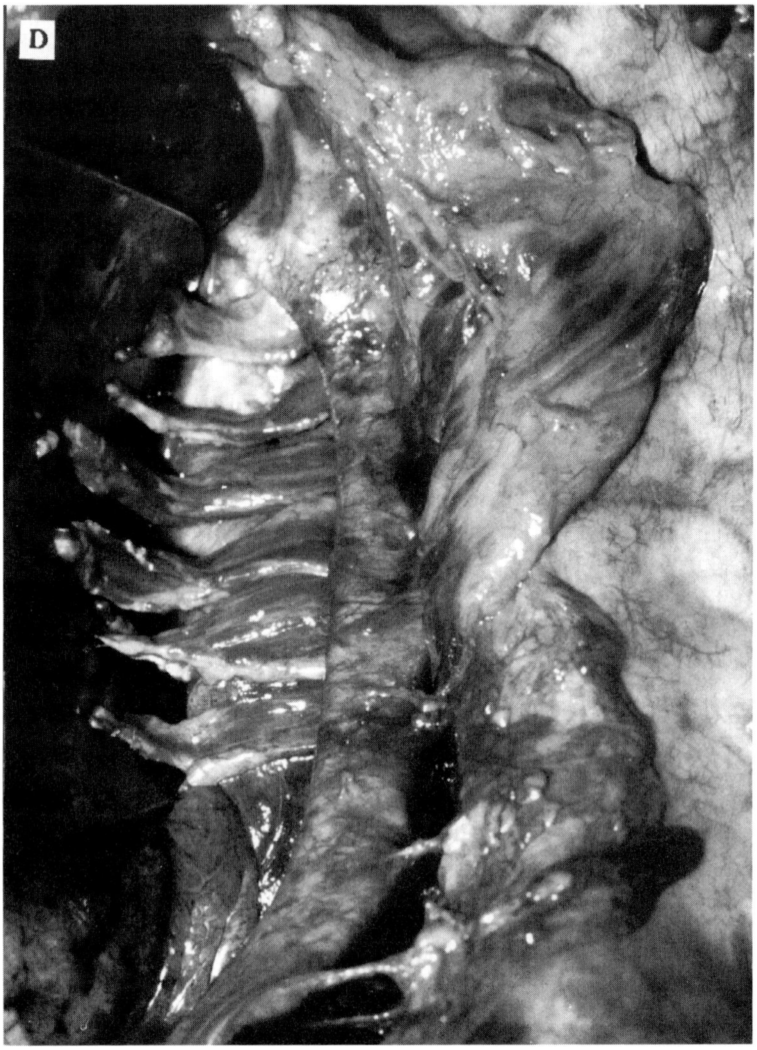


Figure 3D. *Continued.*

## Total Thoracic Aortomyoplasty

The total thoracic aorta from the root to the diaphragm can be entirely wrapped for diastolic counterpulsation with preservation of all aortic branches using the right serratus anterior on the ascending aorta (and optionally the arch), the left serratus anterior on the descending aorta to the eighth or the ninth intercostal vessel origin, and the left LD muscle from that level to the aortic hiatus of the diaphragm.

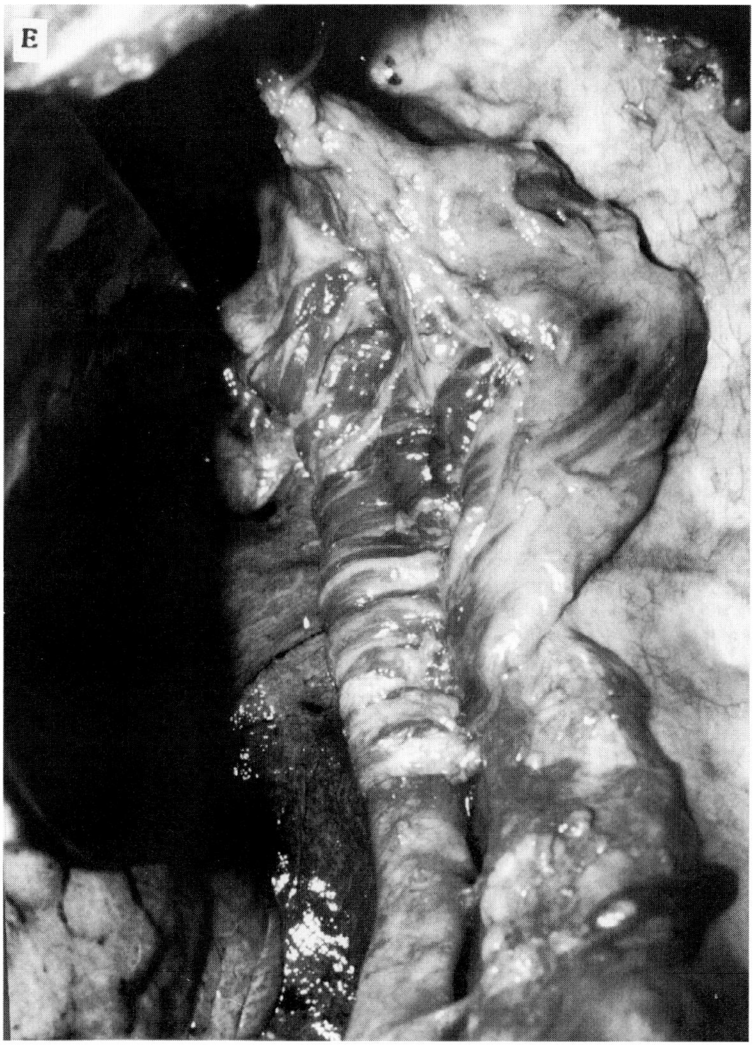


Figure 3E.

## Left Serratus Anterior Proximal Descending Aortomyoplasty

Proximal descending aortomyoplasty (Figs. 3 and 4) is done with the left serratus anterior muscle segments three through the most distal (usually eight or nine). The muscle is transferred as an island on its neurovascular pedicle through a left second rib resection window to the mobilized proximal descending aorta. The muscle is surgically split between adjacent segments to pass between the preserved intercostal vessels. Each muscle segment wraps the aorta at exactly the corresponding level of its in situ position. Thus, the third segment wraps the aorta between the left subclavian and the third intercostal branches, the fourth segment passes between the third and fourth intercostal branch, and the remaining branches are placed in order until all are wrapped. The wrap can be done either from dorsal to ventral (counterclockwise when viewed from above) (Fig. 3) or ventral to dorsal (clockwise when viewed from above) (Fig. 4). Hemodynamic studies will ultimately determine if one orientation is preferred.

## Right Serratus Anterior Ascending Aortomyoplasty

Ascending aortomyoplasty (Fig. 5) is best done with the right serratus anterior. It can also be done with the left serratus anterior, but this motor unit is best reserved for descending aortomyoplasty. The muscle is passed through a right second rib resection window to the mobilized ascending aorta. The wrap is then done in a manner analogous to that described by Chachques et al. for latissimus dorsi ascending aortomyoplasty.[10] As in descending aortomy-

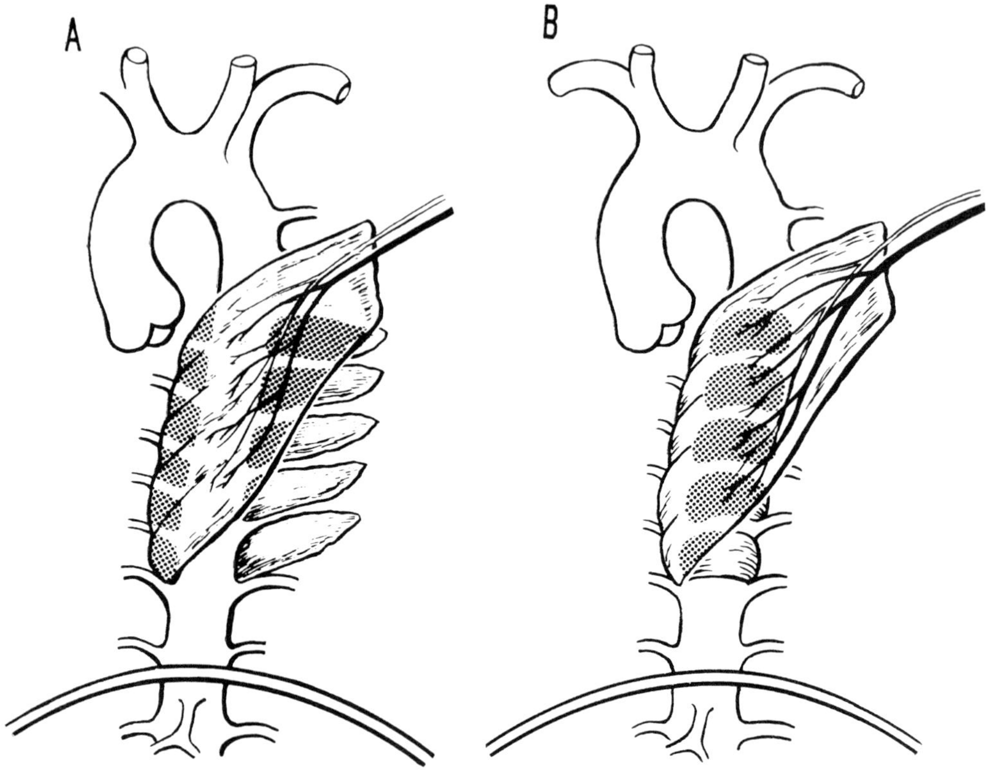


**Figure 4:** *The surgical technique of left serratus anterior descending aortomyoplasty using a clockwise wrap is illustrated in* **A** *and* **B**, *and demonstrated in* **C**, **D**, *and* **E**. *The aorta is mobilized from surrounding structures, preserving the intercostal and other branches* (**C**), *the split serratus anterior muscle segments are passed between these vessels* (**D**), *and the wrap is completed and inset* (**E**). *Continued.*

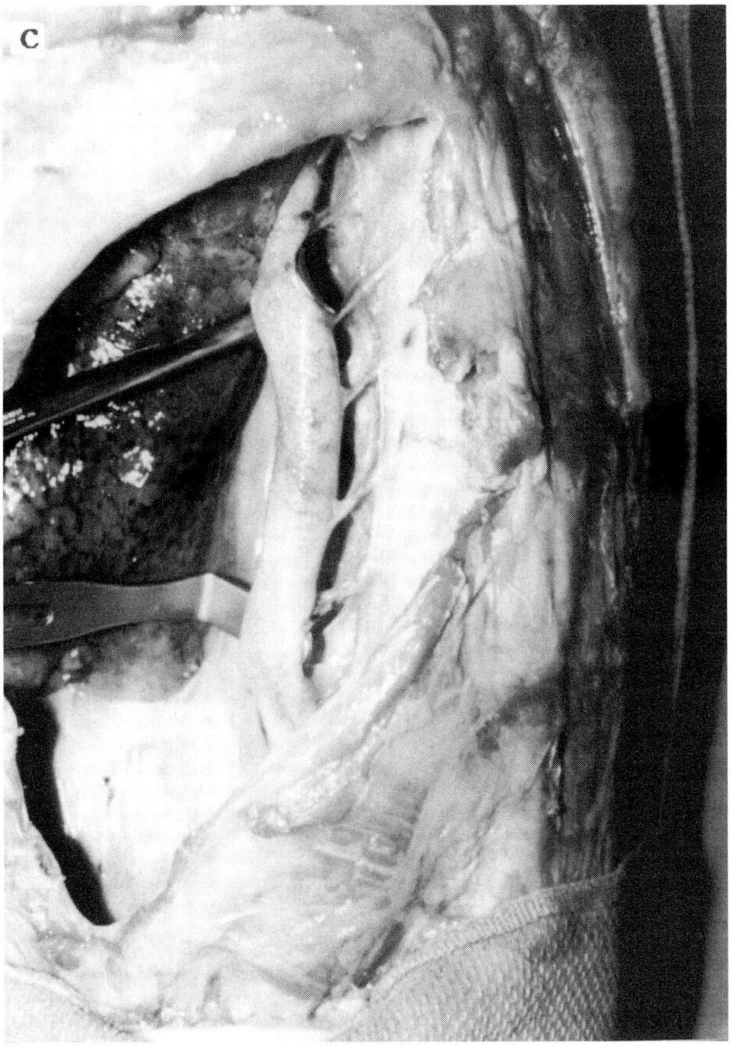


Figure 4C. *Continued.*

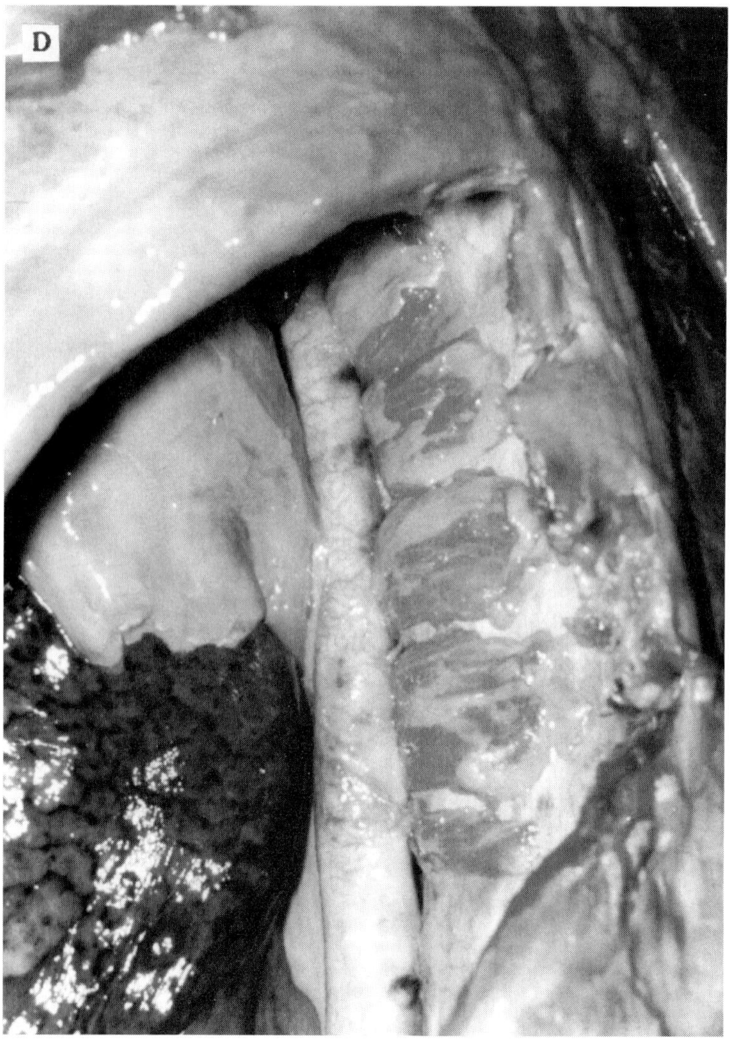


Figure 4D. *Continued.*

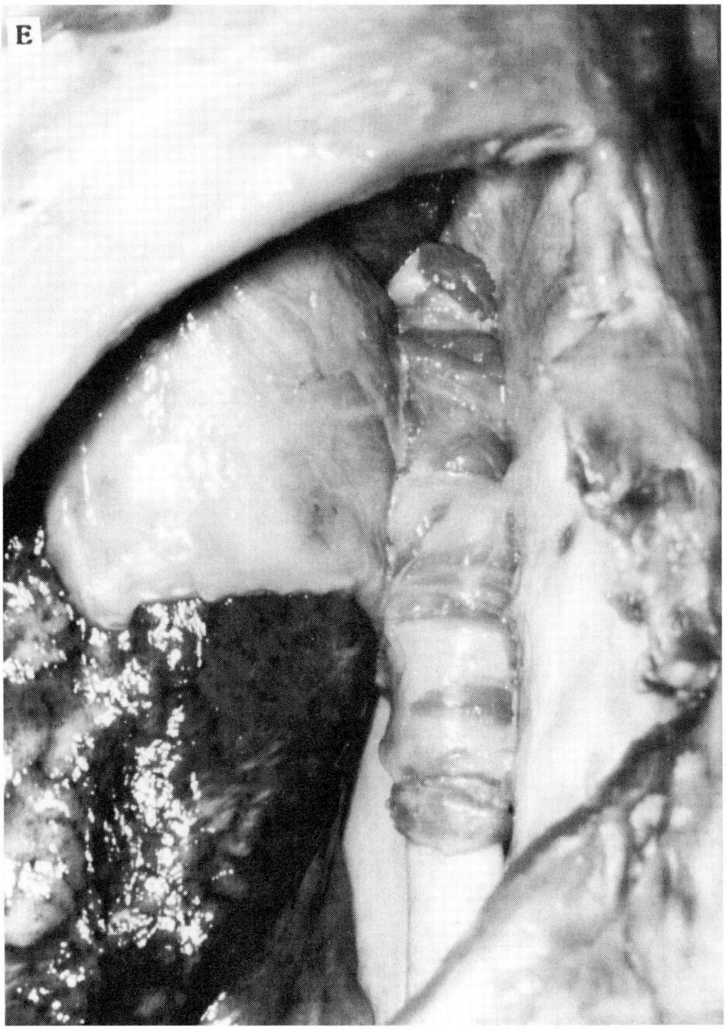


**Figure 4E.**

oplasty, the wrap may be done either clockwise (dorsal to ventral) or counter-clockwise, although the clockwise wrap is technically more straightforward. Optionally, the entire arch or a portion of it may be wrapped by splitting serratus anterior muscle segments to pass between the vessels to the head and upper extremities. Used in this manner, the right serratus anterior covers the arch to about 3–4 cm beyond the left subclavian artery origin.

## Combined Serratus Anterior-Latissimus Dorsi Total Thoracic Aortomyoplasty

The muscle transfers defined in this chapter allow wrapping the entire length of the thoracic aorta for counterpulsation. For total descending aortomyoplasty, the proximal descending aorta is wrapped with the left serratus anterior muscle to the level of the eighth or ninth intercostal vessel origin and the aorta below this level is wrapped to the diaphragm with the left LD muscle. The length of the proximal aortic wrap is determined by the number of serra-

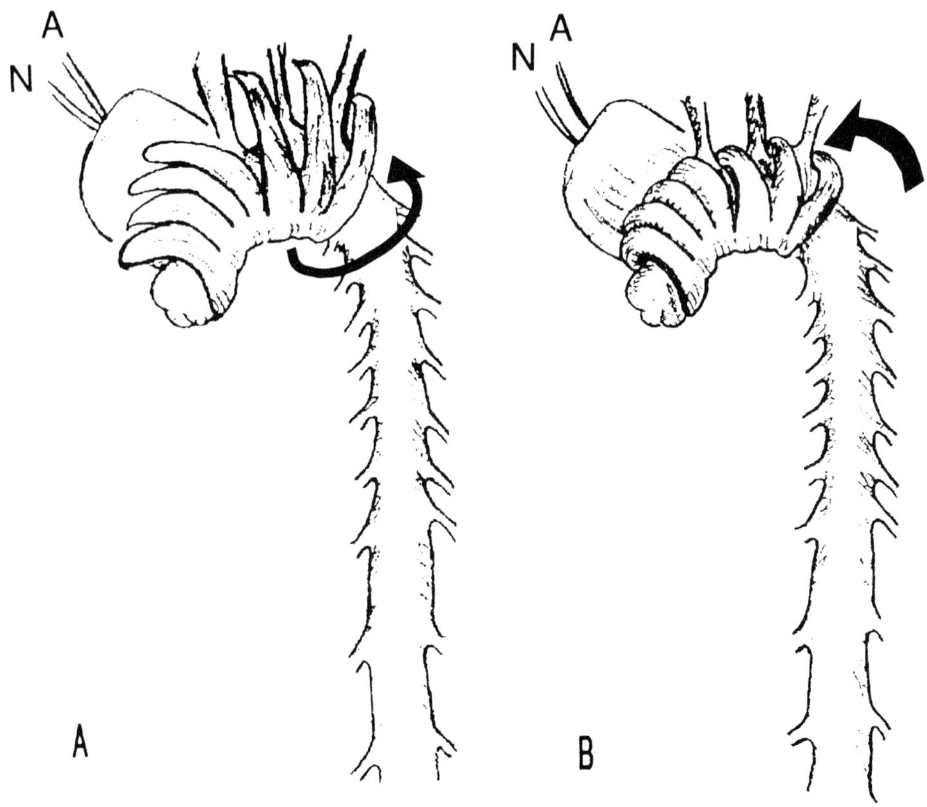


**Figure 5:** *The surgical technique of right serratus anterior ascending aortomyoplasty is illustrated in* **A** *and* **B** *(showing the optional wrapping of the arch), and demonstrated in* **C** *and* **D**. *The muscle is passed behind the ascending aorta* (**C**) *and the wrap is inset* (**D**). *Continued.*

tus muscle segments available. The latissimus dorsi wrap is also surgically split distally to pass between preserved distal aortic intercostal branches. This is customized from patient to patient, as the intercostal vessel origins in the distal descending thoracic aorta have wider spacing and greater variability than in the proximal descending aorta. The proximal intercostal vessels predictably supply each upper rib from 3 through 9 or 10 with an independent pair of aortic branches. In the distal descending aorta, some pairs of intercostal vessels may have common origins with adjacent pairs.

For total thoracic aortomyoplasty, the ascending aorta is wrapped with the right serratus anterior muscle, and the entire descending aorta is wrapped with the left serratus and latissimus (Fig. 6) as described above.

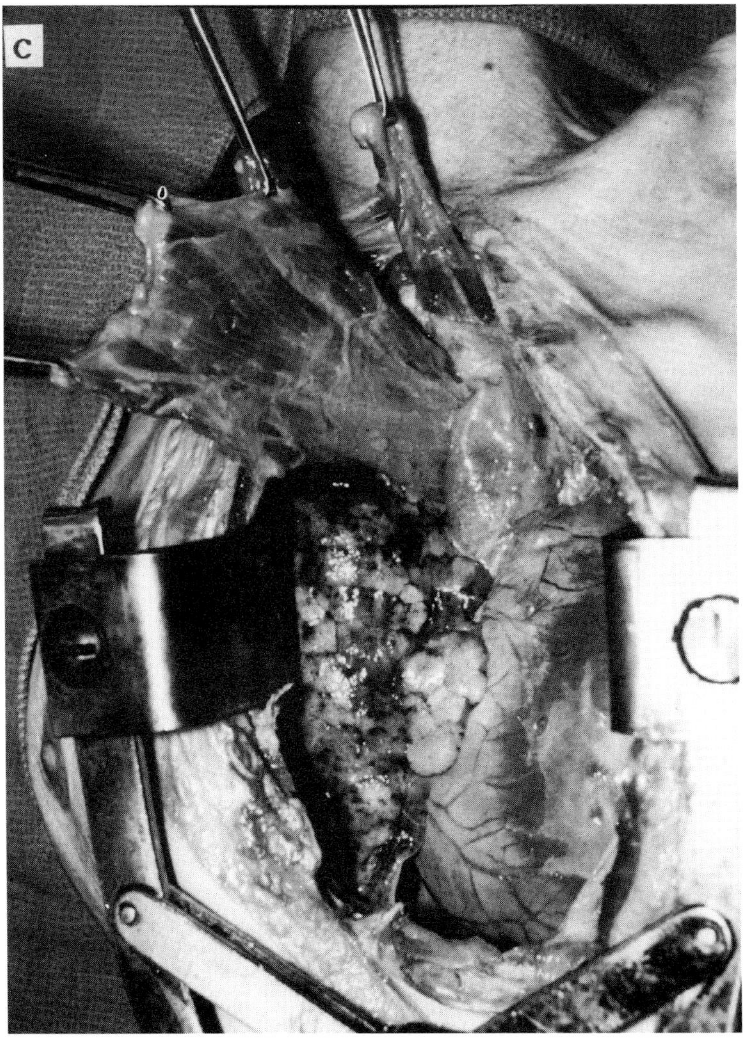


**Figure 5C.** ***Continued.***

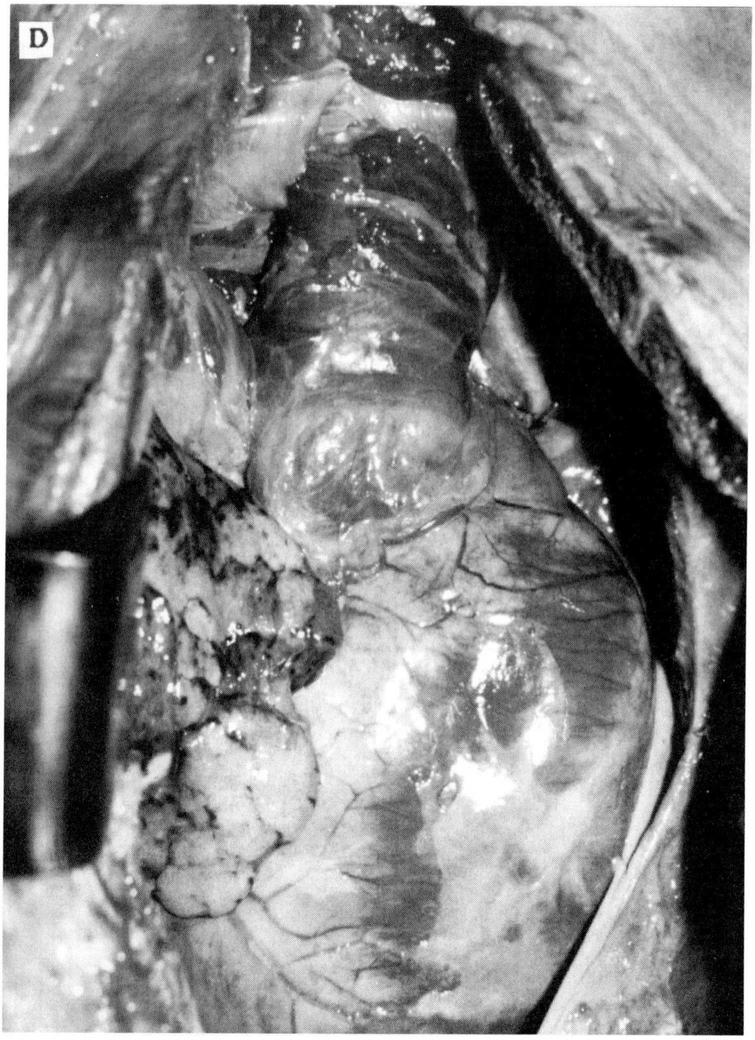


**Figure 5D.**

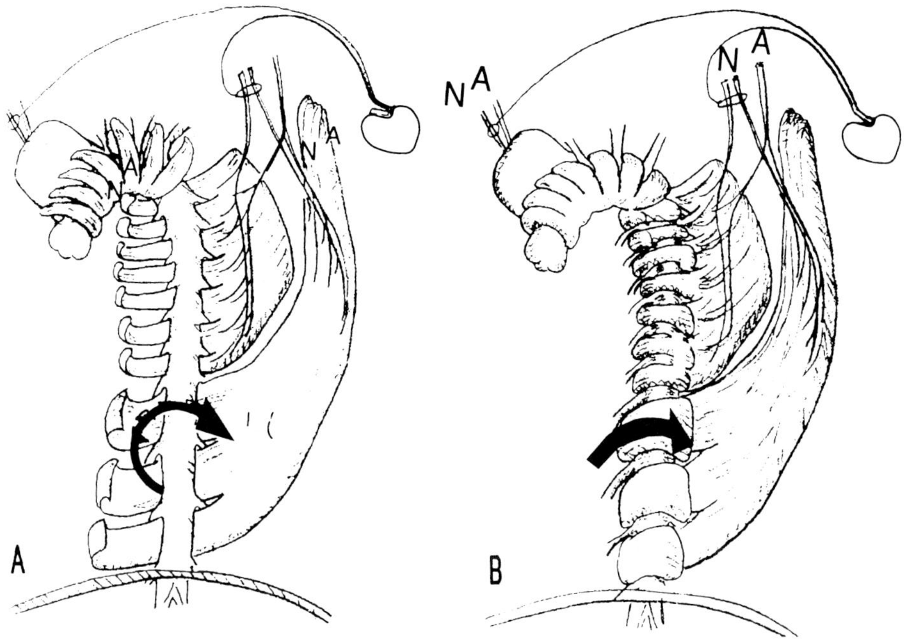


**Figure 6:** *The surgical technique of total thoracic aortomyoplasty is illustrated in* **A** *and* **B** *and demonstrated in* **C** *and* **D**. *The entire thoracic aorta is mobilized circumferentially, preserving all branches and the serratus and latissimus muscles are split for wrapping between these branches. In* **C**, *the split muscle segments are passed between these branches (***A***), and the wrap is completed and inset (***B** *and* **D***). Continued.*

## Cardiomyoplasty

The serratus anterior covers either the dorsal or the ventral surface of the cardiomyoplasty is a double-flap cardiomyoplasty that carries both the left serratus anterior with the left LD muscle on the common thoracodorsal pedicle and uses the serratus anterior to bridge the triangular ventral defect that frequently occurs when either the LD muscle is short or the heart is substantially dilated.

### Serratus Anterior Cardiomyoplasty

The serratus anterior muscle does not have sufficient length to wrap more than half the circumference of the heart. Its use in cardiomyoplasty is as an adjunct to latissimus dorsi wraps, when they incompletely encircle the ventricles because of a short muscle or cardiac dilatation (Fig. 7). In the left posterior wrap, a triangular ventral defect frequently occurs (Figs. 7A and C). The left serratus anterior is carried on the same thoracodorsal vascular pedicle as the latissimus, is placed across the triangular ventral defect, and is inset onto

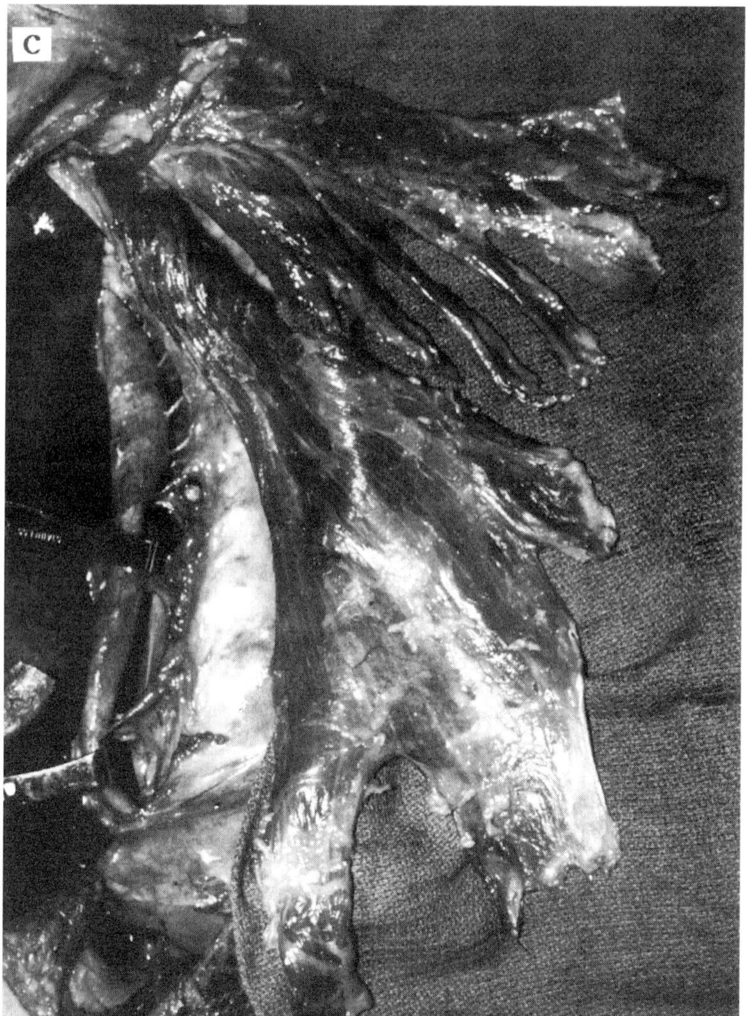


**Figure 6C.** ***Continued.***

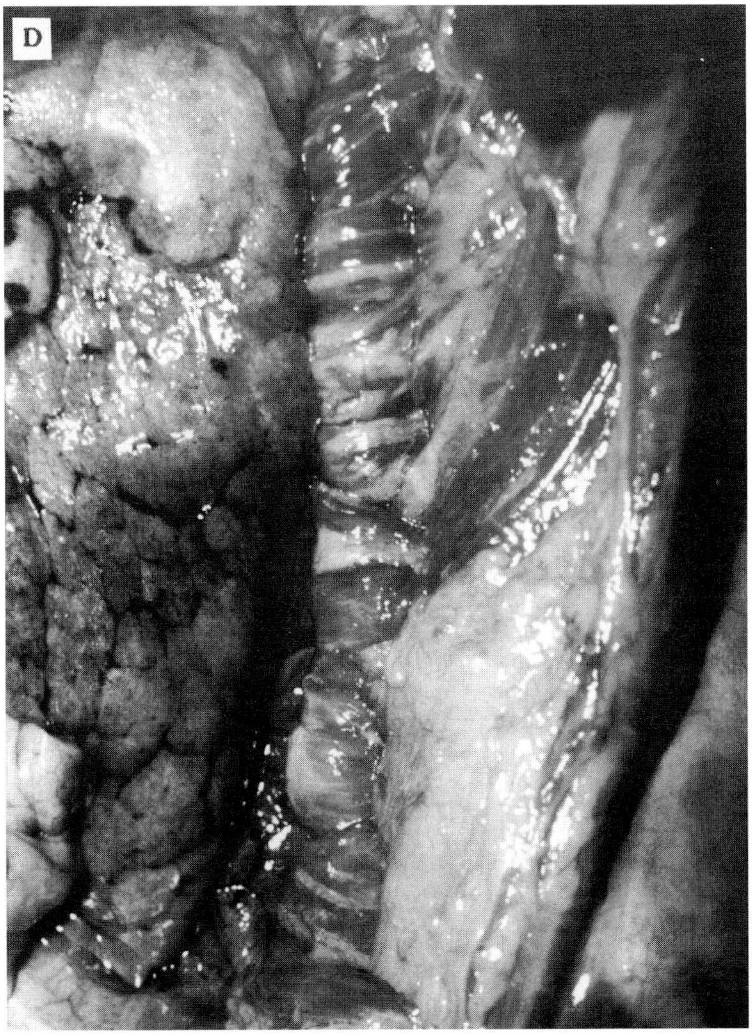


**Figure 6D.**

the latissimus with its fibers oriented in the same direction (transversely to the cardiac axis in left, posterior wraps) to form a contractile muscle cylinder completely around the ventricles (Figs. 7B and D). This avoids the adynamic patch or flap of pericardium previously used.[11] The motor nerves both to the latissimus dorsi and serratus anterior muscles can be paced together for simultaneous contraction.

## Discussion

The concept of cardiac assist with paced skeletal muscle was pioneered by Kantrowitz as a descending aortic wrap with transferred diaphragm.[1] Con-

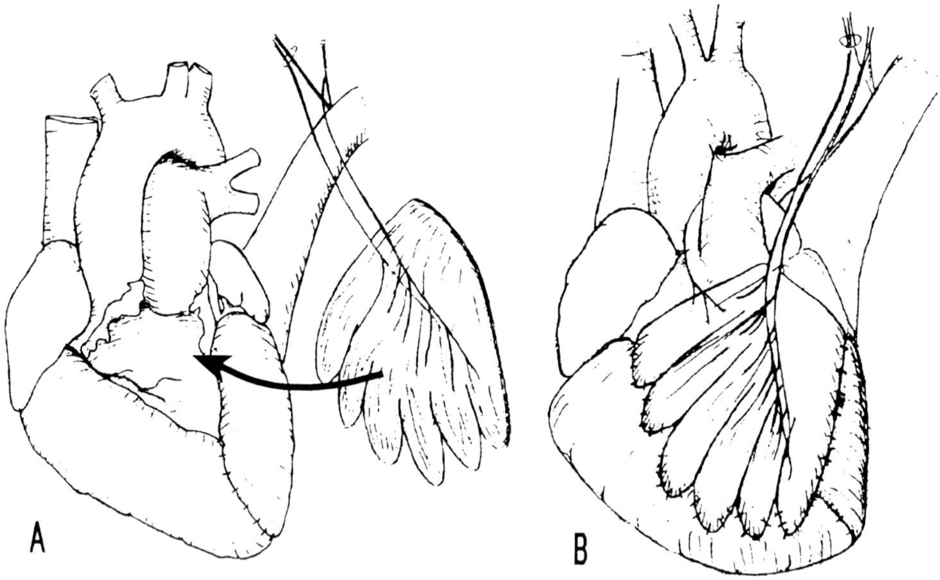


**Figure 7:** *The surgical technique of serratus anterior double-flap cardiomyoplasty is illustrated in* **A** *and* **B** *and demonstrated in* **C** *and* **D**. *A left posterior latissimus dorsi wrap incompletely encircles the myocardium leaving a ventral triangular defect (***A** *and* **C***). The left serratus anterior muscle carried on the same vascular pedicle completes the wrap (***B** *and* **D***). Continued.*

ceptionally, this preceded the first experimental attempts to augment cardiac output with paced LD muscle ventricular wraps.[12,13] LD cardiomyoplasty has been applied clinically by Carpentier and his group[15] and then by others, whereas aortomyoplasty has remained an experimental procedure. This has been primarily because of two major concerns surrounding aortomyoplasty techniques applied to date: (1) small stroke volume because of limited wrap lengths, and (2) the risk of paraplegia following division of aortic intercostal branches that supply the spinal cord. The techniques described in this chapter overcome both of these concerns because of their ability to wrap as much of the thoracic aorta as desired, and their ability to do so without interruptions of intercostal or other branches.

Intrathoracic use of the serratus anterior muscle was pioneered by Arnold and Pairolero.[16] We introduced the concept of segmentally splitting this muscle and have used it clinically for both intrathoracic[7] and mandibular[9] reconstructions.

We have developed experimental models for study of serratus cardiac assist and are currently evaluating the hemodynamic characteristics of these procedures in sheep and goats (Fig. 8). In experimental use of serratus muscle flaps, one must be aware that we have identified no laboratory or domestic animal species with a vascular anatomy exactly like that of man. To date, we have looked at the serratus ventralis (the analogous muscle) in a large number of

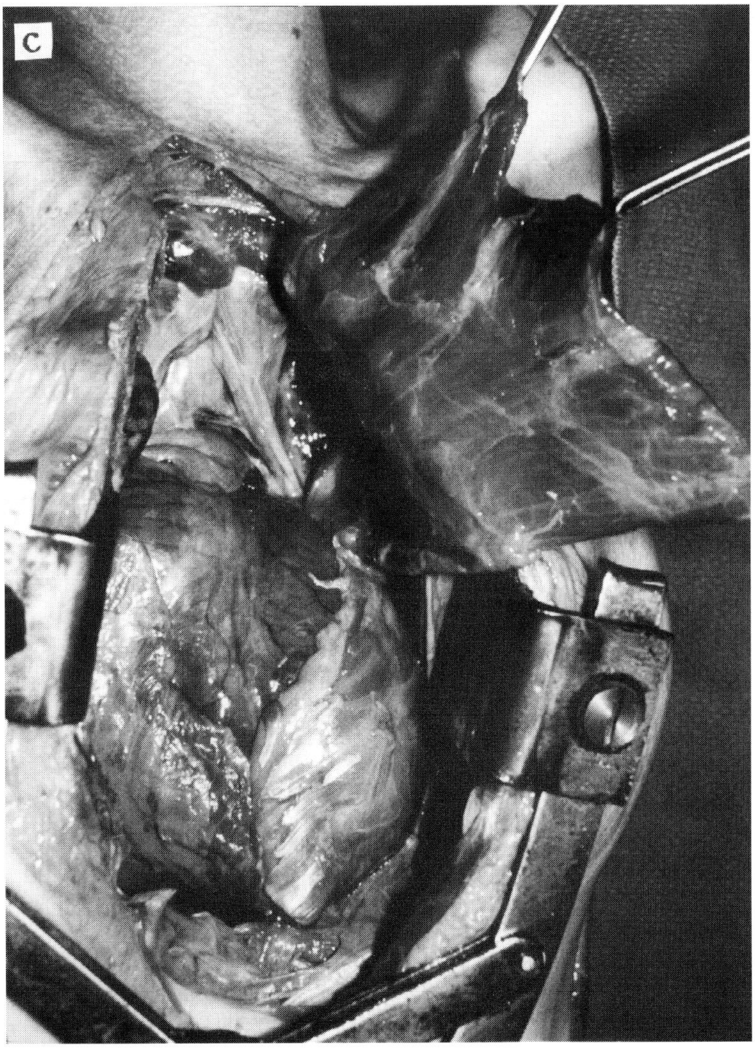


**Figure 7C.** ***Continued.***

nonprimate laboratory and domestic species and have found no examples of vascular pedicles to the external muscle surface as found in man. Rather, the primary vascular supply in these animals comes from the deep cephalic surface of the muscle and runs within its substance. This limits the arc of rotation substantially, but the large size of the serratus ventralis in sheep and goats gives it an arc of rotation comparable to that of humans. Also, this vascular anatomy does not easily permit island pedicle transfers, and it does not allow combined single pedicle serratus anterior-latissimus dorsi transfers, as can be done in most humans. In addition, the serratus in these animals has a distal blood supply from multiple intercostal perforators, unlike the human serratus but similar to the human latissimus dorsi.[8] This requires a delay procedure to

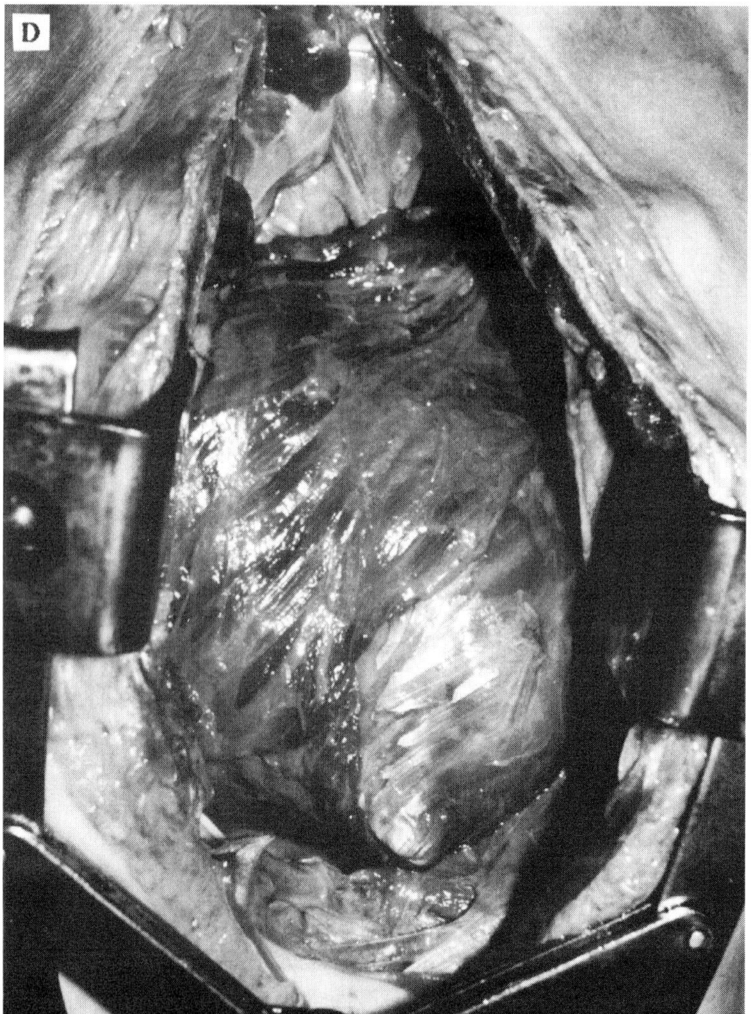


Figure 7D.

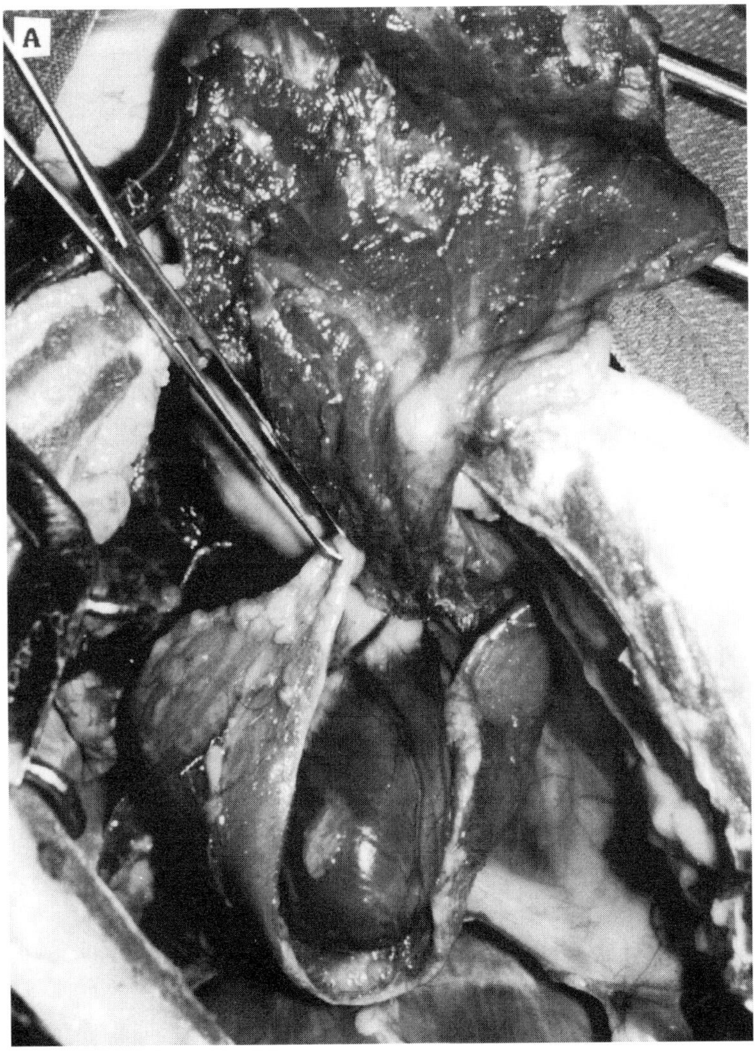


**Figure 8:** *Experimental applications of serratus anterior cardiac assist are shown.* **A** *and* **B** *show serratus ventralis assisted cardiomyoplasty in the goat, which has a short latissimus that incompletely wraps the myocardial circumference* **A**. *The wrap is completed by application of the serratus ventralis across the defect with its fibers oriented parallel to those of the latissimus dorsi (***B***).* **C** *shows experimental total aortomyoplasty in sheep using a serratus ventralis wrap proximally (above) and a latissimus dorsi wrap distally (below) on the descending aorta. The retractor between the two wraps displaces the latissimus muscle pedicle to expose both wraps to view. Continued.*

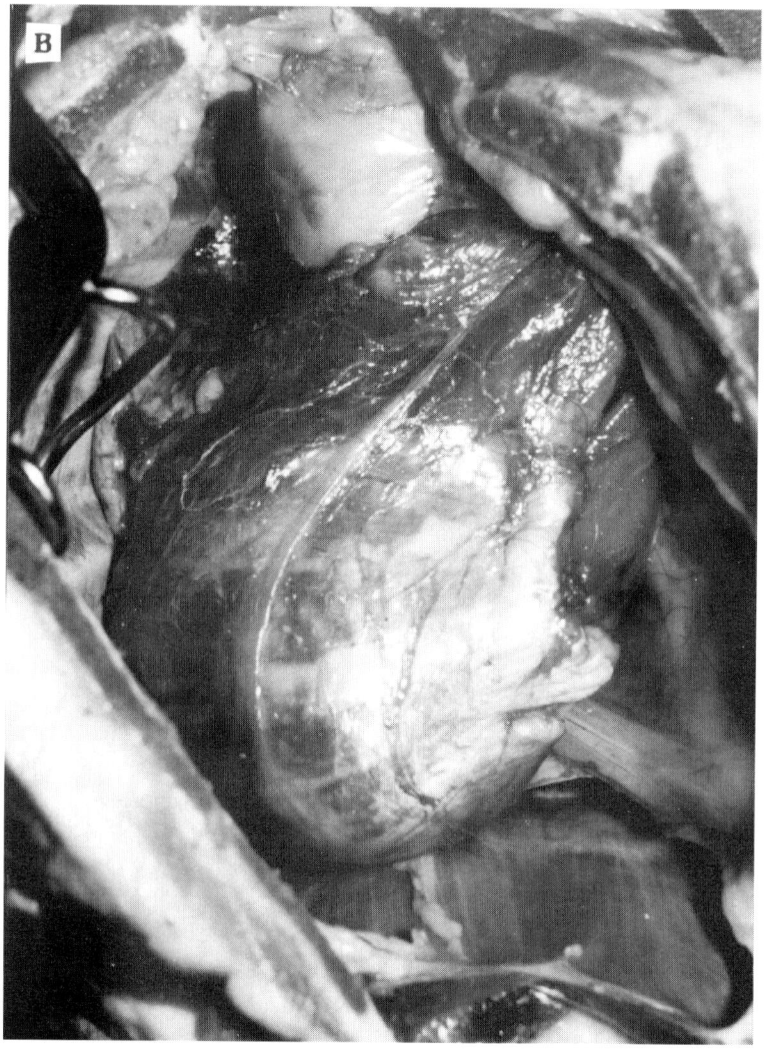


**Figure 8B.** ***Continued.***

avoid distal necrosis of serratus flaps in experimental animals, similar to that required in LD flaps of dogs and probably also of humans.[17]

## Conclusions

This chapter defines the anatomic basis of serratus anterior cardiac assist procedure in humans and introduces applications of serratus anterior motor units to aortomyoplasty and cardiomyoplasty. Serratus anterior aor-

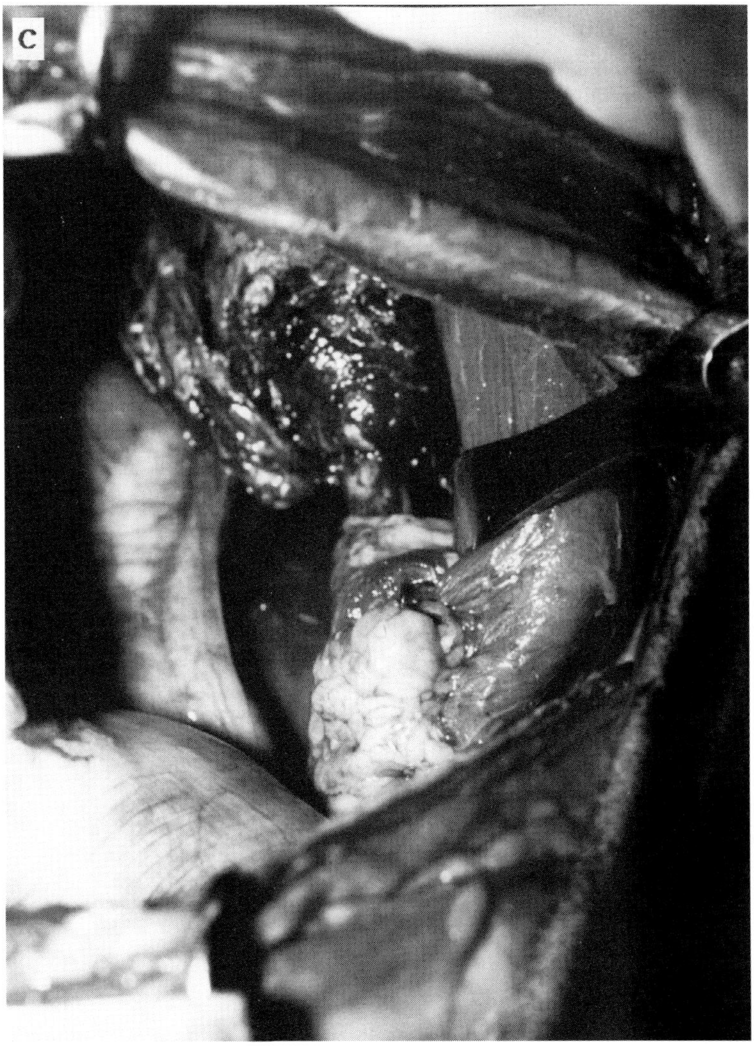


**Figure 8C.**

tomyoplasty has advantages over previously used methods in that the intercostal vessels that supply the spinal cord can be preserved following wrapping of the descending aorta with the segmentally split muscles, and stroke volume is not limited by inadequate wrap length, because the entire thoracic aorta can be wrapped and counterpulsed if needed. The serratus anterior provides a second muscle flap on the same vascular pedicle as the latissimus dorsi for aortomyoplasty of the entire descending thoracic aorta or for double-flap cardiomyoplasty that provides a complete muscle cone encircling the heart.

## References


1. Kantrowitz A, McKinnon W: The experimental use of the diaphragm as an auxiliary myocardium. *Surg Forum* 9:22, 1959.
2. Drinkwater DC, Chiu RCJ, Modry D, Wittnich C, et al: Cardiac assist and myocardial repair with synchronously stimulated skeletal muscle. *Surg Forum* 21:271, 1980.
3. Tobin GR, Gu JM, Tobin AE, et al: The serratus anterior-latissimus dorsi flaps for transformed skeletal muscle cardiac assist: A new technique. In: *Abstracts, The Second Purdue Conference on Cardiac Assistance with Skeletal Muscle.* West Lafayette, IN, Purdue University, 1991.
4. Tobin AE, Hakami A, Barker J, Slater AD, et al: The anatomic basis for serratus anterior aortic counterpulsation in humans. *Surg Forum* 44:657, 1993.
5. Tobin GR, Schusterman MA, Peterson GH, et al: The intramuscular neurovascular anatomy of the latissimus dorsi muscle: The basis for splitting the flap. *Plast Reconstr Surg* 67:637, 1981.
6. Tobin GR, Moberg AW, Dubou RH, et al: The split latissimus dorsi myocutaneous flap. *Ann Plast Surg* 7:272, 1981.
7. Tobin GR: Segmentally split pectoral girdle muscle flaps for chest wall and intrathoracic reconstruction. *Clin Plast Surg* 17:683, 1990.
8. Tobin GR, Gu JM, Tobin AE, et al: The anatomic basis for latissimus dorsi flap loss. In: *Proceedings of the Cardiovascular Science and Technology Conference.* Arlington, VA, Association for the Advancement of Medical Instrumentation 1991, p. 69.
9. Tobin GR, Moberg A, Ringberg A, et al: Mandibular-facial reconstruction with segmentally split serratus anterior composite flaps. *Clin Plast Surg* 17:663, 1990.
10. Chachques JC, Grandjean PA, Fischer EIC, et al: Dynamic aortomyoplasty to assist left ventricular failure. *Ann Thorac Surg* 49:225, 1990.
11. Chachques JC, Grandjean PA, Carpentier A: Latissimus dorsi dynamic cardiomyoplasty. *Ann Thorac Surg* 47:600, 1989.
12. Carpentier A, Chachques JC: Cardiomyoplasty: Surgical technique. In Carpentier A, Chachques JC, Grandjean P (eds): *Cardiomyoplasty.* Mount Kisco, NY, Futura Publishing Co, 1991, p. 105.
13. Termet, Chalencon JL, Estour R, et al: Transplantation sur le myocarde d'un muscle strie excite par pacemaker. *Ann Chir Thorac Cardiovasc* 5:568, 1966.
14. Hume WI: Construction of a functioning accessory myocardium. *Trans South Surg Assoc* 79:200, 1968.
15. Carpentier A, Chachques JC: Myocardial substitution with a stimulated skeletal muscle: First successful clinical case. *Lancet* 8440:1267, 1985.
16. Arnold PG, Pairolero PC, Waldorf JC: The serratus anterior muscle: Intrathoracic and extrathoracic utilization. *Plast Reconstr Surg* 73:240, 1984.
17. Hakami A, Tobin AE, Keelen P, et al: A bipedicle delay enhances latissimus dorsi flap survival. In: *Proceedings of the Cardiovascular Science and Technology Conference.* Arlington, VA, Association for the Advancement of Medical Instrumentation, 1993.

Chapter 35

# *Discussion*

**Dr. Chachques:** How much loss of upper limb function would you anticipate from taking both the serratus anterior and latissimus dorsi?

**Dr. Tobin:** The loss of upper extremity function is surprisingly small. Taking both muscles, one usually sees a winged scapula, but in normal activities the upper extremity has full function. Losses are seen only in the extremes of athletic performance.

**Dr. Chiu:** What did the animal work show?

**Dr. Tobin:** The animal work is still in progress and I think that our preliminary results will correspond closely to those associated with the same techniques that were used for the LD muscle.

Chapter 36

# Double Flap Cardiomyoplasty Using Left Latissimus Dorsi and Right Pectoral Muscles

Juan Carlos Chachques, Michel Pellerin, Marc Radermecker, Michel Tapia, Alain F. Carpentier

## Introduction

The concept of muscle-powered cardiac assistance to improve cardiac function is based on two physiological mechanisms. First, the contractile power of the skeletal muscle is transferred to the ventricle to improve systolic function, and second, the presence of muscle wrap interferes with ventricular diastolic pressure-volume relationship, therefore restoring cardiac reserve and preventing further dilatation. This interpretation is suggested by most experimental studies conducted in heart disease-free animal models, in which cases the latissimus dorsi (LD) muscle flap is always sufficient to allow complete concentric wrapping of the ventricles. This optimal situation, however, is rarely encountered clinically because of the discrepancy between the LD muscle flap surface area and the dilated pathological heart.[1–6]

Several experimental approaches such as maximal dissection of the thoracodorsal bundle, precardiomyoplasty balloon expansion of the LD muscle, progressive denervation, or double flap cardiomyoplasty were studied at Broussais Hospital to correct this problem. The double flap approach is based on the existence of several muscles that can be simultaneously transferred into the chest with the latissimus dorsi flap to optimize the wrapping. In this study, the right pectoralis major (RPM) muscle flap was used in addition to the LD wrap to obtain a circumferential myocardial wrapping. Our experimental approach was designed to establish the technical feasibility of double flap cardiomyoplasty and to study the hemodynamic data in chronic experiments.

From Carpentier A, Chachques JC, Grandjean P: Cardiac Bioassist. © Futura Publishing Co, Inc, Armonk, NY, 1997.

## Methods and Materials

Eight adult female goats (42–49 kg) were used. Initial sedation was obtained by acepromazine 0.5% and anesthesia was induced with IV propofol. The animals were intubated and mechanically ventilated without curarization. Anesthesia was maintained with isoflurane inhalation (2%).

Surgery was first performed on animals in the right lateral decubitus position. A left oblique thoracic incision was performed to progressively dissect the LD muscle and its neurovascular pedicle. Standards for muscle dissection in cardiomyoplasty were strictly observed. Due to the usual excess of LD surface area, the distal part of the LD muscle was not dissected. After pacing electrode implantation (two pacing leads, Medtronic model SP5528), the muscle was transferred into the chest through segmental left second rib resection.

The goat was then placed in the supine position and the RPM muscle was harvested through a median thoracic incision. Two pacing electrodes (Medtronic® model SP5528) were implanted into the proximal part of the pectoral muscle. The RPM and its pacing electrodes were transposed into the chest through a window created by resecting the anterior segment of the right second rib.

The heart was exposed through a median sternotomy. The cardiomyoplasty procedure was performed by wrapping the left ventricle with the LD muscle (posterior to anterior wrapping) and the right ventricle with the right pectoral muscle (anterior wrapping). Sutures were placed between both muscles (Fig. 1).

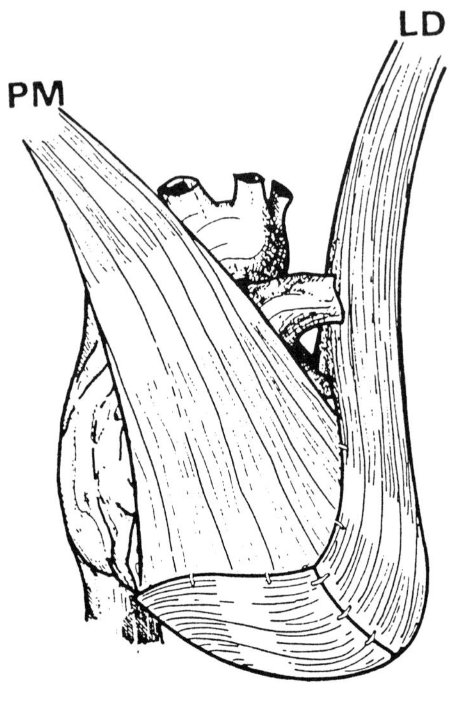


**Figure 1:** *Double flap cardiomyoplasty using the left latissimus dorsi (LD) muscle associated with the right pectoral muscle (PM).*

A sensing intramyocardial lead (Medtronic® Model SP5548) was placed in the right ventricle. The sensing lead as well as pacing leads of both muscles were connected to the cardiomyostimulator (Medtronic® SP1005) using bifurcated Y connectors; the negative leads were coupled and connected parallel to the stimulator. The same procedure was used to connect the positive leads.

## Stimulation Protocol

The usual progressive stimulation protocol developed at Broussais Hospital was used. After a 15-day healing period to promote myocardial adhesion to the LD muscle flap and to permit vascular adaptation, stimulation was delivered and modified every 15 days from one pulse to a burst of six pulses with intermediate steps of two and three pulses. A basic 2:1 mode was chosen.

## Electrophysiological and Hemodynamic Studies

All recordings were done at the time of cardiomyoplasty and 6 months postoperatively. Electrophysiological parameters consisted of muscle impedance, threshold, and full recruitment threshold. The hemodynamic parameters were calculated from invasive pressure monitoring. Central venous pressure and a Swan-Ganz catheter were used to evaluate the cardiac output, mean pulmonary pressure, and pulmonary capillary wedge pressure.

At 6 months, hemodynamic studies (cardiac output, right and left ventricular pressures) were performed before and after induction of acute pharmacological heart failure (propranolol 3 mg/kg, IV), to reduce the cardiac output to a minimum of 50% of the preoperative values. The hemodynamic parameters were recorded with isolated stimulation of the LD muscle flap and during stimulation of both muscles (LD + RPM).

Biopsy specimens of the RPM and LD muscle flaps were analyzed under optical microscopy. Histochemical studies of both muscles were also performed.

## Statistics

Statistical analysis of the data was done with Student's paired *t* test.

# Results

Gross anatomy of the double flap cardiomyoplasty at 6 months showed intact viable muscle wraps. The histological analysis showed normal muscle fibers without inflammation, necrosis, fibrosis, or adipose substitution. ATPase stain demonstrated complete homogeneous distribution of fatigue-resistant type I muscle fibers.

The electrophysiological results (Table 1) emphasize the value of stimulation parameters in the RPM and LD muscles as measured at surgery and 6 months later. The hemodynamic data are listed in Tables 2–4. They demonstrated that at the initial surgery or at 6 months, the stimulated double flap cardiomyoplasty significantly improved ventricular performance.

**Table 1**
Electrophysiological Studies

| | *Intraoperative* | *6 Months* |
|---|---|---|
| LDM 1st contraction (threshold) | 1.2 ± 0.6 V | 1.5 ± 0.4 V (NS) |
| LDM full contraction | 2.1 ± 0.8 V | 2.4 ± 0.5 V (NS) |
| LDM impedance | 414 ± 46 ohms | 315 ± 26 ohms (NS) |
| RPM 1st contraction (threshold) | 1.1 ± 0.7 V | 1.4 ± 0.3 V (NS) |
| RPM full contraction | 2.3 ± 0.6 V | 2.7 ± 0.4 V (NS) |
| RPM impedance | 398 ± 63 ohms | 327 ± 26 ohms (NS) |

All measures were performed through pacing leads. LDM=latissimus dorsi muscle; RPM = right pectoral muscle; V = volts.

**Table 2**
Double Flap Cardiomyoplasty Hemodynamic Results: Cardiac Output (L/min)

| | *(St -)* | *(St +)* | ρ |
|---|---|---|---|
| Baseline | 3.2 ± 0.3 | 3.6 ± 0.2 | <0.05 |
| Heart Failure | 1.5 ± 0.4 | 2.8 ± 0.3 | <0.005 |
| Pectoral Muscle Off | 1.5 ± 0.4 | 2.1 ± 0.2 | <0.05 |

**Table 3**
Left Ventricular Pressure (peak systolic, mm Hg)

| | *(St -)* | *(St +)* | ρ |
|---|---|---|---|
| Baseline | 98 ± 4 | 118± 5 | <0.05 |
| Heart Failure | 42 ± 5 | 76 ± 2 | <0.005 |
| Pectoral Muscle Off | 42 ± 5 | 64 ± 4 | <0.05 |

**Table 4**
Right Ventricular Pressure (peak systolic, mm Hg)

| | *(St -)* | *(St +)* | ρ |
|---|---|---|---|
| Baseline | 29 ±4 | 33 ± 2 | <0.05 |
| Heart Failure | 14 ± 3 | 27 ± 2 | <0.01 |
| Pectoral Muscle Off | 14 ± 3 | 16 ± 3 | NS |

During biventricular heart failure, these benefits were present but depended on the stimulation of the RPM muscle. Synchronous stimulation of both muscle flaps resulted in an 85% increase in cardiac output.

## Discussion

The development of double flap cardiomyoplasty is an interesting alternative to obviate incomplete cardiac wrapping due to the lack of available LD muscle surface area.[7–9] This concept necessitates an anatomic review of thoracic muscle flaps.

Our approach to a double cardiomyoplasty technique was concentrated on thoracic muscle flaps that could be transferred in addition to the homolateral LD muscle flap. This technique uses a left cutaneous incision for LD muscle harvesting and a median thoracic incision to dissect the right pectoral muscle and to expose the heart.

Pectoral muscle as well as latissimus dorsi muscle flaps fulfill the criteria of being easily transposable into the chest (proximity of the heart and adequate neurovascular supply). The human pectoralis major muscle is a thick, triangular muscle that inserts on the proximal half of the clavicle, and originates from the anterior surface of the sternum, from the first to the sixth or seventh costal cartilages, the sternal end of the sixth rib, and the aponeurosis of the obliquus externus abdominis. The muscle converges to a flat tendon (5 cm) attached to the lateral lip of the humeral intertubercular sulcus. The main vascular blood supply of the RPM originates from the pectoral branch of thoracoacromial artery.

The innervation of the pectoralis major muscle is derived from the lateral pectoral nerve, which originates from the anterior division of the upper and middle trunks of the brachial plexus or a single root from the lateral cord. The lateral pectoral nerve fibers originate from the fifth to the seventh cervical vertebrae. It crosses the axillary artery and vein anteriorly, perforates the clavipectoral fascia, and supplies the deep surface of the pectoralis major. It also sends a branch to the medial pectoral nerve, forming a loop in front of the proximal segment of the axillary artery to innervate a part of the pectoralis minor.

Endowed with a major neurovascular pedicle (pectoral branch of the thoracoacromial artery and lateral pectoral nerve), the RPM can be transposed into the chest after division of its distal and proximal attachments. This neurovascular distribution that shows similarities with the thoracodorsal pedicle of the LD muscle allows the implantation of the intramuscular pacing electrodes routinely used in cardiomyoplasty.

Basically, the goat RPM has the same gross anatomic features and was used in this model in association with the left latissimus dorsi to perform a double flap cardiomyoplasty. The usual stimulation system was modified to allow synchronous stimulation of both flaps. This was done through parallel connections of the cathode and anode of both muscles, using bifurcated Y connectors. The Medtronic cardiomyostimulator system was used for simultaneous and chronic electrostimulation of both flaps. The electrophysiological data confirmed the efficacy of the stimulation device with obtention of usual values for threshold, full recruitment threshold, and DC impedance. These values remained stable after 6 months of chronic implantation.

The hemodynamic effects of double flap cardiomyoplasty have demonstrated the benefits of complete heart wrapping. In fact, single LD muscle stimulation improved cardiac output by 45% in an experimental model of heart failure. The synchronous activation of both the LD and RPM muscles resulted in an 85% augmentation. These data confirm the efficacy of the LD muscle wrap in the posterior-anterior cardiocostal wrap in the goat. It also demonstrates that the concept of complete wrapping makes sense and is experimentally superior to partial envelopment of the heart.

Furthermore, this study also demonstrates that the improvement following stimulation is clearly an effect of systolic augmentation and suggests that transformed latissimus dorsi or pectoralis major may produce significant hemodynamic work under basal ventricular filling pressures. The hemodynamic improvement was more pronounced in the experimental model resulting from the induction of biventricular heart failure, which demonstrates the full potential of the cardiomyoplasty procedure.

The histological data obtained from the RPM after 6 months of transposition and stimulation mitigate against any major neurovascular injuries. Microscopic findings have demonstrated that muscles have retained their usual checkerboard aspect without grouping phenomenon, which is a classic marker of denervation-reinnervation as a result of neural damage. There was no evidence of chronic muscle ischemia. This study demonstrates the feasibility of transferring the right pectoralis major muscle into the chest to use it in cardiac assistance.

The muscle fiber orientation of the LD muscle associated with the RPM allows a concentric wrap with two different vectors of force compressing the heart. In fact, both muscle flaps create a biaxial traction from the mediastinum toward the left and right axillary regions, resulting in full compression of both ventricles.[10]

## Conclusion

This experimental study demonstrates the usefulness of a double cardiomyoplasty, connecting the right pectoralis muscle to the left LD muscle as an alternative to incomplete wrapping in cases of major heart dilatation in order to generate maximal hemodynamic support. Pectoral muscle could be used concomitantly with the LD muscle in cases of extremely dilated hearts, or secondarily to supplement an insufficient result of single muscle cardiomyoplasty.

## References

1. Carpentier A, Chachques JC, Acar C, Relland J, et al: Dynamic cardiomyoplasty at seven years. *J Thorac Cardiovasc Surg* 106:42–54, 1993.
2. Chachques JC, Grandjean PA, Carpentier A: Latissimus dorsi dynamic cardiomyoplasty. *Ann Thorac Surg* 47:600–604, 1989.

3. Lorusso R, Zogno M, La Canna G, et al: Dynamic cardiomyoplasty as an effective therapy for dilated cardiomyopathy. *J Cardiac Surg* 8:177–183, 1993.
4. Jegaden O, Delahaye F, Finet G, Van Der Veen F, et al: Late hemodynamic results after cardiomyoplasty in congestive heart failure. *Ann Thorac Surg* 57:1151–1157, 1994.
5. Moreira LFP, Bocchi EA, Stolf NAG, Pileggi F, et al: Current expectations in dynamic cardiomyoplasty. *Ann Thorac Surg* 55:299–303, 1993.
6. Trainini JC, Barisani JL, Varini SD, Roncoroni A, et al: Cardiomioplastia, su perspectiva en el tratamiento de la insuficiencia cardiaca avanzada. *Rev Arg Cardiol* 62:399–405, 1994.
7. Niinami H, Pochettino A, Ruggiero R, Koroteyev A, et al: Canine latissimus dorsi cardio-double myoplasty: acute feasibility study. *J Cardiac Surg* 6:124–131, 1991.
8. Magovern JA, Furnary AP, Christlieb IY, Kao RL, et al: Bilateral latissimus dorsi cardiomyoplasty. *Ann Thorac Surg* 52:1259–1265, 1991.
9. Furnary AP, Magovern JA, Christlieb IY, Trumble DR, et al: Component analysis of bilateral anterior cardiomyoplasty. *Ann Thorac Surg* 55:72–77, 1993.
10. Schaper J, Froede R, Hein S, et al: Impairment of the myocardial ultrastructure and changes of the cytoskeleton in dilated cardiomyopathy. *Circulation* 83:504–514, 1991.

Chapter 36

# Discussion

**Dr. Mikaeloff (Lyon, France):** Would you do this on a patient now that you have proved its efficacy in the animal model?

**Dr. Chachques:** We have electrodes that can be used in patients. I know that Dr. Carpentier has several patients who might need more than a single cardiomyoplasty. He will decide which patient or patients are most suitable for double cardiomyoplasty.

**Dr. Mikaeloff:** Do you need two myostimulators?

**Dr. Chachques:** No, only one with a special adaptor.

Chapter 37

# Effects of Latissimus Dorsi Double Cardiomyoplasty on Left Ventricular Function: Chronic Studies

Ernesto R. Soltero, Lloyd H. Michael, Donald H. Glaeser, Gerald M. Lawrie*

## Introduction

Dynamic cardiomyoplasty has been proposed and is being offered as a therapeutic option for patients suffering from congestive heart failure. More than 500 patients have undergone single cardiomyoplasty procedures worldwide, but the results have been inconsistent.[1–8] The observation has been made that, in many cases, a single muscle may not provide adequate ventricular coverage.

Latissimus dorsi (LD) double cardiomyoplasty has been evaluated experimentally as an alternative to single cardiomyoplasty. In acute studies, double cardiomyoplasty has been shown to provide hemodynamic augmentation,[9–12] but its efficacy has not been tested in long-term studies.

The purpose of this study was to evaluate the effects of double cardiomyoplasty on left ventricular function in a propranolol-induced model of heart failure. Conditioned, fatigue-resistant skeletal muscles were used in these chronic studies.

## Materials and Methods

Eight adult microfilaria-free dogs weighing 15–20 kg were used for this investigation. This animal research protocol was approved by the animal protocol review committee of Baylor College of Medicine (approval number AN-359).

*With the cooperation of Craig J. Hartley, and Nan R. Earle.

From Carpentier A, Chachques JC, Grandjean P: Cardiac Bioassist. © Futura Publishing Co, Inc, Armonk, NY, 1997.

Anesthesia was induced with intravenous methohexital (10 mg/kg). After endotracheal intubation, the animals were ventilated with oxygen using an Ohio ventilator (Ohio Medical Products, Madison, WI) and anesthesia was maintained with isoflurane (1–2% to effect). Normal saline was used for intravenous fluid replacement. Prophylactic antibiotic (cefazolin sodium; Smith Kline and French, Philadelphia, PA; 1 gm intravenously) was administered prior to skin incision.

## Surgical Technique

The left LD muscle was dissected from the chest wall, spinous and scapular attachments; intercostal perforators were ligated and the humeral tendon was transected. The neurovascular pedicle was identified and an arm of a bifurcated pacing lead (Medtronic®, Inc., model #4080) was secured around the thoracodorsal nerve. A portion of the third rib was resected and the muscle was transferred into the chest cavity. The proximal end of the muscle was sutured to the periosteum of the second and fourth ribs to avoid tension on the neurovascular pedicle during stimulation. After closing the incision, the right LD muscle was harvested and transferred to the chest in the same fashion. The animals were then placed in a supine position and the heart exposed through a median sternotomy. The pericardium was incised and suspended with silk sutures. An epicardial pacing lead (Medtronic, Inc. model #6917) was placed in the left ventricular apex to detect the R wave.

The double cardiomyoplasty was performed using the techniques previously reported by our group[12] except that in these chronic animals the LD muscles were not stretched back to resting anatomic length, so that the muscles were not tightly wrapped around the heart (Fig. 1). After completion of the double cardiomyoplasty, the bifurcated nerve stimulating leads and ventricular epicardial sensing lead were connected to the programmable burst stimulator (Medtronic model SP 1005). A subcutaneous pocket was made in the animal's abdominal wall for implantation of the cardiomyostimulator. The median sternotomy was closed with heavy silk suture and the subcutaneous tissue and skin were closed with continuous absorbable suture.

The animals were returned to their cages and allowed to recover from anesthesia. Pain was controlled with parenteral butorphanol tartrate (1–2 mg intramuscularly every 4 hours as needed). Administration of oral antibiotic (cephalexin 500 mg) was continued daily for 1 week. After a 2-week vascular delay period, conditioning of the LD muscles was initiated with the SP 1005 cardiomyostimulator using the training protocol designed for the current clinical trials. The animals were inspected daily and their flanks palpated to assure muscle contraction.

At the end of a 2- to 3-month conditioning program, the final experiment was conducted. The animals were anesthetized and placed in a supine position. A median sternotomy was performed and the ascending aorta was dissected. A custom-made cuffed pulsed Doppler aortic flow probe was placed around the ascending aorta. The right common carotid artery was exposed and a Millar pressure catheter (Millar Instruments, Inc., Houston, TX) was introduced into the left ventricle. The right common femoral artery was exposed and a second

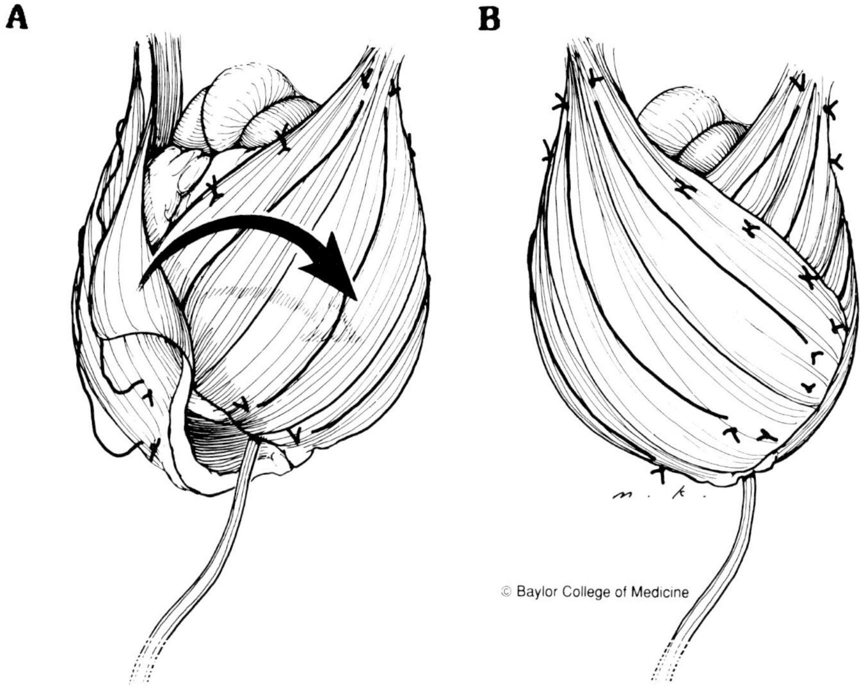


**Figure 1:** *Surgical technique of double cardiomyoplasty. (**A**) Left latissimus dorsi muscle flap suture to RV epicardium; (**B**) right latissimus dorsi muscle flap brought over the LV. Double cardiomyoplasty completed. (Reproduced from Soltero ER, Michael LH, Glaeser DH, et al: New configuration of double cardiomyoplasty based on studies of the length-tension properties of the latissimus dorsi muscle.* J Thorac Cardiovasc Surg *1993, vol. 106, with permission from Mosby-Year Book, Inc.)*

Millar pressure catheter was advanced into the aortic arch. A fluid-filled catheter was placed in the left atrium to measure left atrial pressure.

The animals received a titrating dose of up to 5 mg/kg intravenous propranolol to achieve a steady state of acute heart failure. A state of heart failure was documented by a decrease in stroke volume and left ventricular and aortic pressure.

## Data Acquisition

Data were recorded on a multichannel recorder (Gould, Inc.) and simultaneously captured by a MacIntosh IIci computer (Apple Computer, Cupertino, CA) with a 16-channel analog-to-digital interface, under control of a data acquisition and analysis package (Acknowledge, BioPac Systems, Inc., Goleta, CA). Data were recorded under two different conditions. Following the infusion of intravenous propranolol and stabilization of the failure state, signals were acquired with the cardiomyostimulator off (control protocol). The cardiomyoplasty was then stimulated to contract at a 2:1 ratio (paced protocol).

## Hemodynamic Measurements

In each protocol, an epoch containing contiguous data was sought. In some animals discontiguous segments had to be analyzed due to the occurrence of ectopic beats. In the latter case, both the ectopic beat and its successor were excluded. For the control protocol, 15 beats were selected, while in the paced protocol, 10 complete pacing cycles were analyzed. A pacing cycle consists of a paced and the subsequent nonpaced beat (at 2:1). Parameters of all signals were measured for each beat in the selected epoch.

## Statistics

Within-animal statistics (mean, standard deviation, coefficient of variation) were computed for each protocol using MUMPS (MGlobal International, Houston, TX). These results were then transferred to a VAX 11/750 computer (Digital Equipment Corp, Maynard, MA) for further analysis.

Following preliminary data quality screening, a file was produced for input into BMDP (BMDP Statistical Software, Inc., Los Angeles, CA). Variables in the BMDP file were dog ID and the hemodynamic parameters for the control protocol and each beat of the paced protocol. Transformations performed by BMDP prior to analysis were normalization of the paced protocol values to control protocol and calculation of the cycle average. This was simply the arithmetic mean of the paced and nonpaced beats during the paced protocol.

Since each animal served as its own control, paired $t$-tests were used to assess the statistical significance of the changes observed during the paced protocol. Separate tests were performed for the paced beat, the nonpaced beat, and the cycle average. No adjustment was made for multiple comparison, so $p$ values close to 0.05 need to be considered as marginally significant.

Nonparametric Wilcoxon signed rank tests were carried out simultaneously with the paired $t$-tests. In all cases, the sense of significance agreed between the two tests.

# Results

The hemodynamic parameters measured are shown in Table 1. Stimulation of the double cardiomyoplasty resulted in significant hemodynamic augmentation in the propranolol-induced heart failure model (Figs. 2 and 3, Table 2). Stroke volume increased 20% during stimulation compared to controls. There was a 13% increase in left ventricular pressure during pacing and a 31% increase in left ventricular dP/dt. Peak aortic pressure increased significantly during pacing but the mean aortic pressure was basically unchanged compared to controls (Figs. 4 and 5).

Left atrial pressure was measured in only four dogs. The data obtained in these four animals show that the left atrial pressure increased 10% during electrical stimulation although this difference is not statistically significant (Fig. 5).

**Table 1**
Observed Population Means of Hemodynamic Parameters

| | | | Paced Protocol | | |
|---|---|---|---|---|---|
| | *n* | *Control Protocol* | *Paced Beat* | *Nonpaced Beat* | *Cycle Average* |
| Stroke Volume (mL) | 8 | 10.3 ± 4.2* | 11.9 ± 4.3 | 9.9 ± 4.0 | 10.9 ± 4.0 |
| LV Pressure (mm Hg) | 7 | 78.2 ± 22.8 | 86.0 ± 17.5 | 73.5 ± 22.2 | 79.8 ± 19.7 |
| LV dP/dt (mm Hg/sec) | 8 | 618 ± 225 | 759 ± 227 | 601 ± 260 | 680 ± 238 |
| Peak Aortic Pressure (mm Hg) | 8 | 71.4 ± 28.4 | 75.2 ± 26.0 | 68.4 ± 26.8 | 71.8 ± 26.3 |
| Mean Aortic Pressure (mm Hg) | 8 | 58.0 ± 24.9 | 57.6 ± 23.0 | 55.1 ± 22.8 | 56.3 ± 22.9 |
| Left Atrial Pressure (mm Hg) | 4 | 21.5 ± 9.1 | 22.9 ± 7.5 | 21.3 ± 8.2 | 22.1 ± 7.8 |

Values are presented as mean ± standard deviation. LV = left ventricular.

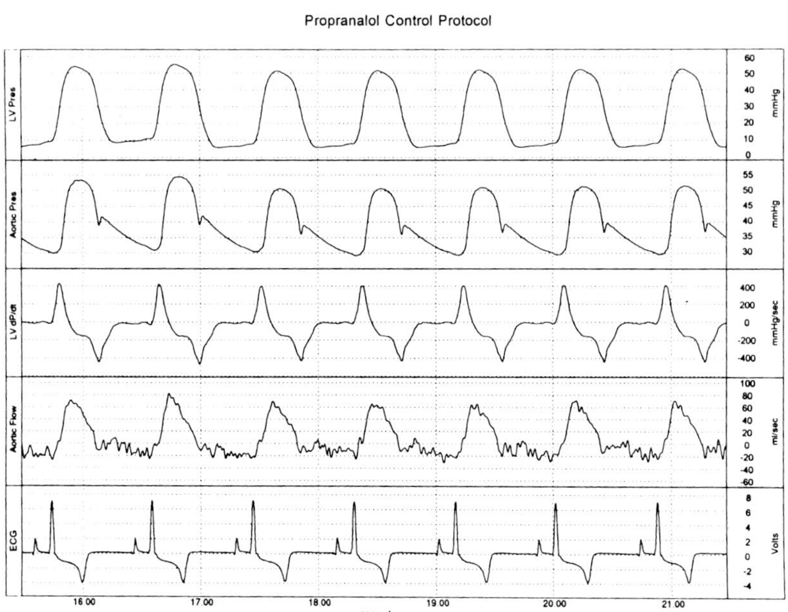


**Figure 2:** *Representative tracings taken from one animal showing hemodynamic parameters during propranolol control protocol. LV Pres = left ventricular pressure; LV dP/dt = left ventricular dP/dt.*

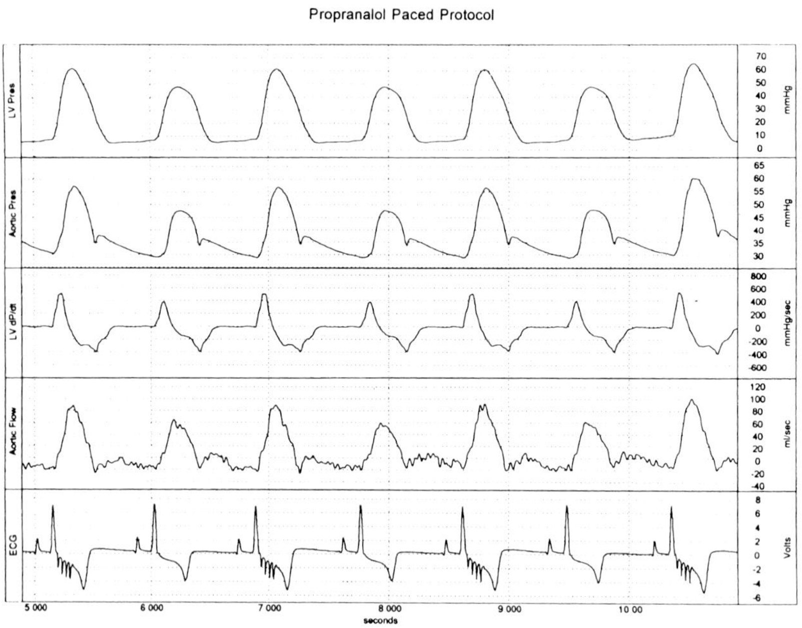


**Figure 3:** *Representative tracings taken from the same animal showing changes in the hemodynamic parameters during the propranolol paced protocol. The animal is being paced at a 2:1 ratio.*

**Table 2**

Effects of Double Cardiomyoplasty Stimulation on Hemodynamic Parameters: Mean Percent Change from Control Protocol

| | *n* | *Paced Beat %* | *p Value* | *Nonpaced Beat %* | *p Value* | *Cycle Average %* | *p Value* |
|---|---|---|---|---|---|---|---|
| Stroke Volume | 8 | 20 ± 20* | 0.0260+ | −3 ± 10 | 0.4 | 8 ± 9 | 0.0286 |
| LV Pressure | 7 | 13 ± 14 | 0.0478 | −6 ± 3 | 0.0007 | 3 ± 7 | 0.2 |
| LV dP/dt | 8 | 31 ± 37 | 0.0493 | −4 ± 4 | 0.0494 | 14 ± 19 | 0.0810 |
| Peak Aortic Pressure | 8 | 8 ± 8 | 0.0249 | −4 ± 7 | 0.2 | 2 ± 7 | 0.4 |
| Mean Aortic Pressure | 8 | 2 ± 12 | 0.7 | −3 ± 9 | 0.4 | −1 ± 11 | 0.8 |
| Left Atrial Pressure | 4 | 10 ± 13 | 0.2 | 0 ± 8 | 1.0 | 5 ± 9 | 0.4 |

*Values are presented as mean ± standard deviation.

+Paired *t*-test, n-1 degrees of freedom.

LV = left ventricular.

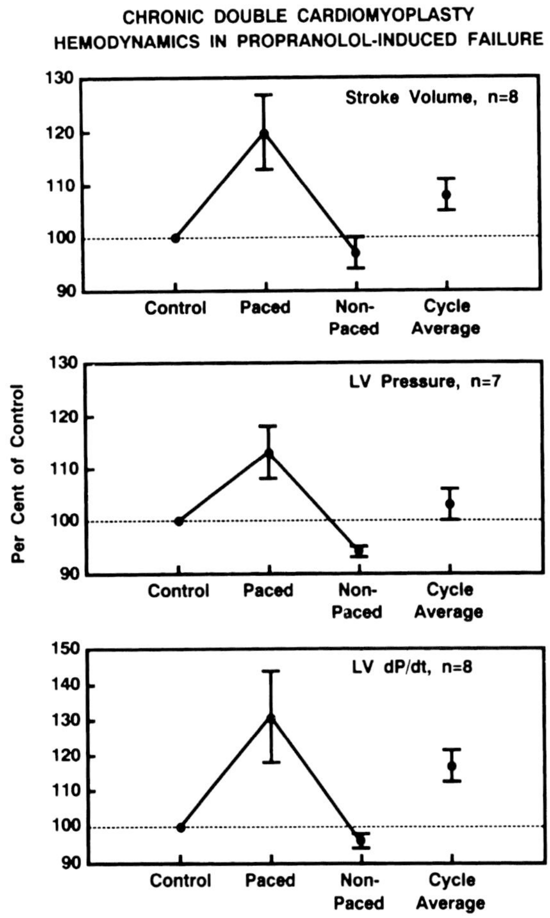


**Figure 4:** *Effect of double cardiomyoplasty stimulation on stroke volume, LV pressure, LV dP/dt in propranolol induced heart failure.*

## Discussion

There is a renewed interest in the use of transformed skeletal muscle for cardiac assist as the incidence of congestive heart failure has continued to increase in recent years. Dynamic cardiomyoplasty represents the first clinical use of skeletal muscle power to provide assistance to a failing heart. The procedure is, at the present time, undergoing an FDA-approved clinical trial in the United States. The inconsistent results observed have generated interest in the pursuit of alternative applications of skeletal muscle power for cardiac assist. Different experimental approaches are being currently investigated, including skeletal muscle ventricles, aortomyoplasty, and several configurations of dynamic cardiomyoplasty using one or two LD muscles.

In our laboratory, we have evaluated an approach for cardiomyoplasty using both LD muscles. The rationale for this approach is the assumption that the double cardiomyoplasty allows for a more complete ventricular coverage

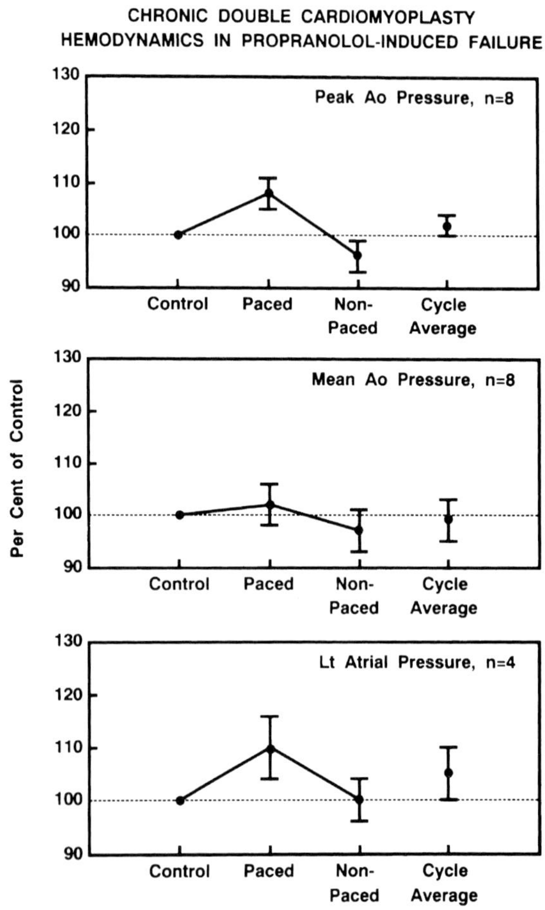


**Figure 5:** *Effect of double cardiomyoplasty stimulation on mean aortic pressure, peak aortic pressure, and left atrial pressure in propranolol induced heart failure*

that may result in greater hemodynamic augmentation than single cardiomyoplasty. In previous acute experiments, significant hemodynamic improvements in left ventricular function during double cardiomyoplasty stimulation have been observed. Niinami and colleagues[9] conducted an acute feasibility study with LD double cardiomyoplasty. They observed an increase in cardiac output of 9.9% with stimulation in a normal heart and an increase in cardiac output of 21.6% in a propranolol model of failure. Magovern and associates[10] performed bilateral LD cardiomyoplasty using unconditioned muscles and compared two different wrap configurations with the conventional left posterior cardiomyoplasty. They observed hemodynamic augmentation with both double wrap configurations and the left cardiomyoplasty, but concluded that the bilateral procedures appear to have greater effects, especially on right ventricular function. Furnary and colleagues[11] compared bilateral anterior cardiomyoplasty with its components, the left anterior cardiomyoplasty and the right anterior cardiomyoplasty in an acute setting. They observed that the bilateral cardiomyoplasty caused a large increase in systolic pressures, but was associated with a significant decrease in baseline function. In their study the left cardiomyoplasty caused minimal changes in hemodynamics with stimulation and they concluded that the right anterior cardiomyoplasty can provide the benefits of the bilateral anterior cardiomyoplasty without the hemodynamic disturbances associated with this configuration. These experiments were conducted using nontransformed skeletal muscles.

In our previous report,[12] we described a new configuration of double cardiomyoplasty based on studies of the length-tension properties of the LD muscle. In this configuration, the LD muscles are tightly wrapped around the heart in an attempt to restore the resting anatomic length of the skeletal muscle. We observed that in the normal heart state, stimulation of the double cardiomyoplasty increased the cardiac output 32%, the stroke volume 39%, and the left ventricular pressure 42%. When acute heart failure was induced with high-dose intravenous propranolol (5 mg/kg), stimulation of the double cardiomyoplasty increased the cardiac output 30%, the stroke volume 28%, LV dP/dt 43%, and myocardial thickening 95%.

Ruggiero and colleagues[13] were the first group to report experience with double cardiomyoplasty in chronic studies. They observed a decrease of 3.7% in cardiac output, a 9.0% reduction in stroke volume, and an increase of 10.6% in left ventricular pressure with double cardiomyoplasty stimulation. In their study the right ventricular pressure was the only parameter noted to improve significantly with cardiomyoplasty stimulation. The differences noted between their acute and chronic studies were attributed to the changes in fiber type that occur during conditioning of the skeletal muscles or to the changes in the contractile force applied to the heart because of intrathoracic adhesions.

In contrast to this latter study where hearts are normal, the studies that we now report were performed after a state of acute heart failure was achieved with intravenous propranolol. Hemodynamic changes associated with chronic dynamic cardiomyoplasty should be more readily observed in animals that have some impairment in ventricular function. Stimulation of the double cardiomyoplasty resulted in a significant increase in stroke volume (20%), left ventricular pressure (13%), left ventricular dP/dt (31%), and peak aortic pressure (8%) compared to controls. These data suggest that a double cardiomyoplasty using conditioned, fatigue-resistant skeletal muscle provides good hemodynamic augmentation in the acutely failed canine heart.

The double cardiomyoplasty configuration used in these chronic animals differs from the configuration previously described in our acute studies in that the shortened LD muscles were not re-stretched to resting anatomic length when wrapped around the heart. We noted early in our experiments with chronic animals that the conditioned, fatigue-resistant skeletal muscles wrapped around the heart shorten. This distorts the anatomic position of the myocardium within the mediastinum, causing significant hemodynamic compromise. Two dogs were lost initially due to this apparent anatomic distortion, and the stretched wrap configuration was abandoned in favor of a nonconstrictive wrap. The major limitation of this study is that the propranolol model of acute heart failure is not clinically significant. Clinically relevant models of heart failure should be used in the future when evaluating double cardiomyoplasty.

Although a double cardiomyoplasty on patients in heart failure will require extensive surgery, the augmentation may be more impressive postoperatively than that obtained from single cardiomyoplasty. We are currently conducting long-term studies comparing different configurations of single versus double cardiomyoplasties in a chronic heart failure model. The information obtained from these studies will be beneficial in evaluating the potential role of double cardiomyoplasty as a means of biological cardiac assist.

## References


1. Chiu RCJ: Dynamic cardiomyoplasty: efficacy and mechanisms. *Cardiac Chron* 6:1–8, 1992.
2. Carpentier AF, Chachques CJ, Acar C, et al: Dynamic cardiomyoplasty at seven years. *J Thorac Cardiovasc Surg* 106:42–54, 1993.
3. Moreira LF, Bocchi EA, Stolf NA, et al: Current expectations in dynamic cardiomyoplasty. *Ann Thorac Surg* 55:299–303, 1993.
4. Furnary AP, Magovern JA, Christlieb IY, et al: Clinical cardiomyoplasty: preoperative factors associated with outcome. *Ann Thorac Surg* 54:1139–1143, 1992.
5. Hill AB, Chiu RCJ: Dynamic cardiomyoplasty for treatment of heart failure. *Clin Cardiol* 12:681–688, 1989.
6. Grandjean PA, Austin L, Chan S, Terpstra B, et al: Dynamic cardiomyoplasty: Clinical follow-up results. *J Cardiac Surg* 6:80–88, 1991.
7. Delahaye F, Jegaden O, Montagna P, et al: Latissimus dorsi cardiomyoplasty in severe congestive heart: The Lyon experience. *J Cardiac Surg* 6:106–112, 1991.
8. Jatene AD, Moreira LF, Stolf NA, et al: Left ventricular function changes after cardiomyoplasty in patients with dilated cardiomyopathy. *J Thoracic Cardiovasc Surg* 102:132–139, 1991.
9. Niinami H, Pochettino A, Ruggiero R, et al: Canine latissimus dorsi cardio-double myoplasty: acute feasibility study. *J Cardiac Surg* 6:124–131, 1991.
10. Magovern JA, Furnary AP, Christlieb I, Kao RL, et al: Bilateral latissimus dorsi cardiomyoplasty. *Ann Thorac Surg* 52:1259–1265, 1991.
11. Furnary AP, Magovern JA, Christlieb IY, et al: Component analysis of bilateral anterior cardiomyoplasty. *Ann Thorac Surg* 55:72–77, 1993.
12. Soltero ER, Michael LH, Glaeser DH, et al: New configuration of double cardiomyoplasty based on studies of the length-tension properties of the latissimus dorsi muscle. *J Thorac Cardiovasc Surg* 106:842–849, 1993.
13. Ruggiero R, Thomas GA, Niinami H, et al: Double cardiomyoplasty: Acute versus chronic results. *Ann Thorac Surg* 56:31–37, 1993.

Chapter 37

# *Discussion*

**Dr. Furnary:** More than a clinically relevant model, you need a hemodynamically relevant model. It is easy to increase a left ventricular pressure of 60. It is much more difficult to increase a left ventricular pressure of 90 or 100 but it is more clinically and hemodynamically relevant. Also, it is misleading to present your data as a percent of control. Your control is actually your second beat or your off beat. I would like you to comment on that.

**Dr. Soltero:** You see a greater increase if you compare the paced beat with the nonpaced beat. We did not compare these here. We compared them to the baseline control protocol. I agree with you about the lack of clinical relevance of this model. We are presently conducting studies with double cardiomyoplasty in the supraventricular tachycardia heart failure model and we will get more information from that.

**Dr. Furnary:** You might do better to put the cardiomyostimulator on 1:4 and measure the 4th beat as compared to the stimulated beat. As you can see from your studies of the off beat, you are robbing Peter to pay Paul; your off beat was much less than your baseline control. We described this in a paper in the *Annals of Surgery*. As you wrap the heart, you depress left ventricular function and you depress the hemodynamic indices, which is the effect of the static wrap. Then you have the effect of the dynamic wrap that happens after you start stimulating the heart. But what you are actually measuring is an increase from the depression you have created by wrapping the heart and it tends to confound your data when you look at it as a percentage of baseline.

**Question from floor:** What happened to the right ventricle?

**Dr. Soltero:** We did not measure right-sided pressures.

**Dr. Mikaeloff:** How can you prove experimentally that the hemodynamic effect is better than with a single flap?

**Dr. Soltero:** We can't in this particular model because we performed a double wrap and there is no way to take the wrap off and then compare it to a single

From Carpentier A, Chachques JC, Grandjean P: Cardiac Bioassist. © Futura Publishing Co, Inc, Armonk, NY, 1997.

wrap. We are conducting experiments now in which we train the muscle in situ and we dilate the heart and then compare different configurations of the double wrap versus the right versus the left wrap. Our preliminary data show that one gets better augmentation with a double wrap. The second best configuration is the right wrap followed by the left wrap.

Chapter 38

# Dynamic Aortomyoplasty for Long-Term Circulatory Support:

## Experimental Studies and Clinical Experience

Juan Carlos Chachques, Marc Radermecker, Pierre Grandjean, François Chaussende, Alain F. Carpentier

### Introduction

Intra-aortic balloon counterpulsation (IABC) is widely used in clinical practice to ameliorate severely altered cardiac function. It has been shown that IABC increases coronary artery perfusion pressure and decreases left ventricle wall tension, thereby optimizing myocardial perfusion and myocardial oxygen consumption.

During the past 5 years, we have reinvestigated the concept of extra-aortic muscle-powered counterpulsation introduced 25 years ago by Kantrowitz et al.[1]

Although these authors have reported moderate diastolic augmentation following the use of paced diaphragm muscle flaps wrapped around the descending aorta, they were hindered at that time by insufficient knowledge of muscle biology and myostimulation. Based on the experimental data that led us to develop the concept of dynamic cardiomyoplasty at Broussais Hospital, we have applied fundamental knowledge of muscle-powered cardiac assistance to perform aortomyoplasty.[2, 3] This surgical procedure consists of the wrapping of an electrostimulated latissimus dorsi (LD) muscle pediculed autograft around the ascending aorta to generate a synchronized diastolic compression. Preliminary work in our laboratory has shown that aortomyoplasty necessitates a patch enlargement of the ascending aorta to optimize its efficacy in such a way as to create a biocompatible reservoir and to eject a larger blood volume. However, in clinical practice, in patients with a large and long

From Carpentier A, Chachques JC, Grandjean P: Cardiac Bioassist. © Futura Publishing Co, Inc, Armonk, NY, 1997.

ascending aorta, it probably will not be necessary to use patch enlargement of the aorta. The ascending aortomyoplasty technique was found to effectively increase diastolic pressure and reduce left ventricular afterload in acute experimental conditions.[2]

However, these early results did not provide any data on the long-term hemodynamic effectiveness of the procedure and on the physiological consequences of chronic external aortic wall compression. The goal of this study was to develop a chronic experimental model and to evaluate the physiological effects of dynamic aortomyoplasty in order to better define future applications in clinical research.

## Materials and Methods

Five adult alpine goats (mean weight, 47 kg) were used for this long-term experiment. Anesthesia was induced with an intravenous injection of propofol (5 mg/kg). The animals were intubated and mechanically ventilated with a Servo Ventilator Siemens 900 C. The anesthesia was maintained with isoflurane 2% inhalation. During the procedure, curariform drugs were contraindicated.

All goats underwent a lateral thoracic incision to provide optimal exposure for careful dissection of the right LD muscle flap. Two pacing electrodes (Medtronic model SP 5528) were implanted into the proximal part of the LD muscle, which was brought into the right chest after a 5-cm resection of the second rib. Great care was taken to preserve the integrity of the thoracodorsal neurovascular bundle.

After closure of the right thoracic incision, a standard median sternotomy was performed, and then the ascending aorta, the aortic arch, and collateral vessels were dissected. The ascending aorta was enlarged with an elliptical autologous pericardial patch treated intraoperatively with a 0.6% glutaraldehyde solution. The patch was implanted after side clamping of the ascending aorta using a 5-0 polypropylene running suture. The mean surface area of the pericardial patch was $253 \pm 24$ mm$^2$. In all animals, the LD muscle flap was positioned posteriorly to wrap the ascending aorta and the aortic arch counterclockwise in order to orient the LD muscle fibers perpendicular to the longitudinal axis of the aorta (Figs. 1 and 2).

The LD muscle electrostimulation protocol was started after an initial healing period of 15 days. An implantable diastolic pulse generator (Prometheus, Medtronic model 6101) was implanted and connected to two sensing myocardial leads (Medtronic model SP 5548) and the LD muscle pacing electrodes. Later, the LD muscle was progressively electrostimulated with 1, 2, 3 pulses per burst and finally with a complete burst of six impulses according to the Broussais Hospital protocol.[3] The parameters used for muscle electrostimulation were the following: pulse amplitude 5 volts, pulse width 210 ms, burst rate of 30 Hz, and burst duration of 185 ms. Diastolic counterpulsation was performed in a 2:1 mode.

The hemodynamic effects were evaluated at 12 months in three goats and at 24 months in the other two goats. The following hemodynamic data were analyzed: left ventricle, aortic and pulmonary artery pressures, and rate of rise of left ventricular pressure (dp/dt) (Gould transducer).

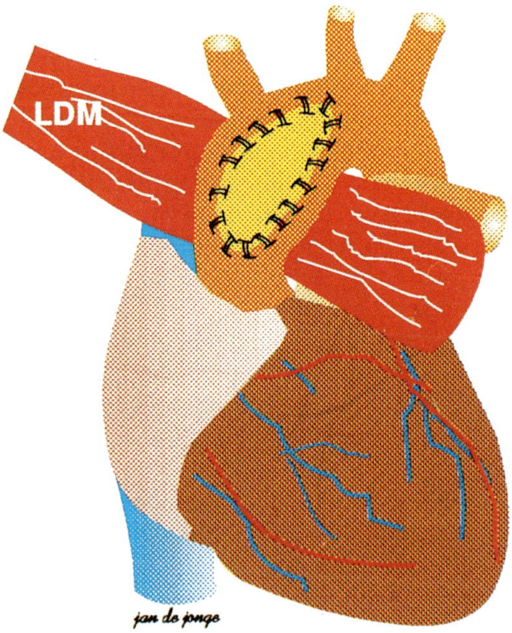


**Figure 1:** *The ascending aorta is enlarged by an autologous pericardial patch. The right LD muscle is positioned behind the dissected aorta.*

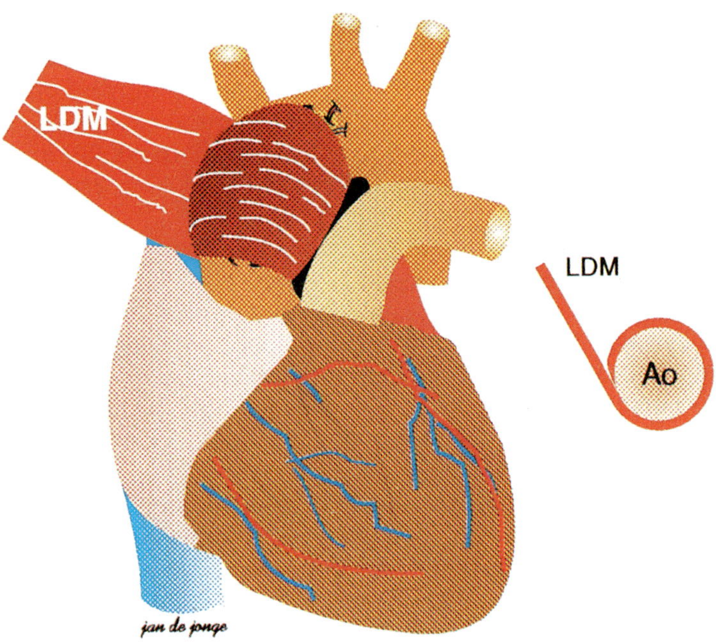


**Figure 2:** *Aortomyoplasty: the aorta is completely wrapped by the right pedicled LD muscle.*

Cardiac output evaluation was performed by the thermodilution technique. The extent of diastolic augmentation was measured by the subendocardial viability index (diastolic pressure-time index/systolic tension-time index). The subendocardial viability index was calculated from superimposed tracings of aortic arch and LV pressure.[4] The variation of this ratio (%) was calculated during assisted cardiac cycles (pulse generator functioning in the 1:1 stimulation mode) and 5 minutes after the device was switched off (basal values). Hemodynamic measurements were performed on healthy animals at baseline conditions and after acute pharmacological heart failure induced with a high dose of propranol hydrochloride (3 mg/kg IV). Tracings were recorded for periods of 60 minutes in order to evaluate the stability of results and also to demonstrate the fatigue resistance of the involved LD muscle flap.

Samples of the LD muscle flap, aortic wall, and aortic valve were processed for histological studies. Anatomopathological analyses of the kidneys, lungs, liver, and spleen were also performed to eliminate the occurrence of thromboembolic events.

Statistical analysis was performed by computer, applying one-way analysis of variance for repeated measures, to determine differences between or within groups. The 95% confidence limit was chosen as the indicator of significance ($p<0.05$).

## Results

All hemodynamic data were collected in long-term experimental conditions before and after induction of cardiac failure. After 12 to 24 months of chronic diastolic counterpulsation, a significant increase of DPTI/TTI persisted at basal state condition, from $1.13 \pm 0.13$ (stimulator OFF) to $1.39 \pm 0.18$ (stimulator ON), $p<0.05$, and after induction of acute heart failure (from $1.10 \pm 0.10$ to $1.40 \pm 0.11$, $p<0.05$) (Fig. 3). During heart failure, aortomyoplasty increased cardiac output from $3.6 \pm 0.5$ to $5.5 \pm 1.04$ L/min ($p<0.05$), and decreased systemic vascular resistances from $1575 \pm 212$ to $1135 \pm 249$ dyne/sec/cm $^{-5}$ ($p<0.05$) (Tables 1 and 2).

Histological studies at 12 and 24 months were performed on: (1) the right LD muscle flap, (2) the wall of ascending aorta, and (3) the interface between the LD muscle flap and the ascending aorta. On gross examination, the LD muscle looked healthy. Tight adhesions developed between the LD muscle and the aortic wall. On histological examination, there was no evidence of neurovascular supply alterations. ATPase histochemical staining technique demonstrated a complete transformation of type 2 glycolytic to type 1 oxydative muscle fibers. The aortic wall consisted of normal intima, media, and adventitia. (Fig. 4). In goats, the elastic fibers of the media are normally segmented. Dense adhesions were found between the LD muscle flap, the ascending aorta (adventitial layer), and the glutaraldehyde-treated pericardial patch. All patches were very pliable and free of any calcification.

The mean diameter of the enlarged aorta was unchanged when compared with preoperative measurements ($20 \pm 2$ vs. $18 \pm 3$ mm). There was no thrombus found in the ascending aorta, and the aortic valves were anatomically and functionally normal.

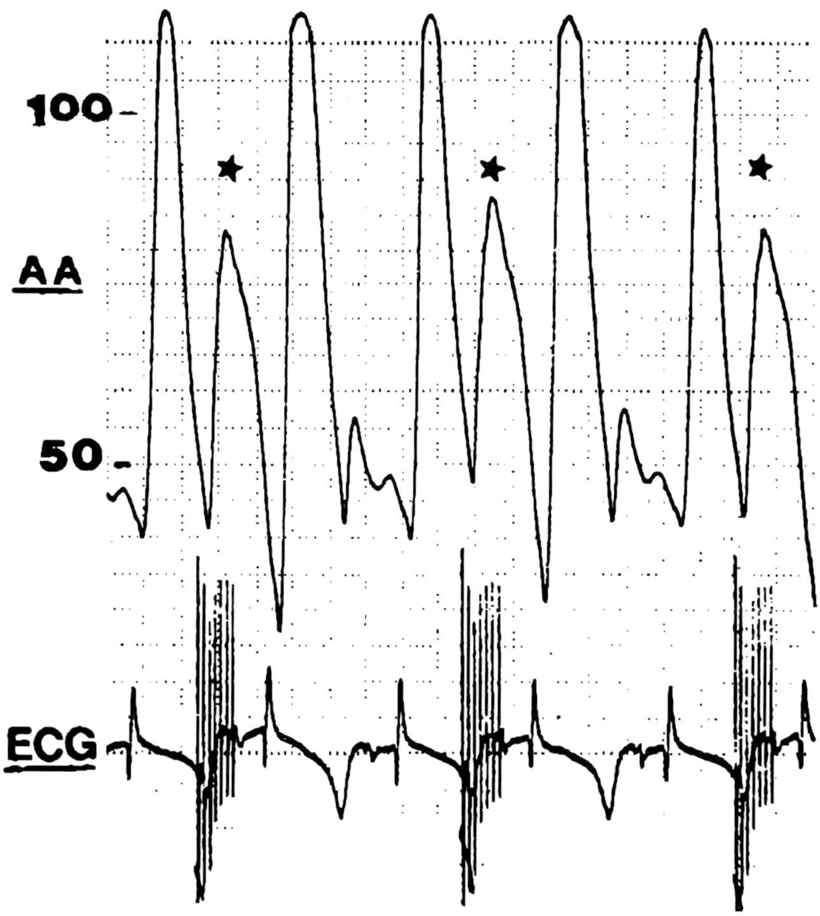


**Figure 3:** *Hemodynamics findings after aortomyoplasty. The stars show the diastolic augmentation, followed by a negative pressure wave corresponding to LD muscle relaxation (this hemodynamic event can be compared with the deflation effect of an IABC). AA = ascending aorta pressure.*

**Table 1**
Hemodynamic Studies Following Aortomyoplasty Basal State

| | *St (−)* | *St (+)* |
|---|---|---|
| LVEDP | 6.8 ± 1.3 | 6.4 ± 0.8 |
| DPTI/TTI | 1.13 ± 0.13 | 1.39 ± 0.18* |
| CO (L/min) | 7.9 ± 1.6 | 7.8 ± 1.1 |
| SVR (dyne/s/cm $^{-5}$) | 897 ± 135 | 903 ± 121 |

* $p<0.05$

LVEDP = left ventricular end-diastolic pressure.

DPTI/TTI = diastolic pressure-time index/systolic tension-time index.

CO = cardiac output.

SVR = systemic vascular resistance (MAP/CO. 80).

**Table 2**
Hemodynamic Studies Following Aortomyoplasty Heart Failure

| | *St (−)* | *St (+)* |
|---|---|---|
| LVEDP | 13.2 ± 1.1 | 11.6 ± 1.5* |
| DPTI/TTI | 1.1 ± 0.10 | 1.4 ± 0.11* |
| CO (L/min) | 3.6 ± 0.5 | 5.5 ± 1.04* |
| SVR (dyne/s/cm$^{-5}$) | 1574 ± 211 | 1134 ± 249* |

* $p<0.05$
LVEDP = left ventricular end-diastolic pressure.
DPTI/TTI = diastolic pressure-time index/systolic tension-time index.
CO = cardiac output.
SVR = systemic vascular resistance (MAP/CO.80).

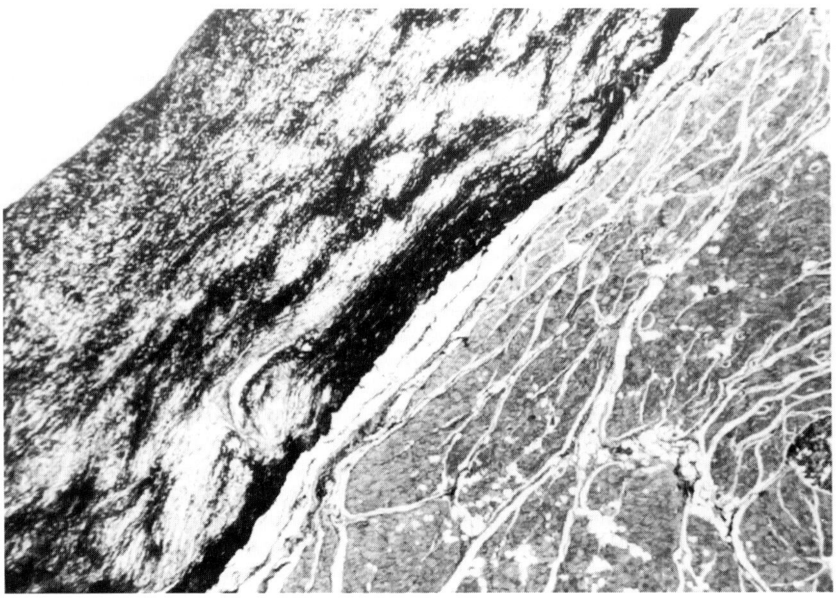

**Figure 4:** *Photomicrograph of aorta and LD muscle. Normal configuration of the aortic wall. The LD muscle shows a preserved myofibrillar structure. Orcein stain; original magnification, × 80.*

## Discussion

Previous publications on aortomyoplasty have demonstrated that, in acute and short-term experimental studies, this procedure can reproduce the two fundamental goals of diastolic counterpulsation: an increase of diastolic pressure and a reduction of left ventricular afterload.[2,5–7] In our experimental approach, we chose the ascending aorta instead of the descending aorta based on three potential benefits: (1) to obviate iatrogenic paraplegia related to the division of intercostal arteries, (2) to take advantage of a larger aortic diameter, and (3) because the closer the coronary ostia and the left ventricle are to the counterpulsator, the more efficient it should be.

In an experimental goat model (presenting a narrow and short ascending aorta), we have shown that patch enlargement of the aorta may improve the efficacy of the procedure. This technique has created a biocompatible autologous reservoir very close to the aortic valve, and continuously washed out by the anterograde left systolic ejection volume. Our study has assessed this model chronically (up to 24 months). This step is a prerequisite to any introduction of this technique as a surgical treatment for chronic left heart failure in humans.

The results obtained in this animal model have shown that, in the basal state in goats, an ascending aortomyoplasty caused a 23% increase of the endocardial viability index (DPTI/TTI) when the stimulator was activated, and a 27% increase after induction of heart failure. A 52% increase in cardiac output was noted in association with a 39% decrease in systemic vascular resistance (stimulation ON) after the induction of acute heart failure. This improvement was documented for at least 1 hour, suggesting that the LD muscle flap had acquired the functional characteristics of fatigue-resistant type 1 myocytes.

These data emphasize that aortomyoplasty can be efficient chronically for cardiac assistance. We also demonstrated that the transformed LD muscle, following a progressive electrostimulation protocol, retained biomechanical characteristics, allowing for an effective aortic counterpulsation.

The duration of muscle electrostimulation was adapted to permit optimal muscle contraction. Similarly, muscle relaxation occurred promptly enough not to interfere with left ventricular systole. This was confirmed by a significant drop of the arterial pressure wave after assisted diastole (Fig. 3). The question of whether or not such circulatory assistance would still be efficient at higher cardiac rates is incompletely answered. It can be expected that due to the reduced speed of shortening and relaxation (characterizing fatigue-resistant muscle fibers), completely slow muscles would be suboptimal at high cardiac frequency. However, since recent data suggest that complete transformation into slow myosin isoform is not necessary for performance, electrical preconditioning of muscle could be used to induce fast fatigue-resistant muscle with advantageous biomechanical characteristics for the purpose of aortomyoplasty.

The histological findings related to the aortic wall have shown an excellent tolerance of the three aortic wall layers, especially the media, to continuous concentrical squeezing. The patch enlargement of the ascending aorta did not lead to aneurysm formation over the long term. These results therefore suggest that aortomyoplasty is an interesting application of muscle-powered left ventricular assistance.[8,9] It might be indicated in patients with contraindications to dynamic cardiomyoplasty such as mitral valve insufficiency or severe dilatation of the heart (e.g., cardiothoracic ratio >60%, LV end-diastolic diameter >75 mm); in these cases, a cardiomyoplasty procedure is generally unsuccessful due to the incomplete cardiac wrapping obtained during surgery. Another indication for aortomyoplasty could be heart transplanted patients, presenting with heart failure due to a graft disease (e.g., coronary arteriosclerosis).[10]

Calcifications in the ascending aortic wall, aortic valve regurgitation, Marfan's disease or any other dystrophic disease of the aorta represent absolute contraindications to aortomyoplasty.

## Aortomyoplasty: Worldwide Clinical Experience

Dynamic aortomyoplasty works to treat chronic heart failure on the basis of diastolic counterpulsation, which is the physiological principle whereby the intra-aortic balloon pump has been shown to support patients with severe hemodynamic deterioration. However, the limitations of the use of this device include: (1) short-term assistance, (2) risk of limb ischemia, (3) presence of intra-aortic prosthetic material, representing a risk of aortic wall injury, thromboembolic complications, and sepsis.

Since November 9, 1992, the date of the first world clinical aortomyoplasty case performed at Broussais Hospital, 28 aortomyoplasty procedures have been performed worldwide.[11–16] Twenty-one male patients and seven female patients have been operated on at: Broussais Hospital – 4; Marseilles, France – 4; London 3; Jedda, Saudi Arabia – 14; and Buenos Aires, Argentina – 3. The mean age of patients was 56 ± 7 years. The etiology of left ventricular failure was: ischemic cardiomyopathy 19, idiopathic dilated cardiomyopathy 8, and Chagas cardiomyopathy 1. An important cardiomegaly was present in most of these patients. The mean cardiothoracic ratio was 68 ± 5% and the mean end-diastolic LV diameter was 82 ± 5 mm (measured by echocardiography). All patients possessed a normal aortic valve function and aortic wall.

Aortomyoplasty techniques consisted of 19 ascending aorta wrappings (in seven cases the aorta was enlarged with a pericardial patch), and 9 descending thoracic aorta wrappings. The right LD muscle was used to wrap the ascending aorta, and the descending aorta was wrapped with the left LD muscle. The distal end of the LD muscle was split longitudinally in seven patients undergoing ascending aortomyoplasty in order to cover the aorta on both sides of the brachocephalic trunk.[2]

Current clinical evaluation (mean follow-up: 10 months) shows a significant improvement of the functional class and the quality of life of operated patients. Hemodynamic and echo-Doppler studies demonstrated diastolic augmentation and compression of the aorta during LD muscle electrostimulation.

Aortomyoplasty offers the following advantages: (1) the procedure can be performed without the need of cardiopulmonary bypass, (2) there are no manipulations of the heart because it is not necessary to open the pericardial sac to wrap the aorta (in this way aortomyoplasty can be considered as a vascular surgical procedure), (3) in cases of reduced diameter of the aorta, enlargement of this vessel can be readily performed using lateral clamping and autologous pericardial patch.

It seems that dynamic aortomyoplasty can be potentially an efficient technique to assist patients with severe refractory cardiac failure. A larger clinical experience and a longer follow-up period is necessary to clearly assess the benefits of this procedure.[17,18]

## References


1. Kantrowitz A, McKinnon WMP: The experimental use of the diaphragm as an auxiliary myocardium. *Surg Forum* 9:266–268, 1959.
2. Chachques JC, Grandjean PA, Cabrera Fischer EI, Latremouille C, Jebara VA, et al: Dynamic aortomyoplasty to assist left ventricular failure. *Ann Thorac Surg* 49:225–230, 1990.
3. Carpentier A, Chachques JC, Acar C, Relland J, Mihaileanu S, et al. Dynamic cardiomyoplasty at seven years. *J Thorac Cardiovasc Surg* 106:42–54, 1993.
4. Buckberg GD, Fixler DE, Archie JP, Hoffman JIE: Experimental subendocardial ischemia in dogs with normal coronary arteries. *Circ Res* 30:67–81, 1972.
5. Pattison CW, Cumming DVE, Williamson A, Clayton-Jones DG, et al: Aortic counterpulsation for up to 28 days with autologous latissimus dorsi in sheep. *J Thorac Cardiovasc Surg* 102:766–773, 1991.
6. Lee F, Hanan SA, Tuchy GE, Rebeyka IM, Yeh T, Borges MR, Abd-Elfattah AS, Wechsler AS: Skeletal muscle extraaortic counterpulsation. *J Thorac Cardiovasc Surg* 102:757–765, 1991.
7. Takahashi R, Yozu R, Kurosaka Y, Kawada S: Assisted circulation using cardiomyoplasty together with aortomyoplasty. *Artif Organs* 17:914–918, 1993.
8. Constance CG, Sabini G, Turi GK, Hines GL: Descending thoracic aortomyoplasty: Effect of chronically conditioned muscle on heart failure. *Cardiovasc Surg* 1: 291–295, 1993.
9. Lazzara RR, Trumble DR, Magovern JA: Dynamic descending thoracic aortomyoplasty: Comparison with intraaortic balloon pump in a model of heart failure. *Ann Thorac Surg* 58: 366–371, 1994.
10. Gonzalez ALF, Herreros JM, Alegria E, Martinez MA, Iglesias I: Dynamic cardiomyoplasty after heart transplantation. *Circulation* 93: 2204, 1996.
11. Chachques JC, Acar C, Farge A, Radermecker M, Berrebi A, et al: Cardiomyoplasty and aortomyoplasty for long-term circulatory support: Clinical experience. *Artif Organs* 17:552, 1993.
12. Mesana T, Mouly A, Caus T, Bauer S, Collard F, et al: Preliminary clinical experience with descending dynamic aortomyoplasty. *Eur JCPE* 6:150, 1996.
13. Raffa H, Memom F, Jabbad H, Kayali MT, Langer J, et al: Aortomyoplasty: A new emerging surgical modality for endstage failure. *Eur JCPE* 6:152, 1996.
14. Trainini J: Aortomyoplasty clinical experience at Buenos Aires, Argentina (personal communication).
15. Yacoub M, Black J: Aortomyoplasty clinical experience at Harefield Hospital, London, UK (personal communication).
16. Pepper J: Aortomyoplasty clinical experience at Royal Brompton Hospital, London, UK (personal communication).
17. Flum DR, Cernaianu AC, Meada R, Lee LA, Salartash K, et al: Descending thoracic aortomyoplasty: A technique for clinical application. *Ann Thorac Surg* 61:93–98, 1996.
18. Chachques JC, Radermecker M, Tolan MJ, Cabrera Fischer E, Grandjean PA, Carpentier A: Aortomyoplasty counterpulsation: experimental results and early clinical experience. *Ann Thorac Surg* 61:420–425, 1996.

# Chapter 38

# *Discussion*

**Dr. Stephenson:** I would like to present some of our work that has been done in dogs. Our diastolic augmentation pressure traces at one year are almost identical. One of the things that held us back from going on to humans is that we still had a problem with rupture when we made the separate skeletal muscle ventricles even though the ones that survived long term seemed to do quite well. What is the next step? When will you go on to humans with this technique and what has to be worked out before you can do that?

**Dr. Chachques:** At Broussais Hospital, we have performed two aortomyoplasty clinical cases so far. The first patient died 3 months following aortomyoplasty due to ventricular fibrillation. The other patient died a few days after the operation. Both patients were in Class IV and had ventricular arrhythmias. This clinical experience showed that patient selection must follow strict criteria.

**Dr. Stephenson:** Did you see diastolic augmentation?

**Dr. Chachques:** Yes, but the postoperative courses of these patients were very difficult with intra-aortic balloon counterpulsation and low cardiac output. They may not have been the best indication.

**Dr. Stephenson:** Was there any compression of the pulmonary artery?

**Dr. Chachques:** No. At autopsy, the pulmonary artery was normal. The skeletal muscle structure had preserved 70% of the muscle fibers.

**Dr. Subramanian (New York):** When working with the intra-aortic balloon, we found that one has to have at least 80% occlusivity in the aorta in order to get a marked diastolic augmentation. Can you tell us how occlusive the aorta became? Also, one of the basics in diastolic counterpulsation is to have an unloading effect. One has to have an active deflation of any counterpulsation mechanism whether it is external or internal. How do you know that you have an afterload reduction with this counterpulsation device?

**Dr. Chachques:** The problem in normal animals is that we have to work with small hearts and normal aortas. We don't have a chronic model of heart failure to study reduction of afterload. In addition, the ascending aorta is very narrow

From Carpentier A, Chachques JC, Grandjean P: Cardiac Bioassist. © Futura Publishing Co, Inc, Armonk, NY, 1997.

and very short, only 3 or 4 cm. The only thing we can say at this time is that we have a diastolic augmentation similar to that of balloon counterpulsation.

**Dr. Subramanian:** How occlusive was it?

**Dr. Chachques:** In animal studies, long-term echographic examinations showed a 40% reduction of the aortic chamber volume. In the early postoperative period, it was 60% to 70%.

**Dr. Subramanian:** That is why your diastolic augmentation was not very marked.

**Dr. Chachques:** It was not small. This animal had normal blood pressure.

**Dr. Cusimano (Toronto):** When you measured your dp/dt ratio, you probably put your aortic line distal to the wrap. What you are really interested in is not the diastolic augmentation to the body but to the heart. If there is a significant amount of contraction of the proximal aorta, what you really want to do is find out what is happening proximal to that wrap and see what is happening to the heart because you may actually be squeezing off the blood to the heart when it contracts. The effect on the distal circulation may be interpreted as an incorrect rise in the diastolic pressure.

**Dr. Stephenson:** With our skeletal muscle ventricles, we plug them in just below the left subclavian, we do measure above and below, and our pressure traces are very similar. My guess is if you could measure the tiny area above the wrap, it would probably be very similar to what you see below.

**Dr. Michael Acker:** Did you get a sense of the diameter initially in the human and then what diameter it was chronically, the patient having lived 3 months? With chronic electrical stimulation and its transformation to a fatigue-resistant aerobic state, skeletal muscle will shrink down. I am concerned that in cardiomyoplasty, you may have a ratcheting girdle. What would be the effect on the size of the passive diameter of the aorta as this muscle is conditioned and shrinks down and gradually constricts?

**Dr. Chachques:** We never found stenosis of the aorta at the level of the latissimus dorsi muscle wrapping. In histological studies, the aortic wall showed a normal structure.

**Dr. Lazarra:** We had the same idea in Allegheny and tried to approach everything through the left chest. Our concern was that there was a large population of clinical patients who previously received an aortocoronary bypass graft and suffered from ischemic cardiomyopathy. Would you consider that to be a contraindication to the way you perform aortomyoplasty?

**Dr. Chachques:** For the moment, we have only three very clear contraindications: aortic calcification, Marfan's disease, and aortic valve regurgitation. We prefer to operate on patients in sinus rhythm because the counterpulsation is more effective in sinus rhythm.

Chapter 39

# Hemodynamic Benefits of Latissimus Dorsi Aortopulmonary Counterpulsation

E.I. Cabrera Fischer, Juan Carlos Chachques, Alejandra I. Christen, Alain Carpentier*

## Introduction

Heart failure is a clinical syndrome in which right and left ventricular assistance are required[1,2] in order to preserve the hemodynamic parameters.

South American trypanosomiasis affects 3.5 million people and diffuse loss of myocardial contractility is found in 20% to 25% of the infected group.[3,4] Moreover, reactivation of *Trypanosoma cruzi* infection has been demonstrated in chronically infected dogs, in which cardiac transplant was performed and immunosuppression induced with cyclosporine A.[5] Thus, mechanical devices, dynamic cardiomyoplasty, and aortomyoplasty have been considered of great interest during the last few years.[6–10] Since none of the available treatments of severe heart failure can be expected to benefit a large number of patients in the near future, new alternative techniques must be developed.[11]

In the last few years, mechanical circulatory assistance systems have been used as alternative treatments to provide recovery support in patients suffering from severe cardiac failure.[12] At present, heart transplantation remains as the best treatment for end-stage cardiac failure, but immunosuppression and scarcity of organ donors restrict this option.[5, 13–15]

Counterpulsation was described as the mechanical removal of blood during systole and the subsequent reinfusion in diastole. This mechanical assistance was also performed by wrapping a diaphragmatic pedicle around the aorta.[16] Furthermore, counterpulsation obtained with the intra-aortic balloon pump is an invasive method with an external power source and can be used only as a temporary device.

*With the cooperation of Marcelo R. Risk, Miguel A. Cierto, and Javier Binstein.

From Carpentier A, Chachques JC, Grandjean P: Cardiac Bioassist. © Futura Publishing Co, Inc, Armonk, NY, 1997.

Cardiac assistance with aortic counterpulsation can be achieved by using the native ascending aorta as a ventricular chamber wrapped by an electrostimulated latissimus dorsi (LD) muscle flap in an animal model of cardiac failure.[10] This would be a useful procedure when cardiac failure is produced by cardiomyopathies associated with severe heart dilatation and/or mitral valve regurgitation. In these cases cardiomyoplastic procedures are contraindicated. On the other hand, biventricular mechanical support of the failing heart is required in order to reverse both right and left ventricular severe failure.[17–21]

The aim of our work was to study the hemodynamic effects of a combined dynamic aortopulmonary myoplasty in an acute animal model of cardiac failure.

## Material and Methods

Eight adult mongrel dogs weighing 22–28 kg were chosen at the beginning of this study, with ages ranging from 24 to 48 months. General anesthesia was induced with sodium thiopentone (20 mg/kg, intravenously), followed by intubation and maintenance of anesthesia with 1% halothane carried out in pure oxygen administered through a Bain tube connected to a mechanical respirator (Bird Mark 8).

In all dogs, a left lateral thoracic incision was performed to facilitate dissection of the LD muscle. The left LD muscle was derived from its insertion on the lateral side of the last four ribs, iliac crest, and thoracolumbar fascia, and it was mobilized proximally as a pedicle flap. Pacing electrodes were implanted (two leads, model SP 5528; Medtronic, Maastricht, the Netherlands) into the proximal part of the LD muscle flap, which was brought into the chest through an opening made by resecting a portion of the second rib. Special care was taken to preserve the neurovascular bundle.

A left lateral thoracotomy at the level of the fourth intercostal space was performed in all animals. The pulmonary trunk, the ascending aorta, the transverse aortic arch, and its branches were dissected. In all animals, the LD muscle flap was positioned behind both the pulmonary trunk and the aortic root. Then, the ascending aorta and the pulmonary trunk were wrapped with the LD muscle flap in a counterclockwise fashion so that its fibers were laid perpendicular to the longitudinal axis of the vascular pedicle (Fig. 1).

Aortic and left ventricular pressures were measured by using two catheters introduced through left and right femoral arteries. A Swan-Ganz catheter was positioned in a pulmonary artery through the right femoral vein. In all animals, blood pressures and cardiac output were measured both before and after cardiac failure induction by using a high dose of halothane (3%).[22] All electrodes were coupled to an external cardiomyostimulator manufactured in our laboratory, and capable of generating a pulse amplitude of 1 to 15 V, a pulse width of 210 ms, a burst rate of 2 to 30 Hz, and 1 to 9 pulses. Diastolic counterpulsation was performed using a delay from the R wave adjusted to provide optimal diastolic augmentation. Short-term cyclic skeletal muscle electrostimulation (3 minutes per cycle) was delivered to allow functional study of dynamic aortopulmonary myoplasty. Synchronization of LD muscle flap stimulation with the cardiac rhythm was achieved by using the R wave of a surface electrocardiogram.

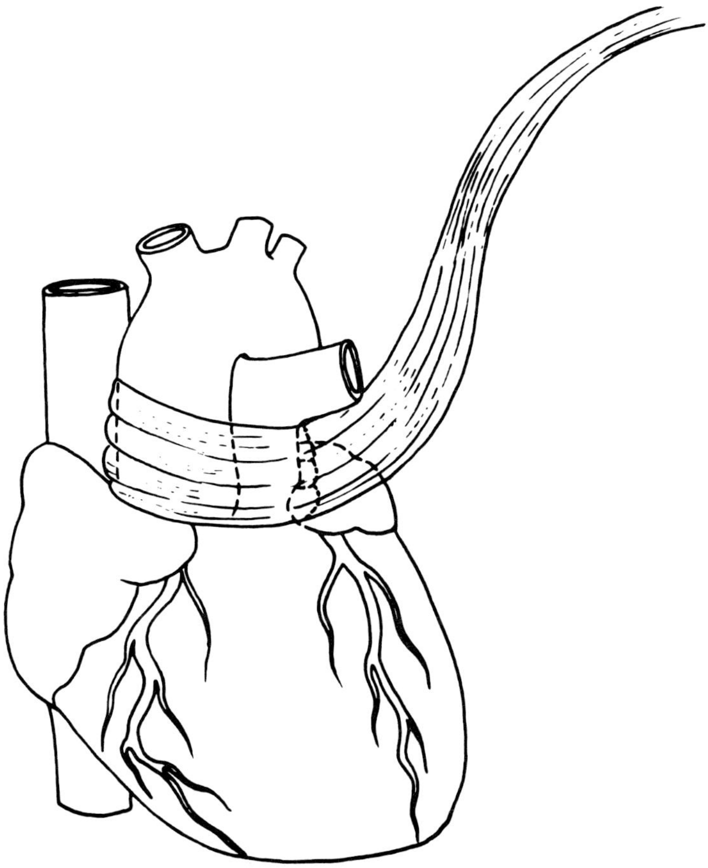

**Figure 1:** *The ascending aorta and the pulmonary trunk are wrapped with the latissimus dorsi muscle flap in a counterclockwise fashion.*

## Measurements

The following hemodynamic studies were performed: measurement of left ventricular, aortic, and pulmonary artery pressures. Left ventricular dp/dt was monitored in all cases. Cardiac output and mean pressures were used to obtain systemic and pulmonary vascular resistance values. The extent of the aortic diastolic augmentation was measured by the subendocardial viability index: diastolic pressure-time index/systolic tension-time index (DPTI-TTI).[23,24] Diastolic augmentation was monitored by the DPTI/TTI index during stimulated and nonstimulated cardiac cycles, before and after cardiac failure. Finally, pulmonary diastolic augmentation was quantified by using the arterial efficiency index that takes into account both diastolic and systolic areas beneath the pulmonary pressure wave.[25]

All animals received humane care in the preoperative period in compliance with the *Guide for the Care and Use of Laboratory Animals* published by the National Institutes of Health (NIH Publication No. 85-23, revised 1985).

## Statistical Treatment

Statistical studies were performed using one-way analysis of variance in order to determine differences between or within groups. The Newman-Keuls test was applied to determine the origin of the differences.[26]

Values reported are expressed as mean ±SD. Pressure values considered here are the mean of five consecutive cardiac cycles; cardiac output values are the mean of three consecutive determinations.

The 95% confidence limit was chosen as the indicator of statistical significance ($p<0.05$).

# Results

No animal deaths occurred during the course of any experimental session, and in spite of the fact that heparin was not administered, no aortic or pulmonary thrombosis was observed.

During the experiments, no aortic or pulmonary regurgitation was observed. No cardiac arrythmias were found during LD muscle flap placement or while electromyostimulation was performed.

Cardiac failure induced by halothane (3%) administration (Table 1) was characterized by a significant increase of end-diastolic left ventricular pressure (from 6.63 ± 1.06 to 13.62 ± 1.06); systemic vascular resistances (from 36.42 ± 5.97 to 57.83 ± 5.71) and pulmonary vascular resistances (from 6.62 ± 1.12 to 8.76 ± 1.62). In addition, a significant decrease was found in systolic left ven-

**Table 1**
Hemodynamic Parameters Obtained with Aortopulmonary Counterpulsation

| | *Control* | | *Cardiac Failure* | |
|---|---|---|---|---|
| | *Nonstimulated* | *Stimulated* | *Nonstimulated* | *Stimulated* |
| MAoP (mm Hg) | 87.75 ± 2.32 | 88.87 ± 2.67 | 71.16 ± 0.91# | 74.83 ± 2.28•& |
| MPuP (mm Hg) | 15.96 ± 0.77 | 14.58 ± 0.71* | 10.62 ± 1.24# | 11.41 ± 0.94& |
| SLVP (mm Hg) | 112.50 ± 4.38 | 111.62 ± 4.24 | 95.25 ± 3.96# | 93.12 ± 2.17& |
| EDLVP (mm Hg) | 6.63 ± 1.06 | 7.13 ± 1.25 | 13.62 ± 1.06# | 11.37 ± 0.92•& |
| CO (L/min) | 2.48 ± 0.50 | 2.46 ± 0.38 | 1.23 ± 0.17# | 1.84 ± 0.32•& |
| CI (L/min/Kg) | 0.11 ± 0.03 | 0.11 ± 0.02 | 0.06 ± 0.01# | 0.08 ± 0.01•& |
| SVR (mm Hg/L/min) | 36.42 ± 5.97 | 37.02 ± 5.19 | 57.83 ± 5.71# | 41.80 ± 7.16• |
| PVR (mm Hg/L/min) | 6.62 ± 1.12 | 6.03 ± 0.81 | 8.76 ± 1.62# | 6.33 ± 0.97• |
| HR (beats/min) | 75.25 ± 4.13 | 75.37 ± 4.31 | 67.12 ± 4.64# | 67.25 ± 4.53& |

MAoP and MPuP = mean aortic and mean pulmonary pressures, SLVP and EDLVP = systolic and end-diastolic left ventricular pressures; CO = cardiac output; CI = cardiac index; SVR and PVR = systemic and pulmonary vascular resistances; HR = heart rate. Values are mean ± SD.

*($p<0.05$) between stimulated vs. nonstimulated in control group.

•($p<0.05$) between stimulated vs. nonstimulated in cardiac failure.

&($p<0.05$) between nonstimulated in control group vs. stimulated in cardiac failure.

#($p<0.05$) in nonstimulated before and after cardiac failure.

**Table 2**
Subendocardial Viability Index (DPTI/TTI) Obtained with Aortic Counterpulsation

| | *Control* | | *Cardiac Failure* | |
|---|---|---|---|---|
| | *Nonstimulated* | *Stimulated* | *Nonstimulated* | *Stimulated* |
| Mean ± SD (mm Hg) | 1.34 ± 0.34 | 1.53 ± 0.32* | 1.22 ± 0.32 | 1.50 ± 0.32• |

Values are reported as mean ± SD.
*(p<0.05) between stimulated vs. nonstimulated in control group.
•(p<0.05) between stimulated vs. nonstimulated in cardiac failure.

**Table 3**
Arterial Efficiency Index Obtained with Pulmonary Counterpulsation

| | *Control* | | *Cardiac Failure* | |
|---|---|---|---|---|
| | *Nonstimulated* | *Stimulated* | *Nonstimulated* | *Stimulated* |
| Diastolic values (mm Hg) | 8.70 ± 1.50 | 10.90 ± 2.53* | 9.00 ± 2.36 | 11.60 ± 2.30•& |
| Systolic values (mm Hg) | 13.87 ± 6.26 | 12.15 ± 3.82 | 12.31 ± 4.39 | 11.61 ± 3.69 |

Values are reported as mean ±SD.
*(p<0.05) between stimulated vs. nonstimulated in control group.
•(p<0.05) between stimulated vs. nonstimulated in cardiac failure.
&(p<0.05) between nonstimulated in control group vs. stimulated in cardiac failure.

tricular pressure (from 112.50 ± 4.38 to 95.25 ± 3.96), cardiac output (from 2.48 ± 0.50 to 1.23 ± 0.17), mean aortic pressure (from 87.75 ± 2.32 to 71.16 ± 0.91), mean pulmonary pressure (from 15.96 ± 0.77 to 10.62 ± 1.24), cardiac index (from 0.11 ± 0.03 to 0.06 ± 0.01) and heart rate (from 75.25 ± 4.13 to 67.12 ± 4.64).

Aortic changes evaluated through the DPTI/TTI index during aortopulmonary counterpulsation by the stimulated LD muscle flap showed a significant increase both in control and after cardiac failure induction as seen in Table 2. Interestingly, values obtained in cardiac failure under LD muscle flap stimulation were not significantly different from those observed during control without counterpulsation.

Pulmonary diastolic pressure values obtained through aortopulmonary counterpulsation with LD muscle flap stimulation showed a significant increase of the arterial efficiency index both before and after halothane 3% administration (Table 3). Systolic pulmonary arterial pressure decreased, though not significantly, when LD muscle flap stimulation was performed both in control and after cardiac failure.

Finally, aortopulmonary counterpulsation monitored on the oscilloscope always showed a high degree of diastolic pressure augmentation (as higher than systolic pressure) as shown in Figure 2.

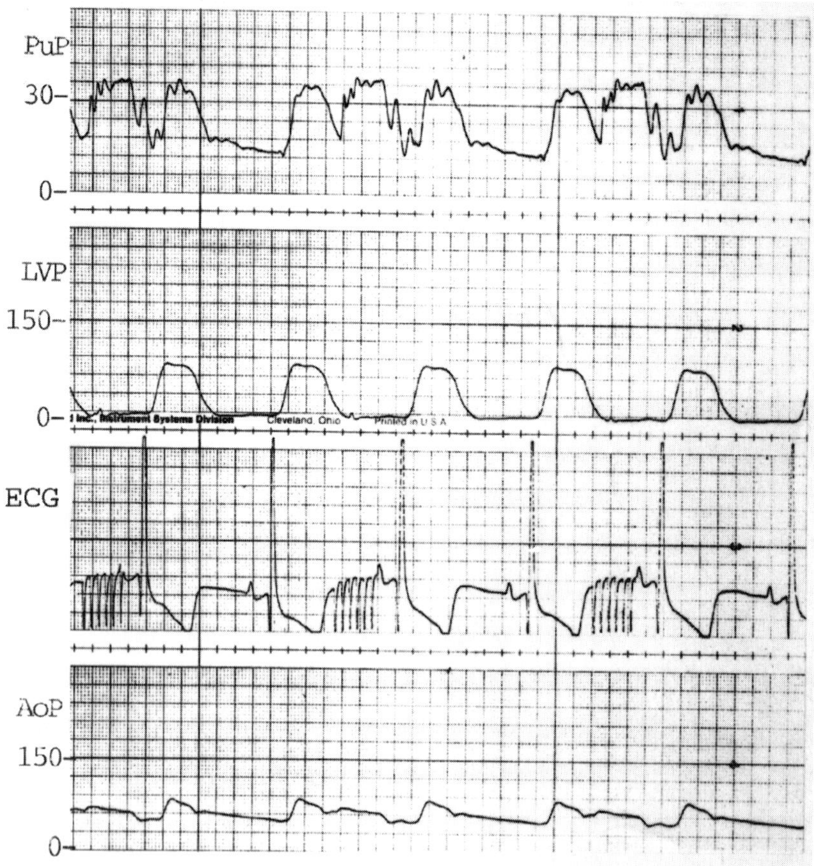


**Figure 2:** *Example of the effect of the latissimus dorsi muscle flap stimulation recorded from a dog. In the first and fourth panel we observe the simultaneous recording of the diastolic pulmonary and diastolic aortic pressure augmentation, respectively, obtained with the pulse trains, 2:1 (see ECG). The second panel shows no changes in left ventricular pressure. Pressure values are expressed in mm Hg.*

## Discussion

Since 1933 when Leriche attempted in dogs[27] the repair of left ventricular aneurysm, the cardiac application of skeletal muscle has undergone major progress to become a clinically feasible procedure. Furthermore, it was demonstrated that skeletal muscles are capable of generating four times the force per cross-sectional area as cardiac muscle does.[28]

Counterpulsation of a vessel created in 1953 by Kantrowitz and Kantrowitz is a method thought to assist cardiac failure.[29] Since then, augmentation of diastolic aortic pressure was considered a useful tool for the treatment of heart failure. In addition, a mechanical auxiliary ventricle was developed with the same purpose in the early 1960s[30] and more recently experiments were performed in order to obtain a biological power source.[10,31] Moreover, diastolic augmentation has also proved to be useful in the treatment of right ventricular failure.[32–34]

On the basis of previous studies,[10,16] the final aim of our work was to obtain simultaneous right and left ventricular support. With this purpose in mind, we designed our protocol to analyze the effects of combined aorto- and pulmonary counterpulsation with autologous LD muscle flap in an animal model of cardiac failure.

The model of heart failure pharmacologically induced used in our experiments was previously developed to mimic as closely as possible human impairment of cardiac function.[35]

As shown in the Results section, instantaneous aortopulmonary diastolic dynamic counterpulsation, obtained with an LD muscle flap synchronized with the cardiac cycle for short periods of time, is capable of restoring hemodynamic parameters in our model of cardiac failure. As expected in this acute experimental animal model, muscle fatigability occurred approximately 5 minutes after induction of stimulation. Therefore, we performed the LD muscle flap stimulation for periods shorter than 3 minutes.

The subendocardial viability index (DPTI/TTI) is a standard method that allows an accurate evaluation of aortic counterpulsation.[23,24] In pulmonary assistance, we used the difference between counterpulsated and noncounterpulsated mean diastolic pressure obtained in each condition, integrating the area beneath the curve. Comparisons of mean systolic and mean diastolic pressure obtained by integration was used previously as an index of arterial efficiency.[25]

The dynamic aortopulmonary counterpulsation described here is a simple method that avoids the possible risk of paraplegia due to the ligation of intercostal vessels, as previously reported for descending aortic wrapping.[36,37] In addition, this method has the advantage of being a bilateral modality for heart failure assistance.

We conclude that in our animal model the synchronized LD aortopulmonary dynamic counterpulsation is an efficient method to assist cardiac failure. More experimental studies would be useful to evaluate the long-term effects of this original technique.

## References

1. Fischer EIC, Willshaw P, Armentano RL, et al: Experimental acute right ventricular failure and right ventricular assist in the dog. *J Thorac Cardiovasc Surg* 90:580, 1985.
2. Cabrera Fischer EI, Chachques JC, Garcia A, et al: Temporary mechanical circulatory support for severe cardiac failure: Experimental study. *Int J Artif Organs* 14:466, 1991.
3. World Health Organization: Chagas' disease: Report of a study group. Series 202. Geneva, World Health Organization, 1960.
4. UNDP/World Bank/WHO (PAHO): Special program for research and training in tropical disease. *VI Programme Reports,* 1981, p 1.
5. Boullon F, Sinagra A, Riarte A, et al: Experimental cardiac transplantation and chronic Chagas' disease in dogs. *Transplant Proc,* 20(Suppl 1):432, 1988.
6. Lee KF, Dignan RJ, Parmar JM, et al: Effects of dynamic cardiomyoplasty on left ventricular performance and myocardial mechanics in dilated cardiomyopathy. *J Thorac Cardiovasc Surg* 102:124, 1991.
7. Chagas ACP, Moreira LFP, da Luz PL, et al: Stimulated preconditioned skeletal muscle cardiomyoplasty: An effective means of cardiac assist. *Circulation* 80(Suppl III):III–202, 1989.

8. Jatene AD, Moreira LFP, Stolf NAG, et al: Left ventricular function changes after cardiomyoplasty in patients with dilated cardiomyopathy. *J Thorac Cardiovasc Surg* 102:132, 1991.
9. Carpentier A, Chachques JC: Myocardial substitution with a stimulated skeletal muscle: First successful clinical case. *Lancet* 8440:1267, 1985.
10. Chachques JC, Grandjean PA, Cabrera Fischer EI, et al: Dynamic aortomyoplasty to assist left ventricular failure. *Ann Thorac Surg* 49:225, 1990.
11. Chachques JC, Grandjean PA, Carpentier A: Patient management and clinical follow-up after cardiomyoplasty. *J Cardiac Surg* 6:89, 1991.
12. Hetzer R, Hennig E, Schiessler A, et al: Mechanical circulatory support and heart transplantation. *J Heart Lung Transplant* 11:S175, 1992.
13. Heck CF, Shumway SJ, Kaye MP: The Registry of International Society for Heart Transplantation: Sixth official report-1989. *J Heart Transpl* 8:271, 1989.
14. Griffith BP: Cardiopulmonary transplantation experience in Pittsburgh. Presented at the International Symposium on Cardiovascular Surgery, 1985, at the Texas Heart Institute, Houston, Texas, Sept 13, 1985.
15. Delahaye F, Jagaden O, Montagna P, et al: Latissimus dorsi cardiomyoplasty in severe congestive heart failure: The Lyon experience. *J Cardiac Surg* 6:106, 1991.
16. Kantrowitz A, McKinnon W: The experimental use of the diaphragm as an auxiliary myocardium. *Surg Forum* 9:266, 1959.
17. Pennock JL, Pierce WS, Wisman CB, et al: Survival and complications following ventricular assist pumping for cardiogenic shock. *Ann Surg* 198:469, 1983.
18. Pennington DG, Kanter KR, McBride LR, et al: Seven years' experience with the Pierce-Donachy ventricular assist device. *J Thorac Cardiovasc Surg* 96:901, 1988.
19. Pennington DG, Lawrence R, McBride LR, et al: Use of the Pierce-Donachy ventricular assist device in patients with cardiogenic shock after cardiac operations. *Ann Thorac Surg* 47:130, 1989.
20. Brugger JP, Bonandi L, Meli M, et al: SWAT team approach to ventricular assistance. *Ann Thorac Surg* 47:136, 1989.
21. Higgins RSD, Elefteriades JA: Right ventricular assist devices and the surgical treatment of right ventricular failure. *Cardiol Clin* 10:185, 1992.
22. van Trigt P, Christian O, Fagraeus L, et al: Myocardial depression by anesthetic agents (halothane, enfluorane and nitrous oxide): Quantitation based on end-systolic pressure-dimension relations. *Am J Cardiol* 53:243, 1984.
23. Buckberg GD, Fixler DE, Archie JP, et al: Experimental subendocardial ischemia in dogs with normal coronary arteries. *Circ Res* 30:67, 1972.
24. Neilson IR, Brister SJ, Kalafalla AS, et al: Left ventricular assistance in dogs using a skeletal muscle powered device for diastolic augmentation. *Heart Trans* 4:343, 1985.
25. Nichols WW, O'Rourke MF: *McDonald's Blood Flow in Arteries: Theoretical, Experimental and Clinical Principles,* third edition. Kent, Great Britain, Edward Arnold, 1990, p 337.
26. Glantz SA: *Primer of Biostatistics,* 1st ed. San Francisco, McGraw-Hill, Inc, 1987, p 287.
27. Leriche R, Fontaine R: Essai experimental de traitement de certains infarctus du myocarde et de l'aneurysme du coeur par une greffe de muscle strie. *Bull Soc Nat Chir* 9:229, 1933.
28. Mommaerts WFHM: Heart muscle. In Fishman AP, Richard DW (eds): *Circulation of the Blood.* Bethesda, MD, American Physiological Society, 1964, p 152.
29. Kantrowitz A, Kantrowitz A: Experimental augmentation of coronary flow by retardation of the arterial pressure pulse. *Surgery* 34:678, 1953.
30. Gradel F, Akutsu T, Chaptal PA, et al: Successful hemodynamic results with a new, U-shaped auxiliary ventricle. *Trans Am Soc Artif Intern Organs* 11:277, 1965.
31. Pattison CW, Cumming DVE, Williamson A, et al: Aortic counterpulsation for up to 28 days with autologous latissimus dorsi in sheep. *J Thorac Cardiovasc Surg* 102:766, 1991.
32. Kimble Jett G, Siwek LG, Picone AL, et al: Pulmonary artery balloon counterpulsation for right ventricular failure. *J Cardiovasc Surg* 86:364, 1983.

33. Spotnitz HM, Berman MA, Rels RL, et al: The effects of synchronized counterpulsation of the pulmonary artery on right ventricular hemodynamics. *J Thorac Cardiovasc Surg* 61(2):167, 1971.
34. Craig Miller D, Moreno-Cabral RJ, Stinson EB, et al: Pulmonary artery balloon counterpulsation for acute right ventricular failure. *J Thorac Cardiovasc Surg* 80:760, 1980.
35. Cabrera Fischer EI, Chachques JC, García A, et al: Effect of cardiomyoplasty on left ventricular diastolic function. *Basic Appl Myology* 1(3):253, 1991.
36. Chachques JC, Grandjean PA, Carpentier A: Dynamic aortomyoplasty. In Carpentier A, Chachques JC, Grandjean P (eds): *Cardiomyoplasty.* Bakken Research Center Series Vol 3, Mount Kisco, NY, Futura Publishing Co., 1991, p 199.
37. Bridges CR Jr, Hammond RL, Anderson DR: Skeletal muscle-powered counterpulsation: I. A critical overview. In Carpentier A, Chachques JC, Grandjean P (eds): *Cardiomyoplasty.* Bakken Research Center Series Vol 3, Mount Kisco, NY, Futura Publishing Co., 1991, p 227.

Chapter 40

# Dynamic Atriomyoplasty

Valeri S. Chekanov, Konstantin V. Shatalov

## Introduction

It is well known that the essential load in the hemodynamic correction of congenital heart diseases associated with tricuspid atresia falls on the anatomically weakly presented right atrium, which has to work with a sharply increased load after the Fontan operation. The idea of using the skeletal muscle for the correction of right atrial insufficiency is very attractive.[1–5] The muscle can be used for the augmentation of right atrial pump function in cases where a conduit is inserted between the right atrium and the pulmonary artery or the right ventricle, or when anastomosis is performed between the appendage of the right atrium and the pulmonary artery. Despite the type of operation performed, the course of the early postoperative period has its own characteristics caused by the absence of an active pumping chamber in pulmonary circulation and the increased load on the right atrium.

The clinical picture usually observed includes the signs characteristic of the right atrial insufficiency: pronounced venous hypertension, hepatomegaly, and ascites.

It seems logical to use the latissimus dorsi (LD) muscle for the improvement of right atrium pump function. But can it be used in clinical situations? If the muscle is not mobilized beforehand, it is very difficult to utilize it after the Fontan type operation has been performed.

So, the dilemma appears. Would it would be better to perform skeletal muscle mobilization before the operation? If so, why must all patients suffer this hard and long injury for muscle mobilization? If the doubts appear after the Fontan-type operation, should the patient be subjected to a new injury, i.e., the LD mobilization and atriomyoplasty during the difficult postoperative period?

The solution to the problem is the use of a diaphagmatic graft. This chapter reports the experimental results obtained with this new technique.

From Carpentier A, Chachques JC, Grandjean P: Cardiac Bioassist. © Futura Publishing Co, Inc, Armonk, NY, 1997.

## Materials and Methods

Experiments were carried out on seven mongrel dogs weighing from 16 to 32 kg. All of the surgical procedures were performed after premedication with ketamine (10–15 mg/kg). Artificial ventilation of the lungs was carried out by means of a Yeager apparatus (Germany) on moderate hyperventilation mode. The hemodynamics were monitored on the Mingograf-7 apparatus (Siemens Elema, Sweden), and an SP-2201 flowmeter (Statham-Gould, USA). Basal anesthesia was maintained by a combination of neuroleptanalgesia and a 2.5% solution of hexobarbital. All hemodynamic parameters obtained by the usual formulas were subjected to statistical analysis by the method of paired comparison of variances.

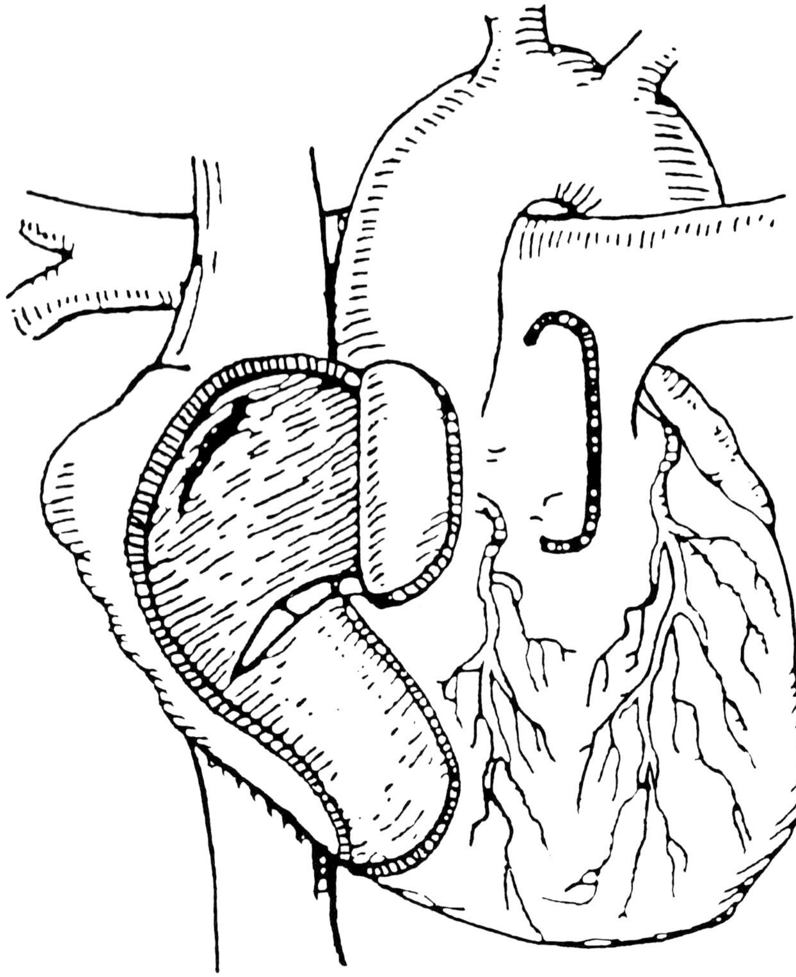

**Figure 1:** *Atriomyoplasty. Two flaps were tailored from the right atrium. The pulmonary artery is opened widely and a C-shaped graft is formed.*

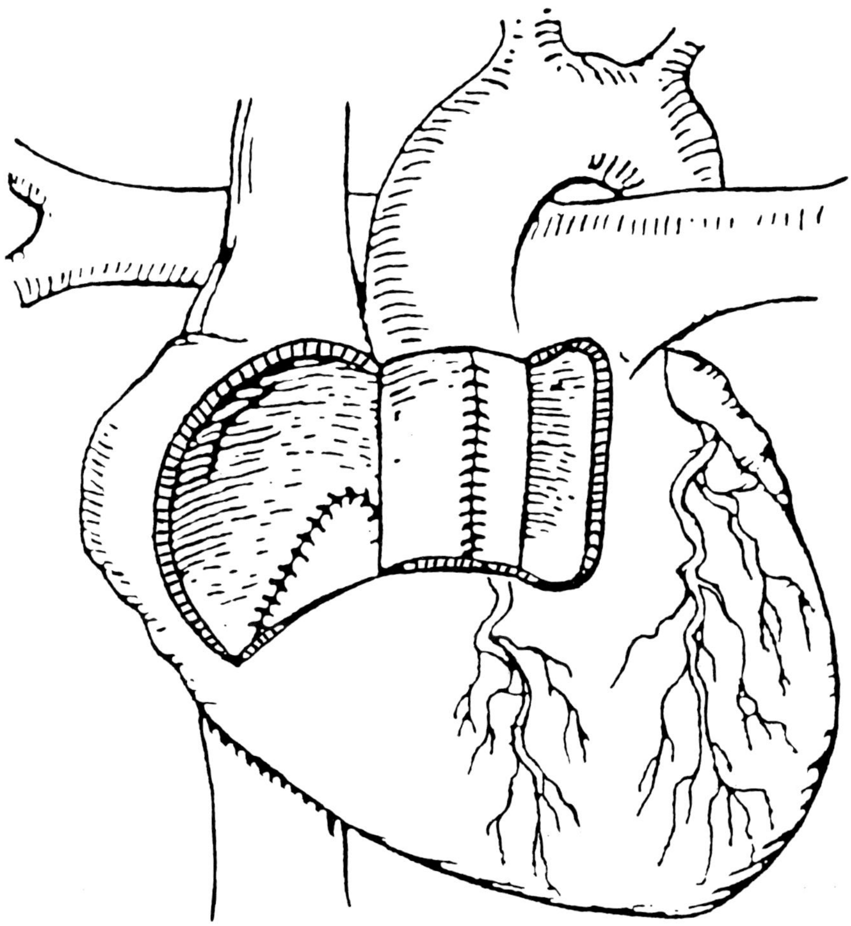

**Figure 2:** *A flap from the atrium and a flap from the pulmonary artery are sutured. The posterior wall of the new chamber is formed.*

The homogenicity of most of the data was confirmed statistically: the standard error for each experiment and for all groups as a whole did not exceed 15%. Multiprogrammed electrical stimulators of the Stiminak type, developed at the Department of Electronics of the Moscow Institute of Physical Instrumentation (I.A. Dubrovskii and A.N. Ryzhikh), were used for the investigation. The course of the operation was as follows.

Two flaps were tailored from the anterior wall and the appendage of the right atrium. The pulmonary artery was widely opened and a C-shaped graft was formed (Fig. 1). The first flap was sutured to the fibrous annulus of the tricuspid valve. As a result, the right ventricle was completely isolated from the pulmonary circulation. After that, we sutured a flap from the atrium and a flap from the pulmonary artery. The posterior wall of the future "new" chamber was formed (Fig. 2). We then tailored a flap from the diaphragm. A piece of pericardium was sutured to the flap. The purpose of this cusp was to

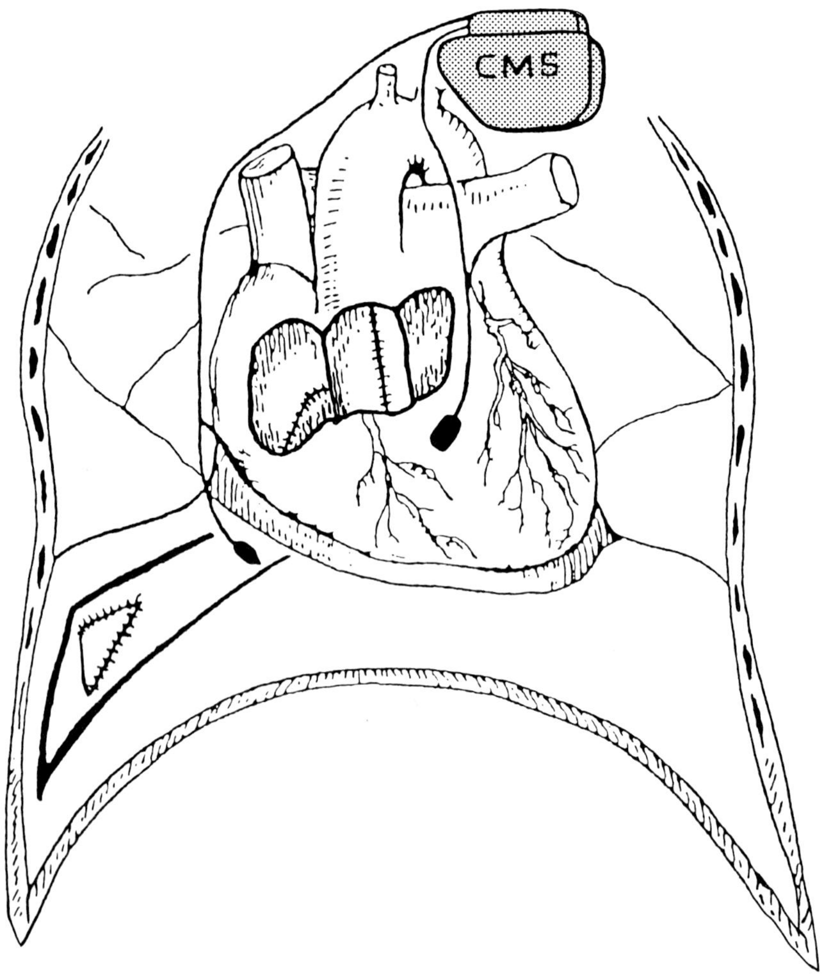


**Figure 3:** *A piece of pericardium is sutured to the flap of diaphragm to prevent blood return from the pulmonary artery into the new chamber.*

prevent blood return from the pulmonary artery into the new chamber (Figs. 3 and 4). Next, the electrodes were connected to the original neurostimulator. A stimulator was used to realize cardioshynchronized stimulation of the diaphragm muscular flap by a burst of impulses with programmed voltage parameters from 3 to 9 V, pulse frequency in the burst from 10 to 100 Hz, impulse duration from 0.1 to 1.8.

## Results

Immediately after the operation, there were signs of right heart failure (Fig. 5). Maximal pressure in the new chamber decreased (15–17 mm Hg) and minimal pressure increased (13–16 mm Hg). The pressure in the arterial

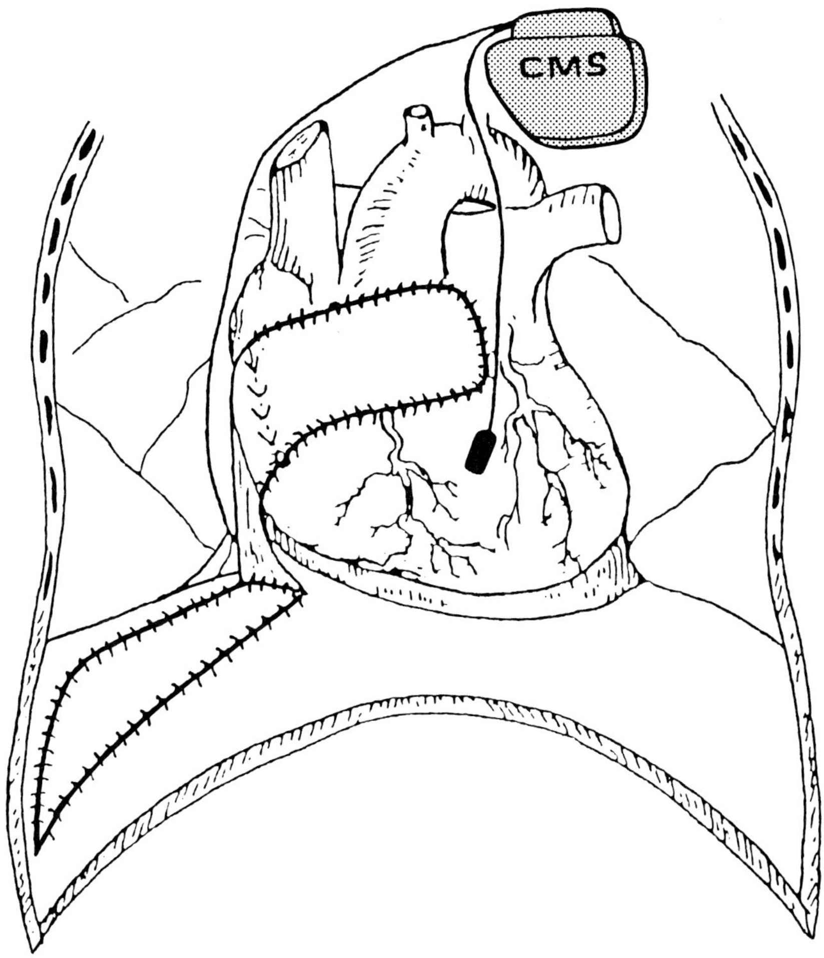


**Figure 4:** *The stimulator and electrodes are connected to the heart and to the flap of the diaphragm.*

system (55–70 mm Hg) and pulmonary artery (14–17 mm Hg) decreased. There was elevated pressure in the interior vena cava (13–16 mm Hg). Cardiac output was sharply reduced (1–2 L/min). All calculated coefficients were unsatisfactory after the operation (Fig. 6). Dp/dt maximum and minimum were sharply decreased (88–98 and 77–87 mm Hg/sec, respectively). Right heart pump coefficient (0.8–1.5 $cm^5$/din sec $M^2$) and right heart power (0.10–0.13 WT/$M^2$) confirmed total inadequacy of the right heart. There was critical right heart insufficiency and the nonviability of the heart was clearly evident.

When we started stimulation, the picture changed. The maximal pressure in the right neoatrium, mean pulmonary pressure, and mean arterial pressure were increased. Pressures in the new chamber and inferior vena cava were reduced. Cardiac output was 3.5–4.0 L/min during the six postoperative hours. Right heart pump coefficient and power also increased 2.5–3.0 times.

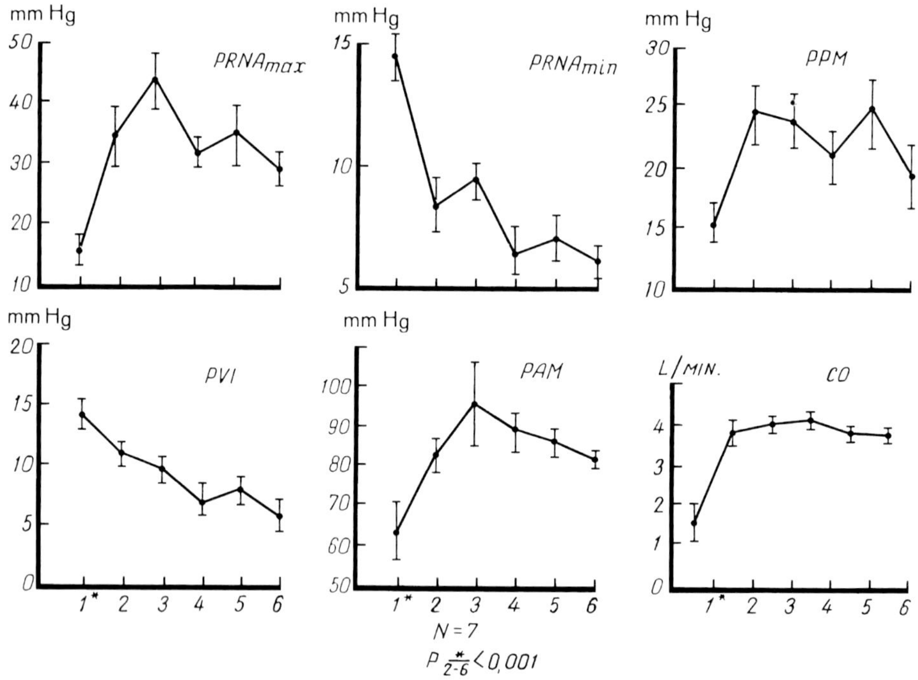


**Figure 5:** *Hemodynamic data 1 hour before operation, and 2, 3, 4, 5, and 6 hours after operation.*

They remained relatively stable during the entire experiment. The indices of contractility increased at first (dp/dt max up to 300 mm Hg/sec and dp/dt min up to 195 mm Hg/sec) but then decreased due to muscle fatigue.

## Discussion

Tricuspid atresia was created in dogs by closing the tricuspid orifice. Pulmonary flow was maintained by a tunnel between the right atrium and the pulmonary artery. To maximize the work of the right atrium we used an electrostimulated flap of diaphragm. The graft was included into the right atrial wall.

Why was the diaphragmatic graft chosen? Its isolation and mobilization after the Fontan operation takes only a few minutes. It doesn't increase the injury created by the operation in general. Anatomically the diaphragm is the most convenient muscle for the application on the right heart. The diaphragm surface is much smoother than any other skeletal muscle's surface, which is very important for thrombogenic prophylactic.

As a result of the performed work, we are able to substantiate hemodynamically the possibility of the use of dynamic atriomyoplasty.[6] We can now recommend this method for the support of atrial work during the first, and most difficult, days after the Fontan operation.

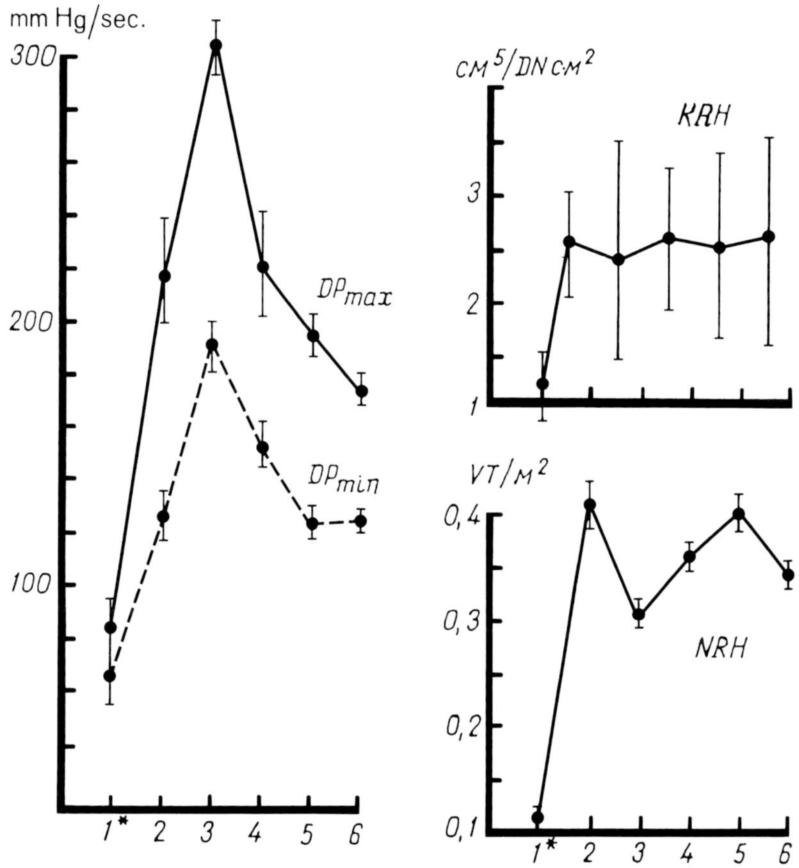


**Figure 6:** *Hemodynamic data 1 hour before and 2, 3, 4, 5, and 6 hours after operation.*

## References


1. Loulmet D, Comtois A, Hollman C, et al: Application of cardiomyoplasty to the Fontan operation: Hemodynamic observations. In Chiu RCJ, Bourgeois IM (eds): *Transformed Muscle for Cardiac Assist and Repair.* Mount Kisco NY, Futura Publishing Co., 1990, pp 247–251.
2. Chachques JC, Grandjean PA, Pfeffer TA, et al: Cardiac assistance by atrial or ventricular cardiomyoplasty. *J Heart Transplant* 9:239, 1990.
3. Loulmet D, Carpentier A, Beaudet RL: Atriomyoplasty in the Fontan procedure. In Carpentier A, Chachques JC, Grandjean P (eds): *Cardiomyoplasty.* Mount Kisco, NY, Futura Publishing Co, 1991, pp 195–198.
4. Chekanov VS, Shatalov KV, Tolmachev MV, et al: Dynamics of atriomyoplasty as a method expanding the possibilities of Fontan's principle in surgical treatment of complex congenital heart disease (experimental study). *J Grudnaja Serdechno-Sosudistaja Chirurgia* 4:11–15, 1991.
5. Krakovsky AA, Chekanov VS: Cardiomyoplasty in Fontan operation. Abstract, 3rd annual meeting of The European Association for Cardiothoracic Surgery, 1989, p 130 (October 9–11, 1989, Munich, FRG).
6. Shatalov KV, Chekanov VS, Dubrovsky IA: Dynamic atriomyoplasty: How do we try to modernize the Fontan's principle? *J Cardiovasc Surg* 32 (Suppl 4):23, 1991.

Chapter 40

# *Discussion*

**Dr. Chachques:** I have only one question regarding your presentation. Why did you choose the diaphragm instead of the LD? In sick patients, taking a part of the diaphragm may lead to severe respiratory insufficiency and may be a most important injury.

**Dr. Chekanov:** You must make a decision, of course, of which one seems to be the best choice: the LD muscle or the diaphragm.

**Dr. Stephenson:** We have published a number of papers, many years ago, reporting on the use of the diaphragm on the right side. Did you stimulate the diaphragm directly or did you stimulate it using the nerve? What we found is that when you stimulated it directly, we get only a small amount of the diaphragm to contract, whereas when we stimulated the nerve we got the entire muscle to contract but we then had some problems with the pedicle blood supply.

**Dr. Chekanov:** We stimulated the diaphragm directly and we did not try to find the nerve. We put an electrode on the pedicle of the flap and when we changed the bursts of the pulse and changed the duration of bursts and voltage, we had good contraction of the flap, but not for a long time. After 5 hours, we did not use a 1:1 mode because the diaphragm fatigued very quickly. We used a contraction ratio of 1:6 or 1:8 and we gave the diaphragm time to rest. In the last experiment, we used an interrupted stimulation to the diaphragm. We stimulated the flap for 10 minutes and rested it for 5 minutes. This increased the working time.

**Sir Magdi Yacoub:** My question relates to the blood supply of the flap. Unlike the LD, the diaphragm has separate neurological and arterial supplies. Would you like comment on how the pedicle had its own blood supply?

**Dr. Chekanov:** We did not study the blood supply of the flap, but in some experiments, we noted that when we took a very big flap, a flap from the periphery, we had quicker fatigue, perhaps due to vascularization problems.

**Dr. Chachques:** In one of your slides, you stated that the diaphragm is less thrombogenic than other muscles. Do you have any data to support that?

**Dr. Chekanov:** No.

From Carpentier A, Chachques JC, Grandjean P: Cardiac Bioassist. © Futura Publishing Co, Inc, Armonk, NY, 1997.

# Part V

## Skeletal Muscle Ventricles

Chapter 41

# Functional Assessment of Skeletal Muscle Ventricle

Hiroshi Niinami, Timothy L. Hooper, Larry W. Stephenson*

## Introduction

Skeletal muscle has been configured in the shape of a pumping chamber by many investigators worldwide to augment the circulation. We refer to these pumps as skeletal muscle ventricles (SMVs). They are constructed from latissimus dorsi (LD) muscle. Similar to the natural heart, this configuration allows translation of linear work into pressure-volume work. SMVs have been evaluated in vitro and in vivo.[1–8] Their potential for left and right ventricular assist has been demonstrated with continued long-term function in vivo up to 27 months in the systemic circulation,[7] and for 4 months in the pulmonary circulation.[8]

To date, SMVs have been evaluated in an extrathoracic position, situated on the chest wall. This approach has proved convenient and also facilitates assessment of SMV function. It is also possible that the vascular supply from the subcutaneous tissue is a good collateral source for the SMVs. However, for SMVs to be applied clinically, it is likely that they will have to be placed within the thoracic cavity. The purpose of the present study was to investigate whether SMV function was influenced by the thoracic position. Furthermore, this study was also undertaken to assess both systolic and diastolic functional characteristics of intrathoracic SMVs and the relationship of these parameters to alterations in muscle stimulation patterns.

## Materials and Methods

SMVs were constructed from the right LD muscle in 10 mongrel dogs weighing between 14 and 21 kg. The care of the animals and procedures in this study complied with the *Principles of Laboratory Animal Care* and the *Guide for the*

*With the cooperation of Robert L. Hammond, Hiroyuki Suga, Hitoshi Koyanagi.

Supported by National Institutes of Health Grant HLBI-34778.

*Care and Use of Laboratory Animals* prepared by the National Academy of Sciences (NIH publication No. 55-23, revised 1985). Anesthesia was induced with intravenous thiamylal (15 mg/kg) and maintained by inhalation of isoflurane (1–2%). Antibiotic prophylaxis was administered, with intravenous cefazolin (1 g) preoperatively, and oral cephalexin (60 mg/kg/day) postoperatively for 10 days. Pain was controlled with parenteral buprenorphine (0.02–0.04 mg/kg).

## Construction of SMV

SMVs were constructed in a manner previously described.[1–4] Briefly, the LD muscle was mobilized completely, apart from its neurovascular pedicle, and wrapped spirally around a tapered mandrel. Mandrel volume was approximately 50 mL. A modified monopolar cuff electrode was placed around the thoracodorsal nerve for subsequent muscle stimulation. A neurostimulator (Model 7421, Medtronic Inc.) was connected to the nerve lead and implanted under the rectus abdominis muscle.

In group A (n=5), SMVs were placed extrathoracically on the chest wall. In group B (n=5), SMVs were placed within the thoracic cavity, following partial resection of the third rib. In both groups, SMVs were left undisturbed to stabilize the vascular integrity for 3 weeks (vascular delay period).[9]

After this delay period, the stimulator was activated to deliver 2 Hz continuous stimulation. The individual pulses were of 210 μsec duration and 2 V amplitude. Stimulation was continued for 6 weeks in order to transform the muscle to a fatigue-resistant form.[10]

## Mock Circulation System

In a second procedure, animals were anesthetized as previously described. The mouth of the SMV was exposed either through an axillary skin incision (group A) or via a median sternotomy (group B), the mandrel removed, and the SMV connected to a mock circulation device. This mock circulation system has been previously described in detail[3,4,6] and is illustrated in Figure 1. Two 5F microtransducer-tipped catheters (Millar Instruments, Inc., Houston, TX) were inserted within the device in order to record preload, afterload, and SMV generating pressures. In group B, a custom-made, 7F 10-electrode conductance catheter (Webster Laboratories, Baldwin Park, CA)[11] was inserted into the SMV to obtain pressure-volume loops of the SMV.

By infusing normal saline into the SMV bladder, using an infusion pump (Model 944, Harvard Apparatus, South Natick, MA), preload was gradually increased at a set rate.

Stroke volume and stroke work were calculated by the derived analytical solution.[6]

## Measurements

Femoral arterial pressure was monitored by a percutaneous catheter connected to a fluid-filled transducer during the measurement and main pulmonary

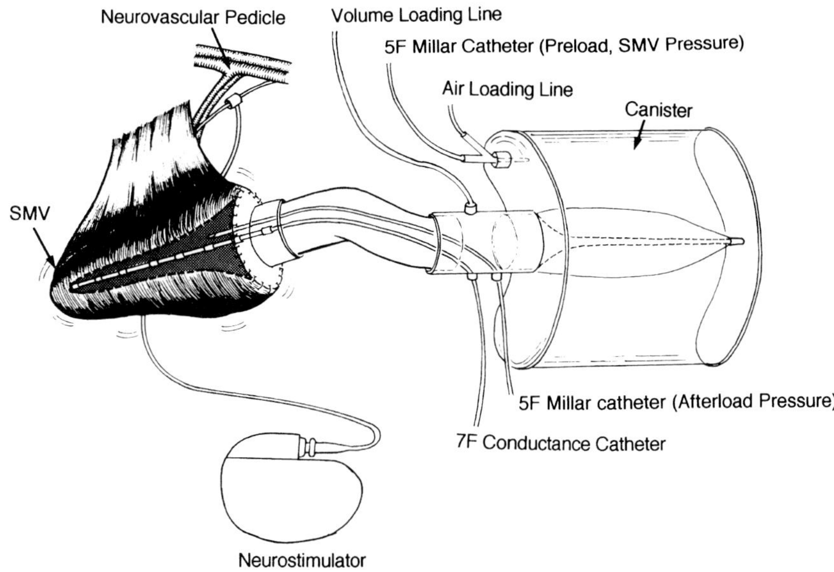


**Figure 1:** *Diagram of mock circulation device showing position of conductance catheter and pressure monitoring lines. SMV end-diastole and end-systole are shown. Afterload is adjusted by injecting air into the rigid cannister, and preload is increased by infusing saline into the closed SMV system.*

artery pressure was measured before the measurement. A 16-mm ultrasonic flow probe (Transonic Systems Inc., Ithaca, NY) was placed around the ascending aorta to measure stroke volume of the left ventricle and cardiac output.

The SMV stimulation parameters were as follows: duty cycle = 310 ms ON, 1.5 sec OFF; voltage = 3 V; pulse width = 210 μsec. Burst stimulation frequency was 25 Hz. SMV preload was increased gradually from 0 to 25 mm Hg at an afterload of 30 mm Hg, to approximate normal right ventricular loading conditions, and 0 to 45 mm Hg at an afterload of 80 mm Hg, to mimic systemic load. Developed pressure was recorded continuously during SMV contractions.

The relationship between SMV pouch pressure and infused volume was recorded during controlled infusion of 0 to 14 mL of normal saline.

Furthermore, in group B, SMV systolic function and diastolic function were analyzed using a volume conductance catheter system. The neurostimulator provided 25 Hz or 85 Hz burst stimuli of 310 ms duration, with a duty cycle of 1,500 ms. The single pulse duration was 210 μsec. The slope of the end-systolic pressure-volume relation (ESPVR), $E_{max}$,[12] was calculated by linear regression of the end-systolic pressure-volume points obtained during volume loading the SMV.

Each measurement took about 20 sec, and between measurements, the SMV was allowed to rest for 5 minutes.

The stroke work of both ventricles was calculated as left ventricular (LV) stroke volume and mean systemic or pulmonary arterial pressure.

### Statistical Analysis

All data given represent mean values ± standard error (±SEM). Statistical comparisons using the paired Student *t* test and multiple analysis of variance were performed using RS-1 statistical software (Bolt Beranek and Newman Inc., Cambridge, MA) and SPSS-PC statistical software (NORUSIS/SPSS Inc., Chicago, IL) on a portable computer (T3200SX, Toshiba, Irvine, CA).

Statistical significance was set at the 5% level throughout the analysis.

### Results

## Comparison of Intrathoracic Versus Extrathoracic SMVs

Dogs in group B with the SMV inside the hemithorax did not exhibit signs of respiratory problems at any time. The two groups did not differ significantly with respect to body weight or mean mandrel volume. The stroke work of the canine right and left ventricles were $0.22 \pm 0.02 \times 10^6$ ergs and $0.81 \pm 0.07 \times 10^6$ ergs, respectively.

Comparative SMV stroke work for the two groups as a function of preload pressure are shown in Figure 2. The respective values for left ventricular and right ventricular (RV) stroke work are also depicted.

At an afterload of 30 mm Hg, SMVs in group B developed greater stroke work at all preloads than those in group A (Fig. 2A) at this afterload ($p < 0.005$). At a preload of 10 mm Hg, the mean stroke work of SMVs in group B was $0.65 \pm 0.06 \times 10^6$ ergs, which was 295% of that of the native RV, compared with $0.21 \pm 0.05 \times 10^6$ ergs in group A.

At an afterload of 80 mm Hg, those SMVs in group B also developed higher stroke work than those in group A (Fig. 2B). These observations reached statistical significance at physiological preloads (5 and 10 mm Hg) ($p<0.05$). At a preload of 10 mm Hg, SMV stroke work was $0.57 \pm 0.14 \times 10^6$ ergs in group B, which was 70% of that of the native LV, and $0.12 \pm 0.04 \times 10^6$ ergs in group A.

Passive diastolic filling curves are given in Figure 3. SMVs in group A were less compliant than those in group B. The differences between groups A and B were statistically significant ($p<0.01$).

## Analysis of Intrathoracic SMVs by Pressure-Volume Curve

Typical pressure-volume loops from one of the SMVs are depicted in Figure 4. End-systolic pressure-volume relation (ESPVR) shifted leftward by increasing burst frequencies as summarized in Figure 5. $E_{max}$, which represents the contractility of the SMV, was $3.44 \pm 0.61$ and $3.45 \pm 0.62$ mm Hg/mL with burst frequencies of 25 Hz and 85 Hz, respectively. These numbers were not statistically different. However, EDPVR was lowered by increasing the burst frequency as summarized graphically in Figure 6. The changes were statistically significant ($p<0.05$). Raising burst frequency resulted in increasing the compliance of the SMVs.

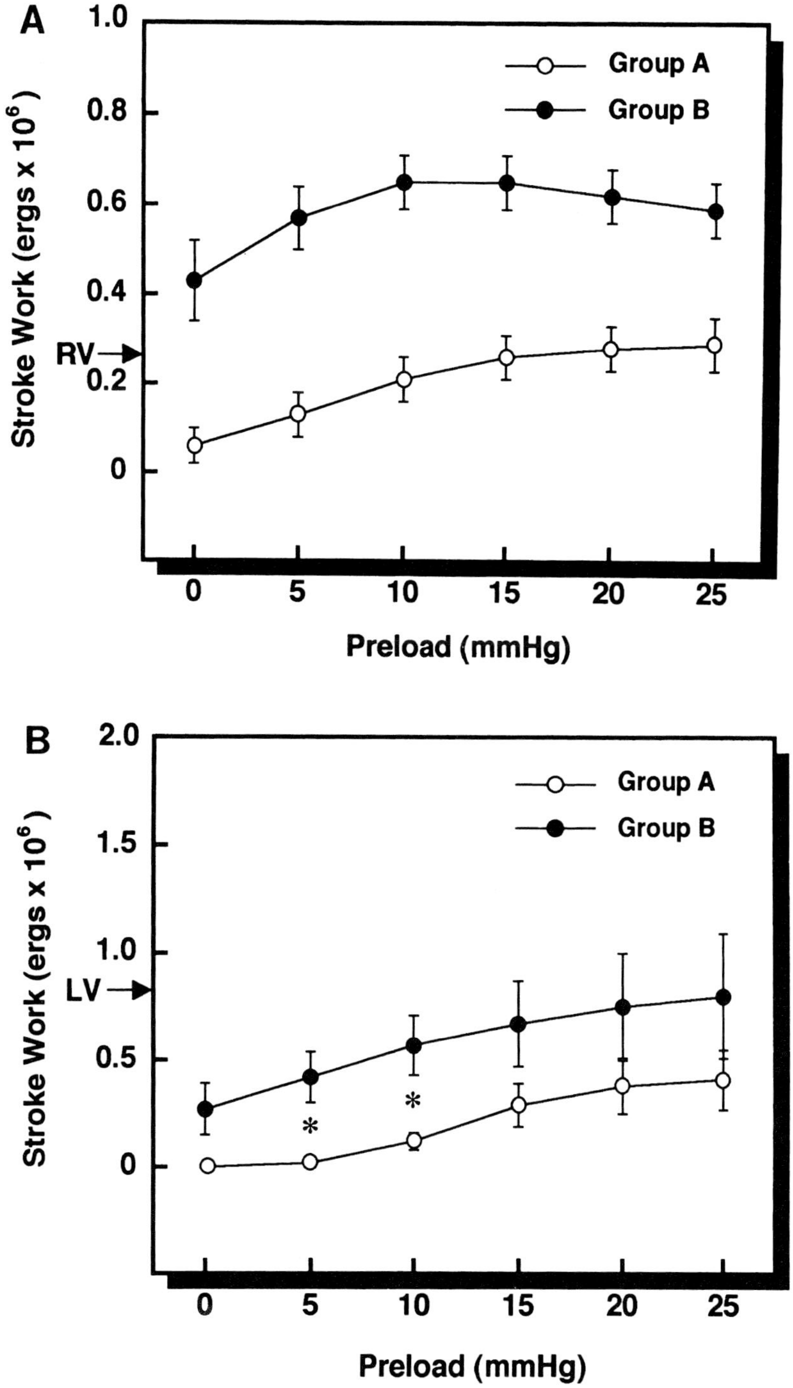


**Figure 2:** *(**A**) Stroke work is plotted versus preload for two groups at the afterload of 30 mm Hg and (**B**) 80 mm Hg. Normal canine right ventricular (RV) and left ventricular (LV) stroke works are shown for comparison. Asterisks indicate statistical difference* ($p < 0.05$).

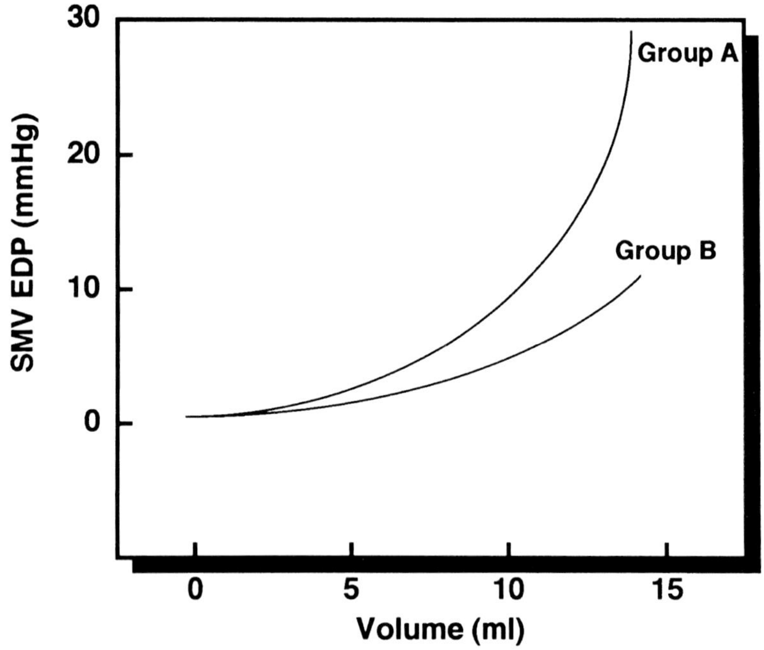


**Figure 3:** *Passive diastolic pressure-volume curves during controlled volume infusion are shown for SMVs in both groups.*

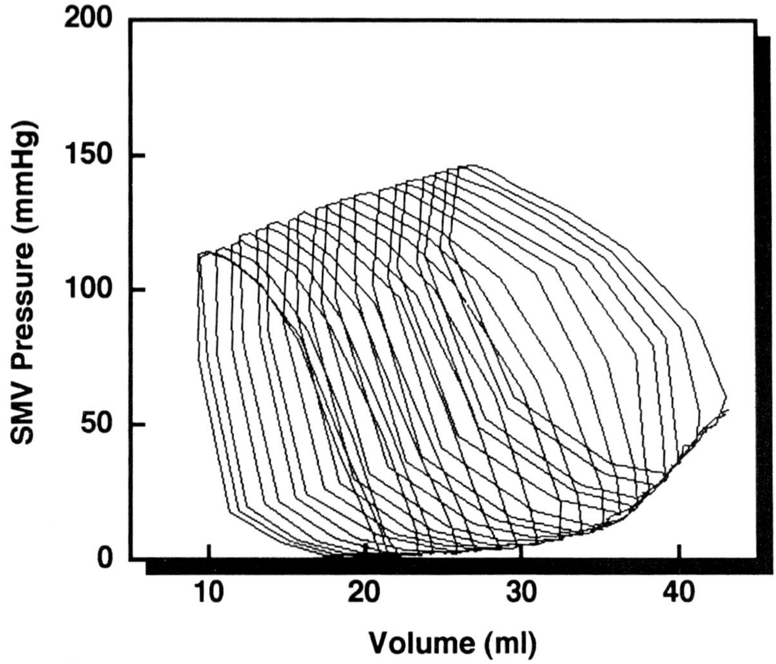


**Figure 4:** *Typical pressure-volume loops tracing obtained from one dog.*

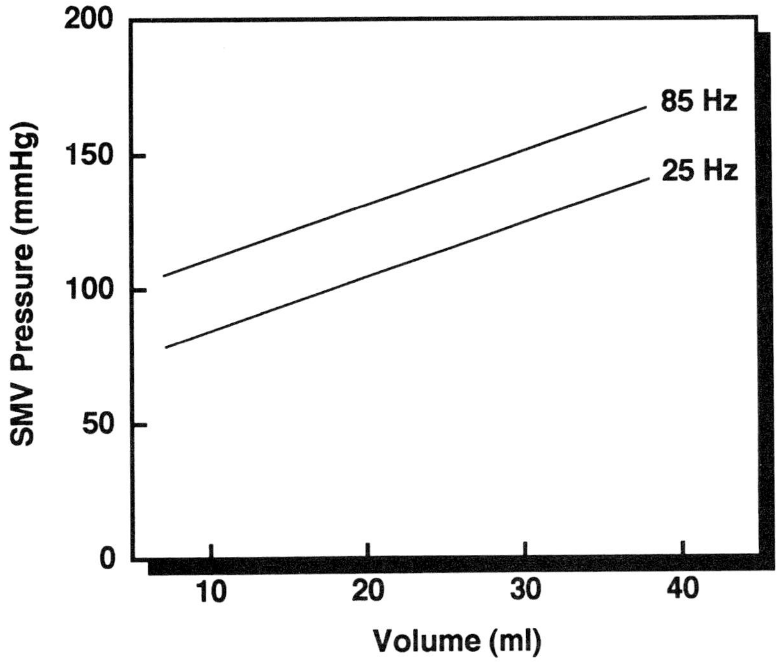


**Figure 5:** *End-systolic pressure-volume relation (ESPVR) during controlled volume infusion are shown for SMVs in two different stimulation frequencies.*

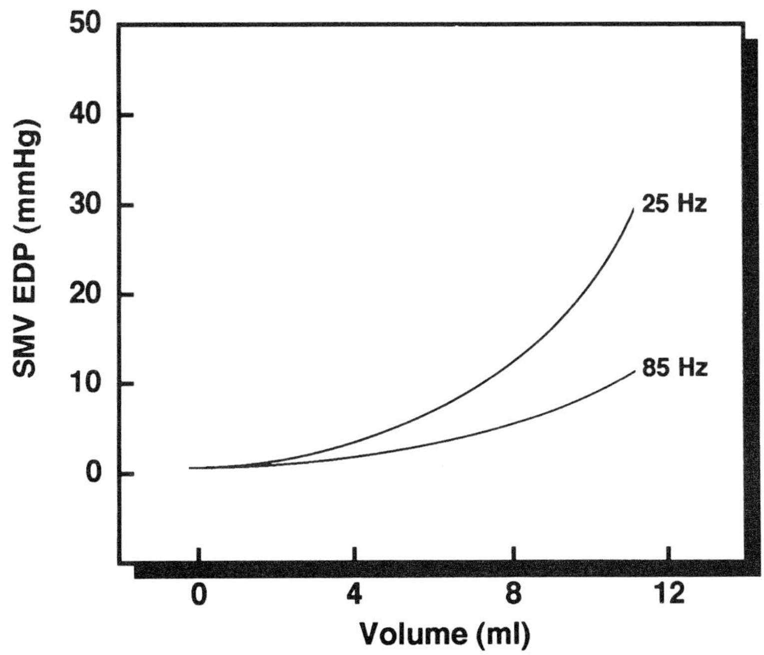


**Figure 6:** *End-diastolic pressure-volume relation (EDPVR) during controlled volume infusion are shown for SMVs in two different stimulation frequencies.*

## Discussion

Ventricles constructed from canine LD muscle have been considered less compliant than those of the heart.[13,14] Consequently, SMVs have required high preloads to achieve optimal performance. Therefore, their previous application in circulation has been mainly to function as aortic diastolic counterpulsators, in which arterial pressure provides the preload.[1,2,7]

To some extent, the diastolic function of SMVs has improved because of attention to certain aspects of SMV design.[6] However, the influence of SMV positioning on subsequent function has received little attention. An extrathoracic situation might be expected to effectively increase SMV wall thickness, since it may be anticipated that the elastic properties of the subcutaneous tissues could adversely interact with diastolic function. This concept appears to be supported by the findings of the present study, which demonstrate better compliance of SMVs placed within the thoracic cavity. An additional advantage of an intrathoracic position is that the SMV is protected from external trauma, and much shorter vascular conduits are required for connection to the circulation. In addition, this could improve the hemodynamic performance of SMVs in circulation by reducing the influence of pressure gradients along the conduits. It is tempting to speculate that in a closed chest model negative intrathoracic pressure may further enhance SMV filling.

However, the reason for superior systolic function of intrathoracic SMVs is unclear. This may relate to the influence on the vascular integrity of the SMV wall. During the vascular delay period, it might be possible that collateral development into the SMV occurs more readily inside the thoracic cavity than it does in the subcutaneous tissues.

In terms of the SMV stroke work, intrathoracic SMVs are capable of performing the work necessary to provide significant left ventricular assist or to effectively supplant right ventricular function, working at the afterloads and preloads of the left and right ventricles, respectively.

Furthermore, in this study, we estimated systolic and diastolic function of the intrathoracic SMV using pressure-volume relationship. The SMV contractility in terms of $E_{max}$ did not change by altering the burst frequency. This means that the effect of raising burst stimulation frequency on the SMV might be different from that of inotropic agents on myocardium. Maximum contractile velocity of skeletal muscle depends on the burst stimulation intensity.[3] Skeletal muscle contractility reflects the intensity of the active state of the muscle. Unlike the heart, which is an electrical and mechanical syncytium, skeletal muscle is modulated by the number and rate at which fibers are activated.[15] It has been demonstrated by Dewar and associates[16] as well as by our group[1] that a single electrical stimulus resulting in a single muscle twitch does not generate enough power to assist the heart. However, rapid repetitive stimuli delivered before the muscle fiber completes its relaxation results in mechanical summation (until fusion occurs), which thereby causes the muscle to generate substantial power.[17] The burst stimulation frequency of the SMV governs the cumulative duration of the active state of the skeletal muscle and was expected to produce an effect similar to contractility of the heart. Increasing the burst frequency of the SMV produces more work.

Curiously, the compliance of SMVs was altered by changing the burst frequency. Increasing burst frequency results in raising the power of muscle relaxation. Skeletal muscle produces work, not only during the contracting period, but also during the relaxation period. This may explain why cardiomyoplasty has been observed to lower the left ventricular end-diastolic pressure during muscle relaxation.[18,19] To obtain sufficient power from skeletal muscle for cardiac assist in terms of the muscle stimulation pattern, a burst of stimuli is better than a single stimulus.[20] When using burst stimulation, skeletal muscle works not only during the contracting period but also during the relaxation period phase of the cycle.

## Summary

This study indicates that both systolic and diastolic function of an SMV is superior with the intrathoracic position when compared to the extrathoracic position. It also suggests that intrathoracic conditioned SMVs from canine LD muscle have pressure-volume characteristics that are similar to the left ventricle and are appropriate for the assist of systemic or pulmonary circulation under physiological conditions. Furthermore, this study exhibits some significant contractile aspects of skeletal muscle that are dissimilar to the heart. These findings should be considered when proposing the use of skeletal muscle for cardiac assist.

## References

1. Mannion JD, Hammond RL, Stephenson LW: Hydraulic pouches of canine latissimus dorsi: Potential for left ventricular assistance. *J Thorac Cardiovasc Surg* 91:534, 1986.
2. Mannion JD, Acker MA, Hammond RL, et al: Power output of skeletal muscle ventricles in circulation: Short-term studies. *Circulation* 76:155, 1987.
3. Acker MA, Hammond RL, Mannion JD, et al: An autologous biologic pump motor. *J Thorac Cardiovasc Surg* 92:733, 1986.
4. Acker MA, Hammond RL, Mannion JD, et al: Skeletal muscle as a potential power source for a cardiovascular pump: Assessment in vivo. *Science* 236:324, 1987.
5. Bridges CR, Hammond RL, Dimeo F, et al: Functional right-heart replacement with skeletal muscle ventricles. *Circulation* 80(Suppl III):III–183, 1989.
6. Bridges CR, Brown WE, Hammond RL, et al: Skeletal muscle ventricles: Improved performance at physiologic preloads. *Surgery* 106:275, 1989.
7. Ruggiero R, Niinami H, Pochettino A, et al: Skeletal muscle ventricles: Update after 18 months in circulation. Artif Organs 15(5):350, 1991.
8. Niinami H, Hooper TL, Hammond RL, et al: Skeletal muscle ventricles in the pulmonary circulation: Up to 16 weeks' experience. *Ann Thorac Surg* 53;750, 1992.
9. Mannion JD, Velchik MA, Acker MA, et al: Transmural blood flow of multilayered latissimus dorsi skeletal muscle ventricles during circulatory assistance. *Trans Am Soc Artif Intern Organs* 32:454, 1986.
10. Mannion JD, Bitto T, Hammond RL, et al: Histochemical and fatigue characteristics of conditioned canine latissimus dorsi muscle. *Circ Res* 58:298, 1986.
11. Baan J, Van der Velde ET, De Bruin HG, et al: Continuous measurement of left ventricular volume in animals and humans by conductance catheter. *Circulation* 70:812, 1984.
12. Suga H, Sagawa K, Shoukas AA: Load independence of the instantaneous pressure-volume ratio of the canine left ventricle and effects of epinephrine and heart rate on the ratio. *Circ Res* 32:314, 1973.

13. Diamond G, Forrester JS, Hargis J: Diastolic pressure-volume relationship in the canine left ventricle. *Circ Res* 29:267, 1971.
14. Spotnitz WD, Spotnitz HM, Truccone NJ: Relation of ultrastructure and function: Sarcomere dimensions, pressure-volume curves, and geometry of the intact left ventricle of the immature canine heart. *Circ Res* 44:679, 1979.
15. Johnson E: Force-interval relationship of cardiac muscle. In Berne RM (ed): *Handbook of Physiology*. Bethesda, MD, American Physiological Society, 1979, p 475.
16. Dewar ML, Drinkwater DC, Wittnich C, et al: Synchronously stimulated skeletal muscle graft for myocardial repair. *J Thorac Cardiovasc Surg* 87:325, 1984.
17. Carson FD, Wilkie DR: *Muscle physiology*. Englewood, NJ, Prentice-Hall, 1974, p 33.
18. Niinami H, Pochettino A, Ruggiero R, et al: Canine latissimus dorsi cardio-double myoplasty: Acute feasibility study. *J Cardiac Surg* 6(Suppl):124–131, 1991.
19. Lee KF, Dignan RJ, Parmar JM, et al: Effects of dynamic cardiomyoplasty on left ventricular performance and myocardial mechanics in dilated cardiomyopathy. *J Thorac Cardiovasc Surg* 102:124, 1991.
20. Grandjean PA: Electrical stimulation of skeletal muscle. In A Carpentier, JC Chachques, PA Grandjean (eds): *Cardiomyoplasty*. Mount Kisco, NY. Futura Publishing Co, 1991, pp 39–62.

Chapter 42

# Dynamic Training for Skeletal Muscle and Its Potential for Cardiac Assist

Norbert W. Guldner, Harald C. Eichstaedt, Peter Klapproth*

## Introduction

Skeletal muscle can be used for cardiac assistance by electrically stimulating it over a period of several weeks. It will then be able to do chronic work with no resulting fatigue. This procedure, however, results in an 80% loss of muscle power and reductions of 60% in muscle mass and 75% in contractile speed.[1–3] The aim of this study was to evaluate a method to train skeletal muscle ventricles that would minimize these disadvantages. Also discussed are the possibilities of using dynamically trained skeletal muscle as skeletal muscle ventricles and a tube cardiomyoplasty for cardiac assistance.

## Material and Methods

Eleven Jersey calves weighing between 61 and 116 kg were used in the study. In all 11 calves, intrathoracic muscle tubes were constructed from the latissimus dorsi (LD) muscle. Nine muscle tubes were dynamically trained as skeletal muscle ventricles (SMVs) and two muscle tubes were used to do anatomical and acute functional studies as a tube cardiomyoplasty.

The SMVs were electrically stimulated during dynamic training using a myostimulator (Medtronic model 7420 and Telectronics model 7220) and electrodes (Medtronic model SP5528 and Telectronics model IML-2). A specially designed training device was used for the elastic training, along with an integrated pressure transducer and a PC.[4] The training device consisted of a noncompliable,

*With the cooperation of Maurice H.J. Tilmanns, Sylvain G. Thuaudet, Bruno J. Messmer, and Peter Bardos

From Carpentier A, Chachques JC, Grandjean P: Cardiac Bioassist. 

central pumping chamber and two very elastic side bladders, which were made of silicone and filled with liquid (Fig. 1).

The left LD muscle was dissected under general anesthesia. The lateral sides of the muscle were folded medially and fixed to a muscle tube, which in turn was wrapped around the central chamber of the training device (Fig. 1), with intrathoracic implantation.

The pressure inside the training device was measured during the contraction of the SMV. It was possible to calculate from these pressure curves the volume of fluid that shifted from the central chamber to the elastic side bladders. From the recorded pressure wave, knowing the time to maximal contraction and the corresponding peak pressure, it was possible to calculate the applied maximal power.[5]

Contractile speed was calculated by dividing the difference in maximal circumference of the central chamber during an SMV contraction by the time of maximum contraction (Table 1).

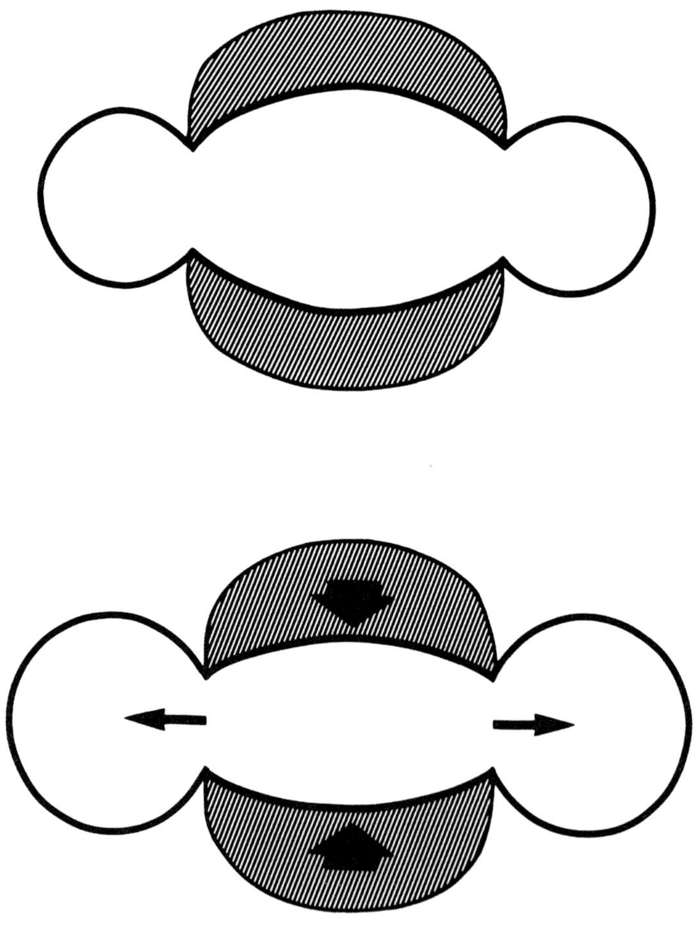

**Figure 1:** *A latissimus dorsi muscle is intrathoracally wrapped around a silicone training device, which consists of a pumping chamber and two elastic side bladders. During dynamic training, the SMV pumps fluid from the central chamber into the elastic side bladders.*

**Table 1**
End-Stage Training Data of Dynamic Trained SMVs

| Calf No. | Stroke Volume (mL) | Contractile Way (mm) | Dynamic Contractile Time (ms) | Contractile Speed [mm/sec] | Power [Watt] |
|---|---|---|---|---|---|
| 6 | 84 | 89.4 | 125 | 715 | 6.8 |
| 7 | 58 | 64.8 | 133 | 481 | 9.6 |
| 9 | 42 | 50.7 | 158 | 321 | 4.9 |
| 3 | 38 | 47.6 | 133 | 358 | 3.1 |
| 5 | 27 | 39.4 | 142 | 277 | 3.9 |
| 8 | 26 | 38.7 | 138 | 280 | 1.5 |
| 4 | 21 | 35.1 | 150 | 234 | 1.3 |
| 2 | – | – | – | – | – |
| 1 | – | – | – | – | – |

SMV = skeletal muscle ventricle.

Dynamic training was performed in two steps. First, a frequency training was done. The rate of muscle contraction was gradually increased from one to around 60 per minute over 3 months. Second, the afterload was increased up to the level of the diastolic pressure.[6] The electrical stimulation, begun intraoperatively, was in pulse trains of 500 ms, frequency of 32 Hz, pulse width of 250 μsec, and an amplitude ranging between 3.0 and 10.5 V.

A tube cardiomyoplasty (Fig. 2D) using the LD muscle was done using the same muscular tube as used in constructing the SMVs (Fig. 2C). The muscular tube muscle was extended by a vascular Dacron bifurcation prosthesis with a diameter of 30 mm (Meadox Mediccus Inc., Oakland, NY). The bifurcation prosthesis was connected with the distal end of the muscle tube and fixed with the 10 mm arms to the pericardium (Fig. 2D) in such a smooth manner that it did not constrict the heart. By stimulating the muscle in heart systole, the musculo-prosthetic wrap compressed the heart. Peripheral blood pressure was measured in the carotid artery.

## Results

The surgical procedure of constructing the SMVs in the nine calves and the tube cardiomyoplasties in the two calves were well tolerated. The first two SMVs failed when a vascular delay was applied. The dynamic training was successfully carried out in the remaining seven calves with SMVs positioned around training devices having no vascular delay. In calf no. 7, however, the training device burst on the 59th day of training after a systolic pressure of 342 mm Hg was measured.

During dynamic training, the systolic pressure in the training device increased up to and above systemic levels between 140 and 340 mm Hg. In calf no. 6, for example, stroke volume increased during training from 20 mL to 84 mL. The maximum output for this calf into the device's side bladders was around 5 L/min. The contractile speed after training varied between 234 and 715 mm/sec (Fig. 3). The power developed by the SMVs varied considerably, from 1.3 to 9.3 Watts due to the quality of training and complications, such as

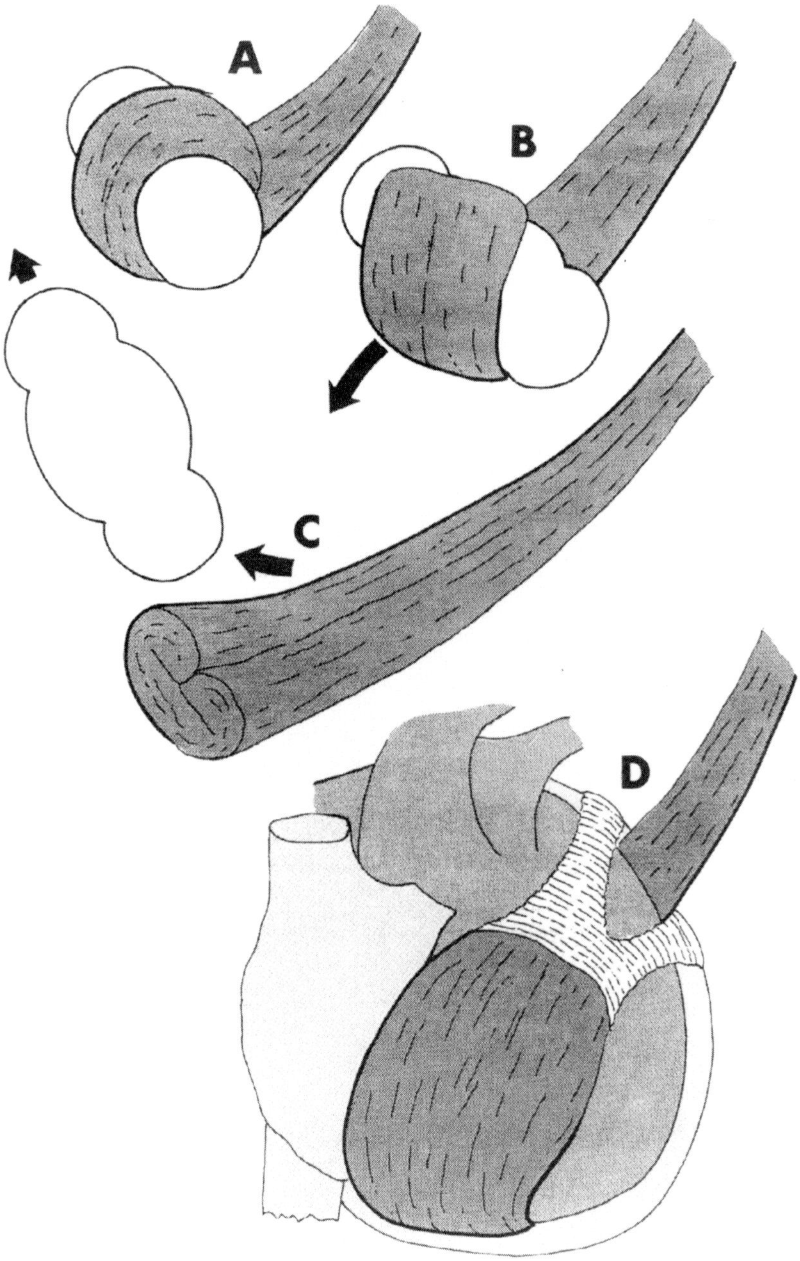


**Figure 2:** *(**A**) Dynamic training of a muscular tube in a skeletal muscle configuration. (**B**) Unwrapping the muscular tube after the training. (**C**) Removal of the training device. (**D**) Performing a tube cardiomyoplasty by help of prosthetic Dacron material and fixation to the left pericardium.*

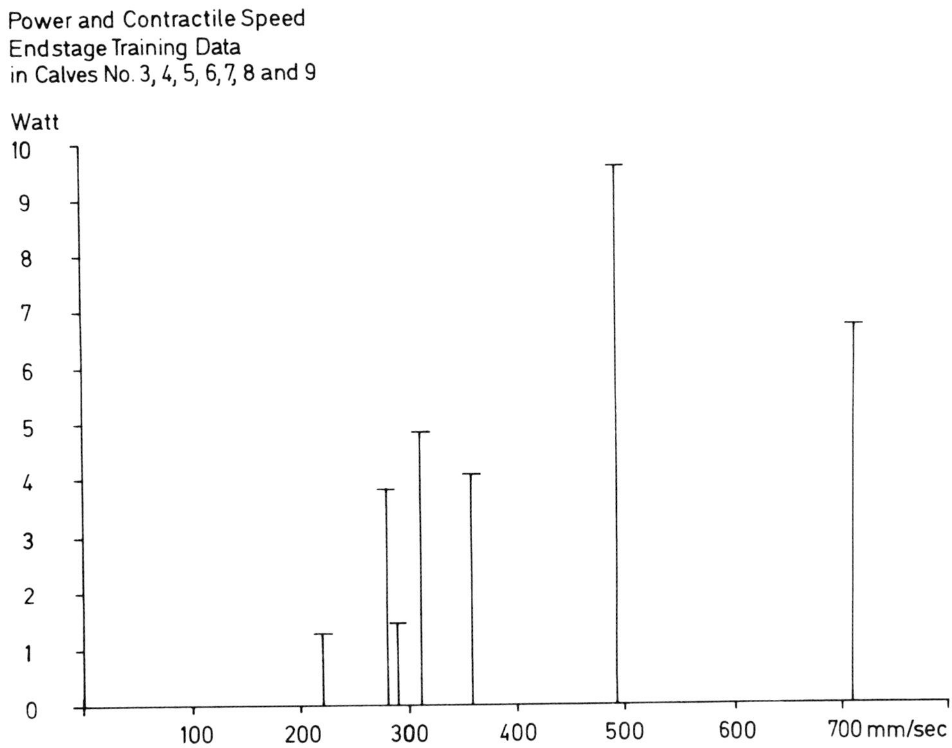


**Figure 3:** *Dynamic training of the skeletal muscle ventricles preserves contractile speed and power.*

electrode fractures in calves no. 4 and 8. In comparison, the maximum power produced by a left human heart ventricle is around 3 Watts and the "average power" is around 1.3 Watts.[7] (The calculations in SMVs presented here correspond to the maximal power results.)

The diameter of the untrained contralateral LD muscle in calf no. 3 was 9 mm compared to 20 mm for the dynamically trained muscle. For calf no. 6, it was 9 mm compared to 28 mm, and for calf no. 9, 14 mm compared to 32 mm.

There were no operative difficulties while constructing the tube cardiomyoplasty prolonged with a vascular bifurcation prosthesis. Burst stimulation to the heart (one synchronous stimulation every six beats) raised the systolic pressure in the carotid artery by about 25–30 mm Hg, from around 105 mm Hg to approximately 105–135 mm Hg in that acute study.

## Discussion

Other clinical trials done using autologous skeletal muscle for cardiac assistance have never used dynamic training.[8–36] They found that electrical conditioning changed a quickly fatigued skeletal muscle into one that was fatigue-resistant but with many disadvantages. There was an 80% loss in power, muscle mass decreased by 60%, and contractile speed decreased by more than 75%.[2,3] If these results are applied to an earlier cardiomyoplasty study,[17] the muscle mass from the LD muscle decreases from 600 g to 275 g and the contractile speed from 500–700 mm/sec to around 50 mm/sec. From the large size of a diseased heart, it is apparent that it cannot develop enough force to have a hemodynamic effect for clinical assistance (Laplace's law). Consequently, it was necessary to develop a method that preserves the contractile speed, power, and muscle mass.

The high power produced following dynamic training (up to 10 W) (Fig. 4) can be explained by the power-velocity relationship, as described by Salmons and Jarvis.[2] High power can be achieved by preserving contractile speed, within certain limits (Fig. 3). Furthermore, the increase in power can be explained morphologically. The largest increase in the thickness of the muscle wall in dynamically trained SMV was found in calf no. 6. It was three times thicker than that of the contralateral side. (The SMV of calf no. 7 could not be examined.)

Four dynamically trained SMVs in circulation represent a small experience. In the atrio-aortic configuration, the SMV contracted like a sphincter and failed. In order to function, the SMV requires an elastic inlay with a rebound force to contain the end-diastolic volume. The first aorto-aortic integrated SMV ruptured on the 16th postoperative day due to the absence of a prosthetic in-

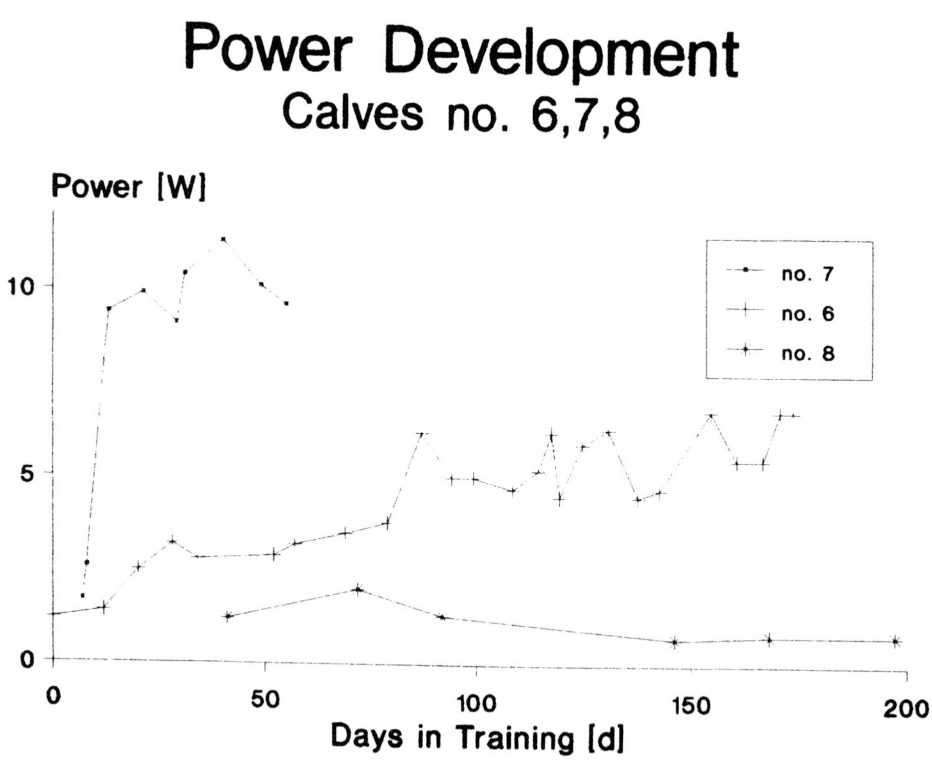


**Figure 4:** *Examples of the different levels of power developed by calves during dynamic training. The SMV of calf no. 7 developed the highest level of power. Its electrodes were placed close to branches of the* nervus thoracodorsalis. *Calf no. 6 developed sufficient power during frequency and afterload training. In calf no. 8, a peripheral electrode fractured, resulting in a low power production.*

lay. Consequently, an inlay was used in the other two SMVs, one of which continued pumping for more than 12 months.

In a study carried out on dogs using the aorto-aortic configuration, approximately 20–25% of left ventricular output was obtained.[12] In acute studies using an apico-aortic configuration done over 3 hours in one dog and over 10

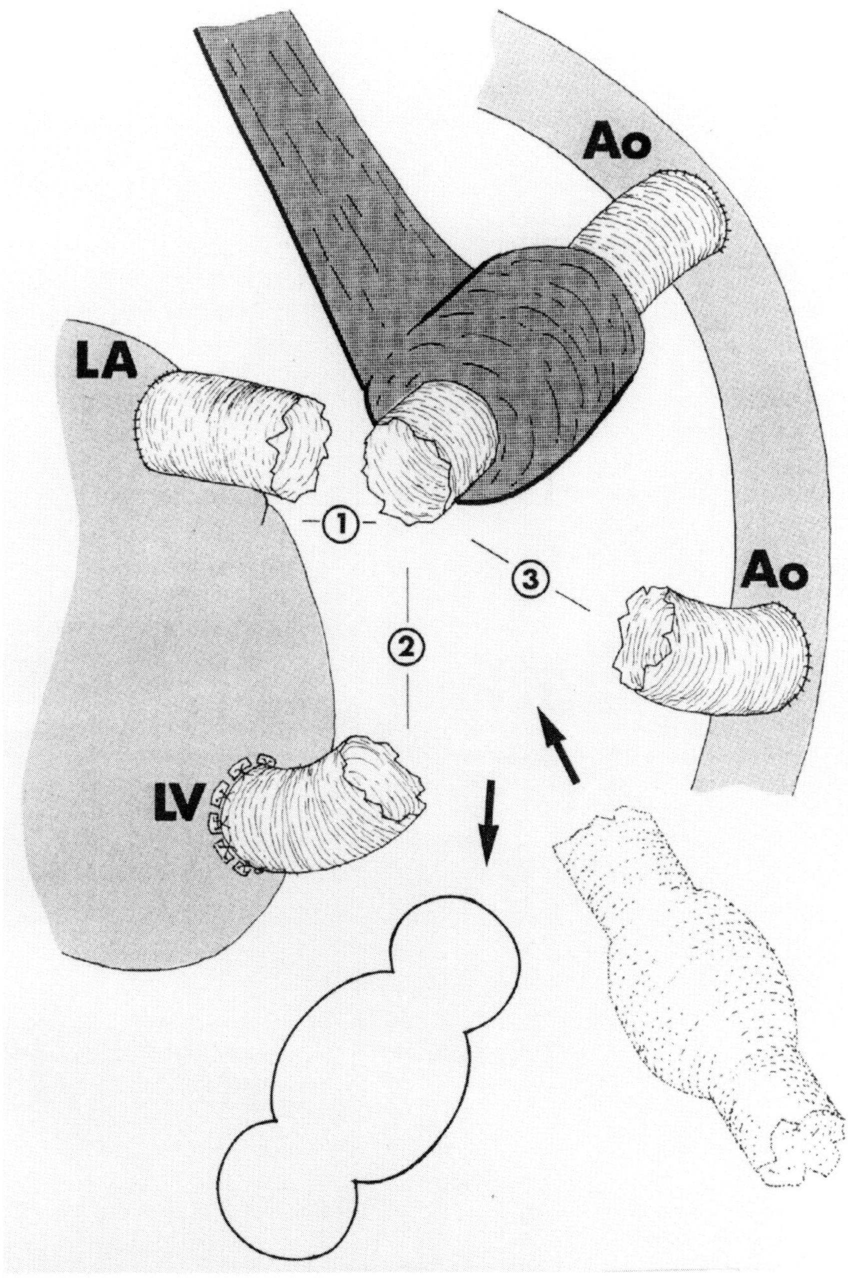


**Figure 5:** *Three different possibilities to integrate a dynamic trained SMV into circulation to assist a failing left heart: 1. atrio-aortal, 2. apico-aortal, 3. aorto-aortal.*

hours in another dog, the left ventricular output was measured at between 40% and 50%.[30] In this present study, power and output data were measured only in the training device and not in the circulation. Even taking into account a large loss of power when integrating the system into the circulation, the dynamically trained SMV is still a powerful, promising technique. Dynamically trained SMVs can be integrated into the circulation as a left heart support, atrio-aortic, aorto-aortic, and apico-aortic (Fig. 5) and as a right heart support in an atrio-pulmonary configuration.

The two experimental tube cardiomyoplasties demonstrate a possible surgical procedure (Fig. 2). They show that in an acute stimulation, systolic peripheral blood pressure could be increased by 25–30 mm Hg. It is assumed that an unfatigued and dynamically trained muscle tube (Fig. 2) could have a potential hemodynamic effect. Muscle-powered assist devices should also benefit from dynamic training.

The dynamic training of skeletal muscles preserves contractile speed and muscular power and increases muscle mass. It is an effective method for autologous cardiac assistance, such as SMVs, cardiomyoplasty, and muscle-powered cardiac assist devices.

## References


1. Guelinckx PJ, Faulkner JA, Essig DA: Neurovascular anastomoses muscle grafts in rabbits: Functional deficits results from tendon repair. *Musc Nerve* 11:745–751, 1988.
2. Salmons S, Jarvis JC: Cardiomyoplasty: The basic issues. *Cardiac Chron* 4:1–7, 1990.
3. Salmons S, Jarvis JC: Cardiac assistance from skeletal muscle: A critical appraisal of the various approaches. *Br Heart J* 68:333–338, 1992.
4. Ruck K, Guldner NW, Tilmans MHJ, et al: The FROG, a device for training intrathoracal skeletal muscle ventricles. *Int J Org* 14:9, 1991.
5. Klapproth P, Tilmanns MHJ, Guldner NW, et al: Fundamentals and development of a computer-programmed evaluation method for performance data assessment of SMVs in training. *Int J Art Org* 14:19, 1991.
6. Guldner NW, Tilmanns MHJ, Klapproth P, et al: Dynamic training of skeletal muscle ventricles. A method to create high performance for muscle powered cardiac assist. 4th Vienna International Workshop on Functional Electrostimulation. Baden/Vienna, September 24–27, 1992.
7. Hurst JW (ed): *The Heart, Arteries and Veins.* New York, McGraw-Hill, 4th ed., 1987, p. 76.
8. Acker MA, Hammond RL, Mannion JD, et al: An autologous biologic pump motor. *J Thorac Cardiovasc Surg* 92:733–746, 1986.
9. Acker MA, Anderson RL, Hammond RL, et al: Skeletal muscle ventricles in circulation: One to eleven weeks' experience. *J Thorac Cardiovasc Surg* 94:163–174, 1987.
10. Anderson DR, Pochettino A, Hammond RL, et al: Autogenously lined skeletal muscle ventricles in circulation: Up to nine months' experience. *J Thorac Cardiovasc Surg* 101:661–670, 1991.
11. Anderson DR, Pochettino A, Hammond RL, et al: Skeletal muscle ventricles in circulation as aortic counterpulsators: Twelve months' update. *J Thorac Cardiovasc Surg* 5:199–203, 1990.
12. Bridges CR, Hammond RL, Anderson DR: Skeletal muscle-powered counterpulsation. In: Carpentier A, Chachques JC, Grandjean P (eds): *Cardiomyoplasty.* Mount Kisco, NY, Futura Publishing Company, 1991, p 233.

13. Carpentier A, Chachques JC, Grandjean P: *Cardiomyoplasty* Mount Kisco, NY, Futura Publishing Company, 1991, 105–122.
14. Carpentier A, Chachques JC, Grandjean PA: Transformation d'un muscle squelettique par stimulation séquentielle progressive en vue de son utilisation comme substitut myocardique. *Cr Acad SC Paris* 301:581, 1985.
15. Carpentier A, Chachques JC: Myocardial substitution with a stimulated skeletal muscle: first successful clinical case. *Lancet* 8440:1267, 1985.
16. Carpentier A, Chachques JC, Grandjean PA: *Cardiomyoplasty.* Mount Kisco, NY, Futura Publishing Company, 1991, p 233.
17. Chachques JC, Carpentier A: Long-term survival and quality-of-life after cardiomyoplasty. *Eur JC PE* 2:197, 1992.
18. Chachques JC, Grandjean PA, Schwartz K, et al: Effects of latissimus dorsi dynamic cardiomyoplasty on ventricular function. *Circulation* 78(Suppl 3): 203, 1988.
19. Chachques JC, Grandjean PA, Carpentier A: Dynamic aortomyoplasty. In: *Cardiomyoplasty,* Mount Kisco, NY, Futura Publishing Company, 1991, 766–773.
20. Chachques JC, Grandjean PA, Serraf A, et al: Atrial cardiomyoplasty after Fontan-type procedure. *Circulation* 82(Suppl IV):183–189, 1990.
21. Chiu RCJ: *Biomechanical Cardiac Assist: Cardiomyoplasty and Muscle-Powered Devices.* Mount Kisco, NY, Futura Publishing Company, 1986.
22. Chiu RCJ, Walsh GL, Dewar ML, et al: Implantable extra-aortic ballon assist powered by transformed fatigue resistant skeletal muscle. *J Thorac Cardiovasc Surg* 94:694, 1987.
23. Chiu RCJ, Bourgeois IM: *Transformed Muscle for Cardiac Assist and Repair.* Mount Kisco, NY, Futura Publishing Company, 1990.
24. Christlieb IY, MacGovern JA, Furnary AP, et al: Considerations on six years of cardiomyoplasty. *Eur JC PE* 2:198, 1992.
25. Desroisiers C, Neilson J, Walsh G, et al: Skeletal muscle-powered counterpulsator. In: Chiu RCJ, Bourgeois IM (eds): *Transformed Muscle for Cardiac Assist and Repair.* Mount Kisco, NY, Futura Publishing Company, 1990, pp 321–327.
26. Grandjean PA, Austin L, Chan BS: Dynamic cardiomyoplasty: Clinical follow-up results. *J Cardiac Surg* 6:80–88, 1991.
27. Guldner NW, Tilmans MHJ, Dehaan H, et al: Development and training of skeletal muscle ventricle with low preload. *J Cardiac Surg* 6:118, 1991.
28. Guldner NW, Tilmans MHJ, Klapproth P, et al: Un ventricule intrathoracique en muscle squelettique: Résultats préliminaires. *J Cardiol* 3:(6) 253–257, 1991.
29. Guldner NW, Tilmans MHJ, Bardos P: Hartinsufficiëntie: Nieuwe perspectieven op heelkundig gebied. *Tijdschrift voor Cardiologie* 4:8, 1992.
30. Huiping LU, Fietsam R jr, Hammond RL, et al: Skeletal muscle ventricles: Left ventricular apex to aorta configuration. *Ann Thorac Surg* 55:78–85, 1993.
31. Mannion JD, Hammond RL, Stephenson LW: Hydraulic pouches of canine latissimus dorsi. Potential for left ventricular assistance. *J Thorac Cardiovasc Surg* 91:534–544, 1986.
32. Moreira LFP, Stolf NAG, et al: Late results of cardiomyoplasty in the treatment of severe cardiomyopathies. *Eur JC PE* 2:198, 1992.
33. Moreira LFP, Stolf NAG, Bocchi EA, et al: Latissimus dorsi cardiomyoplasty in the treatment of patients with dilated cardiomyopathy. *Circulation* 82(Suppl 4):257, 1990.
34. Patisson MB, Cumming DVE, Williamson A, et al: Aortic counterpulsation for up to 28 days with autologous latissimus dorsi in sheep. *J Thorac Surg* 102:766–773, 1991.
35. Pochettino A, Anderson DR, Hammond RL, et al: Skeletal muscle ventricles: A promising treatment for heart failure. *J Cardiac Surg* 1(Suppl):145–153, 1991.
36. Pochettino A, Mocek FW, Lu H, Hammond RL, et al: Skeletal muscle ventricles with improved thromboresistance: 28 weeks in circulation. *Ann Thorac Surg* 53:1025–1032, 1992.

# Chapter 42

# *Discussion*

**Dr. Salmons:** You are doing this investigation in the calf, which is a rapidly growing animal. How many of the changes that you are seeing are due to the normal growth of the animal?

**Dr. Guldner:** It is a weak point to use a growing animal and I realize that. In the future, we should use an adult goat because the reaction of a growing muscle is quite different from the reaction of an adult muscle. While there is an effect of that growth, one cannot explain this increase in muscle mass by this consideration alone.

**Sir Magdi Yacoub:** May I ask you about the model? You said you can alter afterload. When you alter volume, that surely will alter the preload. How can you alter resistance to filling, which is the afterload?

**Dr. Guldner:** With this silicone model, there is a silicone tube outside with a port with which we can add volume. One can increase the pressure in the bladder and then, by inducing a contraction, there is a pressure in the silicone device, perhaps from 10 to 20 to 30 to 40 to 80 up to the diastolic pressure in the aorta. That is our afterload.

**Sir Magdi Yacoub:** You would really need to have a resistance to filling rather than stretching.

**Dr. Guldner:** We do not have it.

**Dr. Jarvis:** We saw some drafts of power output against time. Can you tell me whether you use the same test bursts of stimulation to obtain the power measurements at those various times?

**Dr. Guldner:** We had a burst frequency of about 32 and we had an ontime of 500 ms. That is very long and we took this because we thought that if we had an ontime of 500 ms, we would have another effect of isometric training because we wanted to increase muscle mass.

**Dr. Stephenson:** I just want to reemphasize Dr. Salmon's point. Over the last 6 or 7 years, we have published several papers on dynamic training and we have

From Carpentier A, Chachques JC, Grandjean P: Cardiac Bioassist. © Futura Publishing Co, Inc, Armonk, NY, 1997.

used elastic devices, polyurethane devices, etc. Your results are superior to ours. I think that you have to separate out the growing animals as a variable.

**Dr. Guldner:** You had a mock circulation with an elastic resistance. But in the beginning of your training, the afterload was very high, and I know from your paper the afterload was about 40, 50, and 80 mm Hg from the beginning and that is the point. If you start with an afterload of zero, you have a high contractile speed and then you can start your dynamic training. But if you begin with an afterload of 60 or 80, you don't get this effect.

Chapter 43

# New Efficient Computer Model of Cardiovascular Dynamics

K. Peczalski, A. Peczalski, R.M. Bolman III

## Introduction

Computer modeling of the blood circulation system has existed since the beginning of electronic computer technology. The equivalence between the blood flow and the electrical current was quickly recognized and applied first to the analog computer by Noordegraaf,[1] then to hardware fluid models by Reeve,[2] and finally to an electronic hardware model of the blood circulation system by Babbs.[3]

In this chapter we discuss the operation of the SPICE simulator and the methods to extract the model parameters from experimental and/or clinical data.

## Simulator

The blood circulation system is modeled as an electrical network. Each artery or vein is represented by a combination of resistor, capacitor, and inductor; the heart muscles are simulated with voltage sources and the valves are emulated by diodes (Figs. 1 and 2). The behavior of a common node of two or more branches is expressed by the continuity and telegraph equations. Thus, the circulation system model is reduced to a system of differential equations that need to be solved simultaneously in a time domain. The number of discrete components can be large if high resolution of the model is required. A typical model of the circulation system includes 43 nodes and 86 elements, which translates to a system of 129 differential equations. The boundary conditions are selected by the initial values of blood flow and pressure at each node of the model. For instance, for a circulation model of a healthy adult human (weight 70 kg), the values of pressures were estimated: (a) 128/5 mm Hg for the left ventricle, (b) 120/70 mm Hg for the aorta, (c) 24/2 mm Hg for the right ventricle, (d) 20/14 for the pulmonary artery, and cardiac output (CO) was estimated for 5 L/min. We found that the differential equation can be solved by existing electrical engineering soft-

From Carpentier A, Chachques JC, Grandjean P: Cardiac Bioassist. © Futura Publishing Co, Inc, Armonk, NY, 1997.

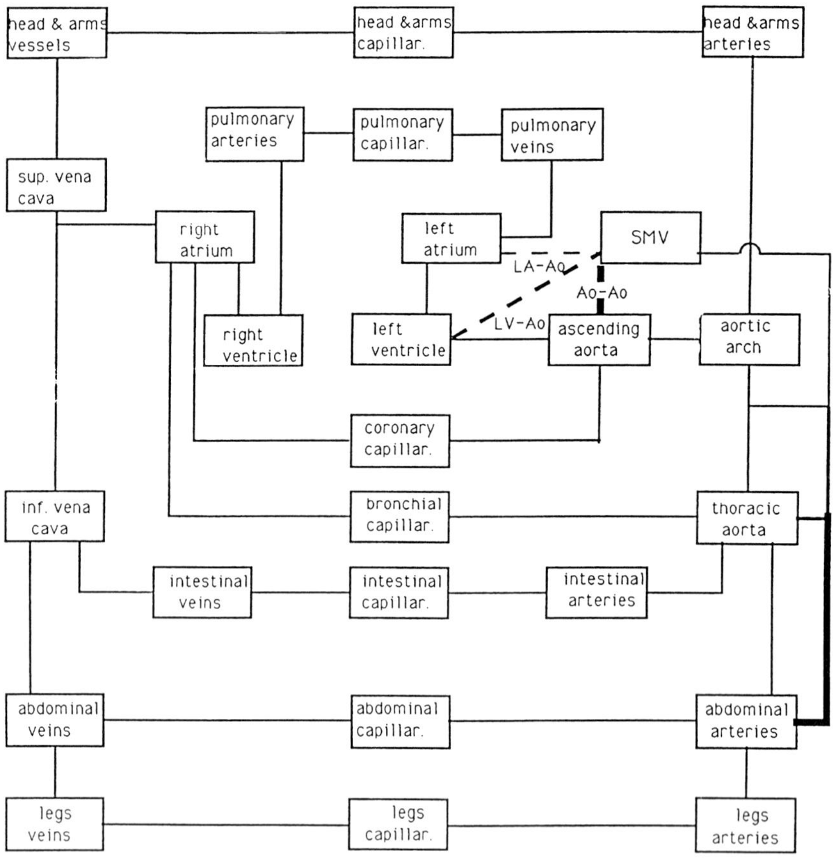


**Figure 1:** *Diagram of cardiovascular circulation.*

ware packages, e.g., SPICE. The SPICE electrical circuit simulator also offers an efficient way of modeling the muscle action (voltage source) and valve (diode) as well as an assist device. As shown above, the number of discrete components can be large if high resolution of the model is required. SPICE can simulate a network with hundreds of nodes. SPICE was first reported in 1973 by Nagel[4] and was fully documented in 1975 by Nagel.[5] SPICE is a digital computer program that simulates the electrical performance of electronic circuits and will determine the quiescent operating point of the circuit or the small signal frequency domain response of the circuit. SPICE contains models for the common circuit components and is capable of simulating most electronic circuits. The original SPICE program consisted of approximately 10,000 FORTRAN IV and COMPASS statements and was then reprogrammed in more efficient C language.

In the model applied in our SMV study, the following parameters were used: (a) elastic properties of the vessels, (b) viscous properties of the vessel walls, (c) viscous properties of blood, (d) inertial properties of blood, (e) dynamic activity chambers of the heart, (f) arteriovenous resistance capillaries, (g) total volume of the blood. The calculation of parameters of circulation elements was done by applying the following equations (used for resistance): $R = \frac{8 \eta l}{\Pi r^2}$, where $\eta$ is

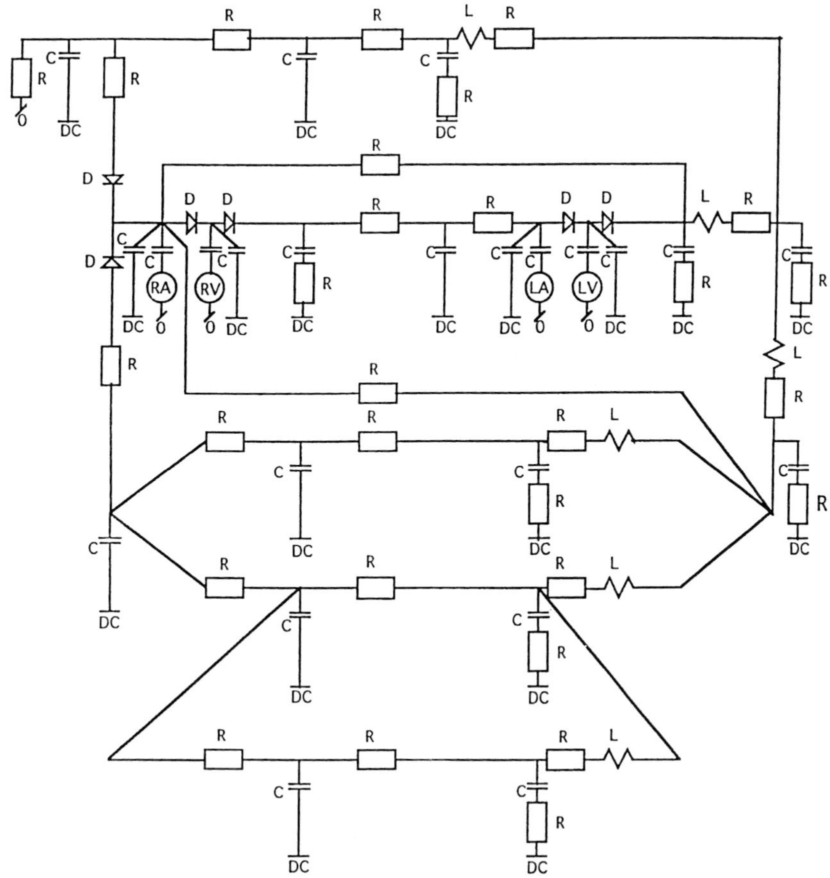


**Figure 2:** *Electric equivalent of cardiovascular circulation. R = resistance; C = compliance; L = inertance; D = diode; DC = voltage source of DC; RV = voltage source for modeling of right ventricle; LV = voltage source for modeling of left ventricle; RA = voltage source for modeling of right atrium; LA = voltage source for modeling of left atrium; 0 = electrical zero.*

viscosity of the blood, l is length of the segment, and r is radius of the segment. These calculated values were transferred to electrical values with the equation: 1 mm Hg/L/min = 1 kΩ. Similarly, the inertance is given as $L = \frac{\rho\, l}{\Pi r^2}$ where ρ is blood density, l is length of the segment, and r is radius of the segment and compliance is $C = \frac{2\Pi r^3}{E\, o\, l}$, where E is wall elasticity modulus, o is width of the wall, l is length of the segment, r is radius of the segment, with the conversion factors $\frac{1\ \text{mL}}{\text{mm Hg}}$ = 60 mF (farad) and $\frac{1\text{g}}{\text{cm4}}$ = 12.59 H (henry) for compliance and inertance, respectively. For completeness, the conversion factor for pressure differences was 1mm Hg = 0.1 V and for blood flow 1 L/min. = 0.1 mA. These values are mutually consistent and applicable to real-time frequency of operation (i.e., 60 cycles/min).

## Simulation of Human Circulation System

In order to demonstrate the predictive and advisory power of the model, we have simulated the hemodynamics of the circulation system in a healthy human and in a circulation system with a congenital defect with and without SMV.

The models of recumbent adults were designed on the basis of the following data (pressures in mm Hg): left ventricle pressure 118, left atrium pressure 7, right ventricle pressure 28, right atrium pressure 2, pulmonary artery pressure 25/12, aorta pressure 116/80, and cardiac output 5 L/min. Figure 1 presents a diagram of human circulation, and its electric equivalent is shown in Figure 2.

Figure 3 presents pressures obtained during simulation of healthy human circulation. The increase of pressure with distance from the aortic valve for the

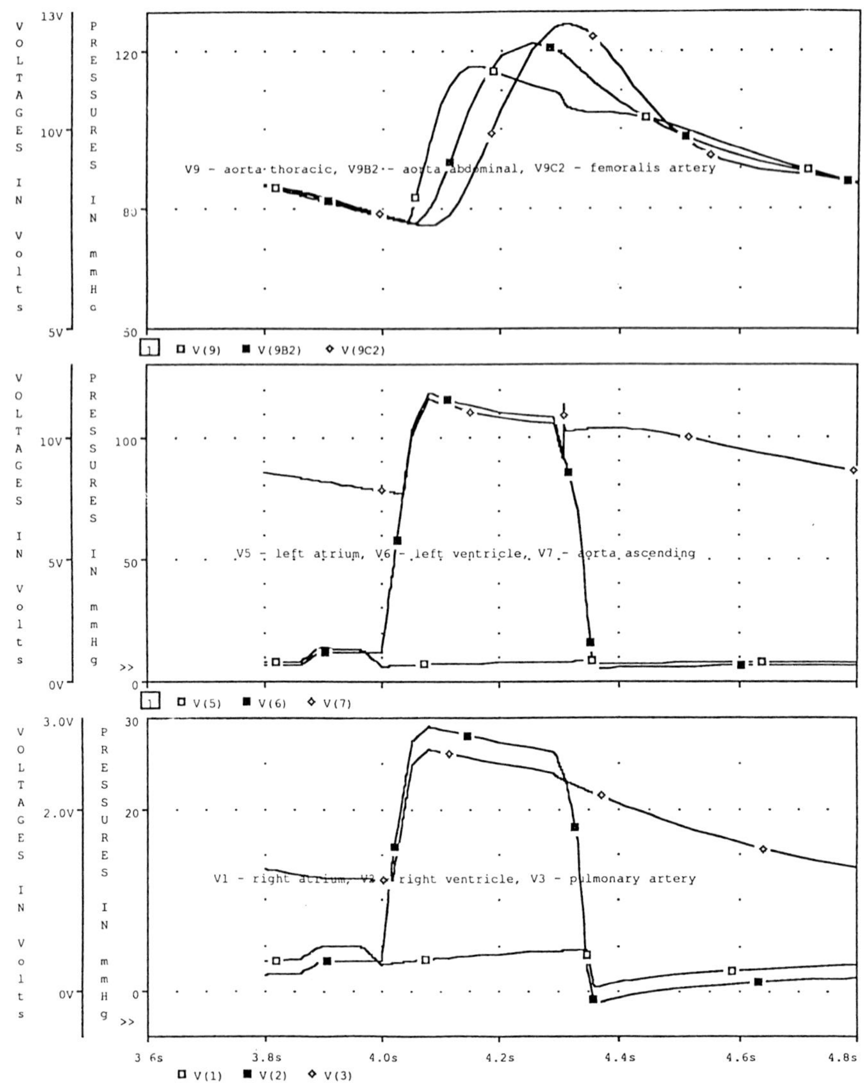


**Figure 3:** *Pressures obtained during simulation of healthy human circulation.*

thoracic aorta, abdominal aorta, and femoralis artery is observed during hemodynamic examination and is also described in many physiological textbooks.

Parameters for simulation of a congenital defect in human circulation were estimated on the basis of published data by Voytik.[6] The following hemodynamic features observed in patients with such defects were incorporated in the model: (a) cardiac output decreased below 3 L/min, (b) redistribution of cardiac output, and (c) venous congestion with increased systemic and pulmonary venous pressure. These effects were modeled by: (a) decreasing voltages of voltage sources

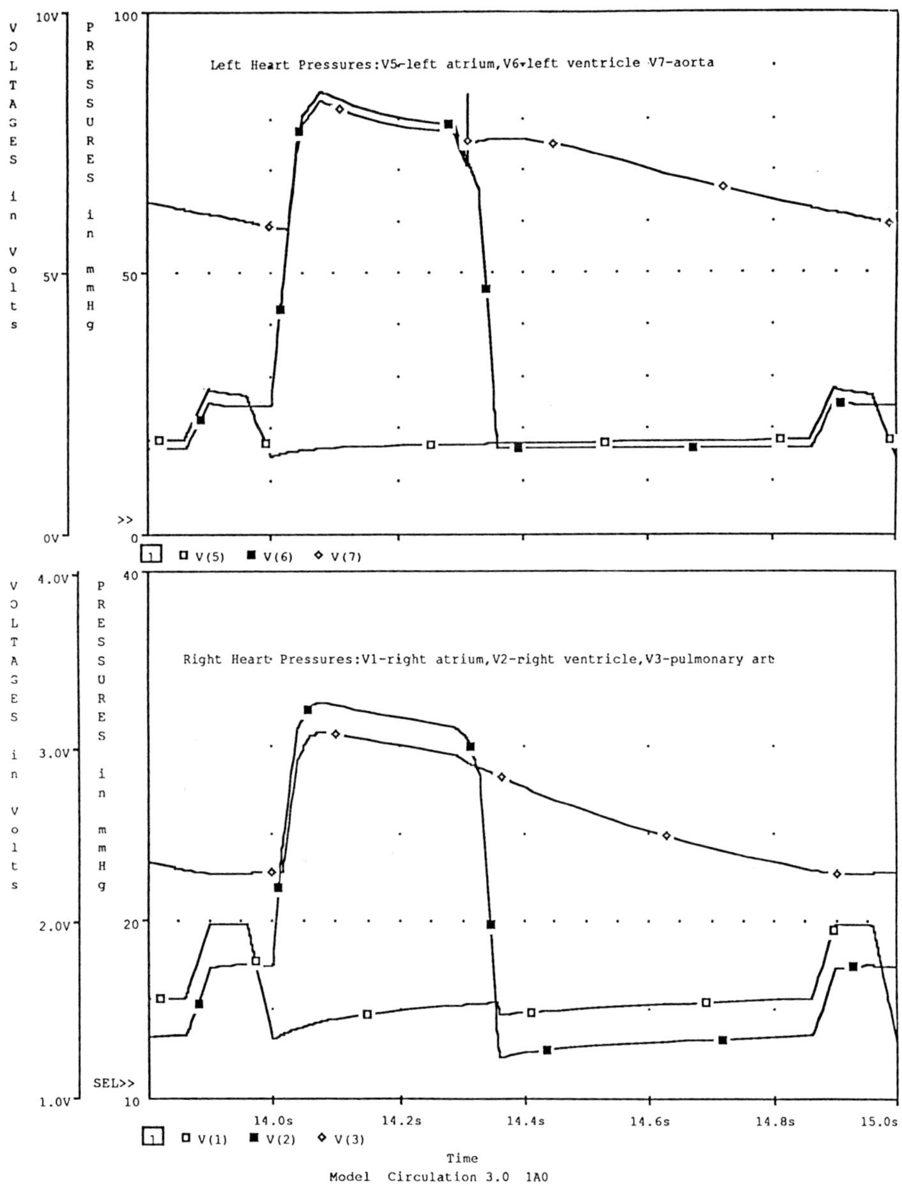


**Figure 4:** *Pressures obtained during simulation of human circulation with congenital defect.*

supplied by active chambers of the heart, (b) changing some numerical values of arteriovenous resistances, and (c) increasing the blood volume (electrical charge) in circulation. Figure 4 presents pressures obtained during simulation of the types of failed human circulation described above.

After designing a mathematical model of SMV and estimating parameters based on experimental data by Ruggiero,[7] simulation of three SMVs of insufficient human circulation was performed. The results of simulation for different SMV configurations (two with a calculated stroke volume of 40 mL with/without valves and one with a stroke volume of 20 mL with valves) in circulation versus results for the same circulation without support or supported by muscle wrapped around the aorta (aortomyoplasty) are presented in Figure 5.

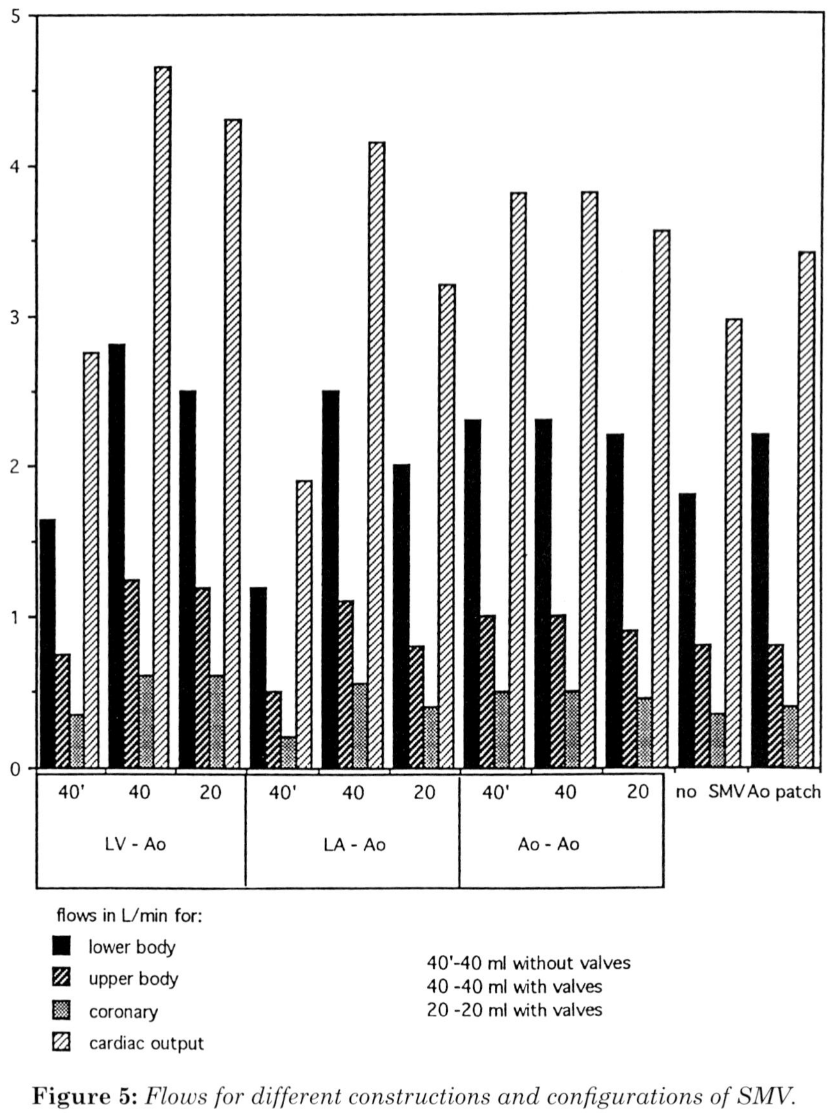


**Figure 5:** *Flows for different constructions and configurations of SMV.*

The simulation was done for SMV constructed for the stroke volume estimated as above, and residual volume, which is equal to two different stroke volumes, i.e., 40 mL and 20 mL, for patients with cardiac output of 2,950 mL/min without assist. The SMV worked in counterpulsation with 500 ms systole in 60 beats/min frequency. The same mode of work was applied for aortomyoplasty simulation.

In SMV of 40 mL stroke volume, with valves in the left ventricle-aorta configuration (LV-Ao), the cardiac output increased from 2,950 to 4,650 mL/min; in the left atrium-aorta (LA-Ao) configuration to 4,150 L/min; and in the aorta ascending-aorta thoracic configuration (Ao-Ao) to 3,800 L/min. The coronary flow increased to 600 mL/min, 550 mL/min, 500 mL/min for the above configurations, respectively, versus 350 mL/min without assist. These results show that the highest increase of flows was found in the LV-Ao configuration. The results of the dynamic aortomyoplasty (Ao patch) simulation without volume

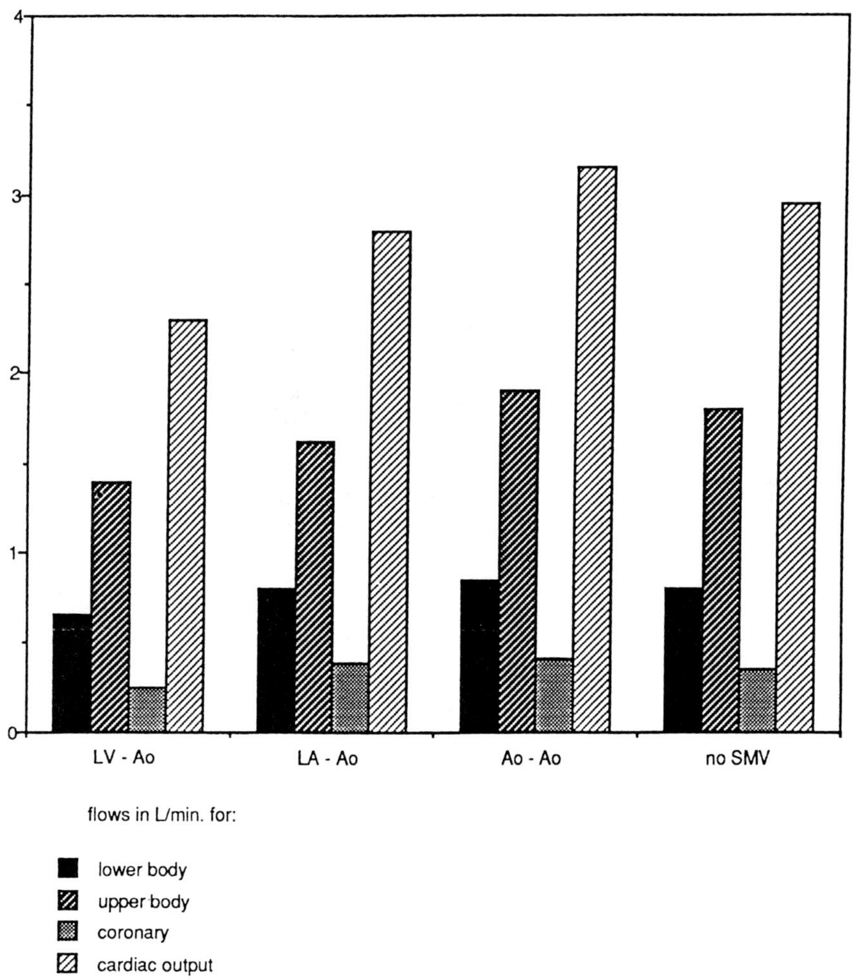


**Figure 6:** *Flows for different configurations of SMV with failed stimulation.*

extension were as follows: (a) the cardiac output increased to 3,4 L/min, and (b) coronary flow increased to 400 mL/min.

All the flow changes for the upper body, lower body, and coronary circulation in different configurations of SMV obtained from simulation are in agreement with the results of our animal experiments and the published data by Ruggiero[7] and Voytik.[6] Another interesting result of the simulation was that for the SMV volumes of 20 mL and 40 mL in aorto-aorta configuration, no differences were found when the chamber was connected to circulation by grafts with or without valves.

Simulation done for the same SMV volumes and configurations but with a failed myostimulator (Fig. 6), i.e., SMV contractility showed the following decreases of cardiac outputs in comparison to 2,950 L/min without assist: (a) for

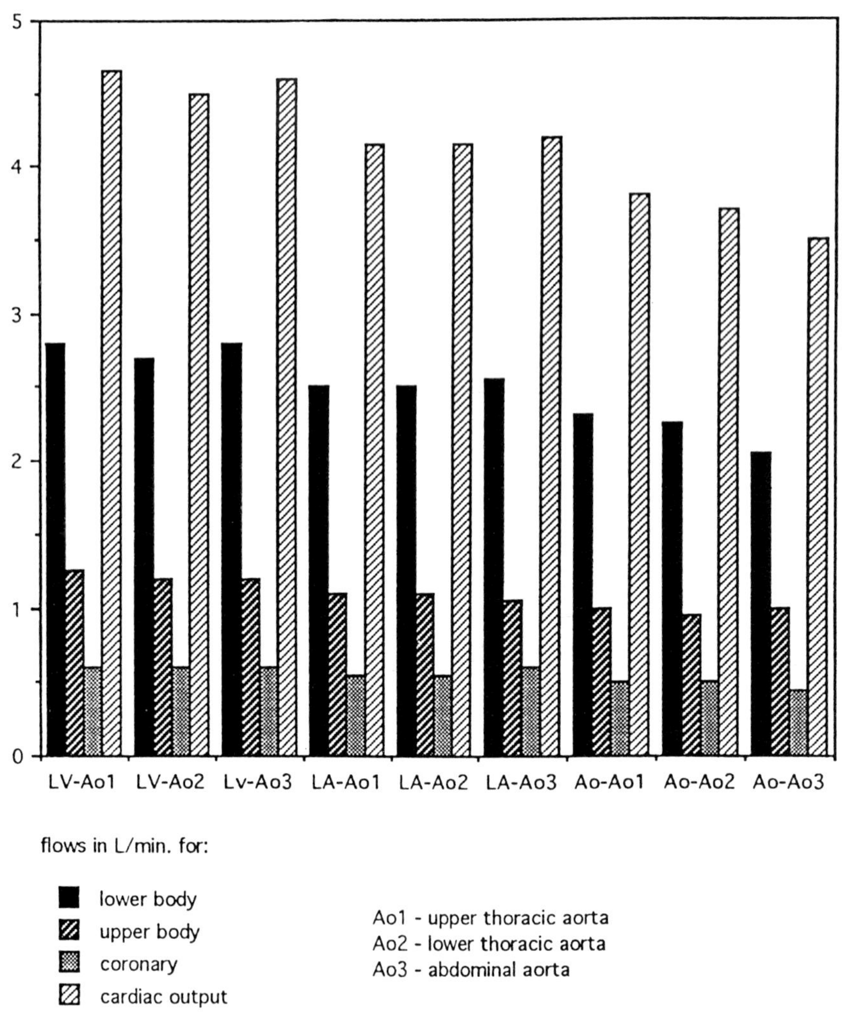


**Figure 7:** *Flows for different configurations of SMV with output connected to different parts of the aorta.*

LV-Ao to 2,3 L/min, (b) for LA-Ao to 2,8 L/min, and a small increase to 3,1 L/min for Ao-Ao. This increase was probably caused by the lower resistance of aorta which was partially bypassed by an MSV system. These simulation results suggest that the application of SMV in the most efficient configuration LV-Ao can be very risky, especially for patients with extremely low cardiac output (assist device dependent).

No significant changes were found for all of the SMV configurations when the output conduit was connected to the lower thoracic aorta or to the abdominal aorta compared to the upper thoracic aorta (Fig. 7). These results are important for designing the options of SMV surgery.

## Conclusions

The computer modeling of the blood system finds increasing applications in planning and interpretation of animal experiments and clinical trials. Obviously the simulation cannot completely replace trials on living organisms because of the many variables and feedback loops outside of the model scope. However, the model can describe the blood dynamics, thereby excluding the need for some experimental configurations and elucidating some confusing clinical and experimental results. Thus, the number of animal experiments and human trials could be decreased. An additional benefit of a good model is its advisory and predictive role during clinical decisions. We have shown that some SMV techniques degrade more gracefully than others. We have also shown that some, but not all, SMVs maintain efficiency even if only half the expected blood output is obtained. The ultimate clinical decision is obviously influenced by the unique clinical picture of the patients. However, the ultimate risk of the SMV predictive selection can be decreased by predictive use of the computer modeling.

## References


1. Noordergraff A, Verdouw PD, Boom, HE: The use of analog computer in circulation model. *Prog Cardiovasc Dis* 5:419–439, 1963.
2. Reeve EB, Guyton AC: *Physical Bases of Circulatory Transport.* Philadelphia, PA, London, England, W.B. Saunders Company, 1967.
3. Babbs CF, Weaver JC, Ralston SH, et al. Cardiac, thoracic, and abdominal pump mechanisms in cardiopulmonary resuscitation: Studies in an electrical model of the circulation. *Am J Emerg Med* 2:299–308, 1984.
4. Nagel, LW, Pederson DO: Simulation program with integrated circuit emphasis. *Proceedings of XVIth Midwest Symposium on Circuit Theory,* Waterloo, Canada, April 12, 1973 (University of California, Berkeley, memorandum ERL-M382).
5. Nagel LW: *SPICE2: A Computer Program to Simulate Semiconductor Circuits.* Manual, May 9, 1975 (University of California, Berkeley, memorandum ERL-M520).
6. Voytik SL, Babbs CF, Badylak SF: Simple electrical model of the circulation to explore design parameters for a skeletal muscle ventricle. *J Heart Transplant* 9:160–174, 1990.
7. Ruggiero R, Niinami H, Pochettino A, et al: Skeletal muscle ventricles: Update after 18 months in circulation. *Artif Organs* 15:350–354, 1991.

Chapter 44

# New Methods in Skeletal Muscle Ventricle Construction

K. Peczalski, W. Jaszcz, R. Bianco, R.M. Bolman III*

## Introduction

The idea of transforming the skeletal muscle into the fatigue-resistant muscle was introduced by Salmons et al.[1] in 1976 and the idea of using the autologous skeletal muscle for improving the failing cardiac function by Kantrowitz et al.[2] in 1959. These combined ideas have become the subject of growing experimental and clinical interest.[3,4]

The originally described cardiomyoplasty evolved into the attempts to construct an additional chamber, the skeletal muscle ventricle (SMV), which would be able to function as a blood pump and replace the mechanical assist device.[5] Indeed, the experimental SMV was constructed, primarily in dogs, and it has proved to develop the sufficient pressure and a continuous work for up to 18 months.[6] The main problems encountered were not adequate mechanical resistance or even rupture of SMV wall.[7]

In order to better preserve the muscle mass and to improve the SMV function, we have introduced the modifications described below in construction of the muscle pouch. The preliminary experiments done on rats and a pilot study on dogs are described in this chapter.

## Material and Methods

The preliminary study was done on three dogs, weighing 28–32 kg. The SMV was constructed from the left latissimus dorsi (LD) muscle by the following two-stage procedure.

The initial surgical procedure of LD separation from the surrounding tissues, with preservation of a portion of contiguous lumbar fascia, was done following the method routinely used in our laboratory. Briefly, after the dissection of muscle free from all insertions except for the humeral tendon, a

*With the cooperation of R. Solien, K. Gealow, and S. Shumway.

From Carpentier A, Chachques JC, Grandjean P: Cardiac Bioassist. © Futura Publishing Co, Inc, Armonk, NY, 1997.

specially designed "cuff" stimulating electrode (Medtronic Inc.) was implanted around the thoracodorsal nerve, approximately 3–4 cm proximal to the trifrucation. This lead was connected to an external pulse generator and the efficiency of stimulation was determined.

The LD was then wrapped around a Teflon mandrel covered with the gelatin sponge, beginning at the distal end of the flap. The wrap was completed by rotating the mandrel 45° every other half turn for approximately two and one-half turns.

A thoracic window was created by resecting approximately 4–5 cm of the anterior portion of the third and fourth ribs. The wrap was inserted into the window until approximately 50% of the wrap was included inside the thoracic cavity. The dorsal, caudal, and ventral borders of the wrap were sutured to the surrounding intercostal muscles, and acute and chronic chest drainage tubes were inserted. Then a pocket was formed for the implantable myostimulator (Itrel, Medtronic Inc.) behind the left rectus abdominis fascia. After 2 weeks of rest, the LD was submitted to 6 weeks of continued electrical 2-Hz stimulation.

The second stage of the surgical procedure was done 8 weeks later. The Teflon mandrel was removed and the muscle pouch was connected to the circulation by conduits with valves, and in one dog by conduits without valves. The epicardial leads were attached and an external SP 1005 Medtronic pacemaker was connected instead of the Itrel myostimulator. Then hemodynamic studies were done during the acute, approximately 4-hour, experiment and the animal was sacrificed.

The removed heart was fixed in a solution of 8% buffered formalin, and 15 samples from various parts of the SMV, including fibrous tissue around the electrode plate, were taken, embedded in paraffin, and submitted for histologic evaluation.

## Modifications of SMV Formation

Modified shapes of Teflon mandrel were introduced in our experiment, namely ovoid and elliptical, with two parallel protrusions creating the inlet and outlet of SMV to which valved or nonvalved conduits were connected during the second surgical phase.

The mandrel was covered with absorbable gelatin sponge treated with 100 USP of heparin, and saturated with 200 ng of TGF-beta (Ultrapure Natural Human TGF-beta 1, Genzyme, Cambridge, MA) diluted in physiological buffered saline containing 1% protein (PBS-P). The mandrel was wrapped with multidirectional layers of LD (longitudinal and latitudinal) instead of conventional unidirectional layers[8] (Fig. 1).

## Histologic Evaluation

Seven morphological parameters were used in histologic examination: (1) acute inflammatory infiltrates, (2) chronic inflammatory infiltrates, (3) presence of granulation tissue, (4) foreign body granuloma, (5) capillary vessels proliferation, (6) fibroblast proliferation, and (7) fibrosis. Each parameter was semiquantitatively evaluated using 0–4+ grades.

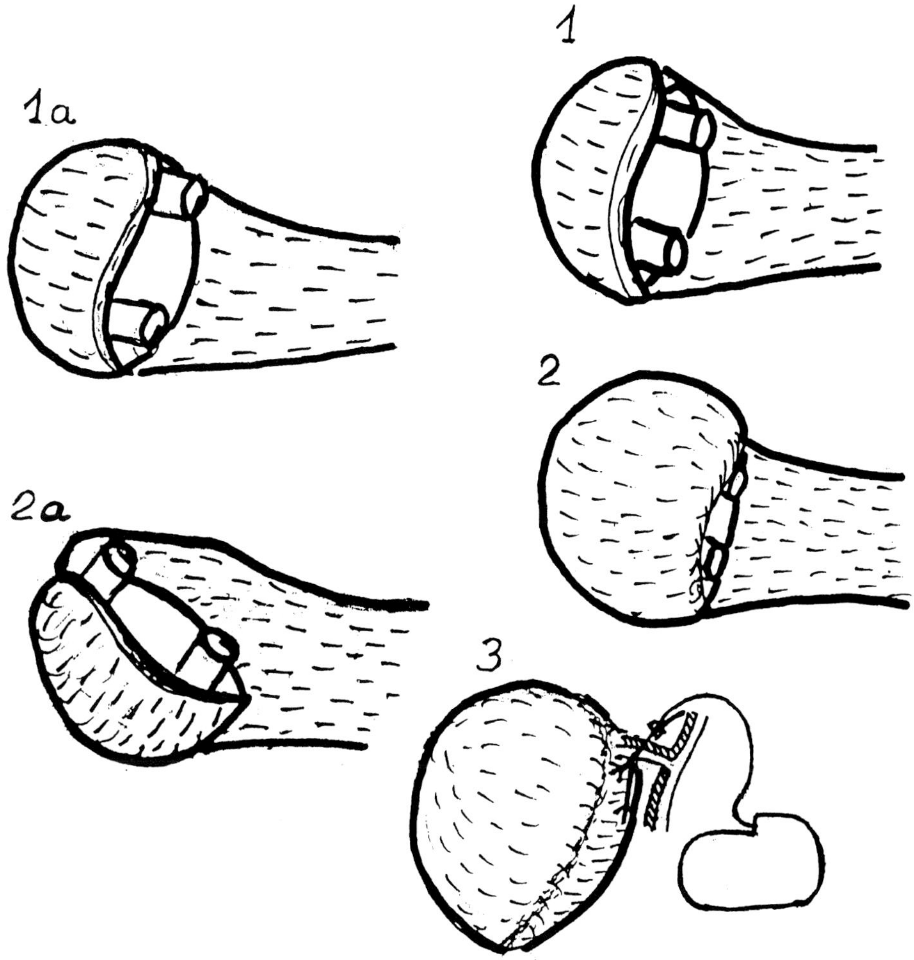


**Figure 1:** *Innovated mode of wrapping LD around the mandrel.*

The same histologic parameters were applied in the initial study done on Lewis rats in order to test the influence of TGF-beta and β-FGF (Human Recombinant Fibroblast Growth Factor, basic, Sigma Chemical Co., St. Louis, MO) on fibrous lining formation in skeletal muscle pockets.

## Results and Interpretation

### Experiment on Rats

The initial study was done on 59 rats; 44 were treated with TGF-beta, β-FGF, or a mixture of both, and 15 control rats received a silicone probe covered with absorbable sponge saturated with PBS-P only. In all of them, the silicone probe, 5 mm in diameter, was implanted under the left and right pectoralis muscles, and secured in place with a single suture. The animals were sacrificed

2, 4, 6 and 8 weeks after surgery. Probes were removed together with pectoralis muscle, fixed in 5% buffered formalin, embedded in paraffin, and submitted for histologic evaluation. Each group consisted of six rats (two of which were controls, all implanted on both sides).

Three different parts of the pocket were studied histologically and semiquantitatively evaluated in three blocks of a given pocket using 0–4+ grades, i.e., 0/0/0 through 0/1+/2+ to 4+/4+/4+. The median score was calculated for each pocket, e.g., 0, 1+, 2+, etc., and then for the whole group of rats.

The inflammatory process was virtually completed after 8 weeks. No granulation tissue, foreign body granulomas, or the remnants of sponge were found. The histologic results are presented in Figure 2.

## Experiments on Dogs

*Dog No. 1*

The SMV was constructed with the ovoid Teflon mandrel covered with gelatin sponge saturated with 200 ng of TGF-beta. It was removed together with the adjacent nerve and the attached electrode used for stimulation of the SMV.

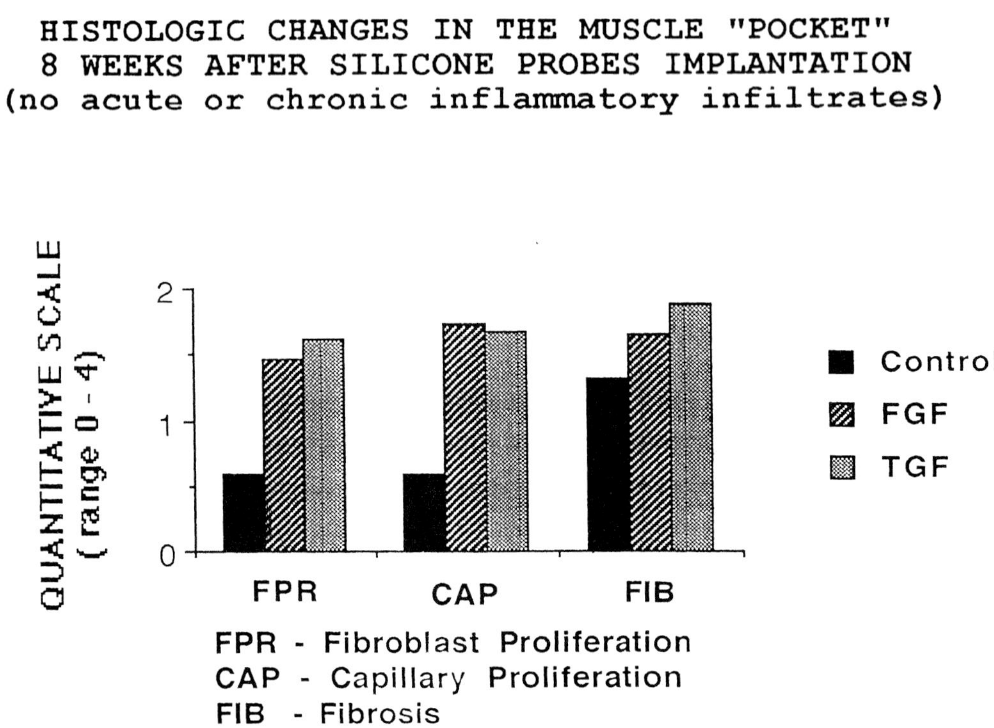


**Figure 2:** *Histologic changes in the muscle "pocket."*

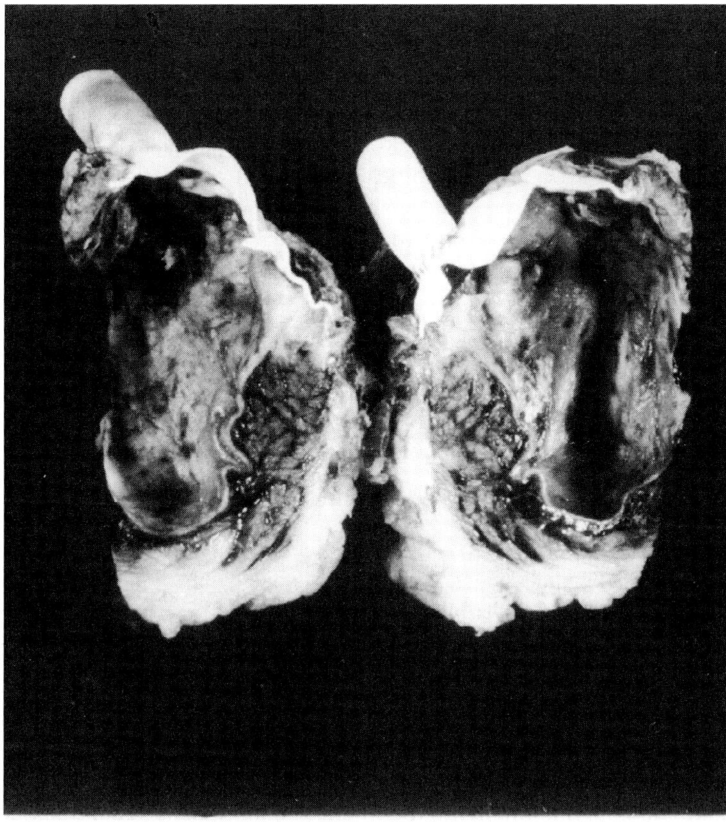

**Figure 3:** *Dog no. 1 (macroscopic).*

On gross (macroscopic) evaluation, the ventricle (cavity) was located in the upper part of the muscular structure. The two conduits and the patch were attached to the basal part of the ventricle. The SMV wall was 10 mm thick in the basal part (close to the attached vessel prosthesis), 15–17 mm in the middle, and 47 mm in the apical part. The internal layer of muscle showed recent hemorrhages. The ventricle was lined with thick and relatively smooth fibrous tissue (Fig. 3).

## Histologic Findings

The fibrotendinous tissue around the electrode plate showed normal blood vessels and a mild perineural fibrosis with some intraneural edema. In five blocks from the apical (thicker) part of the SMV, over 90% of muscle fibers were well preserved with a mild and localized interstitial edema, most likely related to the recent surgery (4-hour acute experiment), as were recent hemorrhages in the internal muscle layer. Only dispersed, isolated muscle fibers showed degenerative changes, mostly myocytolysis, and basophilic degeneration as well as simple atrophy. The similar changes were present in 10 blocks from the middle and basal portion of the muscle wall. In the basal portion of the ventricle where conduits and patch were attached, small foci of intramuscular chronic inflammatory infiltrates were observed.

The most internal layer of the wall (lining) was made of a thick, collagenized connective tissue, well attached to the muscle, showing on the luminal surface the cellular layer comprising proliferating fibroblasts, histiocytes, and few lymphocytes. Vascular proliferation of various intensity was present in all sections and it extended to the internal muscle layer (Fig. 4). In sections with more collagenized fibrous tissue, these vessels were better developed and larger; in areas of intensive fibroblast proliferation, mainly capillary vessels were observed. In none of 15 blocks were the remnants of the gelatin sponge seen.

## Dog No. 2

The SMV was constructed with the ovoid Teflon mandrel covered with gelatin sponge saturated with PBS-P only, without the growth factor. As in dog no. 1, two openings for vessel conduits were in the basal portion, and the electrode was implanted in the apical (caudal) area. The oval ventricle was lined with a thin layer of fibrous tissue, loosely attached to the muscle wall and in some places "detached-looking" with small areas of recent hemorrhages related to the recent surgery. Hemorrhages were also present in the internal muscle layer but they were less intense than in dog no. 1 (Fig. 5). As

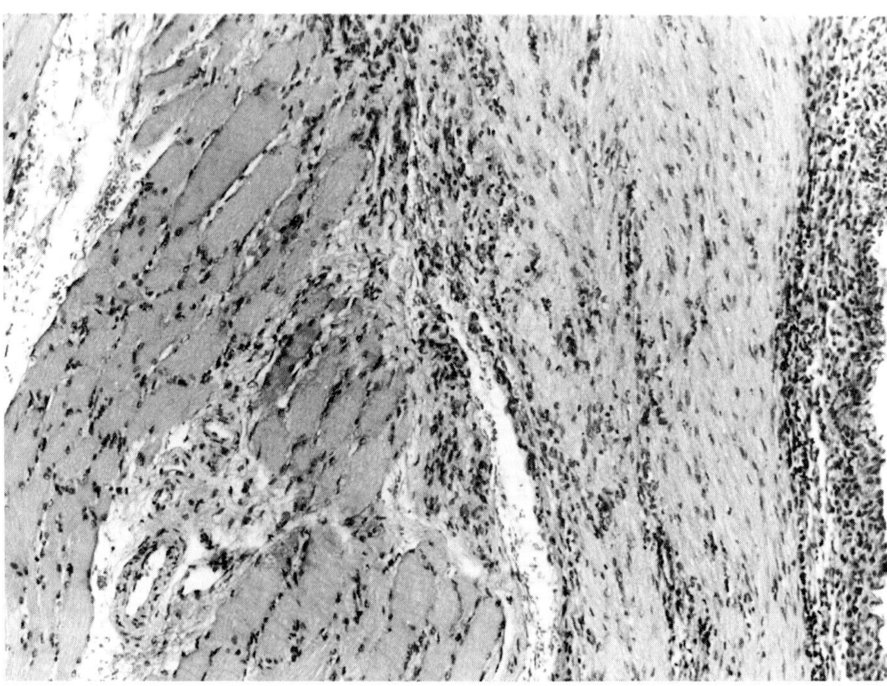

**Figure 4:** *Dog no. 1 (microscopic).*

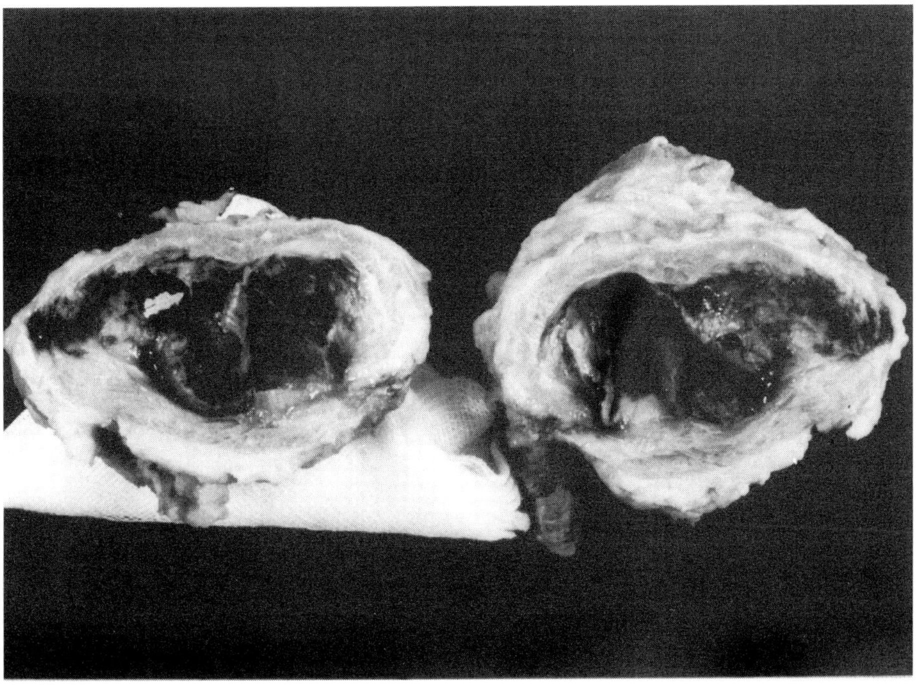

**Figure 5:** *Dog no. 2 (macroscopic).*

in the dog no. 1, multiple blocks from the SMV wall were taken for histologic examination.

Similar to the first dog, over 90% of muscle fibers were well preserved and only two dispersed foci of degenerated or atrophic fibers were seen. Small foreign body granulomas, related to the initial surgical procedure, were present in the attached subcutaneous tissue. The internal, lining layer of the SMV was formed by a relatively thin layer of fibrous tissue with no capillary proliferation and only mild fibroblast proliferation. This most luminal layer was attached to the muscle with a loose connective tissue in which recent hemorrhages were seen (Fig. 6).

## Dog No. 3

The SMV was constructed using elliptical (saucerlike) Teflon mandrel covered with gelatin sponge, inactivated with heparin and saturated with TGF-beta.

On gross examination, there was the electrode implanted in the apical (caudal) part, and the muscle cut through in the basal part, between the vascular prosthesis, in order to remove the mandrel. That area was covered by connective tissue with recent hemorrhagic changes. The SMV was oval, and its internal surface was smooth and lined by a thin layer of fibrous tissue. This layer was thinner than those seen in dogs no. 1 and no. 2, but strongly attached to

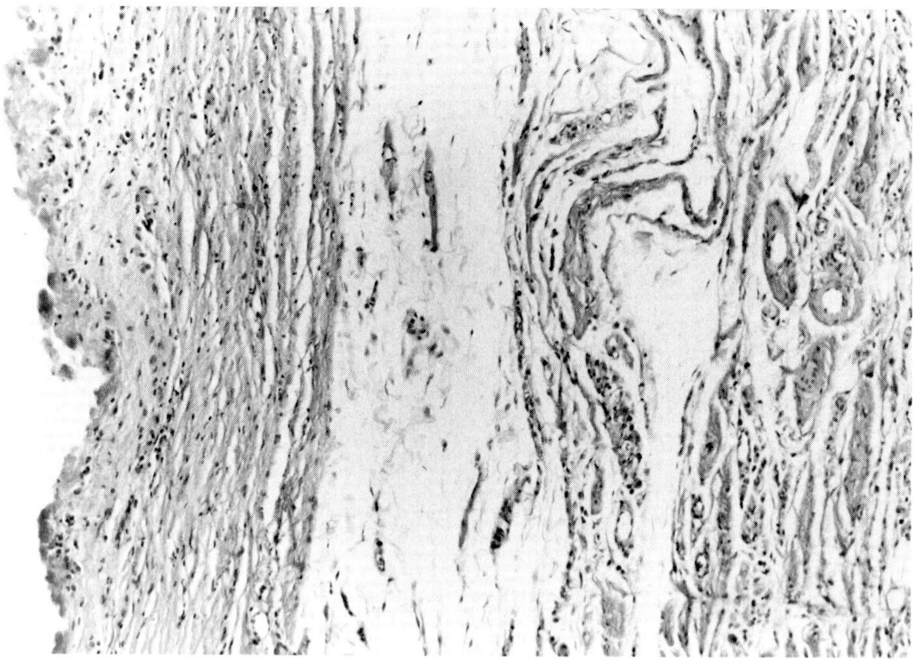

**Figure 6:** *Dog no. 2 (microscopic).*

the muscle as in the dog no. 1. A small portion of the SMV wall was made of a single layer of muscle, and it was 8–11 mm thick. In the remaining SMV wall the double muscle layer was 15–31 mm thick. As in the previous two dogs, the multiple blocks were taken from the various part of the SMV wall including the section of the muscle from the area between vascular prostheses.

Histologic findings in dog no. 3 were quite different from those seen in dogs no. 1 and no. 2. This difference was caused by extensive necrosis of internal layer of the muscle. In a few better preserved portions, there were prominent degenerative or atrophic changes involving 40–50% of muscle fibers. Necrosis also involved the internal lining layer (Fig. 7). The related, reactive changes, or formation of granulation tissue between the outer viable and necrotic inner layers, as well as acute and chronic inflammatory infiltrates around smaller foci of muscle necrosis in the relatively better preserved portion of the inner muscle layer made it impossible to compare dog no. 3 with the first two dogs. However, in the best preserved areas there was formation of lining, "endocardial" stratum showing brisk fibroblast proliferation and prominent vascularization. The degenerative and atrophic changes in the outer muscle layer involved 5–10% of muscle fibers and were comparable to those observed in dogs no. 1 and no. 2.

The cause of such an extensive necrosis may be the discoid shape of the mandrel with more sharp angles on the edge, requiring "bending" of the muscle and compromising the blood supply. Even in such disabled muscle some effective assist of the failed heart (induced by reversible balloon model, Jaworski

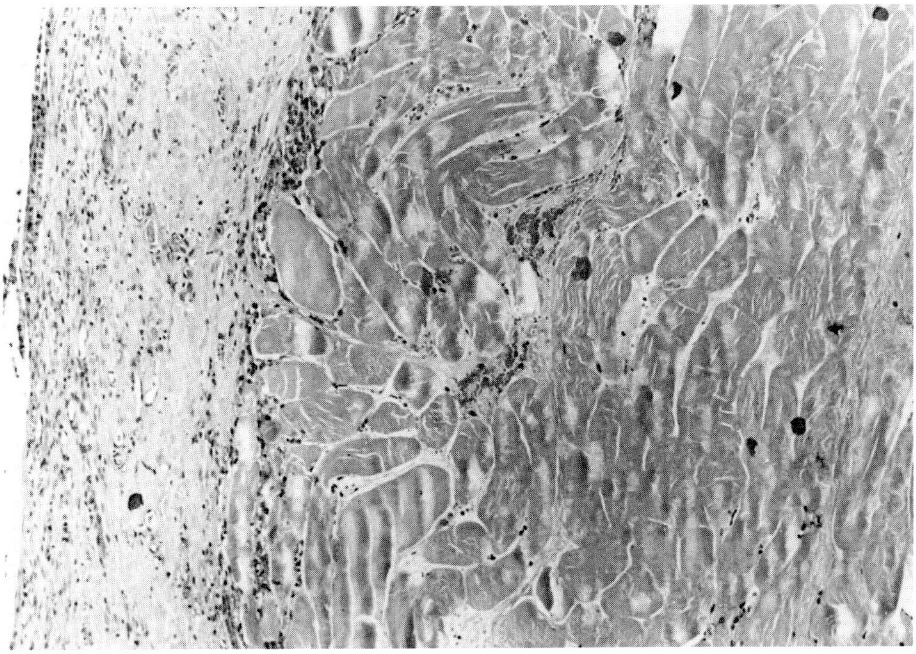

**Figure 7:** *Dog no. 3 (microscopic).*

et al.[9]) was obtained in dog no. 3 SMV, attached to the circulation during the terminal acute experiment. However, high 200 mm Hg pressure was obtained inside of SMV of dog no. 1 with definitely better preserved muscle. In dog no. 2, it was 80 mm Hg.

In spite of the small size of this pilot study, some interesting observations were made. The SMV muscle wall formed around the ovoid mandrel, wrapped by multidirectional layers of LD, was well preserved and looked grossly better than SMV formed by the conventional way of unidirectional wrapping with the LD. We are not aware of the published detailed histologic study on the SMV wall but in our carefully studied dogs the muscle was histologically very well preserved with more than 90% muscle fibers not showing any degenerative or atrophic changes. The 2-month observation is not long enough to draw any definite conclusion but the modified wrapping method seems to be worth further long-term experiments. The blood pressure obtained inside the SMV of the first dog was good and in the other two it was acceptable.

The ovoid shape of the mandrel seems to be superior to the discoid shape. It is risky to draw conclusions from this very small experiment but only the dog that received the elliptical mandrel had massive necrosis and the lowest induced pressure. Two parallel protrusions of the Teflon mandrel covered with sponge saturated with growth factor should increase the thickness of the fibrous inner layer in places where the conduits were attached.

## Discussion

The goal of our study was to increase the integrity of the SMV wall in order to secure its long-term efficient work and to prevent the rupture that was reported to occur predominantly at the sites of conduit attachment. Our hypothesis was that a thicker, stronger internal fibrous layer of SMV wall will increase its resistance to rupture and possibly help in its function. Since TGF-beta and β-FGF increase fibroblast and vessel proliferation, we tried to introduce these growth factors during the first phase of SMV formation. From the preliminary experiments on rats and a pilot study on dogs, it seems that this goal was achieved.

Certainly this inner layer will be restructured after the continuous work of SMV connected to circulation. We expect that this layer made of collagen fibers will acquire more parallel elastic fibers that may largely replace the collagen fibers. It remains to be seen how a fibroelastic layer will influence SMV function and whether it will prevent the rupture of the SMV wall. These questions can be answered only in long-term experiments.

## References

1. Salmons S, Streter FA: Significance of impulse activity in the transformation of the skeletal muscle type. *Nature* 263:30, 1976.
2. Kantrowitz A, McKinnon W: The experimental use of the diaphragm as an auxiliary myocardium. *Surg Forum* 9:266–268, 1959.
3. Carpentier A, Chachques J: Myocardial substitution with a stimulated skeletal muscle. *Lancet* 1:1267, 1985.
4. Magovern GJ, Heckler FR, Park S, et al: Paced skeletal muscle for dynamic cardiomyoplasty. *Ann Thorac Surg* 45:614–619, 1988.
5. Acker MA, Anderson WA, Hammond R, et al: Skeletal muscle ventricle in circulation: One to eleven weeks experience. *J Thorac Cardiovasc Surg* 94:163–174, 1987.
6. Ruggiero R, Niinami H, Pochettino A, et al: Skeletal muscle ventricles: Update after 18 months in circulation. *Artif Organs* 15(5):350–354, 1991.
7. Anderson D, Pochettino A, Hammond R, et al: Autogenously lined skeletal muscle ventricles in circulation. *J Thorac Cardiovasc Surg* 101:661–670, 1991.
8. Hooper T, Niinami H, Hammond R, et al: Intrathoracic skeletal muscle ventricles: A feasibility study. *J Cardiac Surg* 6(3):387–395, 1991.
9. Jaworski J, Granas M, Peczalski K, et al: A new animal model of reversible acute left heart failure for LVAD studies (abstract). *PACE* 11:583, 1988.

Chapter 45

# Skeletal Muscle Ventricle Right Heart Assist:

## Acute Studies after Tricuspid Valvulectomy

Renato Ruggiero, Gregory A. Thomas, Larry W. Stephenson*

### Introduction

During the past several years, we have fashioned canine latissimus dorsi (LD) muscle into the shape of pumping chambers and then connected these muscle pumps to the animal's own circulation. We refer to these pumping chambers as skeletal muscle ventricles (SMVs) and have used them to pump blood in both the systemic [1–7] and the pulmonary circulations.[9–13]

Results with SMVs in the systemic circulation have been good. In fact, SMVs connected to the aorta have functioned effectively as diastolic counterpulsators for more than 2 years.[5,6]

SMVs have also been connected to the pulmonary circulation to either partially or totally bypass the right heart. Although some long-term successes have been achieved, in general, results have not been as good as with SMVs used for left heart assist. Previously, assistance of the pulmonary circulation with SMVs has been attempted in dogs with normal hearts. Right atrial filling pressures may be too low in this situation. The purpose of this present study was to evaluate SMVs pumping blood from the right atrium to the pulmonary artery in a canine model where severe chronic tricuspid regurgitation had been created.

### Materials and Methods

SMVs were constructed using the right LD muscle in six mongrel dogs weighing 20–30 kg. The animals were operated on and treated in accordance

*With the cooperation of Huiping Lu, Hiroshi Niinami, Robert Fietsam, Jr, Hisako Nakajima, Hidehiro Nakajima, Frank W. Mocek, Robert L. Hammond, Agustin Arbulu

Supported by NIH Grant HL 34778.

From Carpentier A, Chachques JC, Grandjean P: Cardiac Bioassist. © Futura Publishing Co, Inc, Armonk, NY, 1997.

with the *Guide for the Care and Use of Laboratory Animals* published by the National Institutes of Health (NIH publication No. 85–23, revised 1985).

## SMV Construction

The right LD muscle was dissected from the subcutaneous tissue and the chest wall. The thoracodorsal neurovascular bundle was identified and protected. All muscle insertions were divided except for the humeral tendon, which was left intact. All collateral blood vessels were interrupted.

A unipolar cuff nerve electrode (Model 6901, Medtronic, Inc., Minneapolis, MN) was placed around the right thoracodorsal nerve. The muscle was then wrapped around a cone-shaped plastic mandrel, the volume of which was matched to the size of the animal size (2.5 cc/kg). A Teflon sewing ring (USCI, Billerica, MD) was sutured at the base of the SMV and used to secure the SMV to the mandrel. A small anterolateral thoracotomy was then made with removal of a short segment of the second rib and the SMV was positioned inside the chest at the apex of the right pleural cavity.

The nerve electrode was connected to a unipolar neurostimulator (Itrel, Model 7421, Medtronic, Inc., Minneapolis, MN) that was placed in a pocket under the right rectus muscle and the wound was closed. After a 3-week vascular delay period that has been shown to be necessary for the muscle to recover from the temporary ischemia that follows dissection, the neurostimulator was activated transcutaneously, and the SMV was electrically conditioned for 6 weeks to achieve fatigue resistance. The protocol of electrical conditioning consisted of single pulses at 2 Hz frequency, pulse duration of 210 μsec, and pulse amplitude of 1–3 volts.

## Tricuspid Valvulectomy

The animals were allowed to recover for about 3 weeks after SMV construction. Two to 3 weeks into the electrical conditioning period, they were taken back to the operating room and underwent median sternotomy and tricuspid valvulectomy. The valve was excised through the right atrium during a brief period of 2 to 3 minutes of caval inflow occlusion; cardiopulmonary bypass was not used. After recovery from surgery, the dogs completed the period of electrical conditioning while being monitored for clinical signs of chronic right heart failure.

## Connection to the Circulation

Nine weeks after SMV construction, and 3 to 4 weeks after tricuspid valvulectomy, the dogs were taken back to the operating room for connection of the SMV to the right side of the circulation. After re-do median sternotomy, the SMV mandrel was removed and the SMV was connected to the right atrium using an 18-mm porcine-valved composite Dacron graft as inflow conduit (Hancock, Medtronic, Inc., Minneapolis, MN). A second 18-mm porcine-valved composite Dacron graft was used as outflow conduit from the SMV to the main pulmonary artery (Fig. 1). Side-biting clamps were used to construct the anastomoses with the animals systemically heparinized. Cardiopulmonary bypass was not used.

After the SMV was connected to the right side of the circulation, the neurostimulator was removed and replaced with an implantable rate-responsive, synchronized, pulse-train stimulator (Prometheus, Medtronic, Inc., Minneapolis, MN). With the pacer delivering 33 Hz burst stimulation at 3–5 volts amplitude, the SMVs were stimulated to contract during cardiac systole at a rate of 1:2 with the heart.

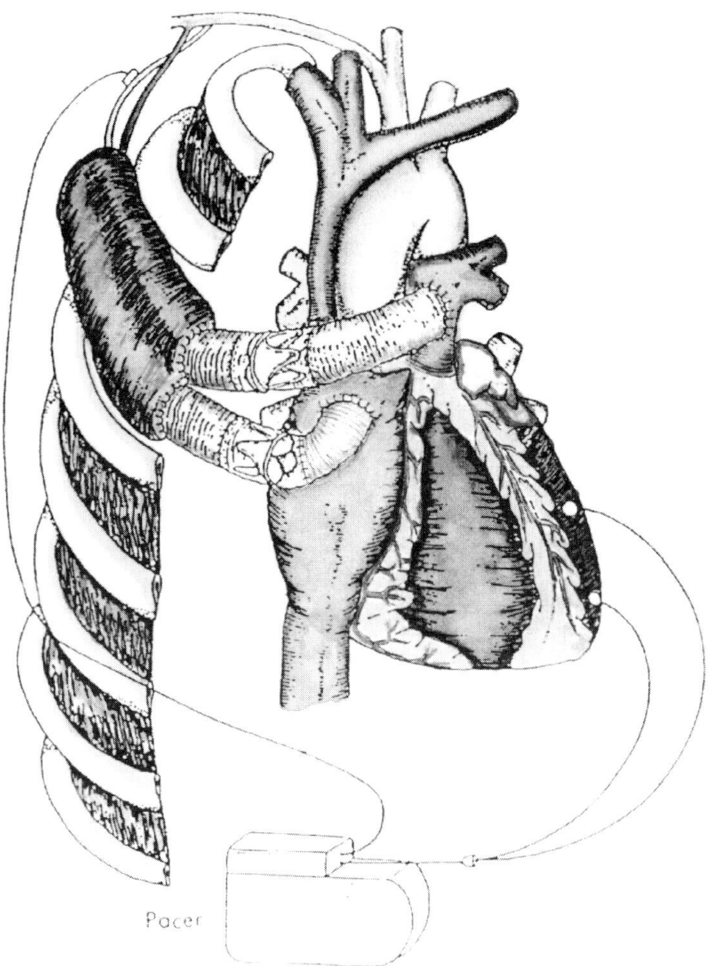


**Figure 1:** *Intrathoracic skeletal muscle ventricle (SMV). Valved inflow conduit from right atrium to SMV. Valved outflow conduit from SMV to main pulmonary artery. Tricuspid valve excised.*

## Measurements

CVP, femoral artery pressure, SMV peak and diastolic pressure, SMV flow, and aortic flow were measured in all of the animals after the SMVs were connected to the right side of the circulation. Pressure catheters were used to measure systemic blood pressure. Microtransducer tip catheters (Millar Instrument, Inc., Houston, TX) were used to measure CVP and pulmonary artery and SMV pressures. Aortic flow and SMV flow were measured with ultrasonic flow probes (Transonic System, Inc., Ithaca, NY) placed respectively around the ascending aorta and around the SMV outflow conduit. During this experiment, measurements with the SMV off and then on were obtained at baseline after connection to the circulation and then every 30 minutes for as long as 3 hours. The SMVs pumped continuously in the pulmonary circulation except for the brief periods when the pacer was turned off for measurements. At the conclusion of data collection, the animals were euthanized. Data were expressed as means plus/minus standard error. Student's *t*-test was performed on paired data with RS/1 software (Bolt Beranek and Newman, Inc., Cambridge, MD) on a portable computer.

## Results

The six dogs entered into the experiment were numbered in the order in which they were operated on. Measurements obtained at the time of tricuspid valvulectomy showed an average increase of central venous pressure from 3 ± 3 mm Hg before valvulectomy to 11 ± 1 mm Hg after valve excision. All animals survived the first two operations. In the postoperative period, during the interval between the triscupid valvulectomy and connection to the circulation, all animals showed evidence of chronic right heart failure manifested by tachycardia, hepatomegaly, and severe ascites that in some cases required treatment with diuretics.

At the time of initial data collection, immediately after connection of the SMV to the right circulation, mean CVP decreased from 16 ± 5 mm Hg with the stimulator off to 14 ± 3 mm Hg with stimulator on. Systemic systolic pressure increased from 91 ± 17 mm Hg with the stimulator off to 96 ± 24 mm Hg with the stimulator on. Systemic diastolic pressure increased from 46 ± 14 mm Hg without stimulation to 50 ± 20 mm Hg with stimulation. SMV peak pressure was 14 ± 6 mm Hg with the stimulator off vs. 31 ± 6 mm Hg with the stimulator on. SMV diastolic pressure decreased from 11 ± 5 mm Hg with the stimulator off to 8 ± 6 mm Hg with stimulator on. Aortic flow was 790 ± 614 mL/min without stimulation and 721 ± 552 mL/min with stimulation. Finally, SMV flow was 0 without stimulation and 357 ± 258 mL/min with stimulation. The ultrasonic flow probe failed to record SMV flow in two animals due to the thickness of the Dacron outflow circuit. SMV pressure and SMV flow increase were statistically significant ($p<0.05$). Hemodynamic data showed slow deterioration of function of the SMV throughout the duration of the experiment.

Hemodynamic measurements obtained at baseline (time 0), at 1 hour, and at 3 hours are summarized in Tables 1, 2, and 3, respectively.

Figures 2 and 3 show SMV output and cardiac output with SMV on and off in the dog with the most significant hemodynamic findings (dog 6).

**Table 1**
Right SMV - Hemodynamics
(Baseline)

| *Dog #* | *HR* | *CVP* | | *Femsystolic* | | *Femdiast* | | *SMV Peak* | | *SMV Dia* | | *Ao Flow* | | *SMV Flow* | |
|---|---|---|---|---|---|---|---|---|---|---|---|---|---|---|---|
| | | *Off* | *On* | *Off* | *On* | *Off* | *On* | *Off* | *On* | *Off* | *On* | *Off* | *On* | *Off* | *On* |
| 1 | 180 | 13 | 13 | 106 | 131 | 64 | 84 | 20 | 27 | 16 | 16 | 250 | 350 | 0 | 200 |
| 2 | 165 | 11 | 11 | 92 | 92 | 44 | 48 | 11 | 32 | 10 | 10 | 1544 | 1536 | N/A | N/A |
| 3 | 120 | 13 | 13 | 68 | 68 | 30 | 30 | 20 | 25 | 17 | 14 | 100 | 100 | N/A | N/A |
| 4 | 150 | 22 | 14 | 94 | 96 | 32 | 32 | 10 | 28 | 8 | 6 | 1200 | 900 | 0 | 262 |
| 5 | 135 | 12 | 12 | 74 | 74 | 44 | 44 | 5 | 42 | 4 | 2 | N/A | N/A | 0 | 193 |
| 6 | 120 | 22 | 20 | 112 | 114 | 62 | 62 | 15 | 33 | 11 | 2 | 858 | 721 | 0 | 771 |
| Mean | 145<br>±25 | 16<br>±5 | 14<br>±3 | 91<br>±17 | 96<br>±24 | 46<br>±14 | 50<br>±20 | 14<br>±6 | 31*<br>±6 | 11<br>±5 | 8<br>±6 | 790<br>±614 | 721<br>±552 | 0<br>0 | 357*<br>±258 |

* = $p<0.05$ on vs. off.

**Table 2**
Right SMV - Hemodynamics
(1 Hour)

| *Dog #* | *HR* | *CVP* | | *Femsystolic* | | *Femdiast* | | *SMV Peak* | | *SMV Dia* | | *Ao Flow* | | *SMV Flow* | |
|---|---|---|---|---|---|---|---|---|---|---|---|---|---|---|---|
| | | *Off* | *On* | *Off* | *On* | *Off* | *On* | *Off* | *On* | *Off* | *On* | *Off* | *On* | *Off* | *On* |
| 1 | 165 | 16 | 16 | 84 | 102 | 44 | 56 | 20 | 24 | 17 | 16 | 150 | 150 | 0 | 0 |
| 2 | 180 | 7 | 8 | 76 | 78 | 42 | 44 | 11 | 25 | 10 | 8 | 322 | 319 | N/A | N/A |
| 4 | 180 | 24 | 19 | 89 | 90 | 34 | 34 | 18 | 25 | 13 | 8 | 700 | 800 | 0 | 200 |
| 6 | 105 | 17 | 15 | 72 | 86 | 42 | 50 | 7 | 24 | 4 | 4 | 731 | 1107 | 0 | 549 |
| Mean | 158<br>±36 | 16.0<br>±7.0 | 14.5<br>±4.7 | 80.3<br>±7.7 | 89.0<br>±10.0 | 40.5<br>±4.4 | 46.0<br>±9.48 | 14.0<br>±6.1 | 24.5*<br>±0.6 | 11.0<br>±5.5 | 9.0<br>±5.0 | 476<br>±286 | 594<br>±439 | 0<br>0 | 250*<br>±278 |

* = $p<0.05$ on vs. off.

**Table 3**
Right SMV - Hemodynamics
(3 Hours)

| *Dog #* | *HR* | *CVP* | | *Femsystolic* | | *Femdiast* | | *SMV Peak* | | *SMV Dia* | | *Ao Flow* | | *SMV Flow* | |
|---|---|---|---|---|---|---|---|---|---|---|---|---|---|---|---|
| | | *Off* | *On* | *Off* | *On* | *Off* | *On* | *Off* | *On* | *Off* | *On* | *Off* | *On* | *Off* | *On* |
| 2 | 165 | 14 | 11 | 82 | 84 | 34 | 34 | 16 | 32 | 15 | 19 | 510 | 523 | N/A | N/A |
| 4 | 150 | 26 | 24 | 90 | 100 | 24 | 26 | 20 | 24 | 14 | 14 | 600 | 600 | 0 | 147 |
| 6 | 96 | 26 | 24 | 105 | 106 | 52 | 52 | 15 | 18 | 5 | 3 | 1105 | 1124 | 0 | 468 |
| Mean | 137 | 22.0 | 19.3 | 92.3 | 96.7 | 36.7 | 38.0 | 17.0 | 24.7* | 11.3 | 12.0 | 738 | 749 | 0 | 308* |
| | ±36 | ±6.9 | ±7.2 | ±11.7 | ±11.4 | ±14.2 | ±13.1 | ±2.6 | ±7.0 | ±5.5 | ±8.2 | ±321 | ±227 | 0 | ±227 |

* = $p<0.05$ on vs. off.

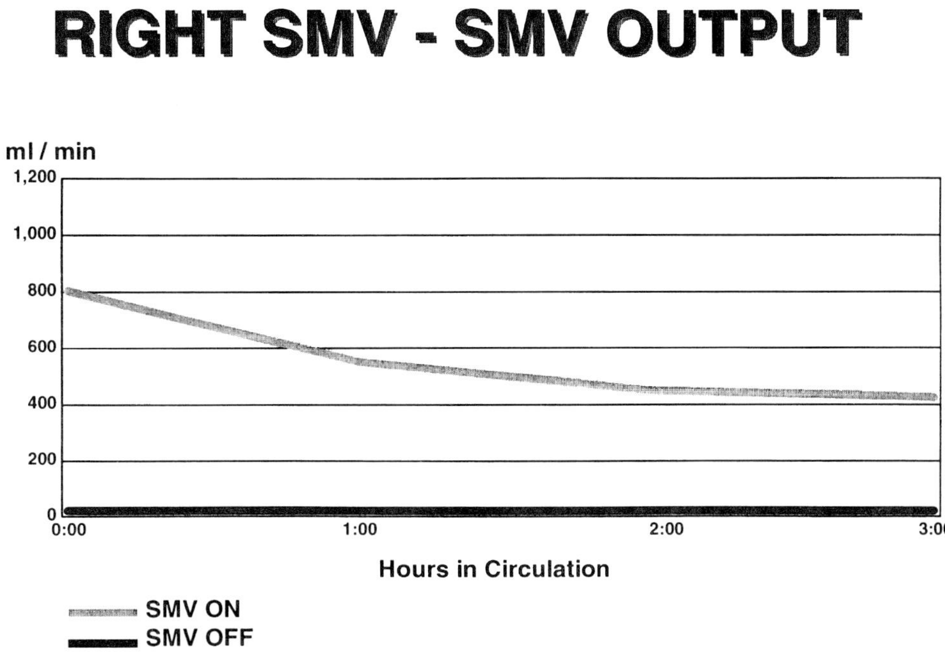


**Figure 2:** *Skeletal muscle ventricle (SMV) output as a function of time, dog 6.*

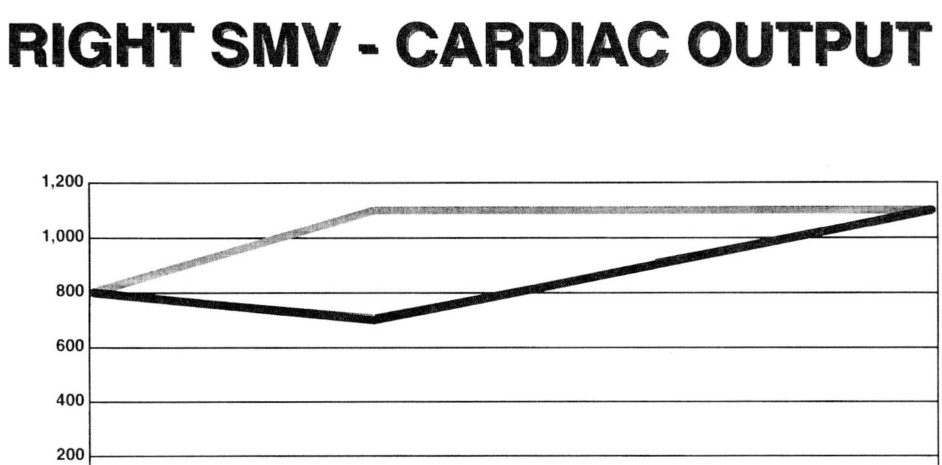


**Figure 3:** *Cardiac output as a function of time with skeletal muscle ventricle (SMV) on and off, dog 6.*

## Discussion

Assistance of the right side of the circulation with SMVs has been difficult to achieve due to low right atrial pressure which provides preload that may be inadequate for optimal SMV function. In this present experiment we used a model of tricuspid valvulectomy to increase CVP in order to obtain higher filling pressure for the SMVs after connection to the circulation. Although there was improvement in some hemodynamic parameters in some animals, in general the results were disappointing.

A few weeks after SMVs were constructed and placed in the thoracic cavity, the tricuspid valve was excised. After tricuspid valvulectomy, signs of right heart failure developed in all animals. The SMVs were then connected to the circulation in parallel with the right ventricle so that blood flow could go either from the right ventricle to the pulmonary artery or from the right atrium to the SMV and then to the pulmonary artery. Tricuspid regurgitation caused elevated right atrial pressure. With the SMV stimulated during systole at a 1:2 ratio with the heart, a small decline in CVP and a small increase in systemic systolic and diastolic pressure were recorded with stimulator on vs. off. However, statistical significance was obtained only for increase in SMV peak pressure and SMV flow.

In previous studies, electrically preconditioned SMVs have been shown to generate significant contractile power for prolonged periods of time.[1–13] The SMVs created for this experiment appeared to contract quite well prior to connection to the circulation. It is not clear why in most animals there were no major hemodynamic improvements after the SMVs were connected to the circulation. All dogs had evidence of severe right heart failure, with ascites, tachycardia (average heart rate at baseline measurements 145 ± 25 beats/min), and mild to moderate cardiogenic shock (average cardiac output 790 ± 614 mL/min). Rapid heart rate in particular is not compatible with optimal SMV performance because it does not allow enough time for adequate filling of the SMV pumping chamber. Careful review of the hemodynamic data shows that at baseline measurement at least one animal was in profound shock (dog no. 3); of the other five animals, the best function was demonstrated in dog no. 6, which did not have tachycardia. In a recent experiment from our laboratory, Thomas has demonstrated that low cardiac output in itself is not the cause of poor SMV function.[7] This study suggests that following tricuspid valvulectomy tachycardia is a problem, therefore induced heart block may be a method to improve this experimental model.

Anderson et al. demonstrated in dogs that SMVs constructed from LD muscle and connected to a totally implantable mock circulation device were capable of generating stroke work and power output 61% and 42%, respectively, of stroke work and power output of the native canine right ventricle, after pumping continuously for 4 weeks at preloads and afterloads similar to the right-sided circulation.[8]

Macoviak tested SMVs in the pulmonary circulation.[9] Using LD muscle, he constructed SMVs in four dogs. After a period of vascular delay and electrical conditioning, the animals underwent a second-stage procedure during which, while on cardiopulmonary bypass, the SMVs were connected with a valved inflow conduit to the right atrium or the inferior vena cava or the proximal pulmonary artery; a valved conduit was used as outflow to the distal pulmonary artery. At the same time the tricuspid valve was excised and the right coronary artery was ligated proximally in an effort to induce acute right heart failure. At a preload pressure of 15 mm Hg and a preload volume of 35 to 40 mL, these SMVs were able to provide pulmonary pressure in physiological ranges for as long as 20 hours until thromboembolic complications developed.

Later on, Bridges constructed cone-shaped SMVs using the left LD muscle.[10] After a period of vascular delay and electrical conditioning, valved grafts were used to direct venous return from the superior and inferior vena cava to SMV and outflow from SMV to pulmonary artery. Total right heart bypass in five dogs and partial right heart bypass in two dogs were obtained for periods as long as 8 hours. In a subsequent study, the same author connected cylinder-shaped SMVs to the superior vena cava and main pulmonary artery.[11] With the SMV stimulated to contract every fourth heart beat, significant increases in systemic arterial pressure, pulmonary artery pressure, superior vena cava blood flow, and decrease in mean caval pressure were achieved for several hours.

Niinami connected SMVs to the right ventricle using a Rastelli-type configuration.[12] In this acute experiment, SMV inflow was obtained with a valved synthetic graft connected to the right ventricle and SMV outflow with a second valved conduit anastomosed to the pulmonary artery. The main pulmonary artery was ligated proximal to the outflow conduit, so that the SMV functioned in series with the right ventricle. With this design, right ventricular pressure was used to generate higher SMV preload instead of relying on central venous pressure. SMVs were stimulated at 33 Hz burst frequency to contract during diastole in a 1:2 mode. When comparing hemodynamic data with the stimulator on vs. off, cardiac output increased by 27% at 1 hour (1437 ± 54 mL/min vs. 1140 ± 64 mL/min) and by 30% at 4 hours (1403 ± 161 mL/min vs. 1074 ± 99 mL/min), systemic arterial pressure increased at 1 hour by 12% (87 ± 5 mm Hg vs. 78 ± 5 mm Hg) and by 13% at 4 hours (81 ± 3 mm Hg vs. 72 ± 3 mm Hg), peak pulmonary artery pressure increased at 1 hour by 35% (28 ± 2 mm Hg vs. 21 ± 2 mm Hg) and by 37% at 4 hours (31 ± 3 mm Hg vs. 23 ± 0.5 mm Hg). Similar data were duplicated in a chronic experiment, with 16% increase in cardiac output and 7% increase in systemic pressure 1 week after surgery.[13] Six dogs had significant right heart assistance for periods between 1 and 12 weeks, with three animals surviving longer than 1 month and two longer than 3 months.

Chiu's group has used skeletal muscle for hemodynamic support in the setting of acute right heart failure.[14] Using a model of acute pulmonary hypertension obtained by injecting glass microspheres into the pulmonary artery, they were able to demonstrate that dynamic cardiomyoplasty is capable of increasing pulmonary flow, systemic arterial pressure, and cardiac output in dogs. It is possible that this model of pulmonary hypertension could be useful in the evaluation of SMVs for right heart assistance.

In summary, previous studies of animals with normal heart function indicated that SMVs can be used for right heart assist. In the present study, although mild improvement in hemodynamics was demonstrated in some animals (SMV off vs. on), in general the results were disappointing. This could be attributed to tachycardia or possibly other unrecognized factors. The model of tricuspid valvulectomy needs future testing, including evaluation in the setting of heart block.

## References


1. Mannion JD, Hammond RL, Stephenson LW: Hydraulic pouches of canine latissimus dorsi: potential for left ventricular assistance. *J Thorac Cardiovasc Surg* 91(4):534–544, 1986.
2. Mannion JD, Acker MA, Hammond RL, et al: Power output of skeletal muscle ventricles in circulation: Short-term studies. *Circulation* 76:155–162, 1987.
3. Acker MA, Anderson WA, Hammond RL, et al: Skeletal muscle ventricles in circulation: One to eleven weeks experience. *J Thorac Cardiovasc Surg* 94:163–174, 1987.
4. Anderson DR, Pochettino A, Hammond RL, et al: Autogenously lined skeletal muscle ventricles in circulation: Up to nine months experience. *J Thorac Cardiovasc Surg* 101:661–670, 1991.
5. Ruggiero R, Anderson DR, Pochettino A, et al: Skeletal muscle ventricles: Update after 18 months in circulation. *Artif Organs* 15:350–354, 1991.
6. Mocek FW, Anderson DR, Pochettino A, et al: Skeletal muscle ventricles in circulation long-term: 191 to 836 days. *J Heart Transplant* 11:S334–340, 1992.
7. Thomas GA, Lu H, Isoda S, et al: Skeletal muscle ventricles in circulation: Decreased incidence of rupture. *Ann Thorac Surg* 61:430–436, 1996.
8. Anderson WA, Andersen JS, Bridges CR, et al: Skeletal muscle ventricles as potential right heart assist or substitute. *Trans Am Soc Artif Intern Organs* 34:241–246, 1988.
9. Macoviak JA, Stinson EB, Starkey TD, et al: Myoventriculoplasty and neoventricle myograft cardiac augmentation to establish pulmonary blood flow. *J Thorac Cardiovasc Surg* 93:212–220, 1987.
10. Bridges CR, Hammond RL, Dimeo F, et al: Functional right-heart replacement with skeletal muscle ventricles. *Circulation* 80:(Suppl III) 183–191, 1989.
11. Bridges CR, Woodford W, Mora G, et al: Use of skeletal muscle power to augment the pulmonary circulation. *Surg Forum* 41:267–270, 1990.
12. Niinami H, Hooper TL, Hammond RL, et al: A new configuration for right ventricular assist with skeletal muscle ventricle: Short-term studies. *Circulation* 84: 2470–2475, 1991.
13. Niinami H, Hooper TL, Hammond RL, et al: Skeletal muscle ventricles in the pulmonary circulation: Up to 16 weeks experience. *Ann Thorac Surg* 53:750–757, 1992.
14. Hill A, Li C, Tchervenkov C, et al: Dynamic cardiomyoplasty for hemodynamic support during acute pulmonary hypertension. *J Thorac Cardiovasc Surg* 103:1200–1206, 1992.

Chapter 46

# Physical and Numerical Simulation of Blood Flow within a Skeletal Muscle Ventricle

A.P. Shortland, F. Iudicello, S. Salmons*

## Introduction

For some years, the surgical treatment of end-stage cardiac failure has been restricted to cardiac transplantation and the temporary use of mechanical circulatory support devices as a "bridge to transplant." The shortage of donors, problems of rejection, and high cost of the transplant program severely limit the number of patients who can benefit from treatment. There is, therefore, a strong case for seeking alternative therapeutic approaches that could be extended to a broad category of seriously affected patients. The discovery of adaptive transformation of fast-twitch skeletal muscle, which includes a marked increase in its resistance to fatigue, opened up the possibility of diverting a skeletal muscle, such as latissimus dorsi, from its normal function to a cardiac assist role.[1,2] Our earlier collaborative work[3] showed that suitably conditioned skeletal muscle was capable of operating continuously at levels within the range of power outputs of normal cardiac muscle.

The most conservative approach to the use of skeletal muscle is to wrap the muscle around the heart, as in the cardiomyoplasty procedure pioneered by Carpentier and Chachques.[4] Although this approach has the advantage of preserving the intima, basic studies indicate that the loading conditions under which such a graft finds itself would be far from optimal.[5,6,19] Despite reported successes,[7] the hemodynamic benefits of this procedure are variable, even in the hands of the originators.[8] In several laboratories,[9–11] progress has been made toward obtaining a counterpulsatory assist by encircling the aorta. The available length and lumen of the vessel limit the flow that can be produced in this way, but the approach may prove beneficial in a carefully selected group of patients. A procedure that has potential for very broad application is that of a separate skeletal muscle ventricle (SMV) used either in a

*With the cooperation of R.A. Black, J.C. Jarvis, F.S. Henry, and M.W. Collins.

From Carpentier A, Chachques JC, Grandjean P: Cardiac Bioassist. © Futura Publishing Co, Inc, Armonk, NY, 1997.

counterpulsatory mode or in parallel with the patient's heart as a true auxiliary ventricle.[1] Such an SMV could sustain indefinitely levels of pumping power similar to those available from the best current generation of mechanical artificial ventricles without the need for an external power supply. In one experimental dog, such a ventricle has pumped blood in circulation for more than 2 years.[12]

Despite its attractions, this approach poses a significant problem: it places a potentially thrombogenic surface in the circulation. Thrombosis can lead to impaired function of the device and put the patient at risk of infarction. If this procedure is to become available to patients who are candidates for long-term circulatory support (an estimated 30,000 per year in the US and 2,000–3,000 per year in the UK), we must be confident that interfacial events inside the SMV do not give rise to thromboembolic complications. For these reasons, characterization of flow in candidate SMV configurations is an important objective.

## Hemodynamic Considerations

The fluid mechanics of a ventricular assist device are particularly complex. The flow of blood through such a device is likely to be highly disturbed, or even turbulent. As a result, the cells within the flowing blood—and those that line the vessel walls—are subjected to a wide range of shear stresses. Turbulent blood flow, in particular, can be detrimental to the blood constituents, causing hemolysis or platelet activation.[13,14] The release of red-cell contents can trigger the cascade of biochemical events that lead to the formation of emboli and mural thrombus. On the other hand, deposition of platelet aggregates and cell debris onto a surface is more likely to occur in regions of flow recirculation and stagnation, where the residence time of fluid is prolonged.[15,16] In the case of a skeletal muscle ventricle, the flow patterns will be dictated mainly by the size and orientation of the connections to the ventricle, the stroke volume, rates of contraction, and the shape of the chamber itself at each stage of the pumping cycle.

Our approach has been to simulate the assisted cardiovascular system in vitro, where the interaction of an SMV with a mock circulation can be assessed under controlled, physiological flow conditions. Modeling of this type offers a number of advantages over in vivo testing:

- The effects on flow of variation in stroke volume, ejection fraction, and timing can be studied in a systematic way.
- The assessment of radically different configurations is relatively straightforward.
- The need for many animal experiments is reduced, as animal studies can be reserved for evaluating configurations that have been selected on the basis of their proven flow characteristics.

In our apparatus, a diagram of which is given in Figure 1, the compliant ventricle is modeled as a thin-walled, translucent rubber ventricle. Function is

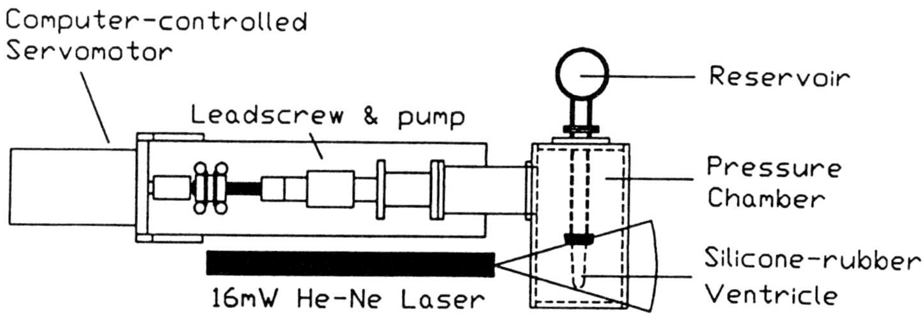


**Figure 1:** *Schematic diagram of the SMV physical model and flow-visualisation apparatus.*

simulated by coupling a computer-driven positive displacement pump to a sealed, fluid-filled chamber that houses the ventricle. The pump can generate any arbitrary flow waveform. Flow patterns within the model SMV are visualized by planar laser illumination and quantitated by particle trajectory analysis. The apparatus is currently being extended so that fluid displaced from the rubber ventricle enters a mock circulation, consisting of a flow circuit with compliance chambers, peripheral resistances, and fluid reservoirs, together with transducers for measuring pressure and rate of flow. In this way, interaction of the SMV with steady and pulsatile flows can be modeled. Full-field flow measurements are made using laser light to illuminate the model SMVs as they are inflated and deflated under the action of a positive displacement pump. We use a state-of-the-art charge-coupled device video camera to capture time-lapsed images; the camera has a "frame integration" facility that enables the movement of particles within the flow field to be recorded over an adjustable time interval (Fig. 2). The resulting images have streak lines that reveal the flow structures within the ventricle, especially areas of flow recirculation and stagnation.[17] The camera can be triggered electronically so that images can be captured sequentially or synchronized to the flow waveform generated by the pump.

This physical model has shown us that:

- Coherent vortices appear to be the dominant flow structure for the two axisymmetric geometric configurations that we have considered thus far.
- These flow structures are dependent on pulse shape, amplitude, and frequency.
- The inlet configuration has a marked influence on the flow structures.
- The stability of the vortices depends mainly on the duration of the filling phase within each cycle.

If cardiac assistance is to be introduced at the earliest possible postoperative stage without fatiguing the SMV, it may be necessary to interpose one or more quiescent cycles between assisted beats. A simulation of such extended quiescent periods at the end of SMV filling has revealed travelling annular vor-

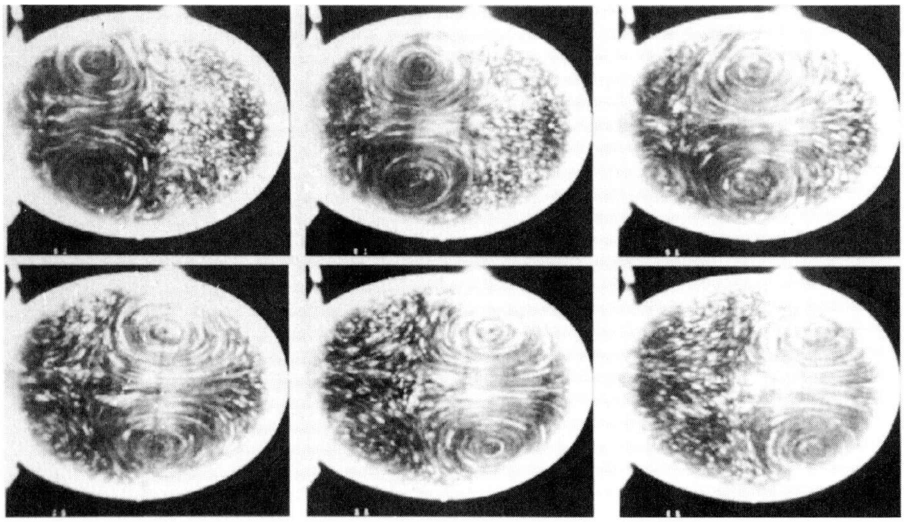

**Figure 2:** *Time-lapse video images of flow patterns throughout a 1-sec quiescent period.*

tices. The video images depicted in Figure 2 are of 3/25 sec duration and were taken sequentially at 1/5 sec intervals during such a quiescent period. Moving vortices are associated with apical thrombus formation in dilated left ventricles.[18] The influence of quiescence is therefore highly relevant to the design of clinical SMVs.

## Numerical Simulation

We have used some of the results to conduct a comparison of flows in physical and computational models of an SMV. Data describing the wall movement of an axisymmetric elastomer ventricle, pumping fluid to and from a reservoir, are used as the input to a corresponding single-block, moving-wall, axisymmetric model, constructed with a commercially available numerical package (FLOW3D, Release 3.2, AEA Technology, Harwell, UK). This multiblock model incorporates a realistic treatment of the rounded end and allows a certain degree of asymmetry in the flow. Four sets of data were transferred, each representing a time history of ventricular wall movements over one cycle. Velocity data from the computational package were then compared to experimental measurements acquired by the semiquantitative flow visualization technique. Comparison of initial predictions with experimental data revealed significant differences, which we suspected were a partial consequence of the size of the time steps used. Since the time step was fixed by the video apparatus, we performed a Fourier decomposition on the data and then regenerated the data with a smaller time step. With this smaller time step, a finer grid, and a more accurate model of the advection terms in the momentum equations, the calculations produced flow fields that were in much better agreement with the experiment (as shown in Figs. 3 and 4).

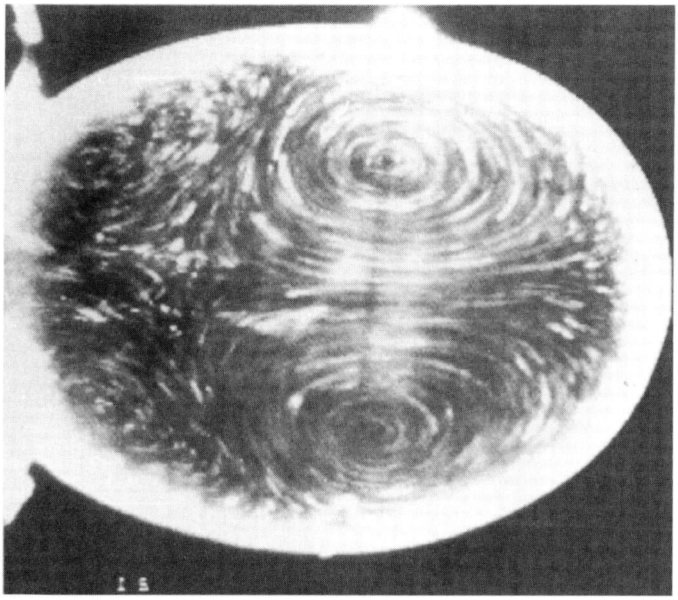

**Figure 3:** *Video image of the flow pattern observed in the physical model during late diastolic filling (time step corresponds to that shown in Figure 2). The particle trajectories confirm that vortex formation is a characteristic feature of the flow in ventricles having a single, axisymmetric inlet.*

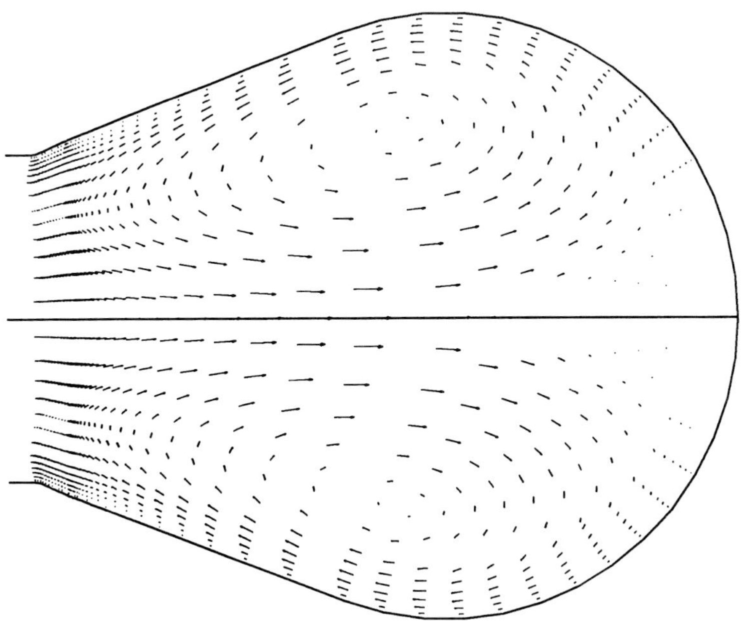

**Figure 4:** *Velocity vector plot of the flow field produced for a single time step using FLOW3D's post-processor, JASPER. Sequences of these plots have been animated and recorded on videotape.*

## Conclusions

The flow visualization system is very powerful and will be used in future studies of the flow characteristics of candidate model ventricles. Although the current physical model is axisymmetric, this may not be the case in future models. We are now planning modifications that will provide a physical simulation closer to the cardiovascular hemodynamics found in the clinical situation. A T-shaped inlet section has been constructed that will allow us to investigate the flow patterns that exist within a model SMV as it modulates the steady flow from a constant head tank. We aim to extend this work to include the modeling of pulsatile flow, with the use of a second servo-motor system that can deliver the range of flow waveforms likely to be present upstream of an SMV in vivo.

The numerical simulation will progress in parallel, the exchange of data with a corresponding physical model enabling us to validate the code at each step. The predictive exercise based on the current multiblock model will be directly comparable with videotaped results of flow fields from the physical model.

Our overall aim is to generate surgical guidelines for the construction of a skeletal muscle ventricle that is not susceptible to thrombus formation. This is an essential step toward implementing this surgical technique in patients with cardiac failure.

*Acknowledgment:* This work has been supported by grants from the British Heart Foundation.

## References

1. Acker MA, Hammond RL, Mannion JD, Salmons S, et al: Skeletal muscle as the potential power source for a cardiovascular pump: assessment in vivo. *Science* 236:324–327, 1987.
2. Salmons S, Jarvis JC: Cardiac assistance from skeletal muscle: A critical appraisal of the various approaches. *Br Heart J* 68:333–338, 1992.
3. Acker MA, Hammond RL, Mannion JD, Salmons S, et al: An autologous biologic pump motor. *J Thorac Cardiovasc Surg* 12:733–746, 1986.
4. Carpentier A, Chachques JC: Myocardial substitution with a stimulated skeletal muscle: First successful clinical case. *Lancet* 1:1267, 1985.
5. Salmons S, Jarvis JC: The working capacity of skeletal muscle transformed for use in a cardiac assist role. In: Chiu RC-J, Bourgeois I (eds): *Transformed Muscle for Cardiac Assist and Repair.* Futura Publishing Company, Inc., Mount Kisco, NY, pp 89–104, 1990.
6. Salmons S, Jarvis JC: Cardiomyoplasty: The basic issues. *Cardiac Chronicle* 4:1–7, 1990.
7. Moreira LFP, Stolf NAG, Jatene AD: Hemodynamic benefits of cardiomyoplasty in clinical and experimental myocardial dysfunction. In Chiu RC-J, Bourgeois I (eds): *Transformed Muscle for Cardiac Assist and Repair.* Futura Publishing Company, Inc., Mount Kisco, NY, pp 179–188, 1990.
8. Hagege AA, Desnos M, Chachques JC, Carpentier A, et al: Preliminary report: Follow-up after dynamic cardiomyoplasty. *Lancet* 335:1122–1124, 1990.
9. Pattison CW, Cumming DVE, Williamson A, Clayton Jones DG, et al: Aortic coun-

terpulsation for up to 28 days using autologous latissimus dorsi in sheep. *J Thorac Cardiovasc Surg* 102:766–773, 1990.
10. Desrosiers C, Neilson I, Walsh G, Kochamba G, et al: Skeletal muscle-powered counterpulsator. In Chiu RC-J, Bourgeois I (eds): *Transformed Muscle for Cardiac Assist and Repair.* Futura Publishing Company, Inc., Mount Kisco, NY, pp 321–327, 1990.
11. Chachques JC, Grandjean PA, Fischer EI, Latremouille C, et al: Dynamic aortomyoplasty to assist left ventricular failure. *Ann Thorac Surg* 49:225–230, 1990.
12. Mocek FW, Anderson DR, Pochettino A, Hammond RL, et al: Skeletal muscle ventricles in circulation long-term: 191 to 836 days. *J Heart Lung Transplant* 11:S334–340, 1992.
13. Stein PD, Sabbah HN: Measured turbulence and its effect on thrombus formation. *Circ Res* 35:608–614, 1974.
14. Sutera SP, Mehrjardi MH: Deformation and fragmentation of human red cells in turbulent shear flow. *Biophys J* 15:1–10, 1975.
15. Karino T, Goldsmith HL: Rheological factors in thrombosis and haemostasis. In Bloom H, Thomson DP (eds): *Haemostasis and Thrombosis.* Churchill Livingstone, New York, Ch. 24, 1987.
16. Richardson PD: Blood flow in prosthetic devices. *Sci Prog Oxf* 69:375–391, 1985.
17. Shortland AP, Black RA, Jarvis JC, Salmons S: Time-lapsed video imaging of disturbed flow (technical note for submission to *ASME J Biomech Eng*), 1985.
18. Delemarre BJ, Bot H, Pearlman AS, Visser CA, et al: Diastolic flow characteristics of severely impaired left ventricles: A pulsed Doppler ultrasound study. *J Clin Ultrasound* 15:115–119, 1987.
19. Salmons S, Stevenson LW: Adaptive capacity of skeletal muscle and its therapeutic applications. In: Rose FC (ed): *Neuromuscular Stimulation.* Demos Publications, New York, pp 203–215, 1989.

Chapter 47

# Skeletal Muscle Ventricles:

## In Search of Thromboresistant Linings

Gregory A. Thomas, Peter I. Lelkes,
Larry W. Stephenson*

### Introduction

A variety of techniques for the use of skeletal muscle for cardiac assistance are currently being explored.[1–4] One method, cardiomyoplasty, involves wrapping skeletal muscle directly around the heart, where it is then stimulated during cardiac systole in hopes of increasing left ventricular performance.[5,6] Another method is aortomyoplasty. With this technique, the muscle is wrapped around the thoracic aorta; the muscle is then stimulated during diastole, providing aortic counterpulsation.[7] An alternative method of skeletal muscle cardiac assist is the construction of separate pumping chambers, termed skeletal muscle ventricles (SMVs).[8]

SMVs can provide hemodynamically effective cardiac assist[8,9] (Fig. 1). SMVs have functioned as blood pumps in the systemic circulation for over 2 years in a canine model.[10] However, unlike cardiomyoplasty, human trials of SMVs for cardiac assistance have not been attempted. One of the problems associated with SMVs pumping blood in the circulation is blood-surface interactions that lead to thrombosis and thromboembolic complications. In contrast, an advantage to cardiomyoplasty and aortomyoplasty is that unless prosthetic or autogenous material is used to repair a ventricular defect or enlarge the aorta, during these two procedures blood remains at all times in contact with autogenous endothelium. While much focus has been directed toward improving SMV hemodynamic performance, we have also directed major efforts toward solving the problems related to blood-surface interactions in SMVs.

---

*With the cooperation of Dawn M. Chick, Robert L. Hammond, Huiping Lu, Hidehiro Nakajima, Susumu Isoda, Hisako Nakajima.

Supported by NIH Grant HL34778, NIH NRSA HL 08384, and by AHA Grant-in Aid, Wisconsin Chapter.

From Carpentier A, Chachques JC, Grandjean P: Cardiac Bioassist. © Futura Publishing Co, Inc, Armonk, NY, 1997.

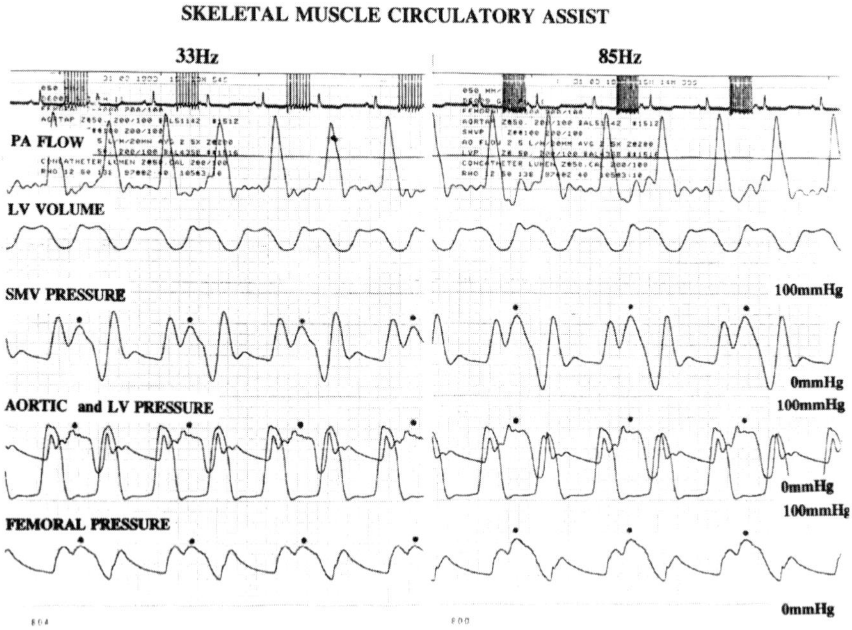


**Figure 1:** *Hemodynamic trace taken from operation with skeletal muscle ventricle (SMV) aortic counterpulsation. An SP1005 Cardiomyostimulator (Medtronic, Inc., Minneapolis, MN) was used to deliver synchronous stimulation at 33 and 85 Hz burst frequencies. Diastolic augmentation is noted by the dots.*

## Skeletal Muscle Ventricles in the Circulation

Acker and coworkers were the first to report on dogs with SMVs functioning chronically in the circulation.[11] They constructed SMVs from the latissimus dorsi (LD) muscle and connected them to the descending thoracic aorta. The muscle was stimulated in diastole to provide aortic counterpulsation. In their series, animals developed renal failure from emboli that came from the SMV lining. Five of these six SMVs were constructed as a tube, with anastomoses at each end, and the SMVs were lined with polytetrafluorethylene (PTFE) (Fig. 2). Thrombus formation occurred at the inlet and outlet orifices of the tube-shaped SMV and these animals died from thromboembolism. The sixth SMV was configured as a blind pouch, and was lined only by the connective tissue reaction that formed around a cone-shaped Teflon mandrel. This dog developed a thrombus at the apex of the pouch on postoperative day 1 by echographic evaluation. This was confirmed on autopsy at day 9.

We have also used skeletal muscle with a pneumatic system to hydraulically transfer the power of muscular contraction to blood pumps lined with polyurethane.[12] SMVs functioned continuously for 3–6 weeks in four dogs. The aortic flow was interrupted in a similar fashion to Acker's model.[16] No dogs died from embolic complications, but evidence of emboli were found in the distal organs of two dogs. The polyurethane lining appeared to have improved thromboresistant characteristics when compared to PTFE, although embolic complications remained problematic.

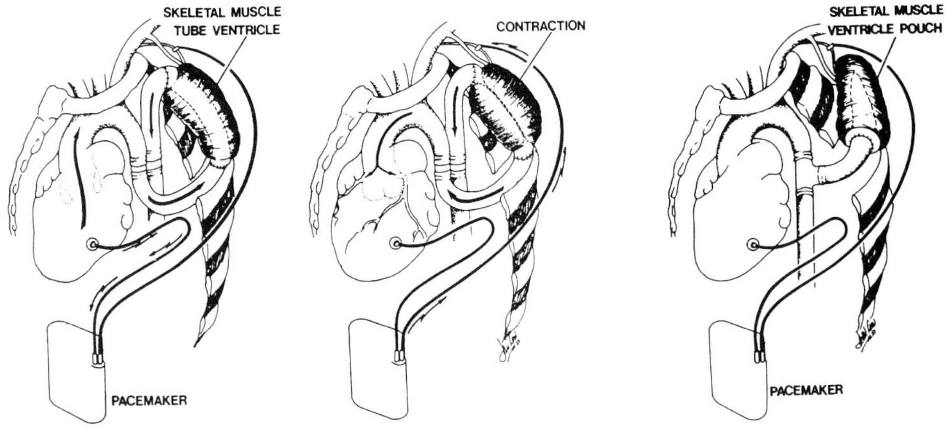


**Figure 2:** *Schematic representation of tube SMV and pouch SMV. During contraction, blood is pumped both toward the heart and distally toward the viscera.*

## Autogenous Linings

Because of this early high incidence of thromboembolism, subsequent investigations focused toward methods to decrease the incidence of this complication in SMVs in the circulation. Complicated anticoagulant regimens were avoided because of potential bleeding complications; for these and other long-term studies of SMVs in the circulation, the only antithrombotic agent employed has been aspirin, 75 mg given on alternate days.

In an effort to provide an even more thromboresistant surface to the SMV, Anderson et al. compared the thrombogenicity of pouch-shaped SMVs lined with the connective tissue lining that formed around the mandrel to those that he lined with either autogenous pleura or pericardium.[13] A pouch shape for SMVs in circulation was chosen in an attempt to improve blood flow characteristics associated with the anastomoses and decrease the rate of embolism. Also, a bifurcated PTFE graft was used and the aorta was ligated between the two limbs of the graft to obligate blood flow into and out of the SMV (Fig. 3). A total of 15 dogs were used in Anderson's study; six SMVs were lined with parietal pleura, four with pericardium, and five by fibrous reaction. Anderson found that thrombus formation occurred in all but three dogs. In the three thrombus-free animals, autogenous pleura was used to line the SMVs. Echographic evaluation demonstrated that thrombus was located the apex of the SMV cavity in the remaining 12 dogs. However, none of these animals had evidence of embolism on autopsy.

Based on these studies, pleural linings appeared to have resulted in improved thromboresistance of SMVs. Additionally, the blind-end pouch design for SMVs appeared to have decreased the rate of embolic complications when compared to the tube-shaped SMV, although adherent thrombus formed frequently at the apex of the SMVs. Long-term studies of SMVs in circulation corroborate these findings. In a report on four dogs surviving long-term, from 6 months to over 2 years, no evidence of embolism was found, even though three of these dogs had laminated thrombus formed at the apex of their SMVs at the time of death.[10]

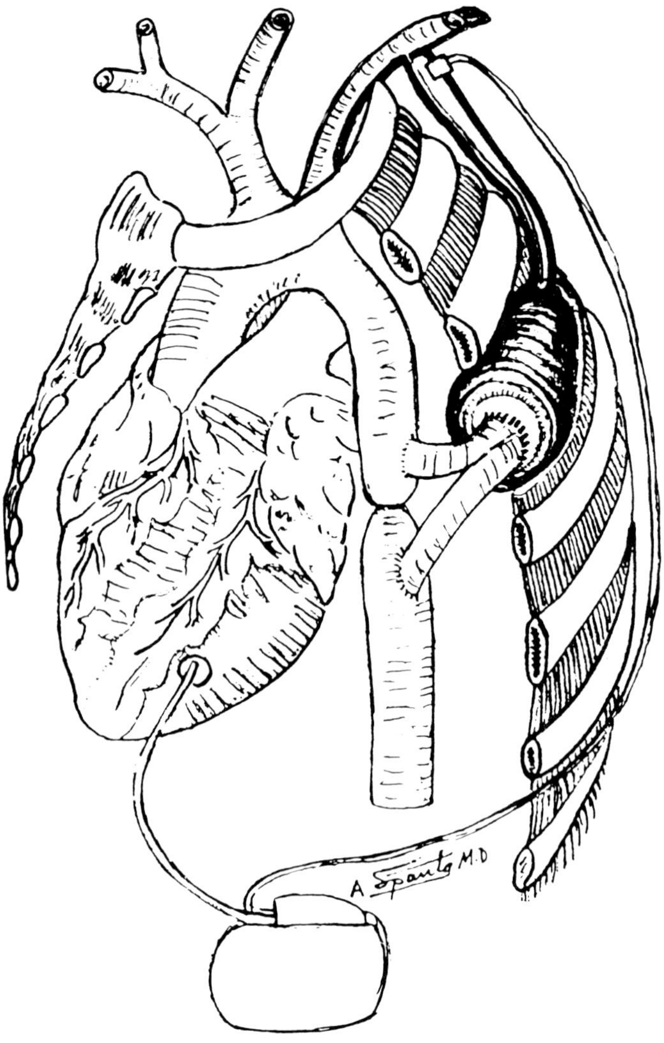


**Figure 3:** *Schematic representation of current aorto-aorto configuration for SMV circulatory assist. The aorta is ligated between the two limbs of the PTFE graft in order to obligate blood flow through the SMV.*

## SMV Design

Although the incidence of embolism is low, further attempts were made to decrease the troublesome incidence of SMV thrombosis. Pochettino and coworkers theorized that the high incidence of apical thrombus formation was due partially to the design configuration of the SMVs.[14] They changed the shape of the SMV mandrel from a conical to an ovoid shape in order to change the blood flow characteristics at the apex and "wash out" stagnant blood with each SMV contraction. No separate autologous lining was used in these SMVs; they were lined only with the fibrous, connective tissue reaction that formed around a Lycra shell mandrel during the several weeks' delay between construction and connection of the SMV to the circulation. Additionally, these SMVs were oriented slightly differently from those in the previous studies, in that the apex of the SMV was constructed using the ventral aspect of the latissimus muscle as opposed to the dorsal aspect as in Anderson's and other previous studies.[13] Thrombus occurred early (before 1 week) in 3 of 12 dogs. Two of these dogs also had evidence at autopsy of renal infarctions. However, in all dogs surviving beyond 1 week, no evidence of thrombus or thromboembolism was noted either on periodic echographic evaluation or at autopsy.

Using similar construction techniques, we have also tested SMVs for right-sided cardiac assistance.[15,16] Niinami evaluated SMVs in the pulmonary circulation, connected between the right ventricle and pulmonary artery, over a 16-week period.[17] Of six dogs surviving more than 1 day, two developed adherent thrombus in the base of the SMV. Although in this study the dogs were also given warfarin postoperatively, it is still a positive finding that none of the animals had evidence of pulmonary embolism after dissection and examination of the pulmonary vasculature.

Recently, Nakajima, et al. completed an extensive histologic evaluation of 44 SMVs that had functioned chronically in the circulation as aortic counterpulsators.[18] These SMVs included those lined with autogenous tissue such as pleura or pericardium, and also those lined only by the fibrous reaction to the mandrel. The overall incidence of thrombosis was 55% for all of the SMVs in circulation. Most of these thrombi were located at either the apex or the base adjacent to the anastomosis of the PTFE conduits of the SMV. Although undocumented, we suspect that these areas most likely represent regions of stagnant blood flow within the SMV. Even though the incidence of SMV thrombosis appears to increase in comparison to Pochettino's study, the amount of thrombus in most of the SMVs was minimal. The presence of thrombus occupying over 5% of the SMV volume occurred in only 25% of animals, similar to Pochettino's study. Only two dogs (4.5%) died from thromboembolic complications.

Further developments in SMV design may still be instrumental in decreasing the rate of thromboembolic phenomenon. Presumably, ligation of the aorta between the two limbs of the bifurcated graft provides for continuous flow of blood in and then out of the SMV through the afferent and efferent conduits during each cardiac beat. This is in contrast to oscillation of blood flow back and forth between the SMV and the aorta that would likely occur with a parallel circuit. Little is known about the blood flow characteristics inside the SMVs. Gamma imaging and other modalities may be useful for studying these characteristics. Computer modeling may provide further refinements in SMV mandrel shape to decrease areas of turbulent and stagnant flow.

## Endothelial Cell Seeding

Although the incidence of thromboembolism remains low in SMVs functioning long-term in the systemic circulation, the overall incidence of thrombosis inside the SMV cavity remains one stumbling block to the clinical application of SMVs. During the past several years while skeletal muscle was being evaluated as a potential power source for cardiac assist, other researchers were investigating methods to provide a thromboresistant lining for vascular grafts. In 1978, Herring, et al. were the first to report endothelial cell seeding of vascular grafts in circulation.[19] They demonstrated improved thromboresistance; 76% of the seeded grafts were thrombus-free compared to a 22% incidence of thrombus formation on the unseeded grafts. Since this landmark study, many others have demonstrated the feasibility of endothelial cell seeding of vascular prostheses, both in animal models and in humans.[20–22] Although this approach has been able to demonstrate improved thromboresistance in small-caliber vascular grafts, endothelial cell seeding is not yet used widely in clinical practice.[23,24]

Thromboembolism has been problematic with assist devices and artificial hearts.[25,26] Because of this, investigators are examining the endothelialization of mechanical blood pumps and artificial hearts.[27,28] While endothelial cells have been seeded onto the material used to line these pumps, prolonged endothelial cell adherence to the artificial surface under shear stress conditions has been a major limiting factor. If successful, endothelial-lined surfaces of mechanical assist devices might markedly increase their long-term applicability.

Recently, Lelkes, et al. have demonstrated the feasibility of seeding endothelial cells onto the fibrous, connective lining that forms around a synthetic foreign body.[29,30] They constructed pouches by placing several silicon mandrels under each LD muscle in six dogs. Autogenous endothelial cells were harvested enzymatically from adipose tissue in accordance with the techniques developed by Williams and colleagues.[31] These cells were then grown in culture and after 4–6 weeks, seeded at high density ($1 \times 10^5$ cells/cm$^2$) back into the latissimus pouches by surgically removing then replacing the mandrel. Four to 6 weeks after seeding, the pouches seeded with autogenous endothelial cells were lined in areas with a single layer of endothelium.

## Techniques for Endothelial Cell Seeding

We have constructed SMVs by exactly the same method that we now use successfully for chronic in-circulation experiments and then seeded these SMVs with endothelial cells.[32] In our first study, 12 SMVs were constructed in dogs from LD muscle using a polypropylene mandrel with a radius of 2 cm and a length of 6 cm with a tapered apex. The volume of the mandrel was 30 ml. The muscle was secured with suture to a Dacron felt sewing ring located at the base of the mandrel. Six to 12 weeks after these SMVs were constructed, nonautologous canine endothelial cells, derived from jugular vein or ventricular endocardium, were seeded at high density into the SMV lumens. The animals were divided into three groups. Group I (n=5) underwent seeding by open extraction of the mandrel and incubation of a cellular suspension of endothelial cells in culture medium. Group II (n=5) underwent seeding by transcutaneous injection of the cellular suspension into the peri-mandrel space. Group III (n=2) remained unseeded as a control. Because nonautologous cells were used, the animals were killed after 1 week in order to examine the inner lining for the presence of an endothelial layer before significant rejection occurred.

Histologic examination using fluorescently labeled endothelial cells revealed the presence of endothelial cells lining the inner surfaces of all seeded SMVs. Several fluorescent labels were used, these included prelabeling endothelial cells with a marker (KLH-2) that is retained over several cell cycles. Additional methods included uptake of diI-acetylated LDL, which is mediated by membrane receptors for acetylated LDL on the endothelial cells.[33] Additionally, antibodies to von Willebrand factor and platelet endothelial cell adhesion molecules (PECAM) were also used to identify endothelial cells by immunofluorescence (Fig. 4). The presence of fluorescence after prelabeling cells with KLH-2 indicates that the cells lining the SMV lumen were mostly derived from the originally seeded cells or their progeny. Only background autofluorescence was noted in the two control SMVs.

The extent of endothelialization of the SMVs varied greatly, from 30–70% of the luminal surface. However, no differences between the two seeding techniques (open versus transcutaneous) were noted in terms of the degree of luminal surface covered with cells or in the morphologic appearance of endothelial cells attached to the SMV. Electron microscopy was also used to examine the nature of the SMV linings. In the control SMVs, an acellular, rough, fibrous surface was present (Figs. 5, 6). In contrast, a smooth, continuous layer of cells was noted on electron microscopic examination of the seeded SMVs (Figs. 7, 8). At high power, ultrastructural analysis revealed Weibel Palade bodies. These are specific to endothelial cells and confirm that the cells lining the SMV lumen are indeed of endothelial origin.

Of concern in this series was the fact that complete endothelialization of the SMVs was not achieved. This may be in part due to the fact that nonautologous canine endothelial cells were used for seeding; decreased cellular coverage is likely due to a combination of decreased growth of cells along with rejection and

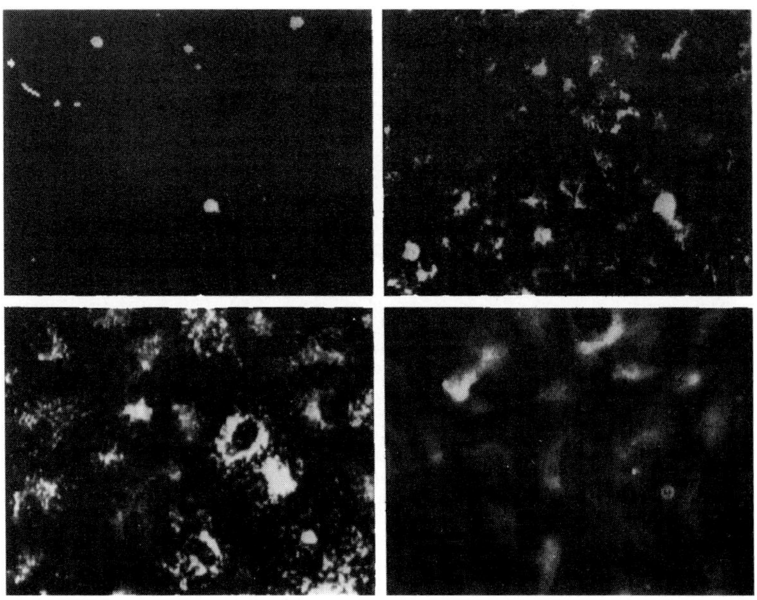

**Figure 4:** *Fluorescent micrograph. Upper left indicates background autofluorescence from an unseeded control. Upper right is staining with von Willebrand factor (Factor VIII-related antigen). Lower left is uptake of fluorescently labeled acetylated LDL. Lower right shows prelabeling with a lipid bound cellular marker (Zynaxis, Philadelphia, PA).*

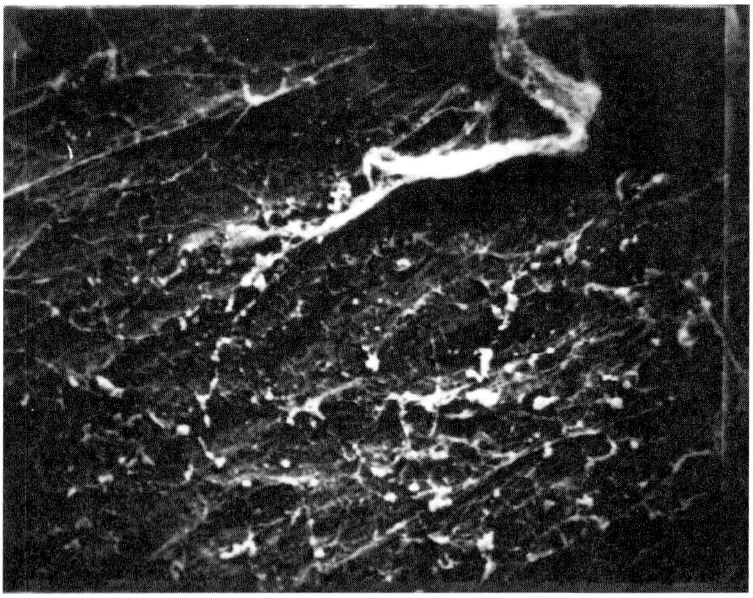

**Figure 5:** *Scanning electron micrograph of an unseeded control SMV. The surface is acellular, and numerous fibers can be seen on the surface.*

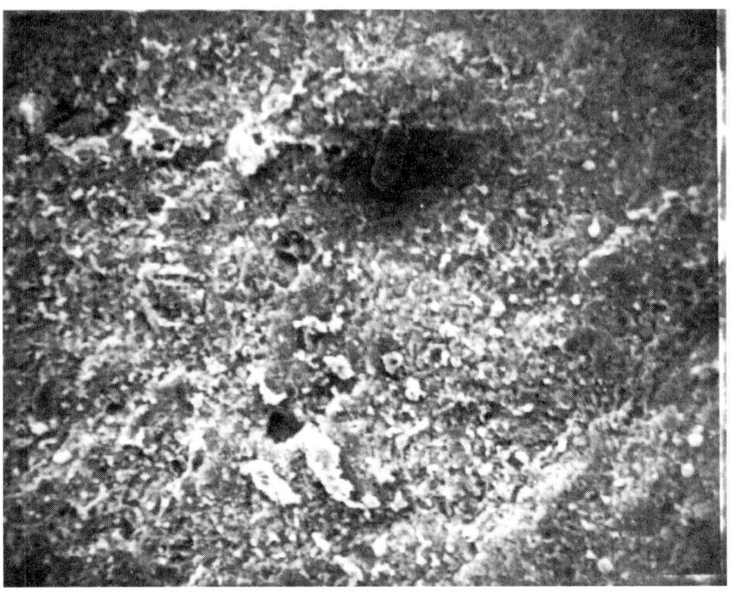

**Figure 6:** *Scanning electron micrograph of a seeded SMV. Although there are a number of blood elements present over the endothelial layer, there is a marked cellularity when compared to the control SMV.*

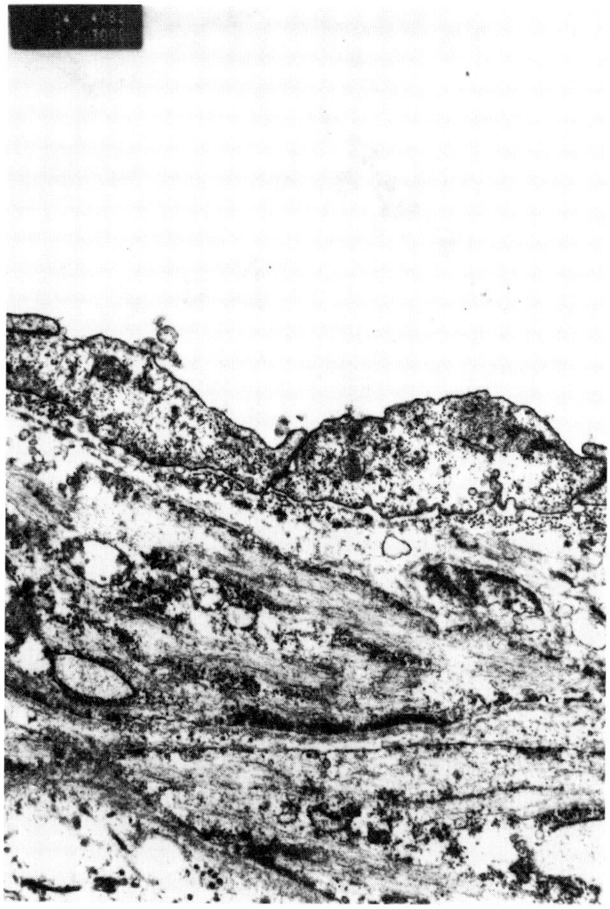

**Figure 7:** *Transmission electron micrograph of seeded SMV. Two endothelial cells are adherent to the luminal wall. There are numerous vacuoles along the basement membrane, and a tight intercellular junction is present between the cells.*

leukocyte-mediated killing of cells that had ahered to the SMV wall. Only 1 week was allowed for the cells to populate the SMV due to the possibility of rejection.

In recent studies, we have used autogenous endothelial cells derived from jugular vein. These cells are harvested enzymatically, then grown in culture. Using the percutaneous method of seeding and allowing 2 weeks for endothelial cell growth, we have been able to achieve 100% coverage of the SMV lumen (unpublished data). Additionally, stimulation of the SMV in situ at 2 Hz for electrical conditioning of the muscle in order to transform it to a fatigue-resistant state does not appear to dislodge the adherent endothelial cells from the basement membrane of fibrous connective tissue.

These experiments show the feasibility of seeding SMVs with a cultured endothelium. In comparison to synthetic, fibrous, or autogenous tissue-lined SMVs, the endothelial-lined SMVs may possess the ideal blood-contacting surface. While the percutaneous seeding technique may have no applicability to-

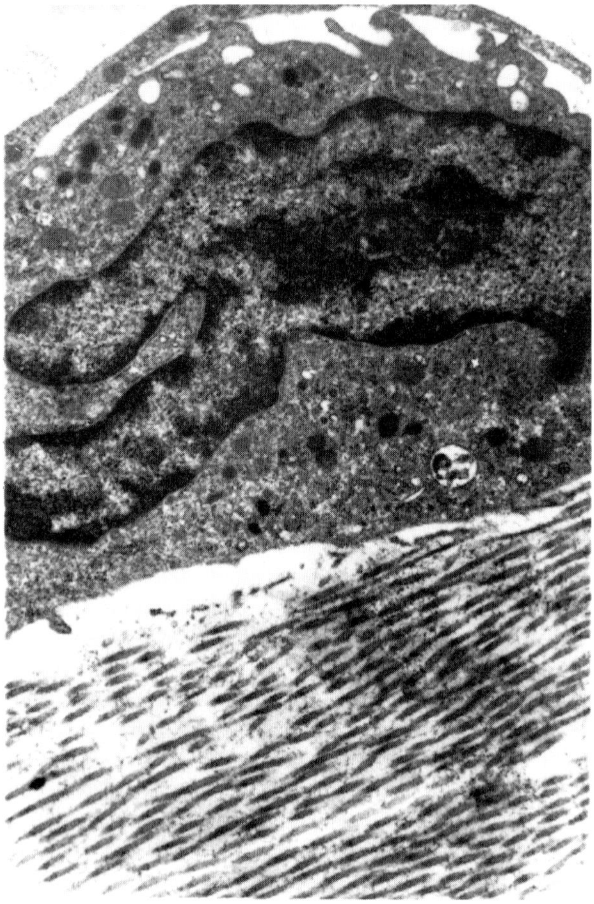

**Figure 8:** *High-power transmission electron micrograph of a single endothelial cell above a layer of fibers, cut partially longitudinally. Only these fibers were present in the unseeded control SMVs.*

ward the endothelialization of other bioprostheses such as vascular grafts, it does simplify the process of seeding SMVs by circumventing an additional operative procedure. In preliminary experiments, we demonstrated uniform staining of the fibrous luminal surface of control SMVs by percutaneous injection of methylene blue. This, in addition to our subsequent results using percutaneous seeding, suggests that this technique is reliable. The exact timing of endothelial cell seeding in the process from SMV construction until connection to the circulation needs to be elucidated. In our experiments, we waited for the induction of a fibrous reaction to the polypropylene mandrel before seeding the SMVs. It may be possible to seed SMVs with autologous endothelial cells at the time of SMV construction and not wait for the fibrous reaction to occur, but it is not yet known whether this will also result in an endothelial monolayer. Additionally, the fibrous layer serves a barrier function, preventing extravasation of blood from the SMV into the surrounding tissues. If the fibrous layer is weak or a small break develops, SMV rupture with exsanguination or pseudoaneurysm formation can occur. Alternatively, SMVs might be seeded with endothelial cells in an open fashion at the time that the SMV is connected to the circulation. Again, it is not known how efficacious this may be in developing a complete monolayer, but single-stage techniques exist for the seeding of vascular grafts.[34] In our hands, transcutaneous injection of the cellular suspension into the extrathoracically constructed SMVs is quick, simple, and apparently effective.

## Advantages of an Endothelial Lining

It remains to be seen whether the endothelialization of SMVs will decrease or eliminate the current incidence of thrombotic complications. A quiescent endothelial monolayer provides the best possible thromboresistant surface. Endothelial cells have been shown to express glycosaminoglycans on their surface that can bind antithrombin III, inhibiting the coagulation cascade.[35] The cells also produce prostacyclin and other factors that inhibit platelet aggregation.[36] However, whether seeded endothelium will exist in a quiescent, antithrombotic state remains to be seen. Recently, numerous studies have elucidated the role of the endothelium in a variety of processes such as the response to inflammation; in vitro work has shown that endothelial cells seeded onto prosthetic vascular grafts express markedly higher numbers of adhesion molecules (ICAM-1, PECAM-1, ELAM-1) on their surface that may contribute to a local, hypercoagulable state.[37] It should still be noted, though, that in vivo studies of small caliber vascular grafts in circulation have shown a decreased incidence of thrombotic occlusion.[41] Therefore, the concept of endothelialization continues to be valid. As the complex interactions between the endothelial cell and other cells become further elucidated, it may be possible to enhance the antithrombotic function of the endothelial cell.

## Retention of Endothelial Cells Under Flow Conditions

It is not clear if an SMV with a seeded endothelial monolayer can withstand the shear stresses of the vascular system. Rosenman et al. showed significant endothelial cell loss from PTFE grafts exposed to in vivo flow conditions.[39] However, pretreatment of graft material with collagen and/or fibronectin increases both the adherence and the retention rates under shear stress conditions.[40, 41] It is likely that the fibrous reaction that is formed around the prosthetic mandrel after SMV construction provides a rich supply of these factors, comprising a much better surface for adherence than artificial grafts. Endothelial cell retention to such a surface under flow conditions remains to be tested.

## Summary

Currently, the incidence of thromboembolism during long-term SMV aortic counterpulsation is low. Although the canine's coagulation system is hypercoaguable in comparison to humans, the risk of embolism due to frequent thrombus formation in the SMV cavity remains problematic. Endothelial cell-lined SMVs must now be tested in the circulation to determine whether this procedure will provide improved thromboresistance. Eliminating thrombus formation inside SMVs represents a major step toward eventual clinical application of this novel form of cardiac assist.

## References

1. Chachques JC, Grandjean PA, Pfeffer TA, et al: Cardiac assistance by atrial or ventricular cardiomyoplasty. *J Heart Trans* 9:239–251, 1990.
2. Chachques JC, Grandjean PA, Fischer CEI, et al: Dynamic aortomyoplasty to assist left ventricular failure. *Ann Thorac Surg* 49:225–230, 1990.
3. Kochamba G, Desrosiers C, Dewar M, Chiu RC-J: The muscle-powered dual-chamber counterpulsator: rheologically superior implantable cardiac assist device. *Ann Thorac Surg* 45:620–625, 1988.
4. Acker MA, Hammond RL, Mannion JD, Salmons S, et al: An autologous biologic pump motor. *J Thorac Cardiovasc Surg* 94:733–746, 1986.
5. Magovern GJ, Park SB, Kao RL, Christlieb IY, et al: Dynamic cardiomyoplasty in patients. *J Heart Trans* 9:258–263, 1990.
6. Hagege AA, Desnos M, Chachques JC, et al: Preliminary report: Follow-up after dynamic cardiomyoplasty. *Lancet* 355:1122–1124, 1990.
7. Chachques JC, Grandjean PA, Carpentier A: Dynamic aortomyoplasty. In Carpentier A, Chachques JC, Grandjean PA (eds): *Cardiomyoplasty*. Mt. Kisco, NY, Futura Publishing Co., 1991, pp 199–208.
8. Pochettino A, Spanta AD, Hammond RL, et al: Skeletal muscle ventricles for total heart replacement. *Ann Surg* 212(3):345–352, 1990.
9. Mannion JD, Acker MA, Hammond RL, Faltemeyer W, et al: Power output of skeletal muscle ventricles in circulation: Short-term studies. *Circulation* 76:155–162, 1987.
10. Mocek FW, Anderson DR, Pochettino A, et al: Skeletal muscle ventricles in circulation long-term: One hundred ninety-one to eight hundred thirty-six days. *J Heart Lung Transplant* 11:S334–S340, 1992.
11. Acker MA, Anderson WA, Hammond RL, et al: Skeletal muscle ventricles in circulation: One to eleven weeks experience. *J Thorac Cardiovasc Surg* 94:163–174, 1987.
12. Anderson WA, Bridges CR, Chin AJ, et al: Pneumatic aortic counterpulsator powered by a skeletal muscle ventricle: 22 to 42 day experience. *Surg Forum* 39:276–277, 1988.
13. Anderson DR, Pochettino A, Hammond RL, et al: Autogenously lined skeletal muscle ventricles in circulation: up to nine months experience. *J Thorac Cardiovasc Surg* 101:661–670, 1991.
14. Pochettino A, Mocek FW, Lu H, et al: Skeletal muscle ventricles with improved thromboresistance: 28 weeks in circulation. *Ann Thorac Surg* 53:1025–1032, 1992.
15. Bridges CR Jr, Woodford EJ, Mora G, Anderson DR, et al: Use of skeletal muscle power to augment the pulmonary circulation. *Surg Forum* 41:267–271, 1990.
16. Niinami H, Hooper TL, Hammond RL, et al: Functional evaluation of intrathoracic versus extrathoracic skeletal muscle ventricles. *J Surg Res* 54:230–236, 1993.
17. Niinami H, Hooper TL, Hammond RL, et al: Skeletal muscle ventricles in the pulmonary circulation: Up to 16 weeks' experience. *Ann Thoracic Surg* 53:750–757, 1992.
18. Nakajima H, Thomas GA, Nakajima HO, et al: Skeletal muscle ventricles as aortic diastolic counterpulsators. *Texas Heart Inst J* 20:105–111, 1993.
19. Herring MB, Gardner AL, Glover JL: A single stage technique for seeding vascular grafts with autogenous endothelium. *Surgery* 84:498–504, 1978.

20. Herring MB, Baughman S, Glover JL: Endothelium develops on seeded human arterial prosthesis: A brief clinical report. *J Vasc Surg* 2:727–730, 1985.
21. Park PK, Jarrell BE, Williams SK, et al: Thrombus-free human endothelial surface in the midregion of a Dacron vascular graft in the splanchnic circuit: Observations after nine months of implantation. *J Vasc Surg* 11:468–475, 1990.
22. Kobayashi H, Kabuto M, Ide H, Hosotani K, et al: An artificial blood vessel with an endothelial monolayer. *J Neurosurg* 77:397–402, 1992.
23. Graham LM, Stanley JC, Burkel WE: Improved patency of endothelial cell seeded long knitted Dacron and ePTFE vascular prosthesis. *ASAIO J* 8:65–73, 1985.
24. Sank A, Rostami K, Weaver F, et al: New evidence and new hope concerning endothelial cell seeding of vascular grafts. *Am J Surg* 164:199–204, 1992.
25. Rokitansky A, Wolner E: Cardiac support and mechanical cardiac replacement. *Internat J Artif Organs* 14:387–392, 1991.
26. DeVries WC: The permanent artificial heart: Four case reports. *JAMA* 259:849–859, 1988.
27. Bernhard WF: A fibrillar blood prosthetic interface for both temporary and permanent ventricular assist devices: Experimental and clinical observations. *Artif Organs* 12:89–111, 1988.
28. Lelkes PI, Samet MM: Endothelialization of the luminal sac in artificial cardiac prosthesis: A challenge for both biologists and engineers. *J Biomechanical Engineering* 113:132–142, 1991.
29. Lelkes PI, Samet MM, Christensen CC, Amrani DL: Factitious angiogenesis: Endothelialization of artificial cardiovascular prostheses. In Maragoudakis ME, Guillino P, Lelkes PI (eds): *Angiogenesis in Health and Disease.* New York, Plenum Press, 1992, pp 339–353.
30. Lelkes PI, Gao H, Edgerton JR, Christensen CW: Endothelial cell seeding of latissimus dorsi muscle pouches. *J Surg Res* 57:460–469, 1993.
31. Rupnick MA, Hubbard FA, Pratt K, Jarrell BE, et al: Endothelialization of vascular prosthetic surfaces after seeding or sodding with human microvascular endothelial cells. *J Vasc Surg* 9:778, 1991.
32. Thomas GA, Lelkes PI, Chick DM, et al: Endothelial lined skeletal muscle ventricles: Open and percutaneous seeding techniques. *J Cardiac Surg* 10:245–256, 1995.
33. Voyta JC, Via DP, Butterfield CE, Zetter BR: Identification and isolation of endothelial cells based on their increased uptake of acetylated-low density lipoprotein. *J Cell Bio* 99:2034, 1984.
34. Williams SK, Jarrell BE, Rose DG, et al: Human microvessel endothelial cell isolation and vascular graft sodding in the operating room. *Ann Vasc Surg* 3:468–475, 1989.
35. Marcum JA, Rosenberg RD: Heparin-like molecules with anticoagulant activity are synthesized by cultured endothelial cells. *Biochem Biophys Res Comm* 126:365–372, 1985.
36. Weksler BB, Marcus AJ, Jaffe EA: Synthesis of prostaglandin I2 (prostacyclin) by cultured human and bovine endothelial cells. *Proc Natl Acad Sci* 74:3922–3926, 1977.
37. Margiotta MS, Robertson FS, Greco RS: The adherence of endothelial cells to Dacron induces the expression of the intercellular adhesion molecule (ICAM-1). *Ann Surg* 216:600–604, 1992.
38. Ortenwall P, Wadenvik H, Kutti J, Risberg B: Endothelial cell seeding reduces thrombogenicity of Dacron grafts in humans. *J Vasc Surg* 11:403–410, 1990.
39. Rosenman JE, Kempczinski RF, Pearce WH, Silberstein WB: Kinetics of endothelial cell seeding. *J Vasc Surg* 2:778–784, 1985.
40. Radomski JS, Jarrell BE, Williams SK, Koolpe EA, et al: Initial adherence of human capillary endothelial cells to Dacron. *J Surg Res* 42:133–140, 1987.
41. Ramalanjaona G, Kempczinski RF, Rosenman JE, Douville C, et al: The effect of fibronectin coating on endothelial cell kinetics in polytetrafluoroethylene grafts. *J Vasc Surg* 3:264–272, 1986.

# Part VI

## Cellular and Molecular Bioassist

Chapter 48

# Cellular and Molecular Cardiomyoplasty:

## New Approaches to Regenerate Lost Cardiac Muscle

Audrius Zibaitis, Ray C.-J. Chiu, Race L. Kao

### Introduction

Congestive heart failure is a major killer in developed countries.[1] This is related to the inability of adult cardiac myocytes to divide and repair damaged heart muscle. An irreversible injury to the heart muscle cells tips over nature's balance between cardiac muscle and nonmuscle cells, causing overload on the remaining myocytes, which finally leads to their demise. Recent basic and applied research in aiding the failing heart has led to a wide array of treatment methods such as artificial heart, mechanical assist devices, and cardiomyoplasty.

In this chapter, we attempt to review the current knowledge and new approaches to regenerate lost cardiac muscle tissue. "Cellular cardiomyoplasty" is an approach to implant cells and grow new muscle fibers in the damaged myocardium that potentially may contribute to the contractile performance of the heart. "Molecular cardiomyoplasty" direction gears toward the induction of cardiomyocytes to reenter the cell cycle, as well as the introduction of myogenic transcription factor genes into nonmuscle cells of the heart with the aim to convert them into cardiac myocytes. Both methods represent novel approaches to combat the problem of chronic heart failure.

### Development of Cardiac Muscle and Myocardial Adaptive Response to the Injury

At the beginning of the third week of human embryo development, some mesenchymal cells from the primitive streak migrate along the notochordal

Supported by grants from the Quebec Heart and Stroke Foundation, the Medical Research Council of Canada, and the National Institute of Health.

From Carpentier A, Chachques JC, Grandjean P: Cardiac Bioassist. © Futura Publishing Co, Inc, Armonk, NY, 1997.

process toward the cranial end of the embryo. Migrating cells meet at the cranial end of the notochordal process where they form a cardiogenic area that becomes the origin of the future heart tissue. At the end of the third week, cardiac myocytes form two parallel endothelial tubes that fuse to form a primitive tubular heart. Soon afterwards, cardiac myoblasts joined by specific desmosomal adhesion sites-gap junctions form a synchronously beating cardiac tissue. Endocardium is formed by endothelial cells, which rest on the cardiac jelly layer and cover primitive heart lumen. Gradual disappearance of cardiac jelly, which is interposed between endothelial cells and myocardium, eventually brings endothelial cells in close contact with the inner layer of the myocardium. The spaces among cardiac myocytes are then invaded by mesenchymal cells, which form intracardial connective tissue.[2] Epicardium is formed by mesodermal cells migrating from the sinus venosus region over the entire surface of the myocardium. This process takes place during the periods of cardiac looping and septation.[3]

Embryonic cardiac myocytes demonstrate a distinct ability to simultaneously combine mitotic and differentiation events. Light and electron microscopy as well as radioautographic studies have demonstrated that cardiac muscle cells with cytoplasmic myofilaments undergo mitotic cell division. However, a few weeks after birth, mitotic activity in ventricular cardiac myocytes ceases and only hypertrophic growth of myocytes along with hyperplasia of nonmuscle cells accounts for the postnatal growth of the heart.[4]

However, not all adult heart muscle cells seem to be under nature's ban on cell division. Radioactive thymidine incorporation studies have shown that adult atrial myocytes, if challenged with an overload due to an injury of the ventricle, enter the mitotic cycle and respond to the increased work demand by myocyte hyperplasia.[5] The Simian virus 40 (SV40) large tumor antigen is also known to be able to initiate a proliferation program in atrial myocytes in vitro and likewise in vivo.[6,7]

Some animals standing on the evolution ladder beneath mammalians appear to have no restrictions regarding the proliferative potential of mature ventricular myocytes. Amphibians, particularly frogs and newts, are capable of restoring functional myocardium following an injury, which in some cases is as drastic as crushing or amputation of part of a ventricle.[8,9]

Mammalian ventricular myocytes respond to an increased load by nuclear division and cytoplasmic growth of the preexisting myocytes. Such processes lead to the appearance of polyploid muscle cells with increased cytoplasmic volume. The degree of ploidity increases in mammalian heart muscle with age, and it has been estimated that close to 80% of adult cardiac myocytes are polyploid.[4] Unfortunately, for yet unknown reasons, enduring hypertrophy of the heart exhausts compensatory mechanisms and eventually evolves into congestive heart failure.

It is of interest that cardiac myocytes, if stimulated by different stimuli such as overload, adrenergic agents, angiotensin II, endothelin-1, and growth factors, will begin to hypertrophy by recapitulating a certain embryonic developmental program. This leads to the ventricular expression of embryonic isoforms of contractile proteins as well as the expression of atrial natriuretic factor,[10] which in the adult heart is restricted to the atria only.[11,12]

Regenerating skeletal muscle, which rebuilds itself from skeletal myoblasts (satellite cells), also expresses embryonic protein isoforms.[13] These observations suggest that certain parts of the embryonic developmental pathway are still available for differentiated tissues, such as striated muscle. Therefore, it is of interest to explore whether it can be possible to manipulate these processes and alter phenotypic expression of striated muscle cells which could have possible therapeutic applications.

## Development of Skeletal Muscle and Skeletal Muscle Myogenic (Satellite) Cells

Skeletal muscle is formed from the embryonic mesodermal cells. In approximately 20-day-old human embryo, mesodermal cells aggregate into the first pair of somites. Cells within the lateral mesoderm follow further division into two planes of somatic and splanchnic mesoderm. The latter will eventually undergo compartmentalization and form three layers dubbed as dermatome, myotome, and sclerotome. It appears that induction of mesodermal cells to form skeletal muscle is influenced by nearby structures, such as the notochord and neural tube.[14] Fibroblast growth factor and transforming growth factor beta families are potent inducers of embryonic cells as well.[15] Cells within myotome are already committed to the myogenic lineage and soon acquire an elongated shape. Limb buds subsequently are populated by myoblasts migrating from the lateral parts of the myotome. There is a mechanistic subdividing of embryonic skeletal muscle cells into primary and secondary myoblasts. Following a few rounds of division within their destination area, primary myoblasts commence a muscle differentiation program, initiate expression of structural muscle isoforms, and fuse to form a sparse network of primary myotubes. This is followed by the secondary myoblast adherence to the primary myotubes, which act as templates for building a bulk of secondary myotubes surrounding primary ones in a concentric fashion. Despite the close contact between both types of myoblasts, there is a specific recognition method in place which favors fusion of the muscle cells allocated to the same subtype.[16]Although at this period of development, a group of cells is intensively dividing and creating a large pool of muscle cells to join myotubes, some myoblasts for yet undiscovered reasons appear to escape the terminal differentiation phase. These cells, which presumably are destined to become satellite cells, adhere to the myotubes and remain in quiescent stem cell phenotype for the remaining time of muscle development.[17,18]

Skeletal myogenic (satellite) cells were first described by Mauro in 1961.[19] Electronmicroscopy revealed that they are situated on the sarcolemma of the mature skeletal muscle fiber and sheltered with basal lamina from outside. Satellite cells are small cells (ca 25-30 μm in length)[20] with a small amount of cytoplasm, and have a relatively high nuclear/cytoplasmic ratio. The paucity of cytoplasmic organelles in satellite cells suggests their dormant status. Rough endoplasmic reticulum is not prominent, suggesting a low level of ribosomal function. The Golgi complex is poorly expressed as well. Nuclei of satellite cells are somewhat more heterochromatic than nuclei propria of the muscle fiber.[21] Another distinct morphological feature of these cells is the presence of caveoli on their plasma membrane, which participate in the uptake of ions and other small molecules. Moreover, these structures are thought to be areas rich in Ca++ pump proteins, and play a role in thyrosine phosphorylation signaling.[22,23] Activated satellite cells dramatically increase the quantity and volume of cytoplasmic organelles, which are essential for these myogenic cells to multiply and repair injured muscle.

It has been estimated that satellite cells comprise about 4% of all nuclei in the muscle fibers.[24] Although these myogenic cells inhabit the whole myofiber, the majority of them reside at the neuromuscular junction sites where they are in close contact with motor end-plates.[25]

Satellite cells remain in quiescent status until their host muscle fiber is challenged with an injury or other factors (cytokines, exercise, etc.).[26,27] Such a disturbance of environment prompts satellite cells to enter a mitotic cell cycle. The regenerative capacity of satellite cells is approaching that of a true stem cell. It is estimated that one skeletal myogenic cell has the potential to produce up to $10^{17}$ of progeny cells.[28]

Localized injury to the myofiber activates satellite cells positioned not only in close vicinity of the damaged area, but also on the distant myofibers as well. Studies on myogenic transcription factors have shown that, in case of injury to the skeletal muscle, the appearance of these early myogenic markers precede the mitotic activity of satellite cells. Furthermore, these factors become expressed even in the satellite cells residing away from the injured site.[29] Some controversies still persist regarding the ability of satellite cells to cross basal lamina which encloses them and thus, it is believed, interferes with the possible myoblast contribution to myofibers other than its own. However, there is a growing collection of data arguing that satellite cells possess the migratory ability that can be a valuable feature in recruiting neighboring myogenic cells to repair injured skeletal muscle fibers.[30,31]

The "repairing" feature of satellite cells is not strictly applied to postnatal myocytes. Satellite cells and embryonic myoblasts recognize each other and fuse together, forming mixed myotubes in vitro.[32] Earlier studies also suggested that myoblasts have a certain degree of willingness to form heterokaryonic muscle fibers. Studies on patients with Duchenne muscle dystrophy showed that skeletal myoblasts of heterogenic origin can fuse with the host's myofibers and contribute to the expression of structural proteins.[33] When myoblasts of genetically different animal species were co-cultured in vitro, muscle cells of both species contributed to the formation of "mosaic" myofibers.[34] The above-mentioned and other observations prompted ideas for exploring satellite cell regenerative potential in restoring damaged cardiac muscle.[35]

## Factors Influencing Differentiation of Myogenic Cells

The major breakthrough in determining the control of the skeletal muscle program came upon discovery of myogenic regulatory factors. So far there are four members known that belong to this family of nuclear transcription proteins. The first member, MyoD, was discovered in 1987 when Davis and colleagues[36] introduced a specific cDNA sequence into the 10T1/2 fibroblasts, and showed that this genetic maneuver can convert fibroblasts into the cells exhibiting a skeletal muscle phenotype. The genomic sequence used was determined by the screening of a distinct mRNA present in 10T1/2 fibroblasts treated with 5-azacytidine, an antitumor agent affecting the DNA methylation process and subsequently gene expression.[37]

The other discovered members of the myogenic determination factor (MyoD) family are myogenin,[38] myf-5,[39] and MRF-4,[40] also known as myf-6 or herculin. All four proteins belong to the ubiquitously present group of helix-loop-helix (HLH) proteins. These molecules have a particular structure that consists of two amphipathic helices situated within the core region, joined by a loop segment.[41] All MyoD family proteins, as well as some other members of the HLH family, have an additional structure, a "basic region," in their N-amino terminal end. Therefore, HLH proteins possessing a basic region are referred to as basic-helix-loop-helix (bHLH) factors. The basic region of bHLH factors has the ability to bind DNA, which gives these molecules the capacity to act as nuclear transcription factors, e.g., activate specific gene transcription programs. Along with the capacity to control muscle cells, myogenic bHLH proteins established themselves as being able to alter the phenotypic fate of non-muscle cells as well. A variety of cells other than muscle respond to the driving force of MyoD factors, which can convert them into the muscle cells.[41]

MyoD members have conserved sequences among vertebrates and many invertebrates which support the ancient ancestry of these genes. Myogenic regulatory genes originating from invertebrates are able to commence the myogenic program in mammalian cells as well. Sea urchin myogenic factor 1, SUM-1, as well as CeMyoD, nematode *Caenorhabditis elegans* myogenic protein, when introduced into the mammalian 10T1/2 fibroblasts, effectively converted them into muscle cells, which subsequently fused and formed myotubes.[42,43] This shows that the muscle gene activation pathway has been well preserved throughout the evolution process.

Basic HLH proteins, including MyoD family members, interact with DNA through association between their basic region and a distinctive DNA site, termed E-box. This DNA sequence, targeted by basic HLH proteins, is present in skeletal muscle genes (muscle creatine kinase, acetylcholine receptor $\alpha$-subunit genes, etc.),[44,45] as well as in other otherwise unrelated genes.[46] It was discovered that all bHLH proteins have the ability to bind E-boxes, but only the MyoD family member interaction with these DNA structures is able to activate the myogenic program.

Myogenic activity of MyoD factors is affected by dimerization with other HLH molecules. Some of them, referred to as E2-proteins, are ubiquitously expressed products of the E2A gene. Similar to the MyoD factors, E2-proteins belong to the bHLH family. Dimerization between bHLH peptides involves joining the helix regions which evokes conformational change in both participating proteins, bringing basic regions together and creating an interface ready for recognition and binding of E-box.[46] Although MyoD factors can bind DNA on their own, the affinity of such an interaction is tenfold lower when compared to similar DNA binding by MyoD and E2-protein complex.[47]

However, not all the members of the HLH group play a role of positive MyoD enhancers. Inhibition of myogenesis is in part attributed to an association of bHLH factors with another HLH member, inhibitor of differentiation (Id). This molecule displays helix-loop-helix structure, but lacks a DNA-binding basic region. Since it has functional HLH domain, it can form heterodimers with E2-proteins. Subsequently, the lack of a basic region on one side abolishes the ability of such a complex to recognize and interact with the E-box. Id proteins, if present in abundance, compete for E2 factors, and in this way heterodimerization partners for MyoD transcriptional factors become depleted. In accordance with this, high levels of Id factor have been detected in proliferating myoblasts, but as differentiation proceeds, the expression of this protein becomes silenced.[48] Therefore, Id might contribute to retaining undifferentiated phenotype in myoblasts.

The question regarding the purpose of extensive redundancy in the myogenic program remains unanswered. A complex view of interrelation among myogenic factors emerges where MyoD members can up-regulate each other's expression as well as its own.

The earliest factor appearing in somitogenesis is myf-5. The polymerase chain reaction technique detected myf-5 mRNA expression even prior to the formation of myotome. Myogenin and MyoD appearance follow shortly after myf-5, and is accompanied by MRF-4 mRNA production which then becomes the most abundant myogenic factor in skeletal muscle.[49,50] Of interest is the fact that data that forced expression of myf-5 in transgenic animals can result in ectopic formation of skeletal muscle tissue.[51] All of these findings argue that myf-5 is the earliest muscle determination factor influencing expression of other MyoD members.

Genetic knockout experiments in mice revealed that despite an appreciable redundancy in the performance of the MyoD family regulators, each member seems to play a distinct role in myogenesis. Homozygous MyoD mutants demonstrated increased myf-5 expression which led to normal formation of skeletal muscle.[52] Likewise, transgenic mice with null mutations of myf-5 gene were able to form muscle tissue as well, perhaps under the influence of intact MyoD.[53] The remaining factors, myogenin and MRF-4, in myf-5 null mice were also absent until the appearance of the MyoD protein which conceivably stimulated their expression.[54] However, in double knockout experiments, mice lacking both MyoD and myf-5 showed no morphological signs of skeletal muscle, and no muscle messenger RNAs along with their encoded proteins were detected.[55] Similar experiments in mice carrying mutations in the myogenic gene did not affect myotome formation, and skeletal myoblast appearance proceeded as usual. Nevertheless the skeletal muscle formation was dramatically affected due to disturbance in secondary myotube genesis. MRF-4 knockout impedes morphogenesis of the ribs, but does not interfere with the generation of skeletal muscle.[56] These discoveries led to the more complex myogenesis concept in which MyoD and myf-5 are interchangeable, but either one is absolutely required for the commitment of embryonic mesodermal cells to myogenic lineage. Myogenin emerged as an essential factor controlling later steps of myogenesis. [57]

There are many more myogenic factors that do not belong to the MyoD nuclear regulator family but can cooperate in MyoD-directed muscle induction through a pathway different from that of E-box. One such representative is a myocyte enhancer factor 2 (MEF-2). It is a member of the RSRF family (related to serum response factor) ubiquitously expressed in mammalian cells.[58,59] Structural muscle gene transcription is regulated by MyoD factor-dependent E-box binding. In addition, binding sites for MEF-2 regulator protein were detected in a few structural muscle genes (muscle creatine kinase, myosin light chain 1/3) as well, and it is most likely to participate in the activation of these tissue-specific genes. [60] Some muscle-specific genes in cardiac and skeletal muscles are influenced mainly by MEF-2 site, but not E-box binding.[61] Furthermore, MEF-2 binding sites were revealed to be within the regulatory elements of MyoD members, myogenin and MyoD.[62] Since these sites and other DNA binding sequences are within close range of each other, they might contribute to the stability of E-box-dependent binding.[63] These data support the view that the muscle differentiation program is under much more complex control involving more nuclear transcription factors than those of the MyoD family alone.

Growth factor effect on skeletal muscle cell proliferation and differentiation is implemented through myogenic regulatory factors. Basic fibroblast growth factor (bFGF) is a potent inhibitor of differentiation and is highly mitogenic to myoblasts. Its effect is thought to be mediated through a protein kinase C (PKC) pathway. This signal transduction enzyme is situated in the cytoplasm, and when activated is able to transfer a signal from the cell membrane receptors to the nucleus.[64] Experimental data with the constitutively active PKC showed that this protein is able to suppress the myogenic program driven by the MyoD regulators. Furthermore, bFGF evoked a phosphorylation process of a specific site in the myogenin basic DNA-binding region. This was implicated in rendering myogenin inactive and allowing myoblasts to continue to proliferate.[65] Alternatively, other bFGF pathways in control of the myogenic program have been proposed in which interaction of muscle transcription factors with other intracellular proteins might influence myogenesis.[27] In particular, myc, ras, fos, jun, and other proto-oncogenes are able to halt or reverse the myogenic differentiation program initiated by the MyoD family.[66,67] bFGF might affect myoblast differentiation through induction of Id. Increased concentration of serum stimulates production of Id, which preferentially associates with E2-proteins, leaving no heterodimerization partners for MyoD.[47]

Transforming growth factor beta (TGF-$\beta$) extends its inhibitory effect on skeletal muscle cells[68] through mechanisms other than these involving PKC. TGF-$\beta$ does not suppress either MyoD production or its capability to bind DNA. Although the exact mechanism of this process is still unknown, the available evidence demonstrates that TGF-$\beta$ repression of MyoD family activity is achieved through interfering with E-box-specific binding by myogenic bHLH proteins.[69] Insulin-like growth factors (IGFs) have a role in controlling myogenic transcription factors as well. Serum withdrawal from skeletal myoblast culture medium induces autoproduction of IGF-I in myoblasts which in turn activates myogenic expression and leads to rapid differentiation events.[70,71]

Extracellular matrix (ECM) elements, especially those involved in structural composition of muscle basal lamina, tremendously influence the development and differentiation events of myoblasts. Laminin is one of the major components of ECM, which signals the cells through engagement of integrins, representing a class of cell adhesion molecules.[72] Some members of the integrin family are shown to participate in myogenesis. $\alpha4\beta1$ integrin and its counterpart, vascular cell adhesion molecule 1 (VCAM-1), play a critical role in secondary myotube formation where primary myotubes serve as a guiding template for building the bulk of the muscle.[16]

Homotypic cell adhesion molecules, such as NCAM and M-, and N-cadherins, mediate cell-cell adhesion processes among myoblasts, and perhaps hold a great deal of control in cell-cell recognition processes during myogenesis and muscle regeneration events.[73-75] Therefore, muscle differentiation is orchestrated by a large array of various factors, and the sum effect of their influence subsequently translates into proliferation or differentiation events in skeletal myoblasts.

## Factors Contributing to Differentiation of Cardiac Myocytes

Although both types of striated muscle (skeletal and cardiac) share many common features, their differentiation programs appear to have a different pathway.

Contrary to the skeletal muscle where MyoD family transcription factors initiate the myogenic program, developmental fate of cardiac myocytes do not seem to be controlled by these myogenic regulators. Analysis of promoters responsible for determining the cardiac muscle phenotype supports this view. It was demonstrated that different regions of the same promoter are required to produce identical contractile protein isoforms in cardiac myocytes as compared to skeletal muscle.[76] Studies performed thus far demonstrated that MyoD proteins are not expressed in cardiac myocytes. Thus, there should be alternative ways for cardiac myocytes to achieve a morphological structure similar to that of the skeletal muscle.

Some of the nuclear factors participating in the transcription of structural muscle genes are the same in both types of muscles. The MEF-2 factor is thought to play a role in the activation of the skeletal muscle program, accomplishing this by cooperating with the bHLH regulatory factors. Muscle isoform of phosphoglycerate mutase (PGAM) enzyme involved in glycolytic reactions in striated muscle is controlled solely by an MEF-2 factor in cardiac as well as in skeletal muscle cells.[61] In addition, MEF-2 participates in transcriptional regulation of cardiac structural genes, such as alpha-cardiac myosin heavy chain and beta-myosin heavy chain.[77]

Homeobox transcription factors controlling embryo body plane specification, as well as migration, differentiation, and proliferation processes in a variety of cells, are also involved in heart muscle genesis.[78,79] Of interest is MHox/Phox homeobox protein which is involved in creatinine kinase M gene regulation, and activates this gene in cardiac and skeletal muscle cells through cooperation with myogenic HLH transcription factors.[80]

Despite the lack of overt evidence for the existence of the MyoD-like muscle regulatory pathway, some experimental data provide a hint for the possible involvement of basic HLH proteins in developmental regulation of cardiomyocytes. The complex of the MyoD family members with E2-proteins is known to bind DNA E-boxes which regulate the activity of the structural muscle genes.

Similar complexes were found to be able to bind cardiac $\alpha$-actin promoter, implying the existence of functional E-boxes within this cardiac regulatory sequence.[81] Another group of investigators demonstrated that antibodies raised against the MyoD1 helix segment reacted with an unknown protein expressed early in the developing chick heart. Moreover, this protein was able to recognize the muscle creatinine kinase DNA sequence containing an E-box.[82] Therefore, despite broad differences in molecular regulatory mechanisms of myogenic programs, heart and skeletal muscles might have similar principles and share similar regulatory factors involved in the implementation of muscle formation.

## Experimental Attempts to Restore Lost Cardiac Muscle Tissue

### Molecular Cardiomyoplasty: Gene Transfer into the Cardiac Cells

It is an attractive idea that instead of replacing the whole heart with a mechanical device, one may bring back to life contractile heart cells that were lost to the disease. Some attempts in this field concentrate on the awakening of the myocardial ability to reenter the cell cycle and thus create a larger pool of muscle cells. There is a strong feeling in the research community that cardiac myocytes have not lost their competence for cytokinesis, but this feature is under negative control of yet undiscovered factors. Experiments with transgenic mice demonstrated that under specific conditions it is possible to induce cytokinesis of some myocardial cells in vivo. The simian virus 40 (SV40) large tumor antigen gene, which has a capacity to stimulate DNA replication,[83] was coupled to a promoter sequence of atrial natriuretic factor, which is constitutively expressed in atrial myocytes. Following the introduction of this genetic construct into fertilized mice eggs, investigators obtained mice that developed atrial hyperplasia. Morphologically, muscle cells looked similar to the normal atrial myocytes and there was no local tumor outgrowth.[6] Similar results in rat ventricles were obtained when ventricular myocytes were targeted with another genomic construct producing SV40 protein.[84] Although these experiments have demonstrated that cardiac muscle cells can be induced to enter the cell cycle, the possibility of uncontrollable growth of oncogene-stimulated myocytes poses a serious risk for a patient and therefore some other methods to activate a replication program should be sought.

Another direction of research concentrating on revitalizing heart muscle has been called "molecular cardiomyoplasty." The concept of this approach is to turn back the altered ratio of connective-to-muscle tissue in favor of the cardiac muscle cells. With the discovery of the myogenic regulatory factors, there has been much interest in the introduction of myogenic master genes into nonmuscle cells of the heart. If successful, such an attempt would transform noncontracting cells into a desirable contractile tissue. In vitro studies have already been done where MyoD gene coupled to a retroviral vector was introduced into primary cardiac fibroblasts obtained from newborn rat ventricles. Nonmuscle cells transduced by this method altered their shape into an elongated one, and following serum withdrawal, fused together forming multinucleated myotubes, a morphological feature specific to skeletal muscle. Immunocytochemical evaluation of the

MyoD-converted cardiac fibroblasts demonstrated the appearance of MEF-2, another myogenic transcription factor, as well as expression of myosin heavy chain protein.[85] Despite the promising results, some questions regarding this approach still remain. There is no knowledge yet of which genes play master roles in directing the cardiac myogenic program. Therefore, there is no suitable candidate yet that can be used for cardiac fibroblast conversion into cardiac muscle cells. Furthermore, a gene delivery system targeting only nonmuscle cells has to be developed.

## Cellular Cardiomyoplasty: Muscle Cell Implantation into the Heart

The cellular cardiomyoplasty procedure has the goal of presenting the cardiac muscle with more myocytes derived from outside of the heart that will eventually be able to contribute to the contractile performance of the failing organ.

Since the fetal cardiac tissue is still in the stage of vigorous cell cycling, it offers the prospect of being used as a source of neocardiomyocytes. Indeed, Field's group working with mice embryonic cardiac muscle cells[86] brought true excitement into the field of myocardial regeneration. They showed that fetal cardiac myocytes grafted into adult mice formed stable long-term implants. More importantly, electron microscopy revealed that implanted cardiomyocytes joined host muscle cells by intercalated discs, thus establishing the likelihood that the implanted fetal myocytes may join the myocardial electrical network. Although technically this approach is very promising, it has serious drawbacks for clinical use, such as the need to obtain human embryonic cardiac tissue and the potential for immunorejection.

To avoid the problem of implant tissue availability, myogenic cell lines have also been used in attempts to restore cardiac muscle. AT-1 cell line is a cardiac muscle cell line derived from SV40 transformed atrial myocytes. When implanted into syngeneic rat myocardium, these cells have developed into a structural cardiac muscle. However, as measured by radioactive thymidine uptake, AT-1 cells retained the quality of uncontrolled proliferation and were not coupled through gap junctions to the syncytium of host cardiac myocytes.[7] Similarly, a mouse satellite cell line (C2C12) was also used in pursuing the objective of restoring cardiac myocytes. Of interest is that these transformed muscle cells formed stable muscle grafts within syngeneic mice myocardium for a prolonged period of observation (3 months). Cells expressed skeletal myosin heavy chain isoform and, following myotube formation, seemingly stopped dividing. Although C2C12 cells were juxtaposed to the host cardiac myocytes, there was no evidence of electrical coupling to the native myocardium.[87] The finding that skeletal muscle cells can survive within the heart is encouraging, and it clearly demonstrates that both types of striated muscle can coexist in the same tissue. Nevertheless, it is more desirable to use primary muscle cells for the intracardial implantation since, contrary to the myogenic cell lines, they are devoid of the risk of developing into tumorigenic tissue.[88]

The third approach in cellular cardiomyoplasty is implantation of primary myogenic (satellite) cells. This approach is currently being pursued by our group. Considering that satellite cells are undifferentiated stem cells of myogenic lineage, we studied the possibility for satellite cells to alter their phenotypic expression under the influence of myocardial milieu. We proposed the hypothesis that satellite cells, when implanted into the injured myocardium, could grow into heart muscle cells and restore compromised contractile performance of the cardiac muscle.

To investigate this conjecture, we explanted canine anterior tibial muscle (Fig. 1) which was then enzymatically processed. Released satellite cells were cultured in vitro (Fig. 2), and passaged a few times to increase the number of myoblasts that were eventually implanted into the injured myocardium. In order to be able to locate implanted satellite cells, they were labeled with either radioactive thymidine or DNA plasmid carrying a gene for bacterial $\beta$-galactosidase. Detailed descriptions of the satellite cell culturing and labeling techniques can be found in our manuscripts published elsewhere.[35,89] Culture myogenicity was demonstrated by allowing satellite cells to fuse and form myotubes containing multiple nuclei (Fig. 3). When the cells multiplied in vitro to reach a sufficient number for implantation (on average, $5 \times 10^6$), they were collected and implanted into the freshly injured left ventricle. The damage to the heart was accomplished by the application of a cryoprobe cooled to $-160°C$ by the circulating liquid nitrogen (Fig. 4). Following the thawing of the frozen left ventricular segment, satellite cells were then immediately implanted into the damaged area (Fig. 5). The choice of inflicting injury to the heart by this method was prompted by the following consideration. Cryoinjury is known to

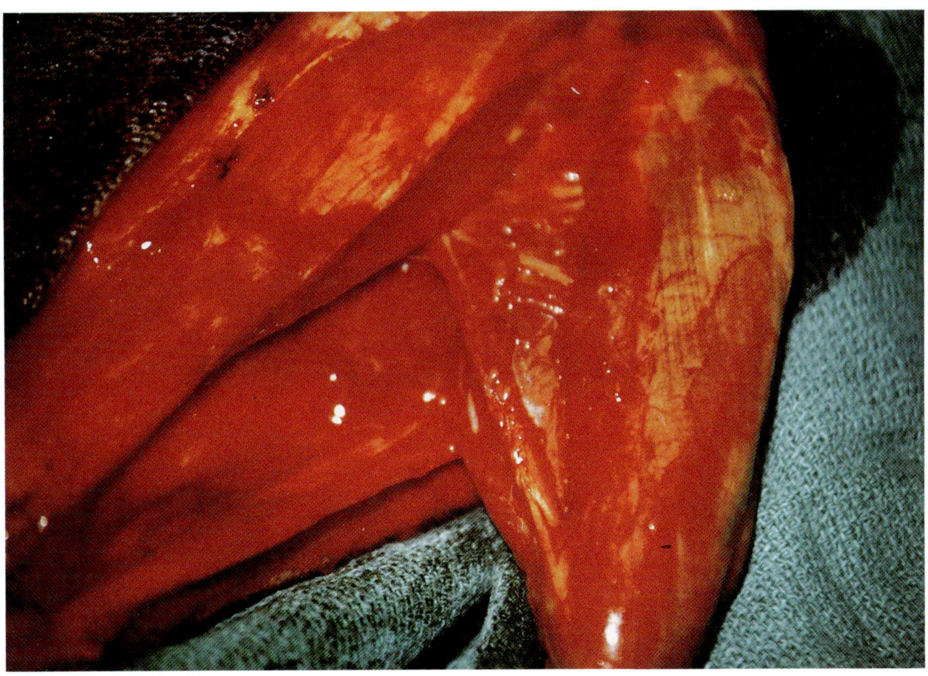

**Figure 1:** *Extirpation of canine m. anterior tibialis to obtain skeletal muscle satellite cells.*

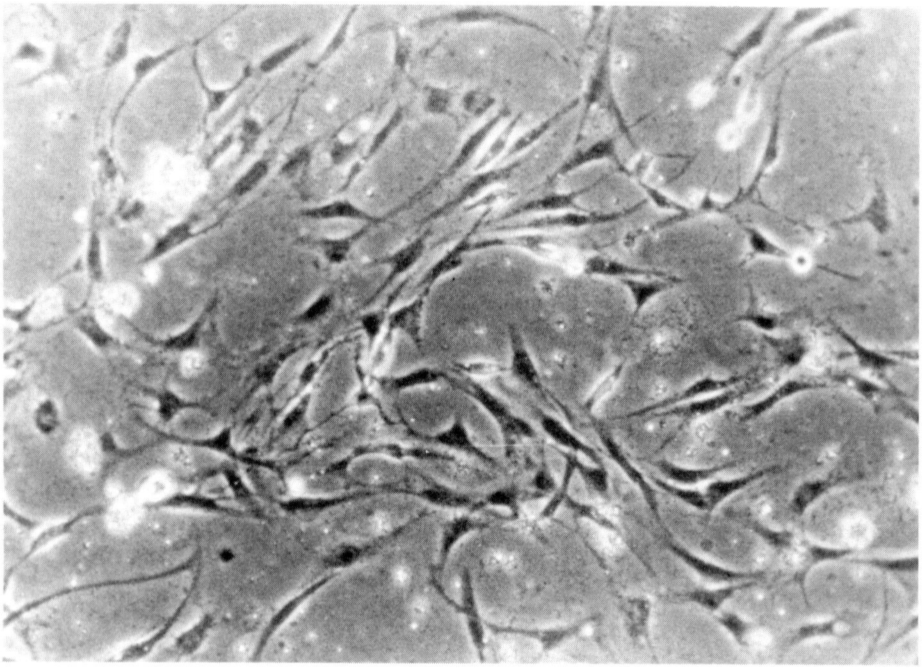

**Figure 2:** *Satellite cell culture in vitro. Magnification 200 ×.*

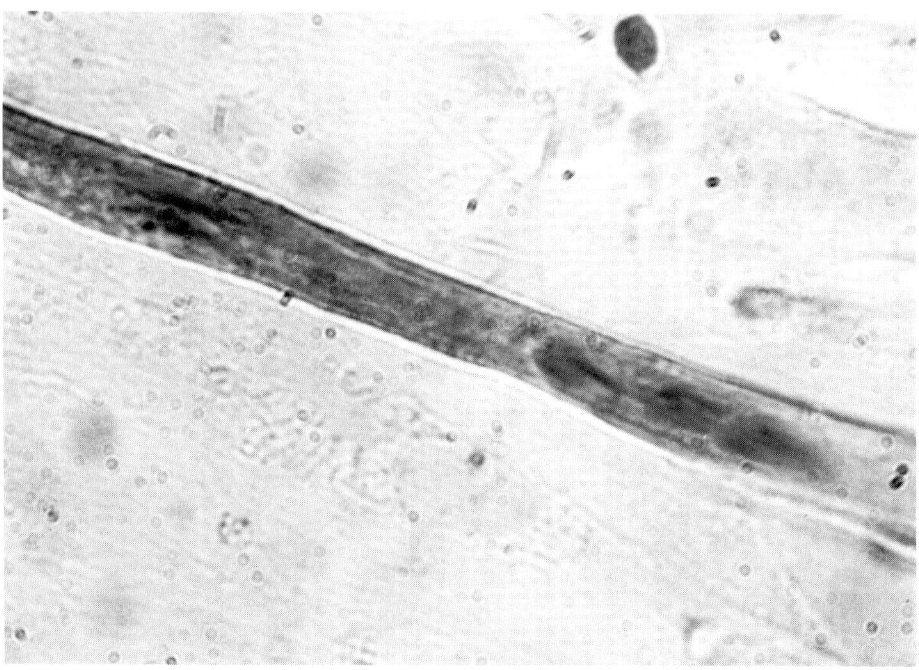

**Figure 3:** *Satellite cell fusion in vitro results in the formation of the multinucleated myotube. Three adjacent satellite cell nuclei (arrowheads) are seen to be incorporated in the myotube.*

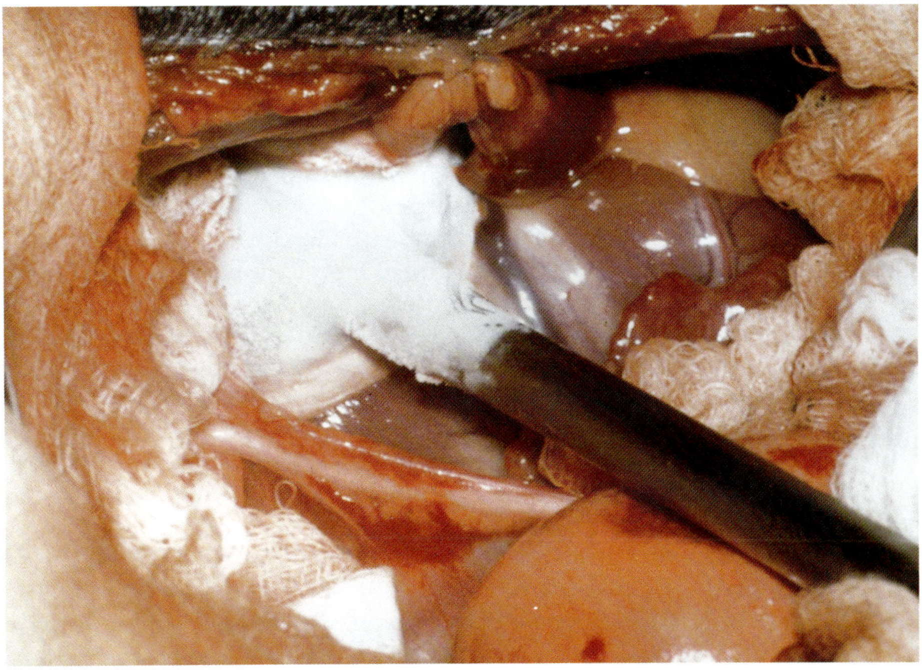

**Figure 4:** *Cryoinjury procedure. Note the cryoprobe applied onto the left ventricle surrounded by a rim of frozen cardiac tissue.*

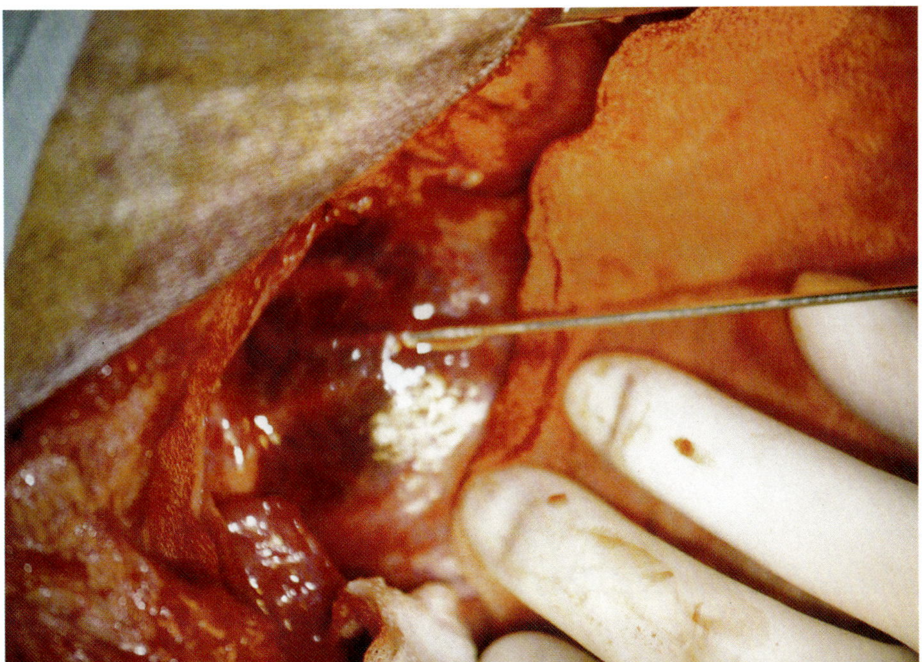

**Figure 5:** *Satellite cell implantation with a 16-gauge intravenous catheter into the cryoinjured myocardium (dark red area).*

create a homogenous scar, completely eliminating viable heart muscle tissue.[90] Furthermore, it spares large blood vessels, leaving a source of blood supply to the injured area. Therefore, after elimination of native myocardium, implanted satellite cells are the only striated muscle cells capable of surviving within the cryodestroyed area of the heart.

The gross and histological evaluation of the implant areas unveiled the presence of striated muscle fibers surrounded by a compact homogenous scar (Figs. 6 and 7). Muscle tissue found within the implant sites had morphological features resembling those of the cardiac muscle. Fibers exhibited cross-striation, centrally located nuclei, and intercalated discs (Fig. 8), which are known to be a particular feature of cardiomyocytes. In addition, cells within the implant region revealed the presence of bacterial $\beta$-galactosidase (Fig. 9), which proved the survival of implanted cells. Thus, our findings are consistent with the proposed hypothesis that the cardiac milieu may influence the differentiation of satellite cells. Further proof supporting these data will be required. Even if the new muscle fails to join the native myocardium, it may be stimulated to contract in synchrony with the rest of the heart by using an appropriate pacemaker, as has been done in dynamic cardiomyoplasty. In our opinion, it could have the potential to become a valuable treatment modality for congestive heart failure. Such an approach would have an advantage over other methods described ear-

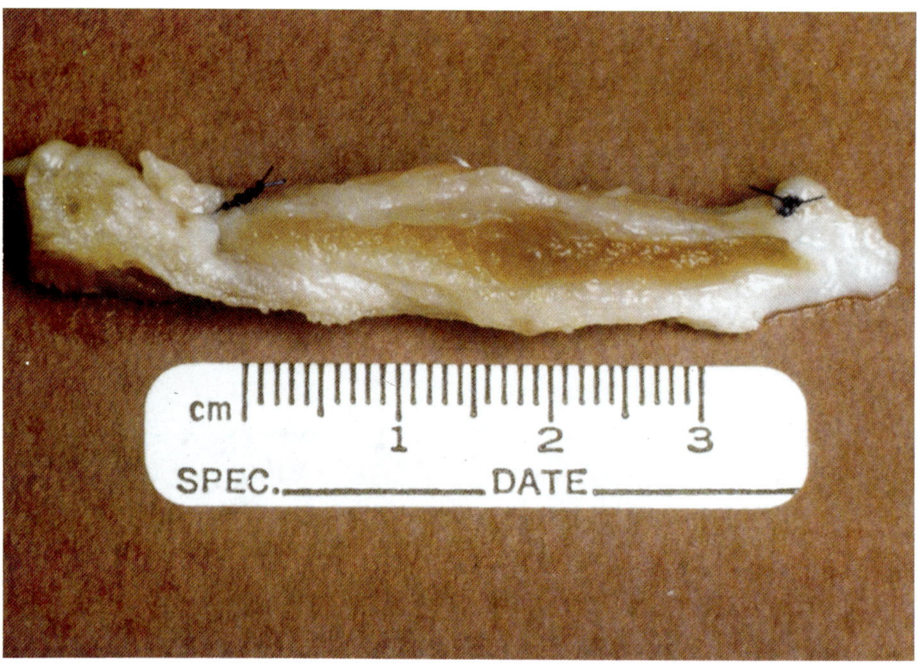


**Figure 6:** *Macroscopic specimen obtained from the experimental site 6 weeks following intracardial satellite cell implantation. Dense scar surrounds the brownish tissue in the area of cell implantation. Prolene sutures at both ends of the specimen were used to close entrance and exit openings of the channel that was created during the injection of satellite cells by the intravenous catheter.*

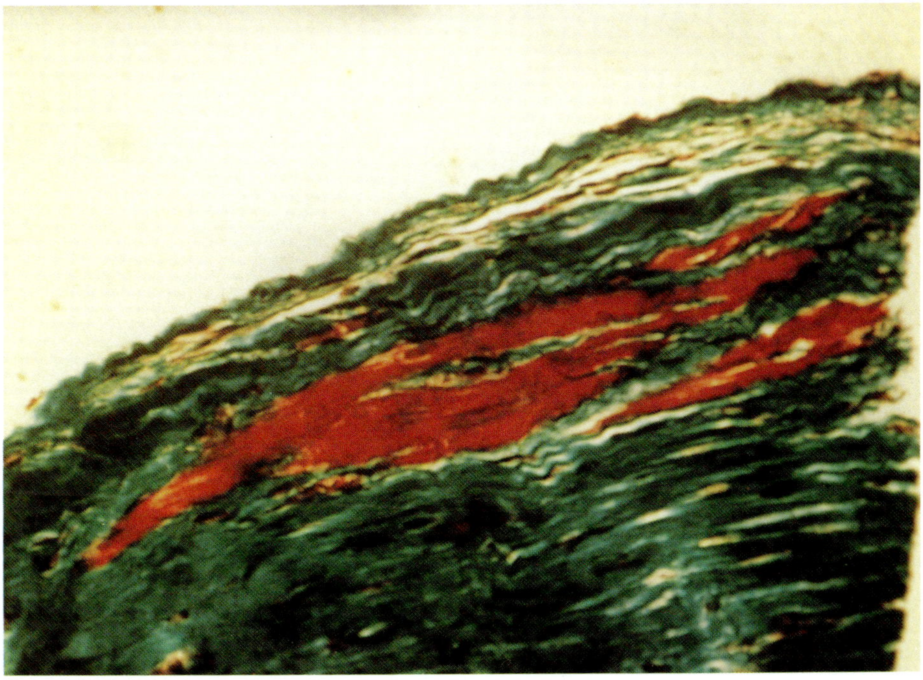

**Figure 7:** *Striated muscle fibers surrounded by a compact homogenous scar.*

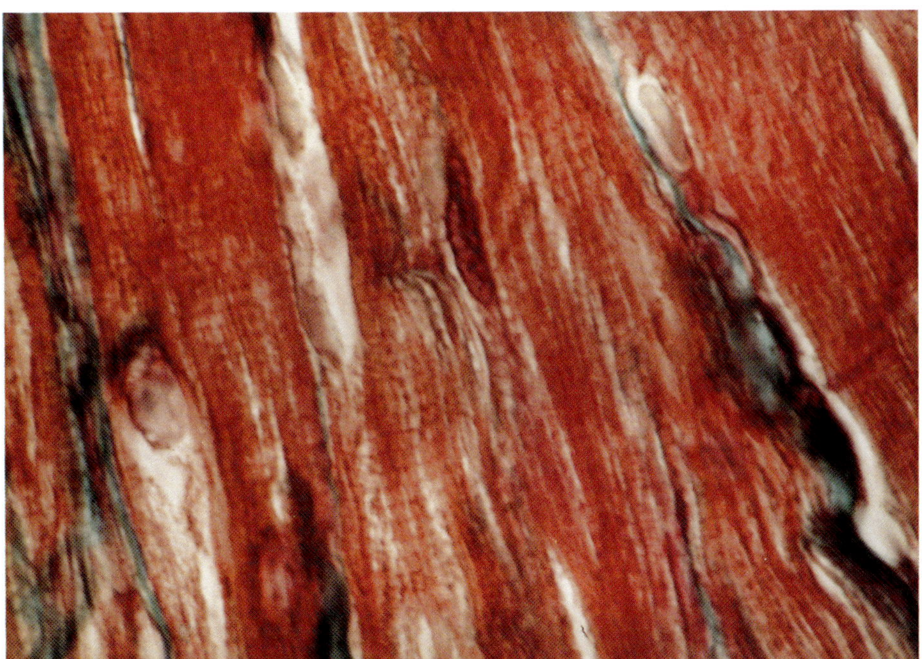

**Figure 8:** *Fibers exhibiting cross-striation, centrally located nuclei, and intercalated discs.*

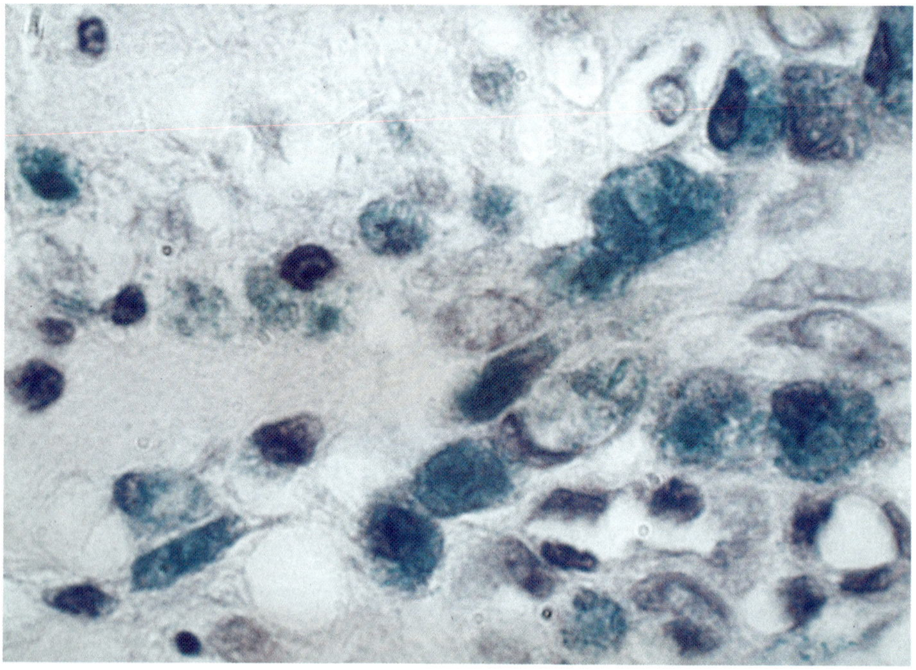

**Figure 9:** *The presence of bacterial β-galactoside is shown in cells within the implant region.*

lier due to the availability of the satellite cell source. As the dynamic cardiomyoplasty procedure has demonstrated, there are some skeletal muscles in the human body, the removal of which does not carry an appreciable handicap to a patient. Furthermore, an implantation of autologous primary myogenic cells would eliminate the risk for allograft or xenograft immune rejection.

## Conclusions

Myocardial inability to restore its lost contractile function often leads to drug-resistant congestive heart failure (CHF). The main obstacle in overcoming this problem is the incompetence of cardiomyocytes to enter the cell cycle in response to injury. For many years, clinical research in CHF focused on replacing the heart with mechanical pumping devices that would achieve a comparable blood flow to that generated by the heart. This exciting new approach was opened with the advent of the cardiomyoplasty procedure, which was based on the idea of using skeletal muscle to enhance cardiac performance. The arrival of new cellular and molecular biological techniques prompted the search for new possibilities to regrow cardiac muscle. An interesting field of molecular cardiomyoplasty has also emerged, applying recent knowledge of myogenic determination factors to regenerate muscle tissue within the heart. Thus, with the growing depth of knowledge in cardiovascular science, tremendous possibilities for their clinical application appear imminent.

## References


1. Kannel WB, Thom TJ: Incidence, prevalence, and mortality of cardiovascular diseases. In Hurst JW (ed): *The Heart, Arteries, and Veins.* 7th ed. McGraw Hill, New York, pp 627–638,1990.
2. Manasek FJ: Histogenesis of the embryonic myocardium. Am J Cardiol 25:149–168,1970.
3. Icardo J: The growing heart: An anatomical perspective. In Zak R (ed): *Growth of the Heart in Health and Disease.* Raven Press, New York, pp 41–79, 1984.
4. Zak R: Cell proliferation during cardiac growth. *Am J Cardiol* 31:211–219, 1973.
5. Rumyantsev PP: Interrelations of the proliferation and differentiation processes during cardiac myogenesis and regeneration. *Int Rev Cytol* 51: 187–273, 1977.
6. Field LJ: Atrial natriuretic factor-SV40 T antigen transgenes produce tumors and cardiac arrhythmias in mice. *Science* 239:1029–1033, 1988.
7. Koh GY, Soonpaa MH, Klug MG, Field LJ: Long-term survival of AT-1 cardiomyocyte grafts in syngeneic myocardium. *Am J Physiol* 264: H1727–33, 1993.
8. Rumyantsev PP: Post-injury DNA synthesis, mitosis, and ultrastructural reorganization of adult frog cardiac myocytes: An electron microscopic autoradiographic study. *Z Zellforsch* 139: 431–450, 1973.
9. Oberpriller JO, Oberpriller JC: Response of the adult newt ventricle to injury. *J Exp Zool* 187:249–259, 1974.
10. Lang RE, Tholken H, Ganten D, Luft FC, et al: Atrial natriuretic factor: A circulating hormone stimulated by volume overload. *Nature* 314:262–266, 1985.
11. Parker TG, Parker SE, Schneider MD: Peptide growth factors can provoke "fetal" contractile protein expression in rat cardiac myocytes. *J Clin Invest* 85:507–514, 1990.
12. Schneider MD, Roberts R, Parker TG: Modulation of cardiac genes by mechanical stress. *Mol Biol Med* 8:167–183, 1991.
13. Matsuda R, Spector D, Strohman RC: Regenerating adult chicken skeletal muscle and satellite cell cultures express embryonic patterns of myosin and tropomyosin isoforms. *Dev Biol* 100:478–488, 1983.
14. Kimelmann D, Christian JL, Moon RT: Synergistic principles of development: Overlapping patterning systems in Xenopus mesoderm induction. *Development* 116:1–9, 1992.
15. Green JB, Howes G, Symes K, Cooke J, et al: The biological effects of XTC-MIF: quantitative comparison with Xenopus bFGF. *Development* 108:173–183, 1990.
16. Rosen GD, Sanes JR, LaChance R, Cunningham JM, et al: Roles for the integrin VLA-4 and its counter receptor VCAM-1 in myogenesis. *Cell* 69:1107–1119, 1992.
17. Armand O, Boutineau AM, Mauger A, Pautou MP, et al: Origin of satellite cells in avian skeletal muscles. *Arch Anat Microsc Morphol Exp* 72:163–181, 1983.
18. Ordahl CP, Le Douarin NM: Two myogenic lineages within the developing somite. *Development* 114:339–353, 1992.
19. Mauro A: Satellite cells of skeletal muscle fibers. *J Biophys Biochem Cytol* 9:493–495, 1961.
20. Banker BQ, Girvin JP: The ultrastructural features of the mammalian muscle spindle. *J Neuropathol Exp Neurol* 30:155–195, 1971.
21. Campion DR: The muscle satellite cell: A review. *Int Rev Cytol* 87:225–251, 1984.
22. Anderson RG, Kamen BA, Rothberg KG, Lacey SW: Potocytosis: Sequestration and transport of small molecules by caveolae. *Science* 255:410–411, 1992.
23. Chang WJ, Ying YS, Rothberg KG, Hooper NM, et al: Purification and characterization of smooth muscle cell caveolae. *J Cell Biol* 126:127–138, 1994.
24. Schmalbruch H, Hellhammer U: The number of satellite cells in normal human muscle. *Anat Rec* 185:279–288, 1976.
25. Kelly AM: Perisynaptic satellite cells in the developing and mature rat soleus muscle. *Anat Rec* 190:891–904, 1978.
26. Darr KC, Schultz E: Exercise-induced satellite cell activation in growing and mature skeletal muscle. *J Appl Physiol* 63:1816–1821, 1987.

27. Olwin BB, Hannon K, Kudla AJ: Are fibroblast growth factors regulators of myogenesis in vivo? *Prog Growth Factor Res* 5:145–158, 1994.
28. Webster C, Blau HM: Accelerated age-related decline in replicative life-span of Duchenne muscular dystrophy myoblasts: implications for cell and gene therapy. *Somatic Cell Mol Genet* 16:557–565, 1990.
29. Grounds MD, Garrett KL, Lai MC, Wright WE, et al: Identification of skeletal muscle precursor cells in vivo by use of MyoD1 and myogenin probes. *Cell Tissue Res* 267:99–104, 1992.
30. Watt DJ, Morgan TE, Clifford MA, Partridge TA: The movement of muscle precursor cells between adjacent regenerating muscle in the mouse. *Anat Embryol (Berl)* 175:527, 1987.
31. Hughes SM, Blau HM: Migration of myoblasts across basal lamina during skeletal muscle development. *Nature* 345:350–353, 1990.
32. Jones P: In vitro comparison of embryonic myoblasts and myogenic cells isolated from regenerating adult rat skeletal muscle. *Exp Cell Res* 139:401–404, 1982.
33. Gussoni E, Pavlath GK, Lanctot AM, Sharma KR, et al: Normal dystrophin transcripts detected in Duchenne muscular dystrophy patients after myoblast transplantation. *Nature* 356:435–438, 1992.
34. Yaffe D, Feldman M: The formation of hybrid multinucleated muscle fibers from myoblasts of different genetic origin. *Dev Biol* 11:300–317, 1965.
35. Chiu RCJ, Zibaitis A, Kao RL: Cellular cardiomyoplasty: Myocardial regeneration with satellite cell implantation. *Ann Thorac Surg* 60:12–18, 1995.
36. Davis RL, Weintraub H, Lassar AB: Expression of a single transfected cDNA converts fibroblasts to myoblasts. *Cell* 51:987–1000, 1987.
37. Taylor SM: 5-Aza-2′-deoxycytidine: cell differentiation and DNA methylation. *Leukemia* 1(Suppl 7):3–8, 1993.
38. Wright WE, Sassoon DA, Lin VK: Myogenin, a factor regulating myogenesis, has a domain homologous to MyoD. *Cell* 56:607–617, 1989.
39. Braun T, Buschhausen-Denker G, Bober E, Tannich E, et al: A novel human muscle factor related to but distinct from MyoD1 induces myogenic conversion in 10T1/2 fibroblasts. *EMBO J* 8:701–709, 1989.
40. Rhodes SJ. Konieczny SF: Identification of MRF-4: A new member of the muscle regulatory factor gene family. *Genes Dev* 3:2050–2061, 1989.
41. Anthony-Cahill SJ, Benfield PA, Fairman R, Wasserman ZR, et al: Molecular characterization of helix-loop-helix peptides. *Science* 255:979–983, 1992.
42. Venuti JM, Morris JH, Vivian JL, Olson EN, et al: Myogenin is required for late but not early aspects of myogenesis during mouse development. *J Cell Biol* 128:563–576, 1995.
43. Krause M, Fire A, White-Harrison S, Weintraub H, et al: Functional conservation of nematode and vertebrate myogenic regulatory factors. *J Cell Sci* 16(Suppl):111–115, 1992.
44. Lassar AB, Buskin JN, Lockshon D, Davis RL, et al: MyoD is a sequence-specific DNA binding protein requiring a region of myc homology to bind to the muscle creatine kinase enhancer. *Cell* 58:823–831, 1989.
45. Piette J, Bessereau JL, Huchet M, Changeux JP: Two adjacent MyoD1-binding sites regulate expression of the acetylcholine receptor $\alpha$-subunit gene. *Nature* 345:353–355, 1990.
46. Murre C, McCaw PS, Baltimore D: A new DNA binding and dimerization motif in immunoglobulin enhancer binding, daughterless, MyoD, and myc proteins. *Cell* 56:777–783, 1989.
47. Weintraub H, Davis R, Tapscott S, Thayer M, et al: The myoD gene family: Nodal point during specification of the muscle cell lineage. *Science* 251:761–766, 1991.
48. Jen Y, Weintraub H, Benezra R: Overexpression of Id protein inhibits the muscle differentiation program: In vivo association of Id with E2A proteins. *Genes Dev* 6:1466–1479, 1992.
49. Ott M-O, Bober E, Lyons G, Arnold H, et al: Early expression of the myogenic regulatory gene, myf5, in precursor cells of skeletal muscle in the mouse embryo. *Development* 111:1097–1107, 1991.

50. Hannon K, Smith CK, Bales KR, Santerre RF: Temporal and quantitative analysis of myogenic regulatory and growth factor gene expression in the developing mouse embryo. *Dev Biol* 151:137–144, 1992.
51. Santerre RF, Bales KR, Janney MJ, Hannon K, et al: Expression of bovine myf5 induces ectopic skeletal muscle formation in transgenic mice. *Mol Cell Biol* 13:6044–6051, 1993.
52. Rudnicki MA, Braun T, Hinuma S, Jaenisch R: Inactivation of MyoD in mice leads to up-regulation of the myogenic HLH gene Myf-5 and results in apparently normal muscle development. *Cell* 71:383–390, 1992.
53. Braun T, Rudnicki MA, Arnold HH, Jaenisch R: Targeted inactivation of the muscle regulatory gene Myf-5 results in abnormal rib development and perinatal death. *Cell* 71:369–382, 1992.
54. Braun T, Bober E, Rudnicki MA, Jaenisch R, et al: MyoD expression marks the onset of skeletal myogenesis in Myf-5 mutant mice. *Development* 120:3083–3092, 1994.
55. Rudnicki MA, Schnegelsberg PN, Stead RH, Braun T, et al: MyoD or Myf-5 is required for the formation of skeletal muscle. *Cell* 75:1351–1359, 1993.
56. Braun T, Arnold HH: Inactivation of Myf-6 and Myf-5 genes in mice leads to alterations in skeletal muscle development. *EMBO J* 14:1176–1186, 1995.
57. Rudnicki MA, Jaenisch R: The MyoD family of transcription factors and skeletal myogenesis. *Bioessays* 17:203–209, 1995.
58. Chambers AE, Kotecha S, Towers N, Mohun TJ: Muscle-specific expression of SRF-related genes in the early embryo of Xenopus laevis. *EMBO J* 11:4981–4991, 1992.
59. Yu YT, Breitbart RE, Smoot LB, LeeY et al: Human myocyte-specific enhancer factor 2 comprises a group of tissue-restricted MADS box transcription factors. *Genes Dev* 6:1783–1798, 1992.
60. Gossett LA, Kelvin DJ, Sternberg EA, Olson EN: A new myocyte-specific enhancer-binding factor that recognizes a conserved element associated with multiple muscle-specific genes. *Mol Cell Biol* 9:5022–5033, 1989.
61. Nakatsuji Y, Hidaka K, Tsujino S, Yamamoto Y, et al: A single MEF-2 site is a major positive regulatory element required for transcription of the muscle-specific subunit of the human phosphoglycerate mutase gene in skeletal and cardiac muscle cells. *Mol Cell Biol* 12:4384–4390, 1992.
62. Kaushal S, Schneider JW, Nadal-Ginard B, Mahdavi V: Activation of the myogenic lineage by MEF2A, a factor that induces and cooperates with MyoD. *Science* 266:1236–1240, 1994.
63. Buckingham M: Molecular biology of muscle development. *Cell* 78:15–21, 1994.
64. Bell RM, Burns DJ: Lipid activation of protein kinase C. *J Biol Chem* 266:4661–4664, 1991.
65. Li L, Zhou J, James G, Heller-Harrison R, et al: FGF inactivates myogenic helix-loop-helix proteins through phosphorylation of a conserved protein kinase C site in their DNA-binding domains. *Cell* 71:1181–1194, 1992.
66. Miner JH, Wold BJ: c-Myc inhibition of MyoD and myogenin-initiated myogenic differentiation. *Mol Cell Biol* 11:2842–2851, 1991.
67. Li L, Chambard JC, Karin M, Olson EN: Fos and jun repress transcriptional activation by myogenin and MyoD. *Genes Dev* 6:676–689, 1992.
68. Florini JR, Roberts AB, Ewton D, Falen SL, et al: Transforming growth factor: A very potent inhibitor of myoblast differentiation identical to the differentiation inhibitor secreted by Buffalo rat liver cells. *J Biol Chem* 35:16509–16513, 1986.
69. Martin JF, Li L, Olson EN: Repression of myogenin function by TGF-$\beta$1 is targeted at the basic helix-loop-helix motif and is independent of E2A products. *J Biol Chem* 267:10956–10960, 1992.
70. Florini JR, Ewton DZ, Roof SL: IGF-I stimulates terminal myogenic differentiation by induction of myogenin gene expression. *Mol Endocrinol* 5:718–724, 1991.
71. Florini J, Magri K, Ewton D, James P, et al: "Spontaneous" differentiation of skeletal myoblasts is controlled by autocrine secretion of insulin-like growth factor-II. *J Biol Chem* 266:15917–15923, 1991.
72. Albeda SM, Buck CA: Integrins and other cell adhesion molecules. *FASEB J* 4:2868–2880, 1990.

73. Lyons GE, Moore R, Yahara O, Buckingham ME, et al: Expression of NCAM isoforms during skeletal myogenesis in the mouse embryo. *Develop Dynamics* 194:94–104, 1992.
74. Rose O, Rohwedel J, Reinhardt S, Bachmann M, et al: Expression of M-cadherin protein in myogenic cells during prenatal mouse development and differentiation of embryonic stem cells in culture. *Dev Dynamics* 201:245–59, 1994.
75. Cifuentes-Diaz C, Nicolet M, Goudou D, Rieger F, et al: N-cadherin expression in developing, adult and denervated chicken neuromuscular system: Accumulations at both the neuromuscular junction and the node of Ranvier. *Development* 120:1–11, 1994.
76. van Bilsen M, Chien KR: Growth and hypertrophy of the heart: towards an understanding of cardiac specific and inducible gene expression. *Cardiovasc Res* 27:1140–1149, 1993.
77. Adolph EA, Subramaniam A, Cserjesi P, Olson EN, et al: Role of myocyte-specific enhancer-binding factor (MEF-2) in transcriptional regulation of the alpha-cardiac myosin heavy chain gene. *J Biol Chem* 268:5349–5352, 1993.
78. McGinnis W, Krumlauf R: Homeobox genes and axial patterning. *Cell* 68:283–302, 1992.
79. Niehrs C, Keller R, Cho KWY, De Robertis EM: The homeobox gene goosecoid controls cell migration in embryos. *Cell* 72:491–503, 1993.
80. Cserjesi P, Lilly B, Bryson L, Wang Y, et al: MHox: A mesodermally restricted homeodomain protein that binds an essential site in the muscle creatine kinase enhancer. *Development* 115:1087–1101, 1992.
81. French BA, Chow KL, Olson EN, Schwartz RJ: Heterodimers of myogenic helix-loop-helix regulatory factors and E12 bind a complex element governing myogenic induction of the avian cardiac alpha-actin promoter. *Mol Cell Biol* 11:2439–2450, 1991.
82. Litvin J, Montgomery MO, Goldhamer DJ, Emerson CP Jr, et al: Identification of DNA-binding protein(s) in the developing heart. *Dev Biol* 156:409–417, 1993.
83. Fanning E, Knippers R: Structure and function of simian virus 40 large tumor antigen. *Ann Rev Biochem* 61:55–85, 1992.
84. Katz EB, Steinhelper ME, Delcarpio JB, Daud AI, et al: Cardiomyocyte proliferation in mice expressing alpha-cardiac myosin heavy chain-SV40 T-antigen transgenes. *Am J Physiol* 262:H1867–76, 1992.
85. Tam SKC, Gu W, Nadal-Ginard B: Molecular cardiomyoplasty: Potential cardiac gene therapy for chronic heart failure. *J Thorac Cardiovasc Surg* 109:918–924, 1995.
86. Soonpaa MH, Koh GY, Klug MG, Field LJ: Formation of nascent intercalated disks between grafted fetal cardiomyocytes and host myocardium. *Science* 264:98–101, 1994.
87. Koh GY, Klug MG, Soonpaa MH, Field LJ: Differentiation and long-term survival of C2C12 myoblast grafts in heart. *J Clin Invest* 92:1548–1554, 1993.
88. Rando TA, Blau HM: Primary mouse myoblast purification, characterization, and transplantation for cell-mediated gene therapy. *J Cell Biol* 125:1275–1287, 1994.
89. Marelli D, Desrosiers C, El-Alfy M, Kao RC, et al: Cell transplantation for myocardial repair: an experimental approach. *Cell Transplant* 1:383–390, 1992.
90. Jensen JA, Kosek JC, Hunt TK, Goodson IIIWH, et al: Cardiac cryolesions as an experimental model of myocardial wound healing. *Ann Surg* 206:798–803, 1987.

Chapter 49

# Molecular Cardiomyoplasty

## A Molecular Restorative Strategy for Treatment of Heart Failure

Stanley K.C. Tam, Wei Gu

### Introduction

Effective therapy for chronic heart failure has thus far proven to be elusive. Overall prognosis remained poor, with 80% and 60% survival at 3 and 12 months, respectively.[1] This is due mainly to the fact that current medical treatment strategies use symptoms relief as the end points. This included inotropic agents[2–7] and vasodilators.[8,9] Clinical trials have shown that most of these strategies in fact increased long-term mortality of patients with heart failure, with the exception of angiotensin converting enzyme inhibitors and nitrates.[10,11] The most fundamental problem of heart failure, that is, power failure due to irreversible loss of functional myocytes, has not been addressed.

### Terminal Differentiation of Adult Cardiac Myocytes

Adult cardiac myocytes from lower organisms such as newts have the ability to proliferate following injury.[12] Although this subject is still controversial,[13] mammalian adult cardiac myocytes become terminally differentiated and lose their ability to undergo mitosis, both karyokinesis and cytokinesis, soon after the newborn period.[14,15] This apparent permanent cell cycle arrest renders the adult mammalian heart incapable of restoration of function by myocyte proliferation after loss of myocytes following injury, for example myocardial infarction due to ischemia. Instead, upon hemodynamic growth stimuli, myocytes become hypertrophic, that is, increase in cell size, along with proliferation of nonmuscle cells, which provides effective short term response.

From Carpentier A, Chachques JC, Grandjean P: Cardiac Bioassist. © Futura Publishing Co, Inc, Armonk, NY, 1997.

However, over the long term, this hypertrophy becomes a maladaptive response that leads to pump failure and "cardiomyopathy of overload."[16]

## Restorative Strategy for Treatment of Heart Failure

A restorative strategy is aimed at solving the fundamental problem of heart failure, as stated earlier, power failure secondary to irreversible loss of functional myocytes. Surgical restorative strategy includes organ transplantation where the pump failure is restored by a functioning organ, cellular transplantation where an attempt is made to restore power by transplanting myocytes,[17] and dynamic cardiomyoplasty which attempts to restore myocardial pump power failure by a heterogeneous organ—skeletal muscle.[18] However, graft rejection and availability of organs and cells are just two of the many problems with transplantation. Dynamic cardiomyoplasty shows promise but the long-term efficacy remains to be shown.[19,20]

## Molecular Restorative Strategy for Treatment of Heart Failure

An intriguing strategy to address the problem of cardiac power failure is to add more endogenous contracting myocytes either by converting nonmuscle cells of the heart into myocytes or by inducing mature adult cardiac myocytes to undergo mitosis, that is, attempting cardiac "regeneration" using molecular interventions. Converting nonmuscle cells into cardiac myocytes requires the identification of a gene or a set of genes that govern the expression of cardiac muscle program. Although extensive research has been done, these gene product(s) termed cardiac myogenic factor(s) have not been identified. Inducing mature mammalian adult cardiac myocytes to undergo mitosis and to proliferate requires the understanding of the molecular mechanisms governing the process of terminal differentiation. Although we have some clues to the process,[21,22] we are far from understanding terminal differentiation, and cannot, at this time, reverse the process.

## Molecular Cardiomyoplasty

Since effecting cardiac regeneration is currently impossible, the next best molecular strategy is to convert nonmuscle cells of the heart to contracting myocytes—not cardiac myocytes but skeletal myocytes. Since the contractile apparatus between skeletal myocytes and cardiac myocytes is essentially the same, it is logical to attempt to convert cells, such as cardiac fibroblasts as in a scar following myocardial infarction, into contracting skeletal myocytes. This conversion is possible because skeletal myogenic factors—the family of basic helix loop helix proteins—exemplified by MyoD, has been well described.[23] MyoD, when expressed, has been shown to mediate the conversion of the mouse fibroblast cell line into stable myoblasts, which could be induced to differentiate into multinucleated myotubes, morphologically similar to skeletal muscle cells.[24] In addition to morphology, these multinucleated myotubes expressed myosin heavy chain and other biochemical muscle differentiation markers similar to skeletal muscle cells. MyoD can be force expressed using a retroviral vector[24] with 95% efficiency in primary cardiac fibroblasts freshly isolated from rat hearts. These molecularly modified cardiac fibroblasts were able to be converted into myoblasts that can subsequently be induced to differentiate into multinucleated cells, morphologically and biochemically similar to skeletal muscle cells.[25] Furthermore, in these in vitro conditions, clusters of these multinucleated cells have been noted to contract, suggesting that these cells may be potentially functional in vivo.

A model of rat myocardial infarction obtained by ligation of the left anterior descending artery has been developed. Currently, the MyoD gene is being delivered into the infarct area of the rat myocardium in an attempt to convert cardiac fibroblasts into myocytes. It remains to be shown whether this "gene therapy" approach for the treatment of heart failure is efficacious.

## Summary

Mortality from chronic heart failure remains high despite what appears to be adequate therapy based on symptom relief. This has led to the reevaluation of the fundamental abnormality in this disease. Molecular strategy is being developed to remedy the fundamental abnormality of pump failure due to the irreversible loss of myocytes and the development of cardiomyopathy of overload. This strategy centers on providing more functioning myocytes either by converting nonmuscle cells of the heart into myocytes or inducing terminally differentiated cardiac myocytes to undergo mitosis. In forced expression of MyoD, a skeleton myogenic factor has been shown to be able to convert primary cardiac fibroblasts into contracting skeletal myocytes in vitro. Further studies with in vivo models are needed to evalute this molecular strategy for the treatment of heart failure.

## References


1. Yamani M, Massie BM: Congestive heart failure: Insights from epidemiology, implications for treatment. *Mayo Clin Proc* 68:1214–1218, 1993.
2. Dies F, Krell MJ, Whitlow P, et al.: Intermittent dobutamine in ambulatory outpatients with chronic cardiac failure (abstract). *Circulation* 74:II-38, 1986.
3. Katz AM. Potential deleterious effects of inotropic agents in the therapy of chronic heart failure. *Circulation* 73(Suppl III):184–188, 1986.
4. Packer M, Carver JR, Rodeheffer RJ, et al: Effect of oral milrinone on mortality in severe heart failure. *N Engl J Med* 325:1468–1475, 1991.
5. Curfman GD. Inotropic therapy for heart failure: an unfulfilled promise. *N Engl J Med* 325:1509–1510, 1991.
6. Feldman AM, Bristow MR, Parmley WW, et al. for the Vesnarinone Study Group: Effects of vesnarinone on morbidity and mortality in patients with heart failure. *N Engl J Med* 329:149–155, 1993.
7. Packer M: The search for the ideal positive inotropic agent. *N Engl J Med* 329: 201–202, 1993.
8. Cohn JN: Introduction: The Vasodilator-Heart Failure Trials (V-HeFT). Mechanistic studies from the VA cooperative studies. *Circulation* 87(Suppl VI):1–4, 1993.

9. Goldstein RE, Boccuzzi SJ, Cruess D, et al. and the Adverse Experience Committee, and the Multicenter Diltiazem Postinfarction Research Group: Diltiazem increases late-onset congestive heart failure in postinfarction patients with early reduction in ejection fraction. *Circulation* 83:52–60, 1991.
10. Pfeffer MA, Braunwald E, Moye LA, et al. on behalf of the SAVE Investigators: Effect of captopril on mortality and morbidity in patients with left ventricular dysfunction after myocardial infarction: Results of the survival and ventricular enlargement trial. *N Engl J Med* 327:669–677, 1992.
11. The SOLVD Investigators: Effect of enalapril on mortality and the development of heart failure in asymptomatic patients with reduced left ventricular ejection fraction. *N Engl J Med* 327:685–691, 1992.
12. Oberpriller JO, Oberpriller JC: Response of adult newt ventricle to injury. *J Exp Zool* 187:249–260, 1974.
13. Quaini F, Cigola E, Lagrasta C, et al: End-stage cardiac failure in humans is coupled with the induction of proliferating cell nuclear antigen and nuclear mitotic division in ventricular myocytes. *Circ Res* 75:1050–1063, 1994.
14. Di Donato RM, Fujii AM, Jonas RA, Castaneda AR: Age-dependent ventricular response to pressure overload: considerations for the arterial switch operation. *J Thorac Cardiovasc Surg* 104:713–22, 1992.
15. Rumyantsev PP: In Carlson BM (ed): *Growth and Hyperplasia of Cardiac Muscle Cells.* New York, Harwood, 1991, pp 3–68.
16. Katz AM: Cardiomyopathy of overload: A major determinant of prognosis in congestive heart failure. *N Engl J Med* 322:100–110, 1990.
17. Soonpaa MH, Koh GY, Klug MG, Field LJ: Formation of nascent intercalated disks between grafted fetal cardiomyocytes and host myocardium. *Science* 264:98–101, 1994.
18. Carpentier A, Chachques JC: Myocardial substitution with a stimulated skeletal muscle: First successful clincial use. *Lancet* 1:1267, 1985.
19. Magovern JA, Park SE, Cmolik BL, Trumble DR, et al: Early effects of right latissimus dorsi cardiomyoplasty on left ventricular function. *Circulation* 88(Suppl): II298–303, 1993.
20. Bellotti G, Moraes A, Bocchi E, et al: Late effects of cardiomyoplasty on left ventricular mechanics and diastolic filling. *Circulation* 88(Suppl):II304–308, 1993.
21. Tam SKC, Gu W, Mahdavi V, Nadal-Ginard B: Cardiac myocyte terminal differentiation: Potential for cardiac regeneration. *Ann NY Acad Sci* 752:72–79, 1995.
22. Gu W, Schneider JW, Condorelli G, Kaushal S, et al: Interaction of myogenic factors and the retinoblastoma protein mediates muscle cell commitment and differentiation. *Cell* 72:309–324, 1993.
23. Olson EN: MyoD family: A paradigm for development? *Genes Dev* 4:1454–61, 1990.
24. Davis RL, Weintraub H, Lassar AB: Expression of a single transfected cDNA converts fibroblasts to myoblasts. *Cell* 51:987–1000, 1987.
25. Tam SKC, Gu W, Nadal-Ginard B: Molecular cardiomyoplasty: Potential cardiac gene therapy for chronic heart failure. *J Thorac Cardiovasc Surg* 109:918–924, 1995.

# Part VII

## Closing Remarks

Chapter 50

# Current Indications and the Future of Cardiomyoplasty

Alain Carpentier, Albert Starr

*This discussion took place at the end of the Second International Meeting on Cardiomyoplasty. This material is still relevant and the following remarks which have been reviewed and updated by Dr. Carpentier and Dr. Starr still give a valuable perspective on the indications and the future development of cardiac bioassist techniques.*

*The Editors*

**Dr. Carpentier:** Dr. Starr, in light of what we have learned, I would like to discuss with you the current indications and the future of cardiomyoplasty although, as Niels Bohr put it, making predictions is dangerous. . . especially about the future!

**Dr. Starr:** Let's take that risk.

**Dr. Carpentier:** As far as the current indications are concerned, there are still important uncertainties due to important variations in the results. These variations result from several causes: the patient's condition, the quality and size of the muscle, the surgical technique, and the underlying cardiac disease. How can we minimize them?

**Dr. Starr:** Biology is neither Newtonian physics nor Einsteinian physics. We are working in a chaotic system. I mean that, in a scientific sense, it is very unpredictable, like the weather.

**Dr. Carpentier:** A chaotic situation may just reflect our incapacity to discern some organized pattern hidden by too many variables or a limited number of facts. Can't we change that?

From Carpentier A, Chachques JC, Grandjean P: Cardiac Bioassist. © Futura Publishing Co, Inc, Armonk, NY, 1997.

**Dr. Starr:** We don't know all the variables. We are trying to make some sense in doing the right thing for the patient at the proper time. As you say, we are dealing with a very broad spectrum of patients at various stages in their disease and therefore we should have different expectations of what our operative interventions can provide.

**Dr. Carpentier:** You are right. The indications of cardiomyoplasty depend on what we expect from cardiomyoplasty: either to increase life expectancy or to improve the quality of life, or both. The answer to that question probably depends on the type of patients, whether high risk or low risk, who are proposed to the surgeon. Let us begin by the first type. These patients may have multiorgan failure, or several risk factors that have been clearly identified in the past years. They have a limited life expectancy due to severe and irreversible myocardial lesions. The aim of cardiomyoplasty in this group is mainly to improve the quality of life.

**Dr. Starr:** As far as patients with multiorgan failure are concerned, they can survive only with early transplantation or with the use of an assist device. I don't think that a myoplasty can address the issue of multiorgan failure; it does not supply sufficient cardiac performance increment to solve that kind of problem.

**Dr. Carpentier:** In other words, you see multiorgan failure as a contraindication to cardiomyoplasty?

**Dr. Starr:** Yes, an absolute contraindication.

**Dr. Carpentier:** I agree. Are there other contraindications?

**Dr. Starr:** I think that another contraindication is an expectation that the operative risk itself is extremely high, for example, if the patient has other risk factors that would make it unlikely that he or she would survive the operation.

**Dr. Carpentier:** Don't we do other operations that carry a high risk whenever there is no other alternative? Wouldn't it be unethical to systematically refuse a cardiomyoplasty to a high-risk patient because we are too concerned with the operative mortality? I have seen surprisingly good results in patients with an ejection fraction below 15%, or a cardiothoracic ratio over 0.6, or elevated pulmonary pressure and even arrhythmias. Let us take a patient with two of these risk factors and repeated episodes of pulmonary edema in spite of adequate medical treatment. If there is no other surgical alternative, how can we refuse to give the patient the opportunity to have this operation?

**Dr. Starr:** Yes, but this is an experimental procedure and we learn nothing from a patient who does not survive the operation. So in a sense, we have to be careful to select patients that we think have a reasonable likelihood of surviving the operation. It should not be a desperate measure. It should be a carefully thought-out plan.

**Dr. Carpentier:** Besides other well-known contraindications such as biventricular failure, severe pulmonary hypertension, and mitral valve insufficiency, would you consider arrhythmia to be a contraindication?

**Dr. Starr:** Yes. In the present state, we are unable, through the regulatory process in the United States, to combine the use of a defibrillator device with a myostimulator. Therefore, if a patient faces a significant risk of death from an arrhythmia, such as recurrent ventricular tachycardia, and is on major drug treatment, then I don't think the patient is a candidate for cardiomyoplasty. Arrhythmia is the most common cause of death in patients with end-stage heart disease.

**Dr. Carpentier:** Would arrhythmia still be a contraindication to cardiomyoplasty in the absence of constraints due to the regulatory process? In other words, do you think it makes sense to combine cardiomyoplasty with a defibrillator?

**Dr. Starr:** Yes. I think it makes a lot of sense, but we have to deal with the artifact of the regulatory process. We are dealing with end-stage heart disease and severe arrhythmias. The patients should receive an implantable defibrillator and this should not preclude myoplasty, but unfortunately in the United States it does.

**Dr. Carpentier:** In France, it is not the regulatory process but the cost that precludes the use of defibrillators in cardiomyoplasty patients. We have to "demonstrate" the benefit of such an expensive procedure. And, before that, many people would like us to "demonstrate" that cardiomyoplasty itself works. They ask for randomized studies. What do you think about randomization?

**Dr. Starr:** I would like to ask the audience if they know of any operation that has been developed through randomization or any single surgical advance that has ever been developed by a randomized series. That has never happened in the past. And it is very unlikely that it will happen in the future. There is perhaps a role for randomization alongside other methods of making surgical advances. As Sir Magdi Yacoub said eloquently this morning, we have to be willing to take a leap forward, and a leap forward cannot be randomized. On the other hand, once the leap is taken and a large number of patients are available for treatment, then randomization can provide some useful information. So I think randomization may be of significance if the operation is extended to very low-risk patients in large numbers. For example, if you combine myoplasty with coronary bypass and expect some improvement in myocardial function from bypass itself, you may want to add myoplasty as an adjunct procedure. That is the kind of question that might be addressed by randomization.

**Dr. Carpentier:** Wouldn't it be desirable to randomize also the low-risk patients without adjunct procedures since in these cases as well an alternative, i.e., the medical treatment, is available?

**Dr. Starr:** Yes, but you have to look at randomization as whether it is the only pathway or an accessory pathway. If the only way a patient can receive the treatment is to be randomized, I think that is a big mistake, because it is possible to do randomized studies alongside of nonrandomized implantations or other operative procedures. So, I wouldn't want to see all low-risk patients for myoplasty randomized but certainly a randomized series would be helpful with other good data kept in a registry.

**Dr. Carpentier:** Surgeons are not well placed for randomization. My patients are referred to me by cardiologists with a specific request. Unless there is an obvious contraindication to cardiomyoplasty, I don't see how I can tell the patient: "You are a good candidate for this operation; I am going to randomize you!" If this patient really needs the operation, he or she is going to see another surgeon who is not a randomizer!

**Dr. Starr:** That is very true and this was a problem in randomized studies of coronary bypass. Can you tell us what are your current indications for cardiomyoplasty in the low-risk group?

**Dr. Carpentier:** Two principles: (1) Keep the operative mortality low, about 5%. (2) Operate at a much earlier stage than in the past, that is, before the onset of those risk factors linked with increased early and late mortality, namely, associated right ventricular involvement, pulmonary hypertension, arrhythmias, mitral valve insufficiency, functional Class IV, and CTR >0.60. For me, the best indications are a progressive enlargement of the heart, or repeated episodes of pulmonary edema in spite of appropriate medical treatment, or the first onset of arrhythmias. One of the two patients I operated on during this meeting illustrated this policy. I was criticized by some people in the audience. But if the operation is going to stop or delay the evolution of the disease and particularly the progressive dilatation of the heart, this is the way to do it. This reminds me of the early days of valvuloplasty. I was criticized to advise early operations in asymptomatic patients with severe organic mitral valve incompetence. Today, this strategy is well accepted and the long-term results are far superior than in patients operated at a later stage and the patients enjoy a much better quality of life.

**Dr. Starr:** It would be very difficult to exercise our clinical choice because now for the first time in the history of cardiac surgery, the regulatory process is involved with a surgical procedure, not just a device.

**Dr. Carpentier:** It is quite a surprising and dangerous evolution. In the past, the regulatory process used to involve only the device itself, and its reliability and safety. Today, it extends to the surgical technique used in combination with a device. Tomorrow, it may pretend to regulate all surgical techniques even in the absence of implanted devices. The regulatory process will guide the surgeon's hand. Surgery will cease to be an art adapted to each individual. We must oppose this evolution, which would be the negation of progress.

**Dr. Starr:** This is very worrisome. During this meeting and for a few years I have had the feeling that we Americans have to look to our European colleagues for some or maybe many of the future advances in cardiac surgery. I must confess that I became somewhat discouraged with cardiomyoplasty, because our series had a very significant late mortality from arrhythmias and we could not demonstrate really significant objective criteria of improved ventricular function although all of the patients subjectively improved enormously.

**Dr. Carpentier:** What have you learned from this meeting and what do you plan to do when coming back to Portland?

**Dr. Starr:** I learned that there were many instances of marked objective improvements in hemodynamics and that the operation of cardiomyoplasty deserves to be more widely used and completely explored in all different phases of dealing with end-stage heart disease. We learned a great deal about the basic science of muscle stimulation and it was marvelous for us as clinical surgeons. On the other hand, I think that the muscle used for artificial ventricles is still in a very early stage and not yet clinically of interest. We plan to do more myoplasties and to expand our animal research projects. I hope that it will be possible to expand the indications to include a randomized study of cardiomyoplasty as an adjunctive procedure in end-stage valvular heart disease and in coronary artery disease with impaired ventricular function. I think it may have a very useful role in dealing with perhaps much larger numbers of patients with those indications than solely with the indications of idiopathic cardiomyopathy. What do you plan to do yourself?

**Dr. Carpentier:** Go ahead. Improve the technique, stimulate companies to incorporate a defibrillator into the myostimulator, convince them to reduce the cost, refine patient selection, understand the mechanisms of action, and further explore aortomyoplasty in high-risk patients. I don't underestimate the difficulties of the task. But as I said, the current situation reminds me of the beginning of ring valvuloplasty. I took me more than 10 years to achieve its full efficiency and 20 years to convince the skeptics. Cardiomyoplasty is twice as complex because it is not only a surgical procedure but also a biological procedure. Therefore, it may take 20 to 40 years to reach the same point of development!

# Index